Healthcare and Biomedical Technology in the 21st Century

George R. Baran • Mohammad F. Kiani
Solomon Praveen Samuel

Healthcare and Biomedical Technology in the 21st Century

An Introduction for Non-Science Majors

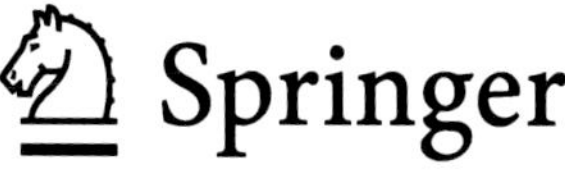

George R. Baran
College of Engineering
Temple University
Philadelphia, PA, USA

Mohammad F. Kiani
Department of Mechanical Engineering
Temple University
Philadelphia, PA, USA

Solomon Praveen Samuel
Orthopedic Surgery Bioengineering Laboratory
Albert Einstein Medical Center
Philadelphia, PA, USA

ISBN 978-1-4614-8540-7 ISBN 978-1-4614-8541-4 (eBook)
DOI 10.1007/978-1-4614-8541-4
Springer New York Heidelberg Dordrecht London

Library of Congress Control Number: 2013947470

Printed on acid-free paper

Springer is part of Springer Science+Business Media (www.springer.com)

Welcome

Dear Student,

Congratulations on having enrolled in this class! We don't know how you feel about engineering and science, or healthcare biotechnology in particular, but our promise to you is that everything you learn here will be useful to you for the rest of your life. It may take you more than one semester to realize that, but the moment will come.

We all know that at some point you or someone you care about will be in need of medical attention and treatment. That will be a difficult and stressful time, made so in part because you probably won't understand everything that's going on. Developments in healthcare technology are also an important contributing factor to the rising cost of healthcare in the United States, which in all likelihood will be a major economic challenge for your generation. We think that what you learn in this course will demystify some of that medical-speak for you and help you to make decisions about your own healthcare options.

We also suspect that from time to time you get involved in discussions about contemporary topics that are somewhat provocative, e.g., should the sale of high-sugar-content drinks be regulated; are genetically modified foods safe to eat. How do you argue your point in an intelligent and educated manner? How do you decide which claims make sense and which are nonsense? We're going to provide you with a framework you can use to analyze science-based arguments and develop well-informed opinions of your own.

In this book, we will introduce you to the healthcare dilemmas facing voters and political leaders everywhere and discuss what makes the scientific method so useful in arriving at decisions based on data analysis. We will expose you to the ethical questions that scientists and policy makers consider when assessing the cost and value of scientific progress, the pros and cons and ethics of performance-enhancing drugs, and how new drugs and devices are developed and approved for sale in the United States, covering topics such as animal testing, human clinical trials, and the patent system.

We will then relive the experience of a visit to a doctor and discuss the various tests and methods used to arrive at a diagnosis, explaining some of the core technologies that enable the sophisticated analytical methods used today. If you or a member of your family has ever needed a tissue or organ replaced, the chapter on implants will provide plenty of background information about the materials used, the way the human body reacts to implants, and you will read case studies that will help you realize how medical treatment decisions are made.

It's likely that someone in your family has suffered from heart disease; in the chapter on cardiovascular devices, we will explore heart anatomy and physiology, and you will learn the how and why of pacemakers, defibrillators, and artificial hearts. We will examine the clever strategies behind the development of new cancer-fighting drugs and how they are to be administered, as well as the techniques used by drug manufacturers to ensure that pills and tablets are designed to get the drug safely to its destination. Our focus on molecules will continue as we discuss the new and emerging field of tissue engineering, when biochemical cues are used to grow human tissue in the lab for eventual use as repair materials, and expose you to the promises and dangers of genetic engineering of crops and animals, and of our own cells to arm them for battle with disease.

In closing, we will describe a visit to the dentist and obtain a better understanding of the tools and procedures used to keep mouths healthy and functional, and how dentists can repair oral tissues when they are lost to decay or require adjustment for other reasons. In the last chapter, we will present an overview of the technology available to aid the disabled live as "normal" a life as possible.

At the end of each chapter, we list what we think are the most important concepts we have presented. These should be helpful to you as you reread and review the chapter and also provide topics for discussion.

We hope very much that your instructor will encourage questions and debate in class. Throughout several chapters we have highlighted questions that we hope will stimulate you to think about these timely topics. Scientists argue all the time, why shouldn't you? It's good practice to question authority and the "accepted" explanation. It will quickly become obvious who can make the stronger case, and arguments will help to clarify your thoughts.

Finally, we realize that science or engineering may not necessarily be your future chosen profession. But, if after finishing this course you leave thinking that the scientific method of rational thinking, evidence-based judgment, and peer review make a lot of sense, then do us all a favor and run for political office!

Preface

Dear Instructor,

We are delighted that you have chosen our book for your course! Let us tell you how the book came to be, and what our guiding philosophy has been during its development.

"Healthcare and Biotechnology in the 21st Century" resulted from our experiences participating in Temple University's General Education curriculum. Every Temple undergraduate student is required to take four courses in subjects outside their major. For example, all non-science and non-engineering majors are required to take two courses in science or technology and two courses in mathematics (numerical proficiency). We decided to institute a new course covering medical technology (our own field of expertise) that would draw on basic biologic, physics, chemistry, and engineering principles, discuss the scientific method, gently underline the value of a quantitative approach to life, and introduce and explain medical technologies that our students or their family members are likely to have encountered as patients.

Our search for an appropriate textbook made us realize that one did not exist. The available biomedical texts were all written for science or engineering majors. We decided to write our own course-pack, and have been using it for several years. The opportunity eventually came along for us to devote some additional time to revising the course pack, and to compile a book on these topics. Discussions with colleagues and publishers were encouraging, and this volume is the product of a recent surge in writing and editing activity.

We want to emphasize that the book is designed for use in an undergraduate-level course taught to non-science, non-engineering majors: students who are likely to have graduated high school convinced that they would never have to take another science course again, who probably did not take more than the minimum number of science courses in high school, and many who may consider their participation in this course to be a waste of time.

In planning this book, we were fully cognizant of research indicating that students not majoring in the sciences or engineering would not profit (learn) from a traditional science or engineering textbook. Instead, we have presented overviews of the developments in biomedical technology, attempting to engage students in scientific and critical thinking. Our reasoning is that although the specific biomedical areas we cover will develop during the students' lifetimes, learning about evidence-based argumentation, peer review, and the inquiry-driven scientific method will stand the students in good stead for many more years.

That's why we have also tried to write the book in a language these students should understand. It's not the language used to communicate with scientists via a manuscript, but students who make an effort to broaden their vocabulary should have little difficulty following the text.

The first portion of the book introduces healthcare policy and its ramifications for the future, discusses how scientists and engineers think and work, shows how science impacts daily life, reveals how medical biotechnology is regulated in the United States, provides an introduction to a few of the technologies that enable modern health care biotechnology, and ends with a description of the events that can occur during a visit to a doctor. In some of the chapters we ask questions designed to encourage student involvement; the answers are not always obvious, and do not require prior scientific knowledge, but provide an opportunity for the instructor to guide discussion according to scientific principles. Feel free to use them or come up with new ones. And yes, we do have a point of view on certain hot-button issues, and that point of view may become obvious to the reader; if you don't agree with it, there's a great opportunity for a classroom debate! We do make an effort to present some alternative views, but emphasize prevailing scientific or data-driven opinions.

That foundation sets the stage for the second portion of the book, where we focus on specific healthcare biotechnologies, with some case histories mixed in to illustrate our points. This is where students will encounter the most "science" information. We realize that each instructor will tailor the amount of material that is taught to the level of the student body. With that in mind, we will advise that portions of Sects. 7.2 and 7.4–7.7 in Chap. 7 may prove difficult for students with poor backgrounds in science and mathematics. Chapters 10 and 12 contain vocabulary that may be unfamiliar to students who have not had prior courses in biology, and the instructor may wish to devote extra time to vocabulary development. Students will need to know the meanings of the words if they are to understand the concepts being presented.

The book is lengthy, and not all the topics can be covered in depth during a typical 14–15-week semester. Feel free to pick and choose according to your interests and your student body, and good luck with the course!

Philadelphia, PA, USA

George R. Baran Ph.D.
Mohammad F. Kiani Ph.D.
Solomon P. Samuel D. Eng.

Acknowledgements

We wish to acknowledge contributions to the text made by:
Ken Boberick, D.M.D.
John A. Handal, M.D.
Thomas K. John, M.D.
Salim Merali, Ph.D.
Bin Wang, Ph.D.

We also thank Ms. Jessica Welhaf for original drawings and illustrations. The contributors of other images are acknowledged directly in the text.

George Baran wishes to thank the staff of The Department of Bioengineering, The Imperial College London, for their hospitality during his leave.

Note: The inclusion of images of proprietary products or citations of specific products or brand names does not constitute an endorsement of these products by the authors.

Contents

1 Is Technology the Cure for Soaring Demand and the High Costs of Healthcare?

> *We live in a society exquisitely dependent on science and technology, in which hardly anyone knows anything about science and technology.*
>
> Carl Sagan

Do you remember the last time you visited your doctor or dentist? During that visit, you came into contact with modern medical technology. At the very minimum, a computer was used to store your personal data and, later, the results of the physical examination, your medical history, and symptoms in the form of an electronic medical record. If you made the appointment because of an injury or pain, additional technological tools were used to help your doctor or dentist make a diagnosis or an assessment of the extent of injury, perhaps blood was drawn for analysis or some type of imaging (e.g., X-Ray, MRI) was ordered. The results of these technologically enabled tests were eventually used to guide treatment.

Virtually all of these technologies have been developed by biologists, biochemists, physicists, or engineers, not necessarily physicians. And yet, few patients receiving treatment have an appreciation of how modern medical tests and procedures work or why they are ordered. In this book, we hope to change that for you! You will see that the healthcare you receive is not only determined by your medical needs, but also by economic factors and government policies influenced by political ideology and religious beliefs.

1.1 Introducing the Problem: Healthcare Statistics and Insurance

In the USA, if an individual is covered by some form of health insurance, availability of treatment for various problems is taken for granted. In other wealthy and middle-income nations, a similar availability of technology for healthcare is also assumed.

G.R. Baran et al., *Healthcare and Biomedical Technology in the 21st Century: An Introduction for Non-Science Majors*, DOI 10.1007/978-1-4614-8541-4_1,

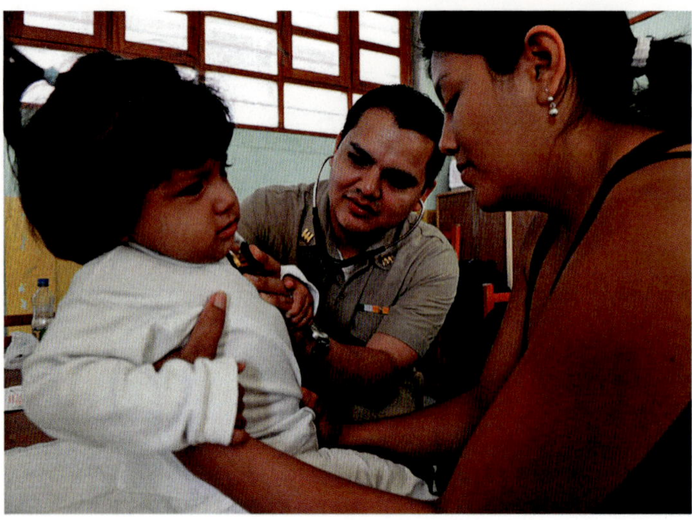

Fig. 1.1 A medical clinic in Mexico where healthcare is paid for from a dizzying variety of sources, including private and government plans. Healthcare providers must contend with diseases of the developing world (malaria, tuberculosis) and diseases of the developed world (diabetes, heart disease, liver disease). Public healthcare spending is approximately $800/year/person

And yet, although technology has been instrumental in improving efficiency and profitability in many economic sectors, healthcare costs continue to climb everywhere and consume an ever-greater portion of national budgets. The Congressional Budget Office estimates that if the current trends continue, in the year 2050 more than 50 % of our economic activity (Gross Domestic Product, GDP) in the USA will be healthcare related and that portion is projected to continue to increase.

Analyses and predictions such as these are partly responsible for the ongoing national debates about healthcare. Should government play a dominant role in healthcare? Is access to affordable healthcare a right or a privilege? Should our goal in the USA be the adoption of universal healthcare coverage (provision of all preventive, curative, and rehabilitative services for everyone)? The costs associated with achieving true universal healthcare in the USA under the current system may be staggering and account to a large degree for the difficulty in achieving a consensus on these questions.

1.1.1 The Global Picture

The twenty-five wealthiest nations of the world, with the exception of the USA, as well as some middle-income countries such as Brazil, Mexico (Fig. 1.1), and Thailand, all have some form of universal health coverage, and many other nations including India, Vietnam, China, and the Philippines are developing their own systems.

This trend toward universal healthcare is global and is considered to be a third great health transition, following (1) the institutionalization of public sewer systems and (2) the development of wide-scale immunization [1]. It also involves the

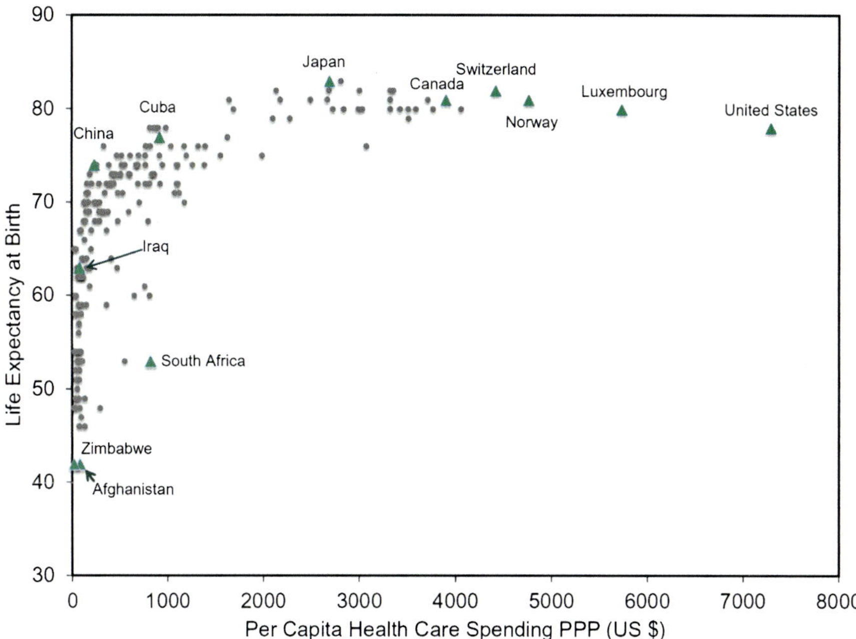

Fig. 1.2 Life expectancy versus per capita healthcare spending with non-OECD countries included

participation and even control by governments, because it is clear to many that spreading the cost of healthcare over a larger population reduces the overall costs and costs per individual.

The USA is the wealthiest country in the history of the world, and yet 60 million of its citizens do not have health insurance. Many studies have shown that access to healthcare is an important determinant of economic growth; for example, the World Health Organization stresses that a decrease of 10 % in infant mortality rates is responsible for an increase of 0.3–0.4 % in economic growth [2]. An easy, but inaccurate, assumption would be that health measures, such as infant mortality rate or life expectancy, are always directly related to how much money a society spends on its healthcare. However, while countries with very low healthcare expenditures do tend to have lower life expectancies, the life expectancy for American citizens ranks number 57 in the world, even though the USA has by far the highest per capita healthcare costs (estimated total $2 trillion annually; $7,000/person in 2008; 17 % of its gross domestic product in 2008; projected to rise to 25 % of GDP in 2025 [3]).

In non-OECD (Organization for Economic Cooperation and Development) countries, countries such as Cuba and Costa Rica have average life expectancies just above that of the USA even though these countries have much weaker economies and spend 1/25 of the amount that the USA does on a per capita basis (Fig. 1.2). It might appear that we are not spending our healthcare dollars wisely and our increasing healthcare costs could be in part responsible for offshoring of jobs, decreases in industrial growth, and dilemmas faced by start-up companies who cannot compete for low health insurance premiums and therefore cannot attract the best workers.

Table 1.1 Annual health insurance premium costs (in US $'s) in industrialized countries

Country	Annual premium (US $'s)	Premium relative to US premium (%)
Australia	2,440	45
Canada	732	13
China	63	1
France	1,773	33
Germany	796	15
Hong Kong	851	16
India	66	1
Indonesia	92	2
Japan	2,249	41
Mexico	634	12
New Zealand	1,035	19
Singapore	87	2
South Africa	200	4
UK	1,200	22
USA	5,429	100

According to the US Chamber of Commerce, healthcare is already the most expensive benefit paid by US employers, with healthcare premiums for workers having risen by 114 % in the last decade (Table 1.1) [4].

1.1.2 Comparing and Evaluating Quality of Healthcare and Its Implications

Discussions about healthcare in the USA have lately taken on a highly ideological tone. When the Obama administration had expanded health insurance coverage (after the George W. Bush administration expanded prescription coverage), many debates began (and continue to this day) about the role of government and the cost of the new programs.

Essentially, some folks believe that the government should not force or mandate employers or citizens to participate in health insurance programs if they do not wish to do so. Also, they see the new programs (loosely defined as "Obamacare") as proof that the USA is becoming more socialistic or liberal and is being turned away from its capitalistic, individualist roots. Insurance coverage is perceived to be a privilege to be earned, and the move into widening coverage is part of an ideological agenda for greater government control of personal lives.

Some folks also argue that the measures of healthcare quality used by the World Health Organization or by the Commonwealth Fund or by the Organization of Economic Cooperation and Development are flawed. Life expectancy is labeled a poor statistic as a measure of quality because it is said to be little influenced by the system; people die in their sleep or in an automobile accident without the healthcare system having any influence on that outcome. Furthermore, the USA has a very diverse ethnic population, and some population members, e.g., African-Americans, have significantly lower life expectancies than other populations. This health statistic is influenced by genetics, lifestyle, diet, income, and educational level, and the healthcare system cannot influence those variables.

Infant mortality rate comparisons can be criticized because not all countries report data in the same way. For example, in Switzerland, an infant must be at least 30 cm long at birth to be counted as living; by that measure, all the premature births who are at greatest risk are not counted. Japan counts births only to Japanese citizens living in Japan, not elsewhere, while Finland, France, and Norway count births to their nationals regardless where they live. Other factors affecting infant mortality include the proportion of single mothers; in the USA, a significant proportion of pregnant women live without a partner and are less likely to receive prenatal care than married women.

In addition, the World Health Organization uses three other criteria to evaluate quality of healthcare: financial fairness (which measures if the financial burden of healthcare costs are primarily borne by those who are better off), health distribution (how equally are a nation's healthcare resources allocate among the entire population), and responsiveness (how equally a nation's responsiveness is spread across the entire population). These three measures are perceived by conservatives to be irrelevant because they imply that the rich should pay more for healthcare.

It is also true that the USA is still a destination for many wealthy foreigners seeking medical treatment and that the medical research in the USA is of the highest quality; by these measures, at least, the USA is still "Number 1."

Folks on the other side of this argument believe philosophically that the fact that there are tens of millions of people in the USA without medical insurance coverage is a scandal for the country with the largest economy in the world and that it is entirely appropriate for the government to get involved because the system has failed many people. They consider access to healthcare to be a right, not a privilege, and view it as appropriate that the wealthiest people pay more for healthcare and that they pay for the less economically fortunate as well. They also point out that the healthcare costs in the USA are so much higher than in the rest of the world that the perceived weaknesses of the quality measures should be overridden by the sheer amount of money being spent. The melting pot nature of the population also means that some groups with a greater than average life expectancy are also included in the statistic. The high rates of obesity in the USA that contribute to lowered life expectancy could be lowered by an aggressive educational program that focuses on health quality rather than on the right of beverage manufacturers to sell their sweetened products.

What do you think? What are the important quality of healthcare outcomes or measures that you think matter most? Should the government be involved in spreading the availability of healthcare, or is that an individual problem?

In any case, everyone agrees that healthcare costs are high and going higher. A great deal of work needs to be done to evaluate not only the quality of healthcare, but the efficiency of healthcare delivery. Critics of widening the pool of those who are covered because everyone will pay more should understand that patients without any insurance whatsoever are routinely treated in hospital emergency rooms (which levy the highest costs), rather than in preventive and health maintenance clinics.

1.1.3 Costs of Healthcare

Why are healthcare costs so high in the USA, and why are these costs always going up? There are many reasons. First, US spending on physicians per capita is about five times higher than in peer countries, and the main reason for that is the high fee structure of specialist physicians [5]. In the USA, we also pay more for procedures such as appendectomies, angiograms, and C-section than in other countries with healthcare systems that allow the payer (in many cases the government) to negotiate prices with providers (physicians, pharmaceutical companies, medical device manufacturers) [6].

Second, according to the Princeton University economist Uwe Reinhardt, the high level of per capita income in the USA is in part driving high healthcare spending. He also includes high pricing for drugs, high administrative costs which result from the large differences in payment plans for different patients, and the nature of our legal system which encourages defensive medical treatment, as other mechanisms responsible for our large healthcare costs [7]. Of course, the fact that no one really knows what surgical procedures cost doesn't help. Attempts to discover what the costs would be for a hip replacement by a group of investigators who called numerous orthopedic hospitals and surgical centers yielded estimates from $11,100 to $125,798 from those institutions who were able to actually provide a bundled price [8]!

Interestingly, the chronically ill is the segment of the population that uses most of our healthcare benefits. This estimated 5 % of the entire population in the USA has five or more chronic conditions such as high blood pressure, diabetes, heart disease, and respiratory illnesses and approximately 21 % of all healthcare spending goes to care for these patients [9]. For Medicare patients (those older than 65), the statistics are more disturbing: 21 % of beneficiaries have five or more chronic conditions and consume 79 % of Medicare spending. These patients see many physicians and visit the hospital often, sometimes relying on the 911 system for care and transport. There is obviously a huge incentive to reduce the number of patients with these chronic illnesses. And even though the care provided to patients in the last years of their lives skyrockets in cost, it is unclear how feasible it would be to find savings in that spending sector; it may be more productive to focus on the reimbursement system, which sometimes seems to reward more care, rather than better care [10]. Assessing which interventions make sense for dying patients has been a flashpoint in the national debate on healthcare, with some politicians referring to plans for committees studying the costs and benefits of end-of-life treatment and care as "death panels" and warning that if the government was in control

What do you think: what could be some effective methods to accomplish a reduction in the cost of caring for patients with chronic disease conditions?

of healthcare, it would intervene to limit access to treatment. Of course, the fact that private insurers often manage treatment options through a combination of co-pay rules, denial of coverage to patients with preexisting conditions and so on is often ignored.

1.2 New Technologies

We all hope that somehow technology will come to the rescue and help to bring down the costs of healthcare. After all, technology gets the credit for making American industry more productive. Is this hope realistic? Will implementation of ever-newer and more sophisticated technologies improve healthcare and bring down overall costs? If you accept the assumption that early detection of a disease or early diagnosis of an ailment reduces eventual costs because intervention can occur earlier, then certainly the advent of new imaging technologies such as ultrasound (Fig. 1.3), which detect brain aneurisms, could reduce the incidence of stroke, a much costlier condition to treat.

Development of lab-on-a-chip technology (Fig. 1.4) has permitted rapid and point-of-care diagnoses.

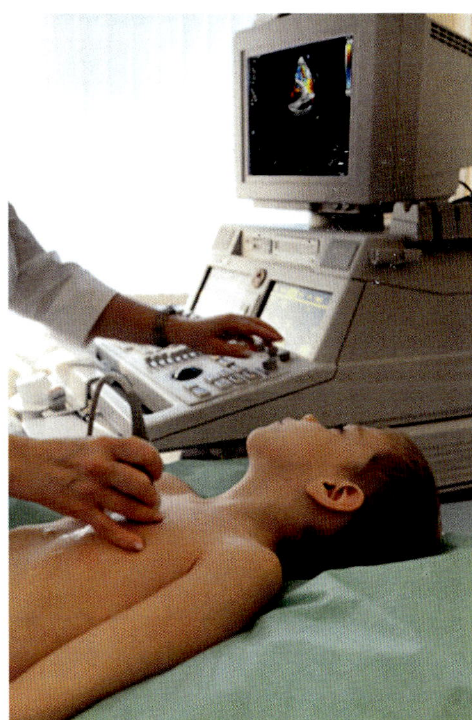

Fig. 1.3 Ultrasound equipment which can be used to image soft tissue such as lymph nodes, the abdomen, and blood vessels. It can also reveal the presence of aneurisms or bulging blood vessels at risk of rupturing and causing a stroke. It is less expensive to treat an aneurism than the aftereffects of a stroke

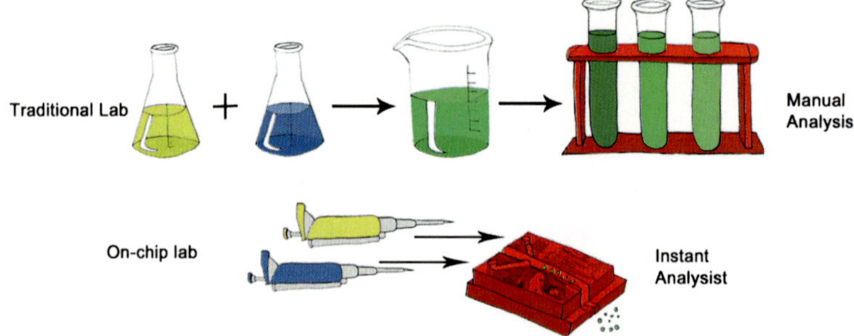

Fig. 1.4 A schematic of the differences between traditional and lab-on-a-chip diagnoses. The traditional analysis requires that the patient travel to a clinical facility to give blood and then wait for a diagnosis. The lab on a chip permits the patient to donate blood anywhere, and if the chip is present, several diagnoses can be obtained quickly. This could reduce the time to treatment and potentially reduce the eventual cost of treatment

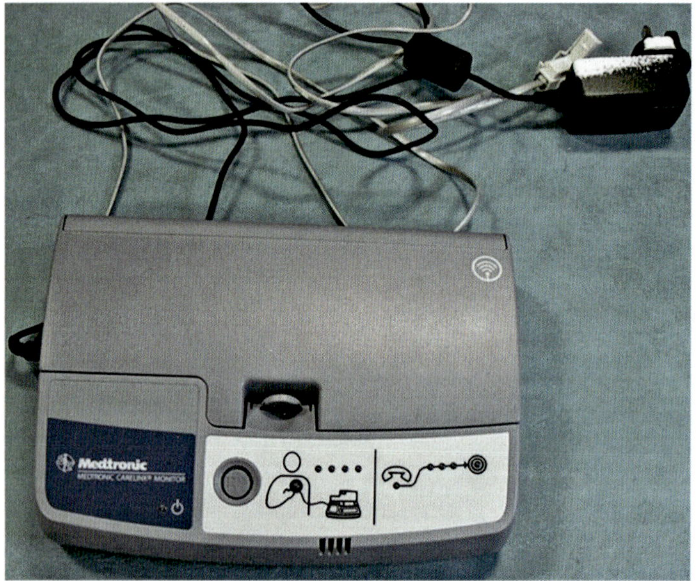

Fig. 1.5 A device for noninvasive heartbeat monitoring. As the label indicates, the sensor is placed over the pacemaker implantation site and is able to download information about pacemaker function and send the data over a telephone line to a diagnostic facility. The patient does not need to travel. Copyrighted by Springer-Verlag London

What do you think: are technologies such as robot-assisted surgery (Fig. 1.6) potential cures for high surgical costs or do they merely represent another expensive gadget?

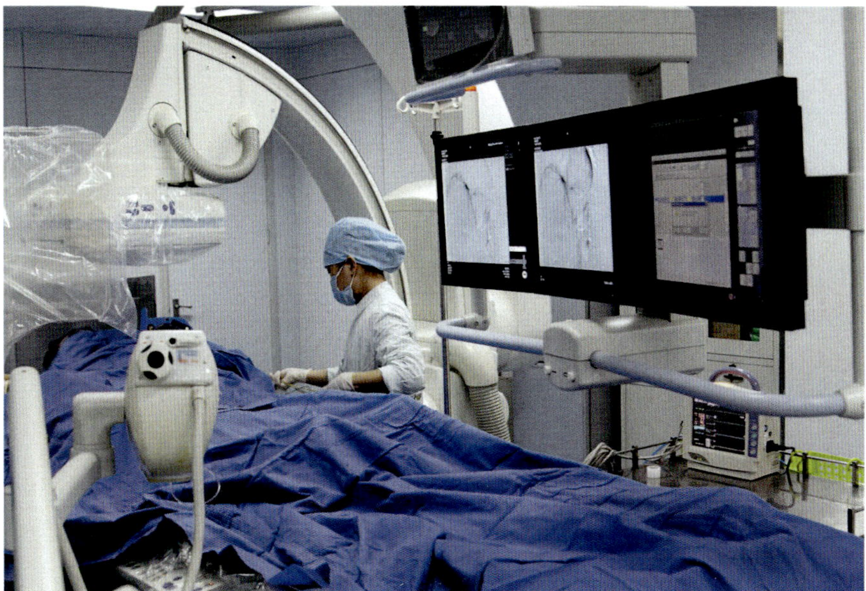

Fig. 1.6 Image and computer-assisted surgical system

New mHealth (mobile health) wireless sensor technologies such as this heart monitor (Fig. 1.5) should also lead to eventual cost savings. A study by the Veterans Administration showed significant savings could result when telehealth technology was implemented in homebound patients.

Technology costs money to develop, market, and maintain, and there is probably a point where the increase in the costs transmitted to the patient or insurer will have to be debated and evaluated.

Even more exciting is a strategy known as "personalized medicine" (Fig. 1.7). If your genetic makeup, your genome, is known to your doctor, then he or she will be able to prescribe a much more effective, personalized dose and type of medication to fight the illness in your body. That's because we are in the process of gathering a lot of data on the responses of individuals to different medications and will eventually be able to better correlate genetic characteristics with the effectiveness of various drugs and doses. In this approach, each patient's medication will be customized!

1.3 Bringing Down Healthcare Costs: Electronic Medical Records

Because so much time and money is spent on healthcare administrative functions, for example, in filing, duplication, taking histories, calling for prior lab and imaging results, any changes to the healthcare system to reduce these tasks should save money. Within the past decade, there has been a push to adopt electronic medical records keeping. The second administration of President George W. Bush called for

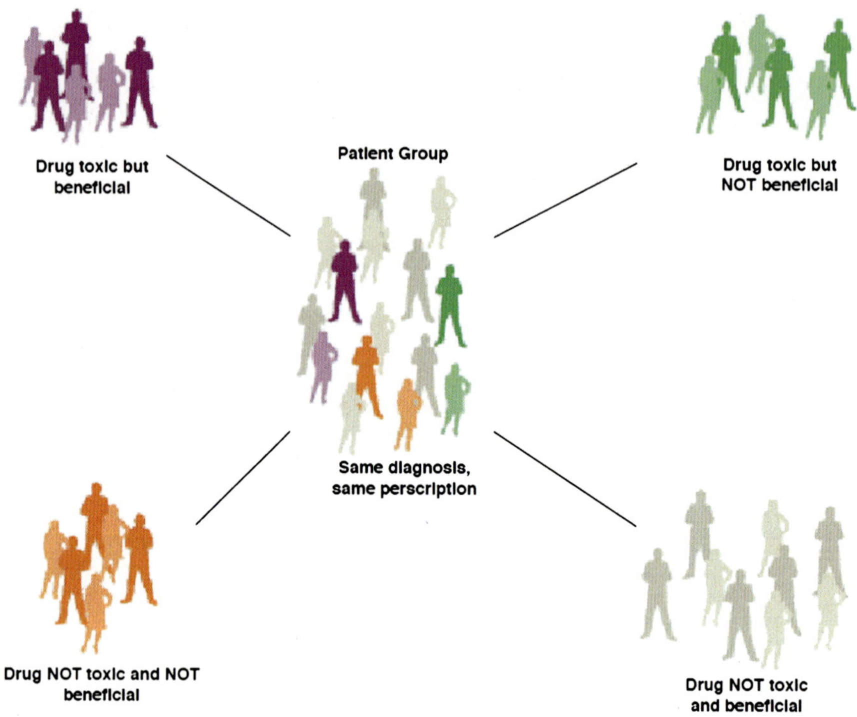

Fig. 1.7 A schematic representation of the strategy and advantages of personalized medicine. As more is learned about the effect of a patient's genetic code on the effectiveness of specific drugs, it may become possible to customize treatment based on a patient's personal genetic makeup

nationwide implementation of electronic medical records by 2014, and the Congress provided nearly $560 million in loans and grants to assist this process. Subsequently, President Obama pledged $50 billion over five years on information technology for healthcare. It will be very costly for hospitals and physician practices to transition to electronic medical records, because of the need for additional data storage, employee training, and network infrastructure [11]. However, if fully implemented, life for patients could be much simpler; it would be unnecessary to have to fill out pages of information for each visit to a physician. There would also be no need to repeat or keep copies of lab results to show to a new physician. Surveys of large hospital systems show that a reduction in costs does occur when electronic records are adopted, because of reductions in drug expenditures, better utilization of diagnostic imaging tests, and easier and more efficient billing [12]. Of course, we all have had the frustration of having to correct inaccurate information that was entered into a computer database on our behalf, so accurate transcription of personal and medical information is very important. Fortunately, it turns out that when experienced personnel work with these systems, transcription errors are not a significant problem [13].

There is another advantage to electronic medical records keeping that may not at first be obvious. If these records could be accessed on a large scale, researchers could examine the effectiveness of drugs and medical devices on large populations and discover which treatments provide the best long-term result. Then, by tunneling down into the records, it will be possible to search for associations between medical conditions and a whole variety of other variables: blood chemistry, weight, blood pressure, etc. For example, one could imagine a scenario where the effectiveness and side effects of a new drug on the whole patient population can be easily studied in a completely digitized medical record system. These types of observational studies could also yield information about the likelihoods of treatment success as doctors don't always know and cannot tell their patients what the chances are of being helped by a specific treatment. It is vitally important that patients, insurers, care providers, and also family members have a good appreciation of the uncertainly associated with treatment options so that the best decisions and best plans can be made.

Some physicians in smaller practices are not enthusiastic about electronic medical record keeping, even though there are financial incentives to convert to paperless systems. They claim that the software is not user friendly, that the software will require frequent and expensive updating, that the pull-down menus do not permit physicians to write customized notes, and that the electronic systems will be used to deny tests that are requested because the system will only approve tests that the insurer will pay. There is also some evidence that in smaller practices, more tests are ordered when an electronic record system is used, perhaps because a simple click of the mouse makes tests easier to order [14].

Still another concern is the security of the records. Although we all sign paperwork mandated by Health Insurance Portability and Accountability Act (HIPAA), which implies that our health data will be kept securely and confidentially, often we hear about hackers who are able to download private information about thousands of people; such a breach of confidentiality with private medical records could have devastating effects [15]. Various means of preserving record security, including use of personal pins, smart cards, and biometrics will need to be evaluated.

Finally, just as investigators uncover fraudulent billing for patient services to federal programs like Medicare, there are concerns that fraud will occur as doctors and hospitals bill the federal government for converting to electronic records. Remember that doctors have an incentive of up to $44,000 per practice to convert to electronic record keeping and the potential payment to a hospital is $2,000,000 in the first year of conversion. Requests for payment of the incentive are submitted to the federal government, but there is currently no audit process to ensure that the conversion has actually been made [16].

1.4 International Aspects of Healthcare Technology Development and Adoption

These fascinating and promising technologies may not be universally accepted by all communities or patients. The World Health Organization, in a survey of the field of medical device technology, reported that "although cutting-edge technologies to develop new medical devices has its place, research in developing current medical devices to

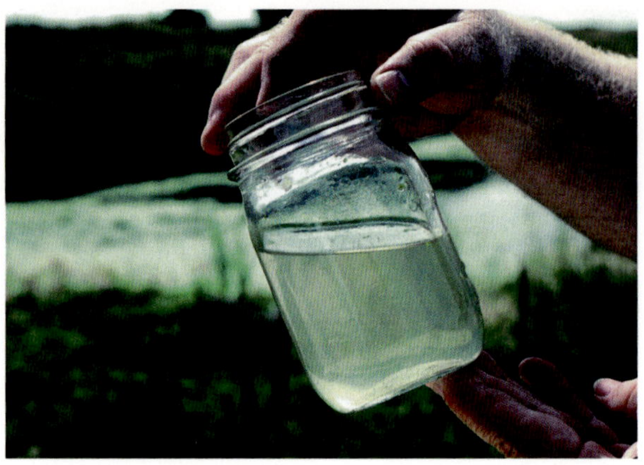

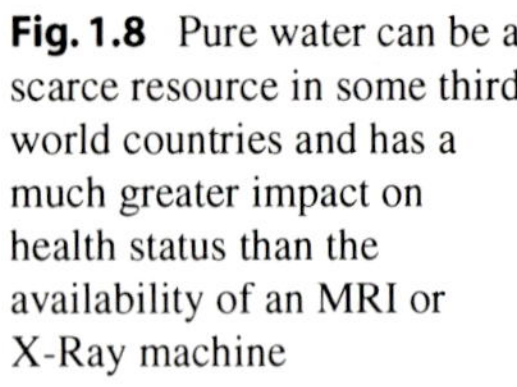

Fig. 1.8 Pure water can be a scarce resource in some third world countries and has a much greater impact on health status than the availability of an MRI or X-Ray machine

make them appropriate to specific contexts, particularly for low-income settings, is also urgently needed." In developing countries, implementation of sophisticated technologies is hindered by the lack of training an adequate number of healthcare personnel and more mundane issues such as the lack of training in maintenance, the absence of reliable power and sanitation, and a scarcity of clean water (Fig. 1.8). For example, in some developing countries, counterfeit or substandard drugs are sold by unscrupulous vendors, leading to injury or death of patients and a subsequent avoidance of medical intervention by many patients. Furthermore, many of the new medical devices being developed in developed countries often require large investments in disposable supplies that represent a huge cost to users in many developing countries.

A related issue is the attitude of some developing countries toward protection of intellectual property, i.e., patent rights. These countries argue that local industry should be permitted to violate patent and trademark rights or receive preferential treatment because the local population cannot afford to shoulder the costs of the protected pharmaceutical products or devices. In response, the holders of these patents point out that protection is needed if new product development is to occur and observe that the lack of research into diseases such as malaria and drug-resistant tuberculosis may in part be a result of not adhering to patent and trade laws. In the period between1975 and 1979, of 1,393 new compounds marketed as medicines, only 16 were meant to treat tropical diseases [17]. Nevertheless, because of political pressures and the demands of global epidemics such as AIDS, the costs of drugs and

What do you think: is it fair that other countries where per capita income is much smaller than in the USA take advantage of medical innovations paid for by the American taxpayer or consumer?

devices in developing countries are lower than in the USA, leading some to claim that the USA subsidizes healthcare in developing countries.

1.5 Progress in Healthcare Technology

As we review the significant progress made in medicine over the past 80 years or so, it becomes apparent that technology has had a significant transformative impact not only on the medical devices that have come into use, but also in the techniques used to develop, characterize, and assess many medical and surgical practices. For example, one of the definitive moments of modern medicine was the discovery of penicillin and the principles by which antibiotics function, which made the development of many antibiotics from 1940 to 1974 possible. It is doubtful that these advances could have occurred without simultaneous progress in, for example, organic and analytical chemistry and clinical trials methodology. Every surgical suite in a hospital is filled with electronic monitors, pumps, imaging equipment, computers, and even robotic surgery equipment, technologies that are empowered and made possible by development in other technology sectors.

Some of the more dramatic developments include life-sustaining machines such as ventilators (a machine used to help a patient breathe when they are unable to breathe for themselves; a tube is placed in the patient's windpipe in a procedure called intubation and connected to the ventilator to supply air to the lungs), kidney dialyzers (machines that filter toxins out of blood for patients whose kidneys no longer function), and cardiac pacemakers (implantable heartbeat stimulators for patients whose hearts beat in an uncontrolled manner).

We also take many diagnostic technologies, including MRI scanners (imaging machines that permit observation of soft tissues such as tendons, ligaments, and the brain in addition to hard tissues such as bone) and CT scanners (devices that obtain a three-dimensional X-ray image of the body) for granted.

Surgical procedures have also been revolutionized by advances in technology including the operating microscope (an optical device that allows surgeons to perform microsurgery as in brain or plastic surgery to repair small bleeding blood vessels) and endoscopes (instruments that allow a surgeon to view and operate in the interior of the body in procedures that can involve the gall bladder, spine surgery, the large intestine, etc.). The particular advantage of an endoscope is that only small incisions need to be made to introduce the device into the body and gain access to the diseased tissue or organ, and therefore, less skin and muscle is cut, simplifying the postsurgical healing process and reducing pain.

1.6 Is Progress in Technology the Best Answer for Improving Health?

The enthusiasm about healthcare technology is not universally shared, even among scientists and policy makers studying these issues. Perhaps the availability of so many diagnostic tests and aids leads to an overprescribing of analyses, because physicians believe that the problem can be surely solved if only it can be clearly identified [18]. If this is true, then technology contributes to an increase in healthcare costs; consider that the prices of recently developed imaging devices, such as PET scanners, are in the $1–2.5 million range and of course the cost is passed on to the consumer and insurer.

It is certainly true that costly technologies drive up the cost of diagnosis and treatment; the prices of most things keep increasing, do they not? But is that the most important measure? Perhaps instead what should be considered is if the use of the expensive PET scanner, for example, identifies a problem that can be treated at an early stage, rather than later when complications arise and the total cost of treatment is much higher. And other overlooked but important measures of healthcare cost-effectiveness include the gain in days worked because of continued good health or total per capita health expenditures over the lifespan of the individual.

What do you think? Would you be able to come up with a dollar figure for the value of extending a human life by one month? By one year? At what point does additional spending on technology begin to yield diminishing returns?

An example of what some regard as the complexities that have arisen as a result of advances in technology is its role in prolonging life even when the patient is experiencing the pain and misery of a terminal illness with no hope of recovery. It is now possible to maintain heart rhythm and blood circulation even if the heart is too weak to do so on its own, to oxygenate the patient by means of a ventilator even if the lungs are not functioning properly, to provide sustenance by means of a feeding tube even if the patient cannot eat on his/her own, and to remove waste through a catheter even if the urinary system is not functioning. Patients may be kept alive, often indefinitely, even as one after another of their organ systems fail and are replaced by technological aids.

If we were all to agree that technology does not contribute unnecessarily to healthcare cost increases, then what other solutions are available to bring down financial burdens on individuals or governments and at the same time increase overall health?

The noncommunicable diseases such as cancers, cardiovascular diseases, diabetes, and chronic respiratory ailments are responsible for about two-thirds of all deaths worldwide [19]. These diseases are also costly to treat in countries with well-developed healthcare systems. Often, the way to achieve disease reduction is obvious: 70 % of all lung cancer deaths in the world are due to smoking; others are due to exposure to asbestos or to coal smoke in poorly ventilated homes (Fig. 1.9). Another type of cancer, that of the stomach, is mostly linked to the presence of a specific bacterium in the gastrointestinal tract. Screening for the presence of this bug and administering antibiotics could significantly reduce this particular cause of death. Cervical cancers are caused by the human papillomavirus, a risk factor that can be avoided with early vaccination.

The risk factors for cardiovascular disease risk are also well known. They include alcohol abuse, high blood pressure and blood cholesterol levels, and high salt intake.

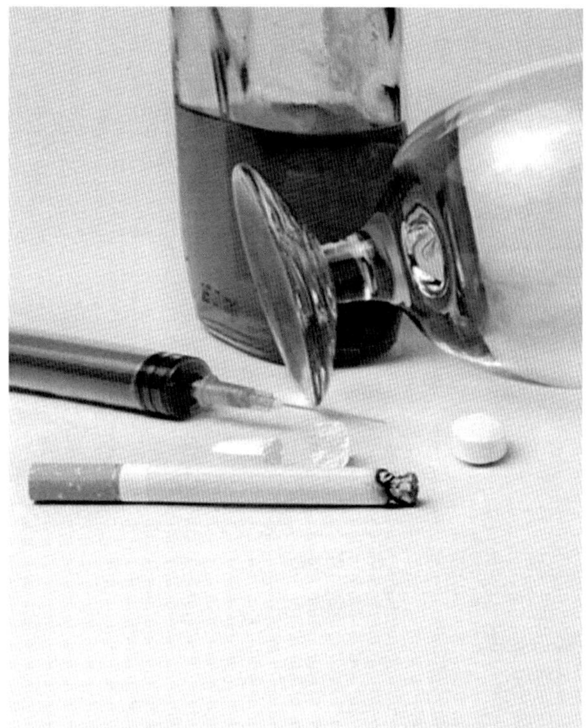

Fig. 1.9 Tobacco, drug, and alcohol abuse contribute to early mortality, yet they are behavioral factors that could be modified

All these factors can be modified or eliminated and do not require an elaborate and expensive system of healthcare technology. Unfortunately, human behavior is not easily modified; many of our actions are automatic, and we make food and behavioral choices without much thought and certainly without first reflecting on the caloric content of that pizza or sugary dessert [20].

Perhaps an important question is to find out if these automatic actions can be modified. The answer appears to be yes, and one way to accomplish this widely is by government regulation. For instance, when government raises the taxes on tobacco and alcohol, there is a measurable decrease in the consumption of these products. We could require fast-food restaurants to post the caloric value of their foods, as is done in the UK and in New York City, or raising additional taxes on high-sugar-content soft drinks as has been tried in Philadelphia and elsewhere. Because these actions reduce the consumption of these foods, there is strong resistance from fast-food chain operators, and from the soft drinks industry, who make the argument that such government actions interfere with freedom of choice, cause loss of jobs, and decrease their profits and taxes that they pay.

What do you think: should governments get involved in behavior modification for our own good? Does your answer depend on who pays for healthcare?

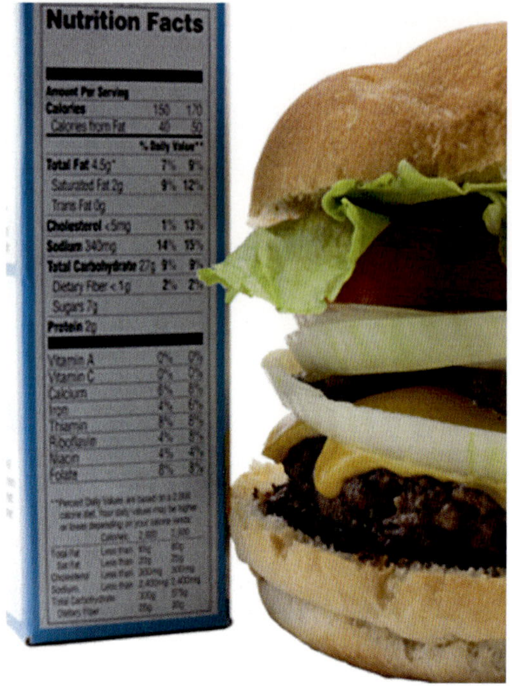

Fig. 1.10 The caloric content of certain foods is high; such foods may contain excessive amounts of fats and sugars, but not enough of the vitamins and minerals the human body needs. An unbalanced diet rich in such foods can lead to obesity, diabetes, and heart disease. Some cities have passed laws requiring such foods to be labeled with their nutritional content identified

Perhaps other approaches would be more easily accepted. For example, we could require that soft drinks must be sold in smaller containers. You have probably noticed within your "consumer lifetime" that many soft drinks have increased in size from 12 to 16 oz, and now 20 oz soft drinks seem to be the norm (Fig. 1.10). Even though the larger sizes are quoted as containing more than one serving, hardly ever does a person limit themself to only half the container. Other subtle ways of cuing changes in behavior, including changes in the size and shape of glasses in school cafeterias (tall glasses result in less consumption), making healthful foods more accessible and unhealthful foods less accessible (increasing the distance required to reach a certain food in a cafeteria line), and slowing down elevators (thereby increasing the likelihood that stairs are used), have been summarized by Marteau et al. [20].

As you continue reading, we will explain how modern health technology works and how it can improve your health (as long as you're covered by good insurance!). Finally, we will discuss what advances are around the corner and how your lives will be influenced in the future by even more sophisticated technologies. Young people, members of Generation X and Generation Y, have a greater stake in the future of healthcare than they often realize: on October 1, 2012, the United Nations released a report estimating that in 2050 there will be two billion people in the world over 60 years of age and that the number of people over 80 will increase to 400 million. These people will need care, for their physical as well as their mental ailments (estimated >100 million people with dementia worldwide); guess who will be paying for that care?

In the chapters that follow, we will also discuss how to think about and analyze medical advertising and the ways in which medical drugs and devices are tested and regulated. We will introduce you to the traditional treatments for conditions such as arthritis and heart disease and then to the new technologies that are being applied in some cases.

Above all, we want to leave you with a sense of being more in control of your healthcare. We want to demystify your visit to the doctor and explain why at sometimes you get an X-ray, and at others, an MRI is ordered. You do want to know more about implants and how sports injuries can be repaired, don't you?

1.7 Foundation Concepts

- The costs of healthcare are growing worldwide and are destined to be the largest component of the world economy within the next 30 years unless changes are made to the way healthcare is distributed and funded.
- The country that spends the most for healthcare (the USA) is not highest ranked in measures of health such as lifespan and infant mortality. Why is that so?
- The high costs of healthcare in the USA are due to an aging population, high physician reimbursement costs, segmented groups of insured individuals without mass purchasing power, and lifestyle issues that contribute to chronic diseases.
- Many new and exciting technologies are being invented to address healthcare costs, including remote medical diagnosis, electronic medical records, and early diagnosis, but the effects of these innovations on costs are not yet evident.
- Many new drugs and devices are less expensive when purchased outside the USA, because other countries' health systems are seemingly able to negotiate lower prices.
- Noncommunicable and chronic diseases such as diabetes, certain cancers, and heart disease have high treatment costs, yet their incidence may be reduced by lifestyle changes.
- The role of government in encouraging and rewarding lifestyle changes that reduce the likely onset of chronic diseases is controversial.

References

1. Rodin, J., & de Ferranti, D. (2012). Universal health coverage: The third global health transition? *Lancet, 380*, 861–862.
2. Commission on Macroeconomics and Health. (2001). *Macroeconomics and health: Investing in health for economic development*. Geneva: World Health Organization.
3. Congressional Budget Office. (2008) *Budget options* (Vol. 1). *Health Care*. Washington, DC.
4. Johnson, T. (2012). *Healthcare costs and U.S. competitiveness*. Council on Foreign Relations.
5. Laugesen, M., & Glied, S. (2011). Higher fees paid to US physicians drive higher spending for physician services compared to other countries. *Health Affairs, 30*, 1647–1656.
6. Klein, E. (2012, March 2). High health-care costs: It's all in the pricing. *The Washington Post*. Washington, DC.
7. Reinhardt, U. (2008, November 14). Why does U.S. health care cost so much? *The New York Times*. New York.

8. Rosenthal, J., Lu, X., & Cram, P. (2013). Availability of consumer prices from US hospitals for a common surgical procedure. *Journal of the American Medical Association Internal Medicine*. doi:10.1001/jamainternmed.2013.460.
9. Emanuel, E. (2012). Prevention and cost control. *Science, 337*, 1433.
10. Wessel, D. (2012, October 4). Looking for savings in health spending. *Wall Street Journal*. New York.
11. Brooks, R., & Grotz, C. (2010). Implementation of electronic medical records: How healthcare providers are managing the challenges of going digital. *Journal of Business and Economic Research, 8*, 73–84.
12. Wang, B., Prosser, LA., Bardon, CG., Spurr, CD., & Carchidi, PJ., et al. (2003). A cost-benefit analysis of electronic medical records in primary care. *American Journal of Medicine, 114*, 397–403.
13. Silfen, E. (2006). Documentation and coding of ED patient encounters: An evaluation of the accuracy of an electronic medical record. *American Journal of Emergency Medicine, 24*, 664–678.
14. McCormick, D., Bor, DH., Woolhandler, S., & Himmelstein, DU., et al. (2012). Giving office-based physicians electronic access to patients prior imaging and lab results did not deter ordering of tests. *Health Affairs, 31*, 488–496.
15. Scope, E. (2009). Virginia public health organization reports EMR security breach. Retrieved from www.ehrscope.com/virginia-public-health-organization-reports-emr-security-breach
16. Abelson, R. (2012, November 29). Medicare is faulted on shift to electronic records. *The New York Times*. New York.
17. Trouiller, P., Olliaro, P., Torreele E., Orbinski, J., Laing, R., & Ford, N., et al. (2002). Drug development for neglected diseases: A deficient market and a public-health policy failure. *Lancet, 359*, 2188–2194.
18. Fanu, J. (1999). *The rise and fall of modern medicine*. New York: Carroll and Graf.
19. Ezzati, M., & Riboli, E. (2012). Can noncommunicable diseases be prevented? Lessons from studies of populations and individuals. *Science, 337*, 1482–1487.
20. Marteau, T., Hollands, G., & Fletcher, P. (2012). Changing human behavior to prevent disease: The importance of targeting automatic processes. *Science, 337*, 1492–1495.

Science, Pseudoscience, and Not Science: How Do They Differ? 2

"There are more things in heaven and earth, Horatio, than you have ever dreamed of in your philosophy."

William Shakespeare, in *Hamlet*

Many news stories related to health and the environment introduce and describe scientific concepts which may be unfamiliar to the reader. Often, the stories draw conclusions based on the scientific or technical concepts that were presented, with the result that the reader is left to rely on a correct interpretation of the concept by the writer. Similarly, many marketing and advertising claims for health-related products rely on anecdotal evidence, rather than on the outcomes of controlled research.

In this chapter, we hope to provide you with the tools to examine stories and claims systematically so that you will become a skeptical and literate consumer of scientific information. That skill should help in real-life situations when you try to evaluate competing claims for optimal diets or nutrition, immunization programs, and even politically charged issues.

2.1 Introduction

Which of these statements are true?

"You should live a chemical-free life."

"Eating seeds is great because every seed is packed with the nutritional energy needed to create a full-grown plant."

"Use only organic beauty products because what goes on your skin enters your bloodstream."

"Why would you inject three diseases like measles, mumps, and rubella (German measles) vaccine into an infant?"

G.R. Baran et al., *Healthcare and Biomedical Technology in the 21st Century: An Introduction for Non-Science Majors*, DOI 10.1007/978-1-4614-8541-4_2,

"Cancer rates are increasing because of the chemicals and growth stimulants we feed animals."

"You should only feed your family food that contains no pesticides or food additives."

It's likely that you have heard at least one of these statements (or one very much like it) at some point in your life and accepted it without much thought because…it sounded right, or "truthy," as the comedian Steven Colbert would say. Did you then act on this so-called advice? If the answer is yes, then you have just provided an unfortunate example of the small role of science in public life.

2.2 Popular Views and Public Perception of Science

What is the usual, commonly held impression of science, scientists, and engineers? If you've known anyone who entered these professions, you probably remember someone "geeky" and studious; the television series "The Big Bang Theory" portrays a group of physicists who fit this popular image of scientists. No wonder that many nonscientists find it difficult to imagine that scientists and engineers actually have something to contribute to daily life!

The news cycle is now on 24 h a day, 7 days a week. We are bombarded by "news" from traditional newspapers, traditional network news programs, cable network news channels, tweets, blogs, e-mail, texts, etc. The concept of news as information is giving way to news as entertainment, and consumers now have so many choices that it is possible to consciously or subconsciously filter out stories that don't fit in with a certain worldview or attitude.

At one time, in the 1960s, physics and engineering were at the top of the news; this was the period when the Western nations worried about the Soviet Union and its space program and atomic bombs, when children in grade school and high school practiced what to do in case of nuclear attack (the trick was to hide under your desk!), and when the Soviets sent up the first orbiting satellite called Sputnik, politicians were ready to fund a variety of science programs. That's when the National Aeronautics and Space Administration (NASA) was organized and President Kennedy called for the USA to land a man on the moon.

Even as scientists and engineers were hailed as heroes when the lunar landing was successful, the more common portrayal of scientists in the media was decidedly one-dimensional and often portrayed scientists as deranged and up to no good. A mad scientist was responsible for creating Frankenstein; another crazed scientist (played brilliantly by Peter Sellars) was responsible for creating instruments of death and destruction in the 1964 movie Dr. Strangelove, which had the subtitle "how I stopped worrying and loved the bomb."

Scientists also seemed to disappoint the public and reporters: where were all those flying cars that were promised? Maybe they didn't quite promise them, but that's what the newspaper stories said. Engineers were supposed to design all sorts of gadgets that would make our lives fun, and instead we get to read about the search somewhere in Switzerland for the Higgs Boson, whatever that is. If scientists and engineers were so wrong about all their promises and predictions, then maybe the nonbelievers in climate are right and there is no threat after all!

Science stories seem to contain words like "wacky," "breakthrough," "scare," and "wasteful" and often have a sensational tone to them; these words don't seem to indicate objectivity on the part of the reporter. One topic has certainly emerged and captured the public's interest: health. Newspapers and television news and entertainment programs routinely feature stories about cancer survival, diet, obesity, new drugs, new kinds of surgeries, and dietary supplements. Dr. Oz has a television show where he talks about medicine in language the ordinary person can understand and a website where he promotes food supplements that can energize you and revitalize your immune system. Another physician, Dr. Joel Fuhrman, is featured on hour-long PBS television programs where he discusses nutrition-based treatments for obesity and chronic diseases. Because these two folks have an M.D. following their names, many people listen...and buy those dietary supplements.

A newspaper headline once stated that bananas are as good as drugs for treating HIV. It completely misinterpreted the results of a study reported in the Journal of Biological Chemistry in 2010. The original article stated that a lectin (type of sugar) found in bananas could interfere with the HIV virus entering cells. However, nowhere in the body of the article was it suggested that eating bananas was an effective treatment for HIV infections.

Still other issues are debated during political elections. Should more nuclear plants, solar cell factories, or wind farms be constructed? Should the government fund research for more energy-efficient cars, or is that a waste of taxpayer money? Should the government fund research that uses embryonic stem cells, or is that morally reprehensible? Is the "fracking" technology for releasing and collecting natural gas safe for the environment? We vote and decide which politicians get elected to make decisions about our future. However, we often don't know what their positions are on these important science-related issues. During the US presidential election in 2012, not a single scientific or technologic issue was debated; yes, the topic of an oil pipeline from Canada to the USA was brought up, but only as it related to "energy independence from the Middle East" and "job creation," not as part of a debate about a sensible energy policy.

Advances in science and technology are single-handedly responsible for the rapid rise in our standard of living over the past 200 years, and politicians and public policy figures all agree that science and technology are keys to future economic development and jobs. However, there seems to be a disconnect between relying on science and technology on the one hand and at the same time minimizing the roles of scientists and engineers in making big decisions. There are so many socio-scientific issues to consider: will additional taxes on high-sugar-content soft drinks influence obesity rates, should the type of materials used to manufacture baby bottles be regulated, should we be teaching evolution or creationism in public classrooms, and should decisions on these topics be made on an emotional basis or on an informed, rational basis?

How can one decide what is true and factual and what is invented or exaggerated by the media to sell advertising? Reading this chapter should help you to separate fact from fiction and turn you into an informed consumer and citizen [1]. We will try to bridge the gap between scientists and nonscientists, so well articulated by C.P. Snow (a physicist, chemist, and writer of some two dozen works of fiction and nonfiction) in his Rede lecture "The Two Cultures" [2]. He and others have lamented the education our secondary and high school students receive, with no realistic discussion of the scientific method, no preparation for how to interpret statistics, to estimate risk, or to evaluate the complexities associated with health and medicine. Instead, science is often taught as a series of individual facts that are barely comprehensible, as if to discourage the greater majority of students from an active and lifelong participation in scientific debates of crucial importance to their lives and futures.

2.3 Student Attitudes About Science

There is disturbing evidence about the state of knowledge regarding science and technology in the US surveys of children in elementary school and in middle school which indicate that kids are excited about science and very much enjoy the hands-on types of science experiences they have as a part of their education, many of which involve animals or the environment: guinea pigs, goldfish, and what can you find in the local pond or stream. Freshmen in high school still maintain a generally high degree of interest in science, but unfortunately, this interest significantly diminishes during the high school years, with physics and chemistry in particular becoming less and less popular.

Gender differences in attitudes to science also appear, though these differences are themselves variable depending on local cultural attitudes. Interestingly, in a science test given to 15-year-old students in 65 countries, girls outperformed boys in Eastern and Southern Europe and in the Middle East; in Western Europe and in the USA, boys outperformed girls [3]. Female students in US high schools seem to enjoy and elect to participate in biology courses, but shun math and physics; it is unfortunate that the early enthusiasm for science and technology shared equally by both boys and girls in elementary education is somehow lost in girls as they continue through high school. Many high school students of both sexes appear to develop a dismissive attitude toward science, reasoning that because the subject matter is of no interest to them, there is no need to learn it and that there will be no further exposure to science in college or in later life. The false notion that geometry, algebra, and calculus have no purpose for a nonscience major in college also becomes widespread. Along with this rejection of science and technology, students lose an ability to interact critically with scientific information. As the science educator Hodson wrote:

> To be fully scientifically literate, students need to be able to distinguish among good science, bad science, and nonscience, make critical judgments about what to believe, and use scientific information and knowledge to inform decision making at the personal, employment, and community level. In other words, they need to be critical consumers of science. This entails recognizing that scientific text is a cultural artifact, and so may carry implicit messages relating to interests, values, power, class, gender, ethnicity, and sexual orientation [4].

It's also curious and alarming that many students believe in certain pseudosciences, and these beliefs appear to persist into adulthood. How many "educated" people are there who believe that ghosts exist, that astrology can explain personalities and predict the future, that aliens regularly visit earth, that wearing jewelry made of certain crystals or metals has an effect on health, or that breaking a mirror brings bad luck (Fig. 2.1)? And even though surveys conducted by the National Science Foundation suggest that Americans are scientifically literate, the 2010 Science and Engineering Indicators report excluded questions about evolution and

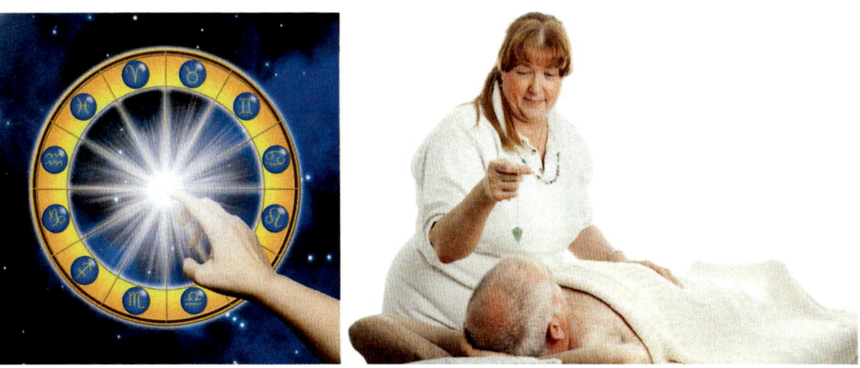

Fig. 2.1 Astrology and new-age crystal therapy hold a fascination for many credulous people, even though no reliable evidence has been presented to support claims of effectiveness

the Big Bang; in other words, we don't really know what Americans think about those two topics [5]. Apparently, the National Science Board thought that Americans would be confused because some of them hold religious beliefs that don't allow them to think independently about scientific evidence.

In order to understand how science differs from pseudoscience, we will first discuss what the scientific method is, how engineers work, and the critical importance of using evidence to support claims made on scientific or technological topics.

2.4 How Science Is "Done"

It's useful to know what the scientific process is, and how scientists and engineers arrive at conclusions, in order to be able to recognize silly or misleading claims and statements. If you adopt some of this thinking and analytical style, you'll be able to make better decisions for yourself, your friends, and family members. You'll learn how to analyze advertising that relies on some random bit of science, how to evaluate many socio-scientific issues that arise during election campaigns, and how to make sense of fad diets claims and food supplement commercials.

Before analyzing the statements listed at the beginning of this chapter and other "controversial" topics, let's discuss how science is done. Let's move away for the moment from emphasizing scientific and technical knowledge that can be memorized (e.g., what is the chemical symbol for arsenic?) to accepting that science is a process fundamentally grounded in asking questions. As questions are asked, evidence-based answers are given; and because not everyone agrees with the answers, a debate begins. This is, fundamentally, what the scientific process is all about: question, answer, debate, verify, and ask further questions.

Science is different from engineering; science attempts to provide answers about events in the natural world, while engineers often use scientific knowledge to modify the world to solve practical problems. How is science done? *Not* as it is done in most high schools.

Students in high school are instructed to follow a certain procedure while performing an experiment. Almost everyone knows what the result will be (they would have heard about it from students in another class); all the chemicals, materials, and equipment for the experiment are listed in the instructions and are conveniently provided. At the end of the experiment, the student is required to write a report that summarizes the activity and explains the result in a way that reinforces a concept found in the book or presented during lecture. In school, there is always a "right" answer, and all other answers are "wrong." That makes grading the report easy.

Does this sound familiar? Do you think that this is the way science is really done? If you think yes, that could explain why you never wanted to be a scientist; after all, why would anyone pursue such a boring, predetermined, repetitive profession? Fortunately, and in point of fact, this is not the way scientists practice their profession.

2.4.1 How Scientific Ideas Beget Scientific Research

Science and technology are professions that demand creativity, and the best scientists are those who are most creative (just as the best writers and artists are usually those who are most creative). A scientist begins work by puzzling over a question; the question may have been assigned by a supervisor or may be one that the scientist has thought of independently. Many scientific questions are based on anecdotal evidence, an informal observation that has not been systematically tested (e.g., people taking the high blood pressure drug Rogaine™ started regrowing hair). The better the scientist, the better the question, because let's face it, some questions are not worth worrying about. As the exact form of the question is formulated, the scientist may do a few experiments to test out his thinking and consult the scientific literature to see if anyone else has worked on a similar problem. It is typical of good science that doing experiments and collecting data are done not to come up with an answer or explanation, but to help decide between any number of competing possible explanations or hypotheses. To be valid, scientific hypotheses must be testable and falsifiable (proven false). A hypothesis is testable if it can be supported or rejected by carefully designed experiments or nonexperimental studies. A hypothesis is falsifiable if it can potentially be ruled out by data to show that the hypothesis does not explain the observations. Statements of opinion and conjectures based on supernatural or mystical explanations that cannot be tested or refuted fall outside the realm of scientific explanation.

Scientists conduct experiments to test hypotheses, but unless experiments are well-planned, the data they yield may be worthless. It is important to use the principles of sound "Experimental Design" when planning, conducting, and analyzing an experiment. We will discuss in some detail the types of experiments (or clinical trials) that involve human or animal subjects in the chapter on "Evaluating and Approving New Drugs and Devices," but here it is worthwhile to introduce some general concepts and ideas that are pertinent to virtually all types of experimentation.

Experiments involve variables: an independent variable or factor is a quantity or value that is set by the experimenter. For example, in an experiment to determine the effect of caffeine on blood pressure, the independent variable could be the amount of caffeine in milligrams consumed within a certain time period. The dependent variable would be the outcome measure; in this case it could be the blood pressure measured 1 h after consumption of caffeine.

In most experiments, it is necessary to have a control group against which the other measurements will be compared; in this experiment, the control group of individuals would be a group that consumes water instead of caffiene, but whose blood pressure is also measured. Because the person constructing the experiment would want to ensure that the control and experimental groups were not somehow self-selected (groups of caffeine-loving individuals all volunteering for the caffeinated group), individuals would be assigned to the control or experimental group at random, perhaps using a random number generator to facilitate the assignments.

Then, when blood pressure is measured, the experimenter would want to ensure that no bias creeps in and would perform the measurements blindly (i.e., would measure blood pressure without knowing if that particular individual had been in the control or in the experimental, caffeine-ingesting group). The experimenter would also realize that measurements themselves involve errors; a systematic error affects the accuracy of the measurement and could result from the measuring instrument not being properly calibrated or by the person making the measurement not knowing how to read the dial indicator. A random error affecting the precision of the measurement would also exist, for example, if the blood pressure value fluctuated during measurement. The effect of random errors can be reduced by replicating the measurement many times.

The common characteristics of "good" experiments include control groups, randomized participating individuals, or specimens, and the data recorder is blinded so that an expectation of a certain result cannot affect the measurement. The precision and accuracy of the measurement technique is known and reported, and an adequate number of replications are performed to reduce the effects of random error. Finally, statistical analyses are performed to determine if differences in results between the control group and the experimental group (or between experimental groups if more than one is involved) are due to a "real" effect of the independent variable or if the differences could be due to chance alone.

The result of all this thinking or experimentation is usually a hypothesis that the scientist formulates as a preferred explanation (Fig. 2.2). Most scientists take pride in coming up with simple explanations or hypotheses (they refer to them as "elegant"). The principle called Occam's razor states that everything else being equal, the simplest explanation is probably the correct one (the razor shaves away unnecessary complications). For example, if you hear hoofbeats, it's likely that horses are galloping by, not zebras; it is more likely that NASA landed a man on the moon than it all being an elaborate hoax and so on and so forth. Think of Occam's razor when you hear wild explanations of how diet pills can make you lose a lot of weight quickly without reducing your food intake or increasing your exercise levels!

Osborne and Dillon list a few examples of great questions that led to experimentation or data collecting, illustrating that the best scientists did not start by collecting all necessary data, but rather used superior intuition to first propose a hypothesis [6]:

- Wegener suggested that because the coastlines of several continents seemed to match or fit together (e.g., western coast of Africa and eastern coast of South America), all continents were joined together at one time and had separated in the process called continental drift (Fig. 2.3). At the time this suggestion was

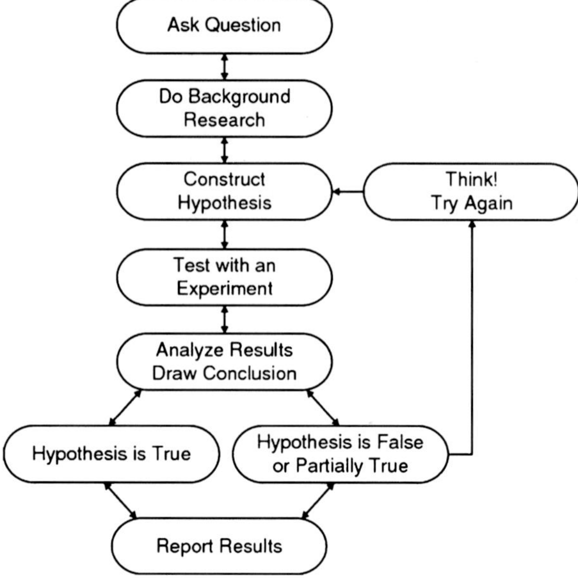

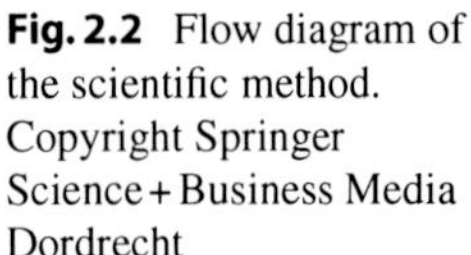
Fig. 2.2 Flow diagram of the scientific method. Copyright Springer Science+Business Media Dordrecht

made (1912), there was no explanation of how this could have happened; only later did seismologic experiments show there are two kinds of earth's crust and provided the evidence validating the theory.

- Louis Pasteur thought that diseases were caused by organisms too small to be seen with the naked eye (the germ theory of disease), that killing such organisms would lessen the chance of milk or wine spoiling (Pasteurization), and that weak forms of disease could be used as immunizing agents against stronger forms of that disease. He was proven right when he "put his money where his mouth was"; he publicly immunized 25 sheep against anthrax and left 25 sheep nonimmunized. All 25 nonimmunized sheep died from anthrax, while only one immunized sheep died. Pasteur later went on to develop a vaccine against rabies.
- Charles Darwin noticed that finches (a type of bird) on isolated islands near South America had substantially different characteristics that depended on the food supply on any given island (e.g., short beaks for eating seeds, long beaks for catching insects). Because all the finches had originally come from the same location (South America), Darwin hypothesized that the birds had evolved characteristics needed for survival on their island homes. This was the beginning of his formulation of the theory of natural selection, a radical departure from accepted dogma, which was that at the moment of creation, all species had been made at the same time. At first he was unsure of proposing this alternative explanation, and he continued thinking and gathering additional data. It was another 20 years before he felt confident enough to publish "The Origin of Species."
- Copernicus showed in a book published in 1543 that the motion of heavenly bodies made sense even if the earth was not the center of the galaxy (the geocentric theory was the accepted version of the solar system at that time). Unfortunately, he had no

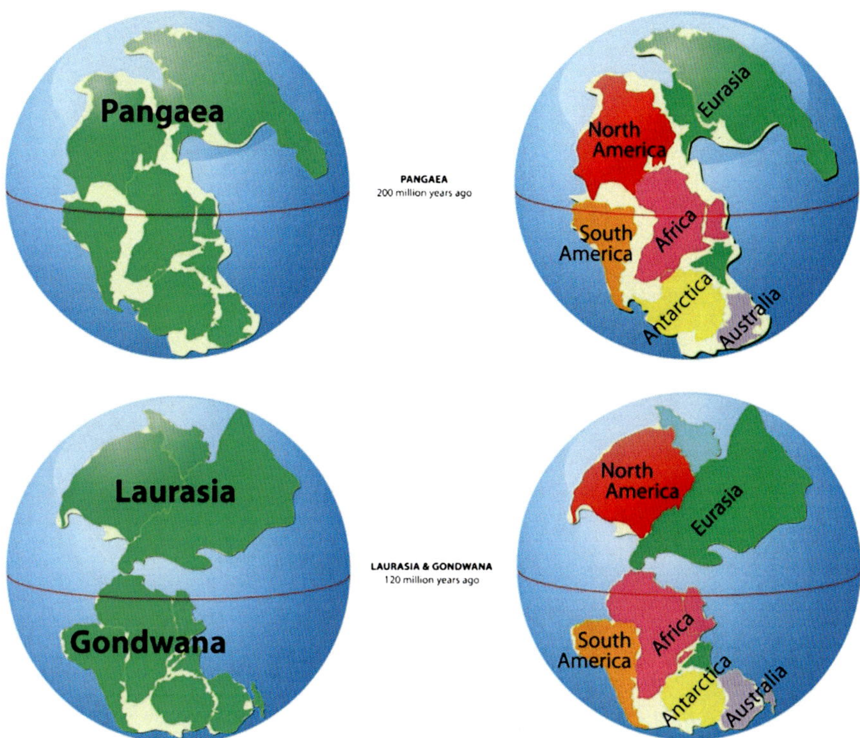

Fig. 2.3 Map showing how all the earth's continents once fit together. At one point, this was only a hypothesis; additional data later confirmed the validity of the hypothesis, lending it the status of a theory

data supporting the idea that the sun was the center of our solar system (heliocentric theory). It took an additional 200 years and work by Tycho Brahe, Johannes Kepler, Galileo, and eventually Isaac Newton before Copernicus's theory was accepted.

During the time a scientist is searching for data to support a hypothesis or to confirm a theory, many complications can occur. Experiments will fail or provide unexpected data that don't fit the scientist's concept; the theory/question is revised and more thinking and experimentation is done. This process of analysis, experimentation, revision of concept, experimentation again, changing the conditions of experiment, etc. is a very different one than that done in high school. There is another critical difference: no one knows the "correct" answer! It's entirely possible to construct an experiment and get a wrong answer, and it happens all the time. This is very central to the way a scientist conducts business, because it's not the way most people are trained to think; it's more comfortable to do an experiment and to accept the answer as the "truth."

Scientists often make their name by proving other scientists wrong by obtaining new data that disproves an established theory or by offering a new interpretation of existing data. They argue about how to interpret evidence all the time in what has been called a process of "organized skepticism" which is the strongest guarantee

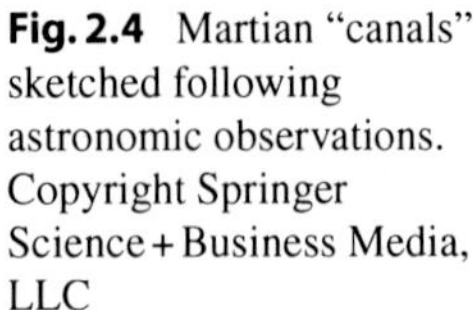

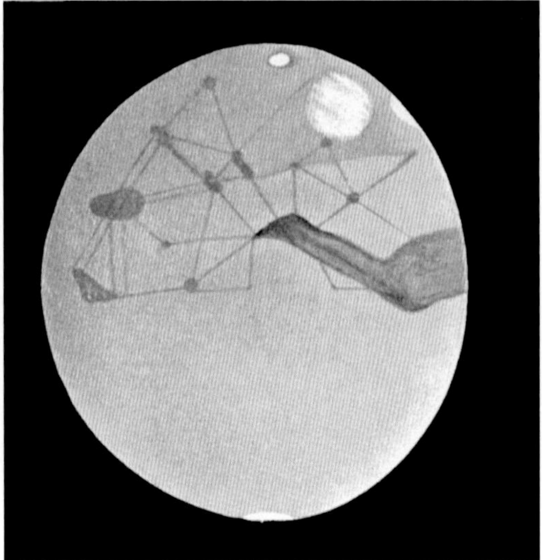

Fig. 2.4 Martian "canals" sketched following astronomic observations. Copyright Springer Science + Business Media, LLC

that the shelf life of any bogus or mistaken explanation or theory will be short indeed. There are many scientific theories that were accepted and popular at one time or another, but were proven wrong as more data became available:

- The existence of a planet called "Vulcan" was believed to be responsible for variations in the orbit of the planet Mercury; many astronomers even claimed to have seen it! This theory was abandoned in 1915.
- The Theory of Spontaneous Generation, formulated by Aristotle, stated that life could start from mud when it was exposed to light. The theory was based on observations of barnacles that seemed to form spontaneously on ship hulls and maggots that would crawl out of a corpse. The theory still had believers in the 1700s!
- Geologic features (Fig. 2.4) observed by astronomers on the surface of the planet Mars led some to theorize that these were canals built by some advanced alien life form; the theory was finally put to rest in the 1960s when NASA sent satellites flying over Mars which transmitted pictures back showing that the features were streaks of dust.

2.4.2 Collecting More Data to Validate a Theory: Who Pays for Science and Engineering Research

As the scientist gains confidence in a theory, depending on the scope of the question and the required amount of additional data needed to answer new related questions, funding is often needed in order to pay for supplies, equipment, and technical support to search for more confirmatory data to support a more expanded theory. The request for funding takes the form of a proposal, in which the scientist describes (with as much specific detail as possible given page limits) the fundamental idea or question, the reason or reasons why it is important to answer the question, what others have done to answer this or a similar question, what preliminary work the scientist has done to answer the question, and the plans the scientist has for further work. (A portion of a real proposal is included in Appendix A.) In order to show a command of the subject matter and to indicate that a great deal of work has already been done, the scientist might propose one or more hypotheses in the proposal. A hypothesis is essentially the best-guess prediction of how the proposed experiments will work out and is based on the current evidence. So, the hypothesis continues to be tested by the experiments proposed by the scientist. It is also true that sometimes a hypothesis is not needed, and with the development of specialized computer algorithms and rapid access to huge amounts of data, it is possible to mine data for correlations without the initial formulation of a hypothesis. At any rate, the hypothesis is tested, and if not supported, it is revised again and again until a conclusion can be drawn that provides at least a partial answer to the initial question.

This proposal, along with several others submitted by other scientists, is evaluated by a group of peers, i.e., other scientists familiar with the field, and given a score. The score is supposed to be related to the originality of the question, the importance of the question, the justification provided for the plans to answer the question, consideration of alternative answers, and finally the plans themselves. The reviewers often evaluate the proposal based on questions such as is the proposed explanation novel, is the hypothesis properly stated, are the experiments properly designed to test the hypothesis, and is the scientific team qualified to conduct this type of research. If the score is good enough, the scientist may receive a grant for a period of a few years to fund the research. Note please that the proposal is reviewed by other scientists who look forward to pointing out what if anything is wrong and silly about the idea and experiments!

Over the next year or two, the scientist will usually choose to disclose the results of experiments in the form of presentations at scientific meetings or publications in peer-reviewed journals and start building a case for a conclusion (answer to the question). If the results or "facts" that the scientist obtains are reproducible, observable natural occurrences, they constitute the evidence the scientist uses to support his/her interpretation of events. Sometimes, the scientist is compelled to draw an inference, which is a conclusion based on the facts but not specifically tested (e.g., if someone walks into your home wearing a wet raincoat, you infer that it is raining outdoors, even though you may not have seen it for yourself).

2.4.3 Announcing Research Results: Scrutiny by Peers

Disclosure of findings from scientific studies will often occur in the form of a manuscript submitted for publication in a scientific journal. High-quality journals will insist on peer review of the submission, which means that two or three other scientists will be asked to read the manuscript and provide a recommendation as to its worthiness for publication as part of a painful exercise called the "peer-review process" (Fig. 2.5). The review is usually done "blind," meaning that the submitting

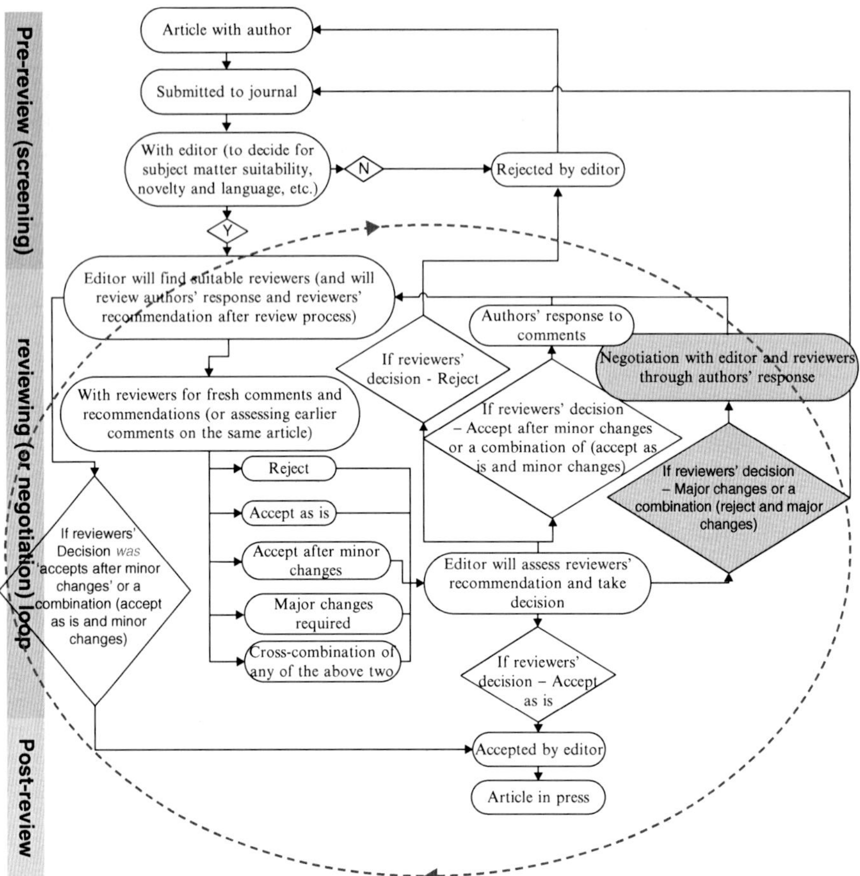

Fig. 2.5 A flow diagram of the peer-review process. The process acts as a safeguard against publication and dissemination of faulty or misinterpreted data. Copyrighted by Springer Science + Business Media B.V.

author does not know who the reviewers will be and often the name and affiliation of the author will be masked from the reviewers. The author will also be asked to disclose any financial considerations that might pose a conflict of interest; for example, a study describing the design of a new hip implant could be influenced by the author owning stock in the company selling the implants.

By the way, this kind of disclosure of a potential conflict of interest is peculiar to scientists. As was documented in the 2010 Oscar-winning movie "Inside Job," economists often write articles without disclosing their work for mutual funds or other investment companies.

The reviewers will consider the quality of the experiments, and their interpretation, realizing all the time that the data *suggest* the answer to a question; data are not absolute facts that state how things are. If the peer review is favorable, the manuscript is published.

Now the real action begins. If the manuscript reports a truly significant or exciting find or explanation (e.g., a cure for the common cold), other scientists get involved. First, questions are asked for more detail about the experiments, and other scientists will try to repeat the experiments to see if they obtain the same results; they will try to replicate the reported experimental results. If not, then the value of the original manuscript is called into question, and an argument begins. The argument may begin even if the experimental results agree, but a different explanation for the observation can be offered by other scientists.

2.4.4 Theories and Laws

At this point you should have recognized one of the main characteristics of the work of science: there is much review and much argument, and it is only after that review and argument is completed that an explanation rises to the level of a theory. And, even after a theory is generally accepted (e.g., the Theory of Relativity), it continues to receive scrutiny because scientists are skeptical by nature. No scientific theory is proven once and for all, and independent testing continuously tests the theory. Remember that no scientific theory can be tested in every possible situation and, as a result, a theory supported by current data is accepted until and unless further testing and data show otherwise.

A famous case in 1989–1990 illustrates this point. At that time, two chemists (Pons and Fleischmann) from the University of Utah claimed to have discovered the phenomenon of "cold fusion," i.e., the ability to fuse two atoms of hydrogen into a single atom of helium. This was tremendously exciting because it was done in an ordinary test tube, and energy was released! Their work suggested the promise of clean, renewable energy everyone had been waiting for. Because of the significance of this discovery, other scientists wanted to learn the details; however, Pons and Fleischmann kept postponing the release of information on the details of their experiments and, eventually, were found out to be sloppy experimentalists at best and frauds at worst.

So, to summarize and define some terms, a theory is an often complex explanation of phenomena that is based on the best available evidence. The evidence offered in support of a theory has been subjected to critical analysis and review by all interested scientists and usually represents the consensus of the scientific community at any given time. Nevertheless, this explanation keeps being retested, and it may be that testing is never completed, e.g., the phenomenon occurred over a time scale not possibly reproducible. For example, how can we do an experiment that replicates the formation of the universe as explained by the Big Bang Theory? Nonetheless, and this is significant to repeat, a theory is based on the best interpretation of the evidence at any given time. Furthermore, a consensus represents the best interpretation of existing data by the scientific community as a whole and does not necessarily mean that all scientists agree with that interpretation at all times. In fact, sometimes those few scientists, who may genuinely disagree with the consensus of the scientific community, may over time be able to change that consensus by presenting new findings or interpretations to falsify the existing theory.

If a theory is an explanation, how can we take advantage of the explanation to invent a better device or develop a new technology? If a law can be formulated, which describes relationships between various bodies and substances in a mathematical way, and these relationships can be confirmed by observation, then the law will provide guidance for utilizing the explanation contained in a theory. For example, Newton's second law of motion states that F = ma, or that the force exerted by a moving object is equal to the mass of the object multiplied by its acceleration. Notice that although this law does not explain why this is true (and it is true, because it has been confirmed by thousands of experiments), it is still a quite useful thing because it becomes a tool to make predictions. For example, an engineer who knows the weight of a bullet and the speed with which it travels can use Newton's second law of motion to calculate the force that bullet would deliver on impact and design a bulletproof vest. Newton's second law also predicts that when catching a fast-moving baseball that would normally hit a baseball glove with a great deal of force, pulling the glove away at the moment the ball hits the glove will reduce the relative acceleration of the ball and reduce the force felt by the fielder's hand.

A scientific law is not necessarily a stronger interpretation of the evidence as compared to a scientific theory, but rather a scientific law has a mathematical form to it while a scientific theory may not.

It is this constant process of review, argumentation, and retesting, all done publically and resulting in the formulation of theories or laws, that distinguishes claims made by science from claims that are belief based without an underpinning of observation or experimental validation. This quote by Carl Sagan may help you understand these issues better: "To be accepted, new ideas must survive the most rigorous standards of evidence and scrutiny."

Cobern and Loving provide an elegant explanation of what science is and what it involves [7]:

> Science is about natural phenomena and the explanations that science offers are naturalistic. The explanations are testable against other natural phenomena, or against other explanations (test of a theory). Science is about explaining, not only about describing. Science also assumes that it is possible to learn about nature, that there is order in nature, and that there is cause and effect in nature.

Science involves criticism, review, and argument, all conducted publically and accepting revisions of explanations and theories. Not all opinions matter, even though that may not seem "fair"; opinions have to be based on relevant and appropriate observations (Fig. 2.6).

It is important to remember the point made in this last paragraph: although everybody is entitled to their own opinion, when it comes to science, not everyone's opinion is relevant, and irrelevant opinions should not be considered in deciding issues that are fact based. Debates and arguments between scientists are not settled by a vote, but by who has the best factual evidence and interpretation of that evidence. As Senator Moynihan once said, "Everyone is entitled to their own opinion, but not to their own facts."

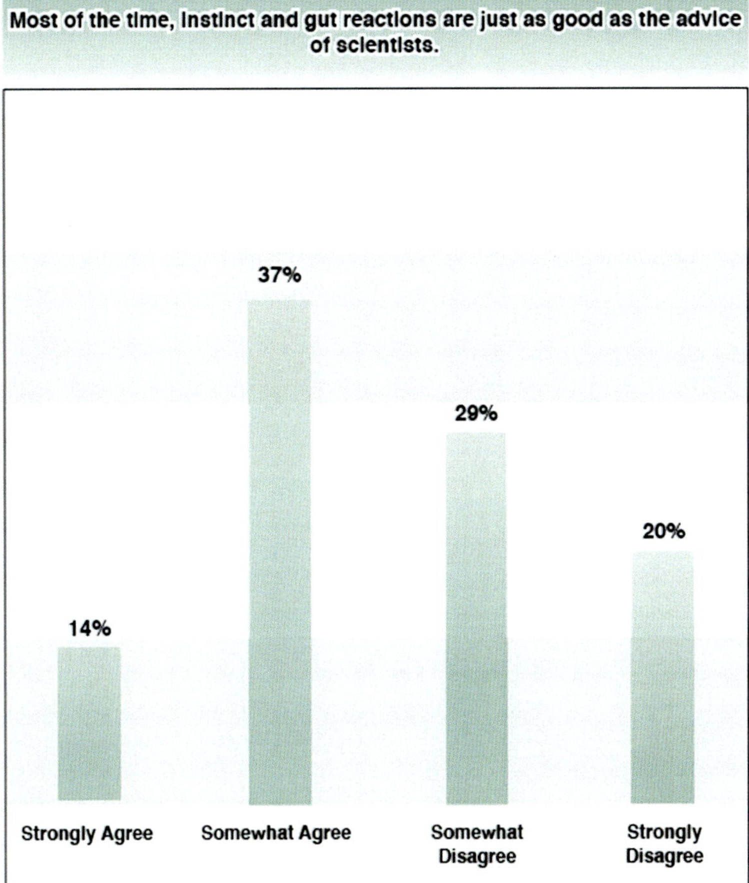

Fig. 2.6 The general public appears to be unaware that scientific advice and opinions are based on training and informed observation and as such are fundamentally different than other uninformed opinions. Data from a University of Texas/Texas Tribune poll of October 2012

2.4.5 What Can Go Wrong in the Scientific Process

Now that we have discussed the ways in which scientists and engineers work hard to devise experiments and theories, and to reach conclusions that will eventually lead to laws that enable design of safe buildings, airplanes, and artificial hearts, it's time to confess that mistakes can be made. Scientists and engineers are human and are influenced by all the same psychological factors that influence everyone else. Furthermore, the scientific process is a human activity and, like most other human activities, can be distorted by many societal factors. Let's see what some of these distorting factors are.

2.4.5.1 Data Distortion

Humans tend to be (and want to be) consistent. That tendency is also responsible for the difficulty we often have giving up a strongly held opinion or reversing an attitude. So, if, for example, a scientist has a strong certainty that a particular bacterium is responsible for a particular disease, there may be a tendency to have more faith in data supporting that opinion than in contradictory data. If a physician comes to think that the patient has a cyst in her breast, then it will be difficult to suddenly reclassify the lump as cancerous.

Once a person makes a decision, he or she is often bound to that decision, and it becomes difficult to revise. This pattern of behavior is common to organizations too, and there have been many large projects that continue to remain active even after it becomes clear to outsiders that the cost are unjustified or the initial design was flawed. There is a particular kind of fantastic optimism that causes project leaders to claim that there will no longer be cost overruns and that the machine will finally work! For example, the US F-35 Joint Strike Fighter program is beset by significant problems. More than 2,400 F-35s were to be bought through 2037, but the total cost of acquisition is now nearly $400 billion, up 42 % from the estimate in 2007; the price per plane has doubled since project development began in 2001. Cost overruns now total $1 billion. On top of it all, the plane's performance was described as "mixed" in 2011. The project continues nevertheless.

Humans (scientists too!) tend to accept or reject evidence based on preconceptions. These preconceptions were likely developed with a good-sized helping of "scientific intuition." It turns out that most people like to think that they have a good sense of intuition, because we all suffer from the human tendency to remember times when our intuition was correct rather than the times when we were dead wrong. Just think of how many times you've played the same lottery number….

This erroneous belief in the power of intuition has many examples. For example, many folks believe that personal interviews are the best way to establish who should be offered a particular position. However, it has been shown that in most circumstances an interview is useless for many reasons [8]. First, an applicant who has a nice personality and is pleasant looking will benefit from the "halo effect" and will be considered to have all the necessary skills for the job regardless of objective measures such as background or experience. Second, the interview is biased by the "primacy" and "contrast" effects; all things being equal, the most recent interviewee is remembered best, and the candidate following a "bad" one will be evaluated too highly, while a candidate following an "excellent" one will be evaluate too harshly [9].

By the way, the halo effect is used to good purpose by the advertising industry; a pleasing name on a product carries over to a pleasing overall impression of the product itself. Do the names Corvette, Viper, Sting Ray, and Jaguar not convey a certain characteristic of the automobiles just because of their names?

Missing or negative data are ignored in favor of data that confirm beliefs or that preserve consistency. It has been shown that the likelihood that a peer reviewer will recommend publication of some manuscript is related to the likelihood of the submitted paper confirming the reviewer's own body of work [10]. Practitioners and believers of holistic medicine often claim that "it's the patient's own fault" if a treatment doesn't work.

On the other hand, evidence may also be overamplified, meaning that even though there may be insufficient evidence, there is nevertheless pressure to proceed to a conclusion. It is sometimes difficult to recognize that evidence is lacking, because people (scientists too!) like to tell stories about what is happening and want to see a cause and effect relationship even when there is none; are you familiar with the phrase "jumping to a conclusion"? That's why it is good scientific practice to first form a hypothesis (make a prediction) and then systematically test the hypothesis with experiment.

Another example of the human desire to tell stories and of our need for consistency is the tendency to see patterns where there are none (or for a scientist to see a connection where there is none). How many of you believe in a "hot streak" even if there is no way that the outcome of a previous event (e.g., a basketball shot going in) could have an effect on the next attempt? Still another sports-related example is the so-called Sports Illustrated cover jinx, which claims that if an athlete or a team is featured on the cover, inevitably the team will suffer a loss or losses, and the athlete will go "cold," i.e., stop performing well. In fact, the jinx is just a manifestation of what is called "reverting to the mean." The team's or athlete's performance is typified by some average performance; an above-average performance is the reason to make the cover, but at some point the team or athlete will have to perform below average, hence the jinx.

But we are programmed to preferentially perceive and pay attention to the outlier and provide exceptional characteristics (good or bad) to the person, fact, or thing that stands out. In part, this habit of ours is what is responsible for ethnic or racial stereotyping. Because members of minority groups stand out more, we endow them with more dramatic traits. If we are member of the majority and meet another who is not, then any characteristics we notice will be exaggerated. So, for example, members of a white majority would often tend to exaggerate the athletic ability (positive characteristic) and the generally lower economic status (negative characteristic) of the black minority.

The tendency to exaggerate is itself even more exaggerated in group settings, when individuals' behavior is influenced by the presence of others; this is called "Groupthink." It turns out that in a group, the thinking and attitudes of the members do not move toward the average attitude, but instead the average attitude becomes more pronounced, more radical. Groupthink is always more extreme than "individual think." This phenomenon could explain the polarization going on in American politics today, when it seems that the divide between the "left" and the "right" is wider than ever, with no apparent common ground in sight.

Because humans are inherently biased, there is a risk that the missing information will be replaced with a biased explanation. One way to avoid this trap is to establish a causal story by gathering what is called covariational information. In this approach, data are obtained while searching for the presence or absence of an effect both when the proposed cause is either present or absent. The questions asked are two: (1) Is there an effect in the presence of the proposed cause? and (2) is there an effect in the absence of the proposed cause?

To borrow an example from Brem and Riss, let's consider the claim that welfare recipients have difficulty getting off welfare because they lack job skills [11]. The explanation (story) might say that job skills improve one's chances of landing a paying job and allows the person to get off welfare. This explanation sounds reasonable and may even be true! But recall the existence of bias…in decades past, explanations involving the role of a "spirit" were assumed to be reasonable. The role of evidence in evaluating the claim made earlier would consist of comparing welfare recipients with job training against welfare recipients without job training. If we find those with training spend less time on welfare than those without, that finding constitutes evidence for the claim. If we also find that those with training obtain well-paying jobs and that those with well-paying jobs are less likely to return to welfare, that is evidence for the mechanism. In real life, of course, these are complex issues, but published research does suggest that if welfare recipients are shown that they can be successful in the labor market (i.e., providing them with job skills), they will show an increased tendency to seek work.

What do you think: how could you evaluate claims that eating more than two helpings of fried foods per day increases blood cholesterol?

2.4.5.2 Other Forms of Bias

It may surprise you to hear that scientists can be biased. Indeed, one of the forms of bias talked about today is based on gender. There are many more male scientists in senior positions than female scientists. Surveys indicate that men and women receive the same number of doctoral degrees in biology, yet at universities, only about 15 % of professors (the highest academic rank) are female. These ratios are somewhat different in other scientific fields; a 2008 survey in the UK found that 25 % of men were employed in science, engineering, and technology versus 4 % of women in those same fields.

There are many potentially accurate explanations for this phenomenon. For example, women have been historically dissuaded from pursuing mathematics and the physical sciences, and indeed there are more women in biologically-intensive science careers when compared to physical sciences-intensive careers. The advancement of women in their careers can be impeded by their traditional child-rearing roles, which can interfere with the single-minded dedication needed at the start of an academic career, when fresh assistant professors are busily pursuing tenure. Whatever the reasons are, folks at various national-level organizations are concerned that large numbers of potentially productive scientists and engineers are being lost to other professions.

What do you think: why are fewer women than men drawn to science and technology careers?

In this chapter, we are more concerned with examining bias and the effects of this slanted gender distribution on scientific practice, rather than on the roots of this form of bias. Two examples serve to illustrate these points. Until recently, the role of men as hunter gatherers was given primacy in studies of the social evolution of mankind; it is only within the past 25 years or so that the role of women as gatherers and toolmakers has been recognized and their importance accented. In another instance, craniologists (folks who measure the size of the skull) used to maintain that the ratio of men's skulls to their body mass "proved" men to be more intelligent than women. A later reexamination of the data showed that the skulls selected for measurement were not randomly selected, and if they had been, the opposite conclusion would have been reached using that line of reasoning (women are more intelligent than men). Other examples of bias include racial bias: claims that whites are more intelligent than blacks, that society could be improved by selective breeding, and that restricting immigration from southern Europe (e.g., Italy) would improve American society's genetic pool.

It is important to understand that bias not only may be used to promote the idea of someone's inferiority, it could also be used at times to promote the concept of a particular ethnic groups superiority in one field or another. In all such instances, extremely careful examination of data to search for evidence of bias would be called for.

Bias does not only occur as the result of gender or race. In some cases, it can occur for political reasons. In the Stalinist Soviet Union (1921–1953), Trofim Lysenko was director of Soviet biology and developed a theory of genetics that claimed an "environmentally acquired inheritance," rather than the more widely accepted genetic theory derived from the work of Mendel. This theory coincided with the communist thinking of that time, which was that organisms (including people) could be easily and quickly remade under controlled environmental conditions. Lysenko's theory became popular in the Soviet Union and formed the basis of its agricultural policy in the mid- and late 1940s. Scientists who dissented from this prevailing theory were imprisoned! Because the theory was based on questionable and even fraudulent data, crop yields in the Soviet Union plummeted, causing severe hardships. Tragically, Lysenko's theory was also responsible for helping justify Mao Tse-Tung's great leap forward in China in 1958, a disastrous experiment believed to have caused the deaths of 20–40 million people from starvation.

Although it is doubtful that scientific fraud on this scale is practiced today, it is important to know that it can occur on a smaller scale, as the result of what may be called the "my-side" bias. That is, a scientist examining data may be tempted to exclude data that does not support his/her working hypothesis and may instead be tempted to interpret the data to support his/her working hypothesis. Studies of human behavior have shown that we all practice the "my-side" bias on a daily basis, though perhaps not scientifically, when we often choose to hear or see only those events and things that coincide with our view of the world.

In keeping with the theme of bias in science, some folks maintain that the science and health technology we have is biased in favor of the West. That is, because most scientists and healthcare professionals are trained and do research in Western Europe or the USA, the current scientific understanding has a bias against those who have not been dominant in science. To reverse this discrimination, some argue that more indigenous or native or traditional notions of science should be included in science curricula. And in fact, there is no reason to exclude multicultural knowledge about the real world, as it has been accumulated over many years and served the needs of various indigenous peoples. However, while recognizing and appreciating the bounty of experience-derived knowledge, we should not confuse folklore with science. The folklore we celebrate enabled a culture to develop new technologies and to survive by successfully solving everyday problems, but it does not bear scrutiny through our definition of the scientific method. That is, traditional or indigenous or aboriginal notions of science and technology should be probed to discover does the technology have a theoretical background, does the theory permit updating and revision, is systematic experimentation part of the development of the knowledge, is the knowledge formalized, and can further research be done on it? Much of the folklore accumulated by native people is generally useful only in the contextual framework of the life of those people and past times; it loses applicability when it enters a setting that is different from where and when it was developed. For example, the use of certain plants to cure or aid those who are ill will work only where those plants grow; knowledge of the key ingredient is lacking, so the knowledge cannot be spread universally. Often too the knowledge has been protected, available only to certain practitioners and their acolytes, and not generally available for all to read, see, and discuss, i.e., not conformable to our definition of science.

2.4.6 Pseudoscience

The strength of the scientific approach relies on the continued scrutiny of data and interpretations of those data and in the peer-review approach to reviewing manuscripts and research. Above all, however, it is the acceptance of the idea that our current understanding of things may be wrong, and if new knowledge is acquired, theories are amended. There is no system of beliefs that is able to make such a claim and that is where science and religion diverge.

You may recall that at the beginning of this chapter, a series of provocative statements were made. If you spend enough time in the early morning hours watching cable television, particularly the infomercial variety of programs, you may encounter even more such statements. Some promise to cure an affliction like baldness, psoriasis, or dementia; others promote all-natural new treatments that are only available by mail order or strange combinations of ingredients only recently discovered to help resolve various health problems (Fig. 2.7).

Some of the ads may seem comical, but you surely think that they must be at least somewhat effective, otherwise no one would be buying television time to advertise. So how should listeners react, who presumably want to find an effective remedy (but not fall victim to misleading advertising such as shown in Fig. 2.8)?

There are explanations for why many of these claims "sound" reasonable, and we can think of reasonable rules that can be followed in examining them. First, news of newly discovered cures are often exaggerated for purposes of a sensational headline, and many of such stories are based (loosely) on very early studies that have not been tested by other scientists. Second, be wary of trying unproven remedies if the advertising is suggesting that since nothing else has worked, what do you have to lose? You could lose even more good health, your time, and certainly some of your money. Patients and their families who may be desperate for a cure are

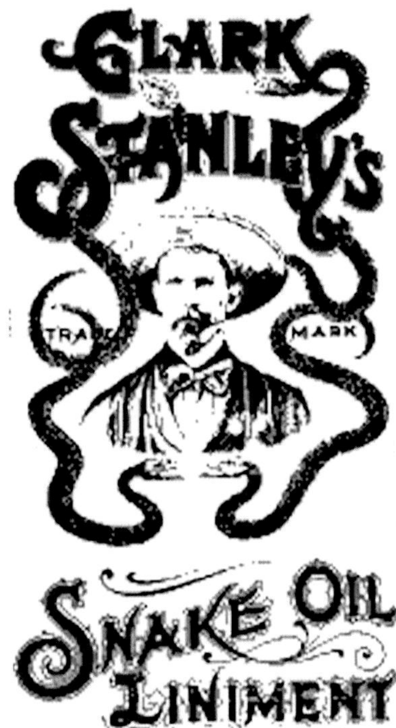

Fig. 2.7 At one time, there were fraudsters selling snake oil as a cure-all in the American west. Snake oil has been replaced by food supplements, cures for baldness, aids for impotence, or pills for extra energy as the next must-have curative substance

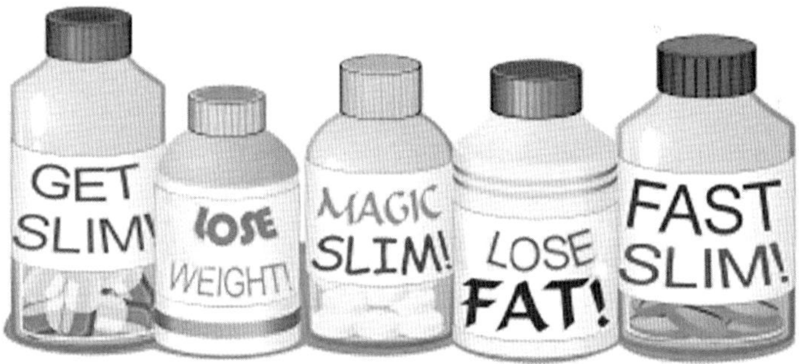

Fig. 2.8 People like to believe in miracle cures

particularly vulnerable and sometimes travel to clinics around the world where licensing and truth in advertising laws are poorly enforced [10]. Third, the reason that dramatic claims of cures are made is because we know that dramatic and sensational news is most easily remembered. Finally, testimonials (when truthful) are only provided by people whom the treatments helped. Recall that in the absence of a controlled study, it is not possible to determine if these improvements came as the result of the placebo effect or not, and in any case, there are no testimonials from people for whom the treatments did *not* help.

As noted above, scientists tend to be very skeptical of even their own claims, and a good helping of skepticism is helpful; remember that extraordinary claims require extraordinary proof, that any causal claim must have relied also on a control group, and that the burden of proof is on the person seeking to overturn the accepted treatment mode.

A few years ago there was a lot of discussion about a compound called beta-carotene that was found in fruits and vegetables. Several laboratory studies, animal studies, and results of observations showed that this compound was protective against cancer. Then, the results of three clinical trials were published, which showed that the compound did *not* work as promised. Infomercials marketing beta-carotene diet supplements would show a stack of laboratory studies on one side, and three clinical studies on the other, and ask "which do you believe?" In this case, the consensus of the scientific community was that the clinical trials had the last word, and while eating fruits and vegetables is definitely a good idea for many health reasons, it does not help to protect against cancer [12].

Regardless of all that we are taught and have read about science and engineering, various pseudosciences maintain their popularity in our society: acupuncture, astrology, homeopathy, etc. All these schemes have advocates who provide testimonials as to the effectiveness of these treatments or beliefs. A survey conducted in 2007 by the National Institutes of Health (NIH) reported that 38 % of Americans use some form of complementary and alternative medicine (CAM). The NIH, under pressure from politicians who believe in alternative medicine, has formed an organization called the National Center for Complementary and Alternative Medicine. The objectives of this institute include the study of alternative medical practice such as the use of herbal medications, dietary supplements, probiotics (e.g., yoghurt), meditation, yoga, spinal manipulation, qigong, tai chi, movement therapies such as Pilates and Rolfing, energy field manipulation such as Reiki and magnet therapy, Ayurvedic medicine, and traditional Chinese medicine. It is of interest to note that on its web page, the NCCAM states that "rigorous, well-designed clinical trials for many CAM therapies are often lacking; therefore, the safety and effectiveness of many CAM therapies are uncertain." Also, "information provided by NCCAM is not meant to take the place of your primary health care provider's medical expertise." There are a number of other warnings about credentials of CAM practitioners, including the fact that dietary supplements have not been tested on pregnant women, that the mechanisms of action of the supplements are unknown, and that standards for ensuring dosage and purity of botanicals and dietary supplements do not exist.

Let's consider acupuncture (Fig. 2.9). A frequent comment made about this practice is "we know it works from thousands of years of experience." The "acupoints" that are described as areas with concentrations of nerve endings and blood vessels have never been found by any microscopic or biochemical techniques. A study reported that during acupuncture, certain brain activity was reduced, which corresponded to lower pain perception in the volunteers taking part in the study. What does that mean, exactly? Was the effect causal or coincidental or was it due to the placebo effect? Many reviewers of homeopathic practice believe that the placebo

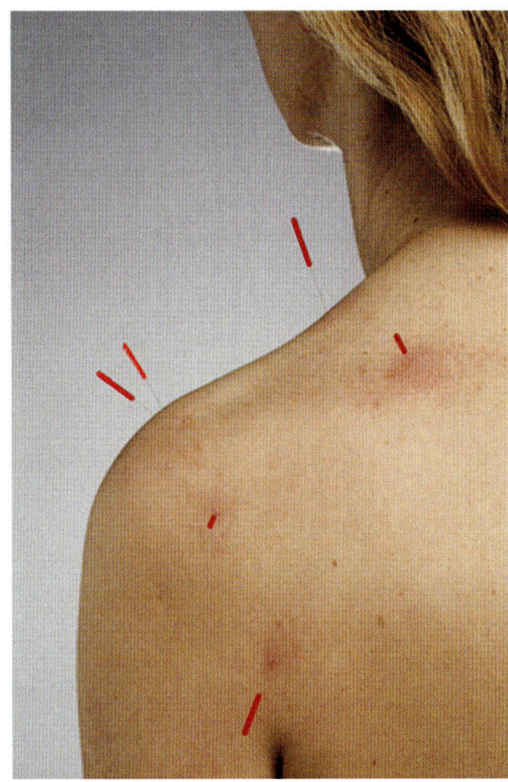

Fig. 2.9 The process of acupuncture. Scientific studies have shown that acupuncture does not work

effect is responsible for the outcomes of treatment and that studies purporting to show it to be effective are improperly designed and do not use the proper controls.

Homeopathy is a type of treatment that is reputed to be effective for treating a number of ailments including arthritis, asthma, depression, headaches, and insomnia. Testimony for its effectiveness is available from the many celebrities who are users, including Paul McCartney, Tina Turner, and Jennifer Aniston, though within the traditional medical community it is considered to be quackery. It has evolved into an industry including a professional trade association (The Society of Homeopaths), whose members are trained in preparing the medications. Homeopaths believe that by choosing a substance that causes the same symptoms as the disease afflicting the patient, and having the patient ingest a very dilute preparation of that substance, the patient will recover. For example, if the patient has a runny nose, the homeopath might take some onion juice (which also causes a runny nose), dilute it in water, and shake the solution in a special way called succession. The dilution of the active ingredient is extreme:

> *What do you think: what questions should be asked when considering an alternative medical approach?*

a common dilution is called 30C, which is achieved by taking a drop of the active substance, diluting it in 100 drops of water, then taking one drop of the first dilution and diluting it again in 100 drops of water, and so on until the dilution has been made 30 times. What are the chances of any of the active substance still remaining? Homeopaths claim that the water "remembers" the active substance even though none may be left and that the memory of the substance is more potent than the substance in its original strength [13]. Again, no scientific proof of any of these claims is provided by their proponents.

So how can you tell science apart from pseudoscience? The answer lies not so much in the specific topic under discussion, but rather in what type of work or process was involved in formulating the new explanation or theory. If the answers to these questions is "no," it is likely that the explanation is pseudoscientific.

- Was the scientific method used?
- Were hypotheses constructed and carefully tested?
- Are mechanisms proposed that explain the phenomenon?
- Did statistical methods and analyses provide evidence of patterns or estimates of certainty or is the idea presented as dogma and unchangeable?
- Were alternative explanations considered and evaluated?
- Has the explanation developed and changed over time as new evidence became available?

2.5 Engineering Methods

At this point it may be relevant to introduce the distinction between science and engineering. After all, almost all the medical devices we will discuss in this book have been designed and manufactured by engineers (Fig. 2.10).

It is interesting that the word engineer may be used both as a noun and as a verb. When used as a verb, e.g., "he engineered a solution," it conveys the idea that someone used their skill, experience, and knowledge to find a more or less perfect answer to some problem. It implies that there was some estimation, guesswork, and trial and error involved. Aren't these actions consistent with what we believe indigenous and ancient peoples had to do? In fact, this behavior to some degree still characterizes the practice of engineering. The engineering method is "the strategy for causing the best change in a poorly understood situation within the available resources" [14]. Consider some of the famous engineering projects: building the Suez canal, tunneling under the English channel to provide a train link between England and France, and the man into space program. All these problems were initially poorly defined, the resources that would be needed had not been accurately estimated, the length of time needed to achieve the goal was unknown, and the side effects of achieving the goal could not be imagined. President John F. Kennedy called for the USA to land a man on the moon within 10 years, but no one at the time had any idea of how to do that exactly. Also, the materials, electronic components, and available resources all changed throughout the duration of the project. Engineers solved that

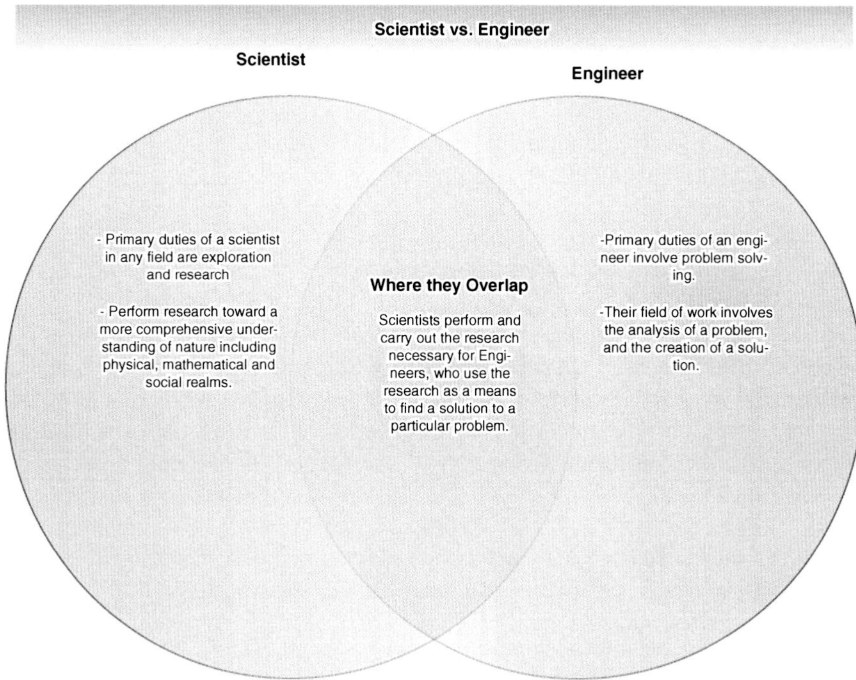

Fig. 2.10 Scientists and engineers have somewhat different perspectives and interests, but their work is complementary

problem, because seeking the best solution while surrounded by uncertainty and change is the engineer's specialty.

The work of an engineer involves design: a new biomaterial put together from available raw materials, a new type of engine, and a new kind of scaffolding for rebuilding a broken bone. At the outset of all exercises in design, the engineer, or more likely the engineering team, has a sense of how to start or pick up a series of hints as to how to find a solution. They also have a set of tools: equations that describe the behavior of some mechanical or electrical system or software that permits rapid calculations to be made. Recall that scientists proceed to gain new knowledge by thinking of new theories or explanations and conducting experiments to test those theories or hypotheses; engineers also have a set of procedures they follow that are somewhat different from those used by scientists.

Engineers will follow the general principles of first, proposing several design solutions. Then, they will estimate the needed resources and compare with the resources that are available. They will then seek to identify the best estimate design and discard the alternatives, and proceed to solve the problem by successive approximations, getting closer with each attempt. The "weakest link" will be identified, and a safety factor developed that will depend on the confidence in the design, the expected lifetime, and the cost of failure. Everything that is learned in the course of solving the problem will be expressed quantitatively, including graphs, tables, and mathematical equations.

Perhaps now it is clear why the engineering approach is so absolutely useful for solving healthcare problems; they are poorly understood, the outlook for stable resources is dim, and new knowledge is constantly being provided by scientists… exactly the environment familiar to engineers.

2.6 Science and Religion (Nonscience)

Because science is a discipline that depends on evidence and religion mostly relies on belief in the absence of physical evidence, conflicts between science and religion are almost inevitable. On occasion, the conflicts become obvious, particularly during a political race or when curriculum choices for public K through 12 education are being debated. In recent years, a good example of the different approach to teaching science offered by strict religious followers has been the discussion about the teaching of theory of evolution versus creationism (a variety of creationism is called "intelligent design"). In general, the followers of creationism believe that the origin of the universe is due to a Creator (or "intelligent designer"), that the theory of evolution is inadequate in explaining the variety of life forms on our planet, that adaptive change only occurs within tightly defined limits, that apes and human do not share a common ancestor, and that the earth is between 6,000 and 10,000 years old. In North, Central, and South America and in Western Europe, these beliefs correspond to a literal interpretation of the Judaeo–Christian bible. Most adherents of orthodox Islam also believe that the origin of the universe is due to a Creator and that apes and humans do not share a common ancestor. However, followers of other religions, e.g., Hinduism, often have radically different views of the origins of the world.

The arguments proposed by creationists include suggestions that creationism is actually more aligned with the requirements of science than is evolution; for example, if evolution is valid, why can't we observe event or processes that support it? Why are there gaps in the fossil record that could show us the transitional species predicted by evolution? Is not the wealth of species and nature observable to us today not a commonsense affirmation of a sublime and powerful Creator? Isn't evolution just a theory anyway?

Let's examine some of these arguments. Taking the last one first, it is a common mistake for nonscientists to minimize the amount of supporting data, other theories, and logic required for a hypothesis to rise to the level of a theory. Scientists, as we have already discussed, are inherently skeptical, argumentative, and tentative and would never claim that a theory has been proven true once and for all. Rather, they argue that the overwhelming weight of available evidence and the interpretation of that evidence support the present formulation of the theory, *until proven otherwise*. Scientists regard this attitude with pride, not as evidence of weakness.

The issue of the missing fossil record is due to a fundamental misunderstanding of the evolutionary theory. Creationists note that the fossils for "missing link," the jump between apelike and man, have not been found. Evolutionary biologists

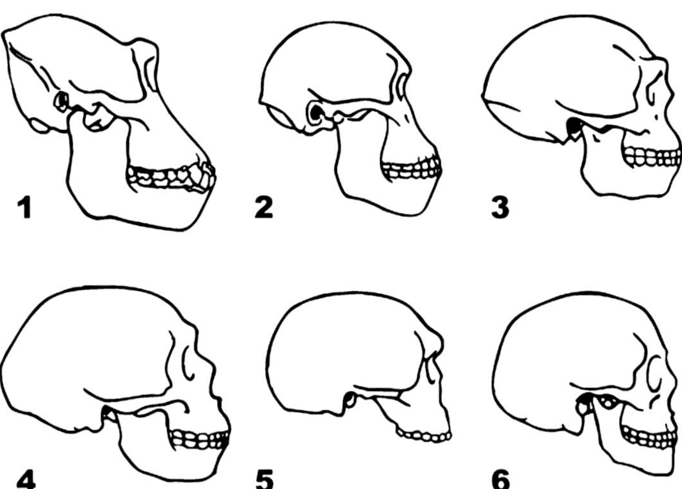

Fig. 2.11 Reconstructions of human skull development with time based on the fossil record

respond by emphasizing that evolution progresses not up a ladder with distinct steps, but rather with many branches splitting off, and species sharing a common ancestor (i.e., man and ape) have gone on along different branches. Also, the conditions for fossil preservation are not easily met. Consider how many hundreds of millions of animals have inhabited our planet; should we not be inundated with fossils if it were that easy to preserve a fossil? The large number of animals that lived in muddy environments, and whose bones were covered and preserved in sediment, are most likely to leave us with fossils, and in addition humans did not live in such environment, and there were few of them to leave a fossil record. However, we have been able to find skulls and other bones of the ancestors of present-day mankind, and those fossils have been used to construct a map of how we evolved (Fig. 2.11).

It turns out that we can in fact observe processes that are indicative of evolution, which is after all a theory stating that the organisms who survive are those best adapted to the environment. A survey of animals on isolated islands, e.g., the Galapagos and others, will show that individual islands are populated by a very non-diverse number of species, all surviving because they are well adapted to their environment. The larger the island, and the greater the variety of habitat, the larger the diversity of species. The ability to analyze DNA has now clearly shown that many genetic mutations have spread in the last few thousand years and have changed the way people digest food, store fat, grow hair, and fight disease. Examining the physiology of Tibetans living at higher elevations, for example, shows that some Tibetans have much greater oxygen-carrying ability in their blood than others and that women with this ability had more surviving children than women with lower oxygen-carrying ability. Therefore, evolution favors those better at surviving a low-oxygen environment in the Himalayan mountains. We have all heard about bacteria that have mutated and are able to resist antibiotics; evolution explains that bacteria able to adapt to antibiotics survive and pass on that characteristic to their progeny, while those bacteria unable to withstand antibiotic challenge die off.

Although some creationists abide by a strict interpretation of the Judaeo–Christian bible, believing that the Creator had completed work within 6 days and the world is only a few thousand years old, others have an amended philosophy called intelligent design (ID). Unlike creationists, proponents of ID do not dismiss radioactive carbon dating (used to establish that many fossils are millions of years old) as a trick, accept the age of the earth as being approximately 4.5 billion years, agree that some evolution occurs, and that natural selection has a role in determining which species survive and transmittal of successful traits. However, they argue that all this is evidence of the intervention and participation by a Creator, not simply evolutionary biology. Nevertheless, ID is inconsistent with our current scientific understanding of the natural world on a number of fundamental issues, including the central role of randomness in natural evolution, and has been declared as a variation of creationist conjecture by the US federal courts.

This is not to suggest that religious belief is necessarily incompatible with scientific method. There have been many active, prominent scientists who were devout Christians and practiced both their faith and profession without apparent contradiction. Francis Collins (director of the National Institutes of Health), William Phillips (corecipient of the 1997 Nobel Prize for Physics), and most interestingly Georges Lemaitre (Belgian priest who proposed the Big Bang Theory) are just some examples. Peter Higgs, the physicist who predicted the existence of a subatomic particle now called the Higgs boson and a nonbeliever himself, has been quoted as saying that:

> The growth of our understanding of the world through science weakens some of the motivation which makes people believers. But that's not the same as saying they're incompatible. It's just that I think some of the traditional reasons for belief, going back thousands of years, are rather undermined.…Anybody who is convinced but not a dogmatic believer can continue to hold his belief [15].

Should creationists and proponents of intelligent design be allowed to have their own opinion? Yes, of course; and if they wish, they should discuss it and attempt to convince others that their view is correct. Should creationism and intelligent design be taught as and considered to be as scientifically and objectively valid as evolution? No, of course not! Those beliefs do not rise to the standard demanded of science. They have no research agenda, because anything not explainable is ascribed to a supernatural authority. Creationism and intelligent design do not propose new research, nor are they capable of modification or falsifiable as new knowledge is uncovered. These attitudes seek to overturn accepted explanations of natural events rather than changing their own underlying principles.

The argument over what (creationism vs. evolution) can or should be taught in public schools has been played out in the courts in the USA. In 1925, the State of Tennessee sued a high school teacher named John Thomas Scopes for violating the state's Butler act, which made it illegal to teach evolution in schools. The Scopes trial was sensational and followed by newspapers from all parts of the USA. Scopes was found guilty and fined $100, but the conviction was later overturned on a technicality. A movie "Inherit the Wind" was made about the Scopes trial.

In approximately ten subsequent law cases, in states ranging from Arkansas to California to Louisiana to Minnesota to Pennsylvania, the courts have consistently ruled that the state may not require that teaching be tailored to the principles of a particular religion, that teaching evolution does not limit the free exercise of religion, that a "balanced treatment" teaching both evolution and creationism was not constitutional, that a school district may prohibit a teacher from teaching creationism as science, and that teachers could not be told to read a disclaimer before teaching about evolution. In the most recent case in 2005 in York County Pennsylvania, the judge ruled that the school district's attempt to maintain an "intelligent design" teaching policy in the schools was unconstitutional.

2.7 Science and Politics

Just as science topics sometimes run afoul of strict religious doctrines, so do politicians on occasion decide that scientific opinions conflict with political or economic necessity. It is sometimes believed that this occurs because few scientists or scientifically trained individuals choose to run for political office. And it is true that there are very few practicing scientists in the US Congress; in 2011, there was 1 physicist, 1 chemist, 1 microbiologist, 6 engineers, and 22 people with medical training among the 435 members of the House of Representatives. As has been mentioned once already, in the 2012 presidential campaign, there were no scientific policy issues questioned or debated.

On the other hand, having a certain background is no guarantee of being open to scientific ways of thinking. In 2012, representative Paul Broun of Georgia, who is a physician, referred to evolution, embryology, and the Big Bang Theory as all coming "straight from the pit of Hell" [16]. Congressman Akins from Missouri (another member of the House Science and Technology Policy Committee at the time the statement was made) stated in the summer of 2012 that women who are raped cannot get pregnant and that therefore rape should not be grounds for abortion; his belief in the immorality of abortion probably influenced him to make a groundless and false statement about a scientific issue.

In 2009, there was a terrible earthquake in L'Aquila, Italy, as a result of which one small village was devastated and 297 people died. Italian seismologists had warned that the town lay on a fault line, and tremors were felt in the days prior to the main earthquake. The scientists stated in the days before the earthquake that a major earthquake was unlikely, but did not discount the possibility. In 2012, the scientists were put on trial for being "falsely reassuring," convicted, and sentenced to 6 years in jail [17]. It appeared that the local government was trying to find a scapegoat for the disorganized renovation efforts following the earthquake, because given the state of the art in earthquake science, no one is capable of predicting the magnitude of an earthquake!

President George W. Bush instituted a program called the President's Emergency Plan for AIDS Relief (PEPFAR), identifying $15 billion to be spent in 2003–2008 to combat the spread of AIDS primarily in Africa. However, because of the influence of Christian conservatives, the legislation creating PEPFAR included the mandatory provision that none of the money would go to charitable groups that enable abortion. Unfortunately, because many charitable groups include contraception, birth control, and abortion counseling among their activities, they could not be funded, in part because the PEPFAR program promotes abstinence as a birth control and HIV control measure. Although portions of these provisions were repealed in 2009 by President Obama, confusion still exists among the many charitable organizations working in Africa, with the result that they do not apply for funding.

The junior senator from Florida, Marco Rubio, identified by some political pundits as a potential nominee for president by the Republican Party for the 2016, was asked in an interview how old he thought the earth is (Senator Rubio is also a member of the Senate's committee on Science and Transportation). He answered by stating that he was not qualified to answer that question because he was not a scientist, that it was one of the great mysteries, and that it is currently a dispute among theologians [18]. What sort of worldview does this influential and potentially powerful political figure have if he states that the age of the earth is a theological question? Is it not a scientific question that has been settled a long time ago?

These examples of political influence on issues that ought to be discussed and decided based on evidence suggest that American voters should insist that candidates for political office should clearly express their views on issues such as teaching evolution and climate change so that the public can judge the suitability of these candidate for becoming policy makers. Of course, American voters themselves should also be better educated about science and public policy or at least apply scientific reasoning skills to complex problems.

2.8 Scientifically Based Arguments

It is likely that you will witness arguments on scientific topics, whether it be on television news covering political or school board meetings, at the supermarket when debating the safety of genetically engineered foods, or at the preschool when parents discuss the pros and cons of immunization.

To illustrate how disagreements may be settled in a rational and scientific manner, let's consider climate change, a topic that is currently controversial. Essentially, the argument is between those who claim that the earth's climate is showing signs of warming and that greenhouse gas emissions resulting from human activity significantly contribute to this trend and those who tend to dismiss such claims as alarmist, deny the trend, or attribute the trend to natural causes. How should this question be argued?

The first structure of an argument is the claim. At this time, in 2012, all relevant international scientific bodies agree that there is a significant man-made contribution to global warming. Parenthetically, it should be noted that the USA and China, who are the largest producers of greenhouse gases, do not view the potential damage caused by global warming as seriously as do other nations in Western Europe, India, and Japan. Various groups affiliated with carbon energy producers (e.g., large oil companies) make the claim that there is no global warming and that, even if there is such warming, industrial processes play no role in that process.

The next step in constructing an argument is to present data, i.e., evidence in support of the claim. Evidence cited by deniers of climate change includes indications that global warming has not occurred over the past 10 years, that the warming that has occurred over the past 22 years is smaller than predicted by current models, and that the carbon dioxide emitted by fossil-fuel burning industry is not a pollutant but is in fact good for agriculture. Scientists have been accused of colluding to alarm the public because they obtain grants to study the phenomenon and deniers of climate change also claim that some government bureaucrats wish to use the fear of global warming as an excuse to raise taxes.

On the opposite side of the argument, scientists show data that the polar ice caps are shrinking, land surface air temperature is increasing, sea surface temperatures (measured since 1850) are increasing, air temperature over oceans is increasing, ocean heat content is increasing, the sea level is rising, the increased carbon dioxide levels is acidifying the oceans, specific humidity is increasing, and for more than 19 consecutive years, there has been a loss of ice from glaciers worldwide.

After data are presented, a scientific argument will proceed to a step called a "warrant" that explains or justifies the relationship between the data and the claim. Global warming naysayers point to the discrepancies between models of climate change and actual changes in temperature, suggesting that the models are erroneous. However, we don't know if the discrepancy falls within the margin of error permitted by the model. The naysayers also point out the "positive" aspects of global warming, i.e., that additional carbon dioxide released to the atmosphere will allow more plant life, and the nations that have affordable energy from fossil fuel are more prosperous than those without.

In order to still better examine the data and conclusions drawn, we proceed to the "qualifier" portion of the scientific argument to help us decide if the conclusions are reliable. Unfortunately, within the context of this book, we cannot examine in detail the data themselves, nor read the very large body of literature published in this area.

Instead, we will turn to the "backing" for the argument, where we examine additional assumptions that support the validity of the argument. It turns out that most of the folks who publically denounce global warming as a hoax are not climate scientists. Although an opinion piece on January 27, 2012 published in the Wall Street Journal disputing the evidence for man-made global warming was signed by 16 scientists, it was later pointed out that the signers had no expertise in climate science, that two had once to worked for Exxon, and that six others worked for think tanks funded by industries including Exxon. Subsequently, on February 1, 2012, the Wall Street Journal published a letter by 40 other scientists including prominent climate change experts who pointed out that 97 % of researchers who actively publish on climate science agree that climate change is real.

So we may summarize as follows: the consensus of the scientific community as expressed in the opinion of scientific societies and national academies of sciences in developed countries is that global warming is occurring and that the man-made contribution is significant, that there are some discrepancies between the exact predictions of the computer models used to predict global warming and the measured temperatures, and that the majority of the folks arguing that global warming is a hoax publish in venues affiliated with politically conservative opinions and have a high probability of being affiliated with fossil-fuel producing industry. Similar to arguments put forward by creationists, a favorite strategy used by climate change doubters to equate the validity of both sides of the climate change debate (e.g., great majority of climate scientists on one side, a few scientists, and many business leaders on the other) is to portray the issue as "controversial" and one where there is still "doubt" about the extent (if any) of climate change. These references to controversy and doubt are meant to imply that perhaps the majority of scientists are wrong, and so it would not be prudent to act on their recommendations to reduce carbon emissions.

This systematic approach, i.e., of claim, data, warrant, qualifier, backing, and rebuttal, is the preferred method by which consensus is arrived in science. It should be readily apparent that the discussions (not just the climate) can get pretty heated on these issues!

2.9 Analyzing Pseudoscientific Claims

Let's now return to the questions asked at the beginning of this chapter.

Should you live a chemical-free life? Impossible, we are made of chemicals, we eat and breed chemicals, and we live in a world made of chemicals. Maybe you should live a synthetic chemical-free life? That has become increasingly difficult since the dawn of civilization. After all, almost everything we wear, material we use for shelter, and even our food contain synthetic components. And, most synthetic materials are perfectly safe when taken properly (e.g., artificial food coloring, artificial flavoring, anticaking additives), and some natural products are not to be consumed under any circumstance (e.g., poisonous mushrooms). As we discuss in Chap. 10, when it comes to toxins, it is all a matter of the type and concentration. In most cases our bodies can safely deal with low concentrations of most synthetic or natural compounds; higher concentrations can be harmful.

Does eating seeds provide a maximum benefit? In order for this to be true, our body would have to be able to process the raw materials in seeds in the same way that the growing plant does. The plant harnesses sunlight, water, and nutrients from the soil that are important catalysts that enable a seed to transform into a healthy and nutritious food for humans.

> Remember that dietary supplements are not regulated by the FDA, so folks who might have a financial interest in selling such supplements are free to claim all sorts of benefits without having to prove any of them! The marketing schemes are subtle and usually involve a bit of truth and a bit of science. For example, a statement can be made that "studies have shown that ingredients found in this supplement boost the immune system." Analysis of this statement would start by first asking about the study: who conducted it, what was the form in which the ingredient was provided, who were the subjects, what were the controls, and was the study replicated by others. And even if the ingredient "boosts" the immune system, that is a long way from being certain that the amount and the form of that ingredient in the supplement will be effective; chances are there are no studies supporting that exact supplement.

Furthermore, just because an ingredient found in a supplement is beneficial, what's to say that more of that ingredient in your diet will be more beneficial? The human body maintains itself in "homeostasis," a kind of equilibrium that balances all the complicated biochemical processes occurring in the body in the liver, kidneys, neural system, etc. A disturbance to that equilibrium (e.g., eating too much cabbage because it contains iron and sulfur, both ingredients that the body requires) will produce well-known and unpleasant gastric effects as the body seeks to expel the excess ingredients.

How about dietary supplements that contain plenty of antioxidants? Here's where the bit of truthful science gets in: free radicals damage DNA; this is of course bad, so eating foods with plenty of antioxidants may reduce the amount of free radicals if the body absorbs this extra amount of free radicals. Of course...free radicals are also involved in killing harmful bacteria in your body; still sure you want to get rid of them?

Antioxidants are found in fresh leafy green vegetables, and it's been found that folks who have a diet rich in such vegetables are usually in better health than those who do not. Is this adequate proof of the value of antioxidants? Here is where the issue of "confounding variables" comes in. It turns out that the folks who eat lots of fresh vegetables are typically better well-off, which implies that their overall diet is better balanced and their economic situation allows them to obtain regular healthcare. Their lives are also probably less stressful than the lives of poor people, who often do not have local sources of fresh vegetables or access to regular healthcare. In this case, therefore, all these other variables (economic status, healthcare, reduced stress) are likely to influence the state of health, and in this way they confound the simplistic interpretation that a green leafy diet alone is responsible for improved health because it eliminates free radicals. To further add to the potential confusion, it is rare that all the studies ever done on dietary ingredients agree with each other.

Use proteins or other natural ingredients in skin creams because these go into your bloodstream? In order for this to be true, the ingredients have to be able to penetrate the skin and tunnel through the walls of veins or arteries to enter the bloodstream. As discussed in Chap. 10 on Targeted Drug Delivery, only particles with low molecular weight and high lipophilicity can be absorbed into the blood stream by transdermal delivery. In fact the size of collagen and related molecules are large enough to prevent them from penetrating the skin; they simply lie on top. If the collagen is able to entrap some water, this can benefit the skin by preventing it from dehydrating. However, petroleum jelly (Vaseline™) is even better at preventing dehydration.

What are the magical ingredients of face creams? First, they often contain a vegetable protein (aloe vera, cucumber extract, etc.). The molecules that make up proteins are often long chains of different atoms bonded together, and they do not penetrate the skin. Instead, they lie on top of the skin, and as the moisture in the cream evaporates, the protein molecules shrink: that's how they produce that pleasing tightening effect on the skin, and in the process skin wrinkles are pulled together yielding a smoother complexion.

What about substances that are claimed to revitalize or rejuvenate or stimulate collagen production? It is true that collagen is important; after all, collagen accounts for about 25 % of all the protein in the human body. So, does it seem that your body would need help in making more collagen if it has already produced so much of it? Not likely, and the substances in facial creams have no route by which they would be incorporated into the cells that make collagen.

Vitamins, particularly vitamins A and D, are also found in facial cosmetics. Unfortunately, the amount of these vitamins it would take to do your skin any good would not be tolerated by your body [13]. Vitamin A, also known as retinol, may be found in amounts up to 2.5 % in facial creams. It is important to note that the acne-fighting ingredient retinoic acid is *not* the same thing as retinol or Vitamin A.

Other ingredients include waxes or oils. Their functions include serving as a vehicle for the fragrances, colorants, and ingredients discussed above, but they also have the important task of protecting skin from loss of moisture (drying out). One of the most effective moisture barriers is petroleum jelly, but the greasy feel of this substance makes it unpopular for direct use.

Avoid immunization because it introduces diseases into your baby's body. It is true that immunization sometimes introduces the viruses or proteins from these viruses that cause disease into the body; however, these viruses have been treated to render them very weak or more often ineffective. They still retain enough of their original character to stimulate the body to create antibodies, so that the organism will be prepared in the event of later contact with a full-strength virus. Also, even babies have an active immune system provided to them free of charge by their mothers. And while we're on this topic, there is a lot of publicity today about the "link" between immunization and autism. Some young parents are fearful of immunizing their infants against measles, mumps, and rubella (the MMR vaccine) because of a report in 1998 appearing in the UK claiming that the vaccine irritated the bowel and permitted harmful proteins to enter the blood stream and damage the brain. Fortunately, the scientific process we've been discussing took over, and when other researchers could not replicate the experimental results, the report and its author (Dr. Wakefield) were scrutinized even more closely. It turned out that his research was funded by lawyers seeking evidence to use in court cases against vaccine manufacturers and he had not disclosed this conflict of interest. He was permanently barred from practicing medicine in the UK, and the original article was retracted in 2010.

Stop feeding animals chemicals and growth stimulants because these are responsible for increasing cancer rates in humans? The rise in incidence of cancer is primarily a result of the gradual aging of the population. Cancer is typically an older person's disease, so if the percentage of the population that is older is increasing, so too is the cancer rate. There is a relationship between food and cancer to be sure, but that relationship has to do with overeating; obesity is associated with increased risks of cancer of the esophagus, breast (in postmenopausal women), endometrium (lining of the uterus), colon, rectum kidney, pancreas, thyroid, and gallbladder. So, as the number of people classified as obese increases, so too will the number of people with cancer. By the way, did you know that 35.7 % of adults and 16.9 % of children in the USA are considered to be obese (defined as having a body mass index greater than 30; overweight means having a body mass index between 25 and 30) and that if the present rate of increase continues, by the year 2030, 44 % of all adults will be considered obese? The Centers for Disease Control projects that this rise in obesity will result in as many as 7.9 million new cases of diabetes/year (compared to 1.9 million/year in 2012) and 6.8 million new cases of chronic heart disease and stroke/year, all adding $66 billion in annual medical costs.

What do you think: perhaps the most effective healthcare cost controls we can implement would be those targeting harmful behavior; if so, perhaps some of the money spent on new technology should be diverted to research on how to change people's behavior.

Table 2.1 provides a handy way of calculating your body mass index. Maintaining a normal weight by paying attention to diet may be the single most effective way (rather than use of dietary supplements) the normal individual can minimize the risk of developing illnesses such as diabetes and heart disease.

Should we avoid eating foods grown using pesticides and other additives? There is certainly nothing wrong with eating foods not grown with pesticides, but if we were to do that universally, then our food choices in the supermarket would be dramatically reduced. First, the amount of "quality" fruits and vegetables would be lowered, because many more of these items would have perished from insect pests. Second, because some additives are used to delay ripening, the available foodstuffs would have to be sourced locally, because transporting mature fruits and vegetables to the table prior to them spoiling would be difficult or impossible. Third, the additives used have been extensively studied and shown to be safe. The environmental concerns over the use of pesticides may be valid but is outside the scope of our discussion. But a related topic is the use of radiation to destroy food-borne bacteria.

Treating food with ionizing radiation (e.g., gamma or X-ray radiation) from a small reactor has the advantage of killing bacteria, viruses, and insects that could be dangerous to humans. Every year there are reports of salmonella (a bacterium found in animal feces) poisoning that kills people consuming raw vegetables that have not been properly washed or contaminated eggs that were consumed partially uncooked. Each year, more than 300,000 people in the USA become ill from food-borne illnesses. Irradiating food would provide a more secure way of distributing non-contaminated food. Low radiation doses are used to inhibit ripening; medium doses reduce the numbers of harmful bacteria (salmonella, *E. coli*, campylobacter) in meat, poultry, and seafood; and high doses are able to sterilize packaged meat, poultry, and their products.

Would you purchase and consume irradiated food? In the USA, supermarkets now stock imported foods such as fruit, spinach, flour, spices, and ground meat that have been irradiated. Although food irradiation is permitted by 50 countries, the types of food which may be treated vary from country to country. Evidence has been collected by the Food and Drug Administration for more than 40 years, and no danger to the consumer from irradiated foods has been identified.

So, when you hear claims being made that sound a bit funny or hard to believe, go ahead and exercise your brain a bit. Look into the evidence, the source of the evidence, and the type of "study" that might have been done to support the claim; does someone stand to make a profit if you believe the claim? And if you're still not sure, go ahead and ask some tough questions; you might be surprised at the answer, and it will give you all the information you need (Fig. 2.12).

Table 2.1 A way of calculating the body mass index (BMI) to estimate if an individual may be classified as obese

	Normal						Overweight					Obese										Extreme obesity		
BMI	19	20	21	22	23	24	25	26	27	28	29	30	31	32	33	34	35	36	37	38	39	40	41	42
Height (ft-in.)	Weight (pounds)																							
4′10″	91	96	100	105	110	115	119	124	129	134	138	143	148	153	158	162	167	172	177	181	186	191	196	201
4′11″	94	99	104	109	114	119	124	128	133	138	143	148	153	158	163	168	173	178	183	188	193	198	203	208
5′00″	97	102	107	112	118	123	128	133	138	143	148	153	158	163	168	174	179	184	189	194	199	204	209	215
5′01″	100	106	111	116	122	127	132	137	143	148	153	158	164	169	174	180	185	190	195	201	206	211	217	222
5′02″	104	109	115	120	126	131	136	142	147	153	158	164	169	175	180	185	191	196	202	207	213	218	224	229
5′03″	107	112	118	124	130	135	141	146	152	158	163	169	174	180	186	191	197	203	208	214	220	225	231	237
5′04″	110	116	122	128	134	140	145	151	157	163	169	175	180	186	191	197	204	209	215	221	227	232	238	244
5′05″	114	120	126	132	138	144	150	156	162	168	174	180	186	192	198	204	210	216	222	228	234	240	246	252
5′06″	118	124	130	136	142	148	155	161	167	173	179	186	192	198	204	211	216	223	229	235	241	247	253	260
5′07″	121	127	134	140	146	153	159	166	172	178	185	191	198	204	211	217	223	230	236	242	249	255	261	268
5′08″	125	131	138	144	151	158	164	171	177	184	190	197	204	211	217	223	230	236	243	249	256	262	269	276
5′09″	128	135	142	149	155	162	169	176	182	189	196	203	210	216	223	230	236	243	250	257	263	270	277	284
5′10″	132	139	146	153	160	167	174	181	188	196	202	209	216	223	230	236	243	250	257	264	271	278	285	292
5′11″	136	143	150	157	165	172	179	186	193	200	208	215	222	229	236	243	250	257	265	272	279	286	293	301
6′00″	140	147	154	162	169	177	184	191	199	206	213	221	228	235	242	250	258	265	272	279	287	294	302	309
6′01″	144	151	159	166	174	182	189	197	204	212	219	227	235	242	250	257	265	276	280	288	295	302	310	318
6′02″	148	155	163	171	179	186	194	202	210	218	226	233	241	249	256	264	272	280	287	295	303	311	319	326
6′03″	152	160	168	176	184	192	200	208	216	224	232	240	248	256	264	272	279	287	296	303	311	319	327	335
6′04″	156	164	172	180	189	197	205	213	221	230	238	246	256	264	272	279	287	295	304	312	320	328	336	344

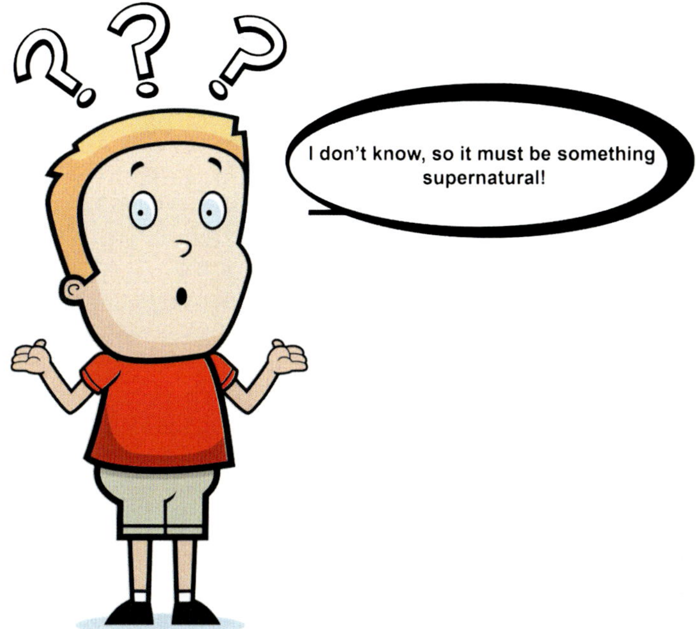

Fig. 2.12 For some reason, folks often want to believe bizarre explanations (e.g., aliens, ghosts, conspiracies) rather than assuming there is a logical and physical explanation that can be found with a little probing

2.10 Summary

Any impartial observer will admit that scientists and engineers continually discover and invent new tools that improve and influence the daily lives of humans. It is likely, given the large number of scientists and engineers being trained in developing countries and the ease with which new knowledge is distributed over the Internet, that the pace of discovery and change will increase. Employment opportunities will arise not only for folks who are practitioners of science and technology, but also for those capable of understanding and utilizing innovations in original ways. Industrialization, made possible by implementing technology, is still the best hope for the poor masses in parts of Asia, Africa, South America, and the Middle East to rise out of poverty.

The daily impact of science and technology is felt in the foods and medicines we consume, the jobs we gain (or lose), the waste we create, and medical care we receive. Scientists and engineers are thinking ahead; as C.P. Snow said, they "have the future in their bones"! Society benefits greatly from encouraging debate and dialogue, without any one particular authority prevailing in all arguments. In other words, we need informed and rational consumers and political leaders who can balance the enthusiasm of scientists and engineers with broader societal concerns. We hope that you will be such informed consumers and citizens!

2.11 Foundational Concepts

- Scientists and engineers are often perceived as "geeks" who know little about the "real" world, and their opinions on everyday matters may not be taken seriously. The popular press often misrepresents scientific findings in the interest of attention-grabbing headlines.
- The way science is done in real life, with creativity, argument, reappraisal, and uncertainty, is different from the way science is taught in school; perhaps that's why so many students don't go on to careers in science.
- The scientific method is a rigorous template for arriving at an explanation for observable natural phenomena. It relies on a fundamental knowledge base, creativity and curiosity, posing hypotheses, experimentation, data analysis, and, perhaps most important, close scrutiny by other scientists.
- Great scientists make great discoveries because of novel and intuitive explanations of well-conducted observations.
- Science is often self-correcting, because of the peer-review system in place for reviewing research proposals and publications.
- Theories are statements and explanations of phenomena made on the basis of a commonly accepted best explanation of observed phenomena; they may be changed when new observations are made or when a better-fitting explanation is provided. Laws are mathematical formulations that describe how events occur, but do not explain those events.
- There is a disproportionate amount of males in science and engineering when compared with females, and this may be the result of gender bias and other cultural factors.
- Scientists are human and are capable of bias in interpreting the results of experiments. That is why the peer-review process is so important, because it can identify this type of bias.
- Pseudoscientific claims are *not* peer reviewed and may also be distinguished from science by a lack of replicated studies, vague or nonexistent experimental design, no control groups, and fuzzy logic.
- Engineers work to provide best solutions to problems in the absence of much needed information and use successive approximations to arrive at an answer.
- Science deals with observable, verifiable, repeatable phenomena; religion relies on other-wordly explanations that cannot be tested or evaluated and has no peer-review system.
- Some politicians are strangely reluctant to base policy decisions on scientific information.
- Scientific arguments must be grounded in factual data. The strength of a scientific view or position may often be evaluated by considering the quality and objectivity of supporting data.

References

1. Osborne, J. (2010). Science for citizenship. In J. Osborne & J. Dillon (Eds.), *Good practice in science teaching* (pp. 46–67). Maidenhead, UK: McGraw Hill Open University Press.
2. Snow, C. (1959). The Rede Lecture: The two cultures.
3. Fairfield, H., & McLean, A. (2012, February 4). Girls lead in science exam, but not in the United States. *The New York Times,* New York.
4. Hodson, D. (2009). *Teaching and learning about science*. Rotterdam, Netherlands: Sense Publishers.
5. Board, N. S. (2010). *Science and engineering indicators*. Arlington, VA: National Science Foundation.
6. Osborne, J., & Dillon, J. (2010). How science works. In J. Osborne & J. Dillon (Eds.), *Good practice in science teaching* (pp. 20–45). Maidenhead, UK: McGraw Hill Open University Press.
7. Cobern, W., & Loving, C. (2001). Defining "science" in a multicultural world: Implications for science education. *Science Education, 85*, 50–67.
8. Schmitt, N. (1976). Social and situational determinants of interview decisions: Implications for the employment interview. *Personnel Psychology, 29*, 79–101.
9. Sutherland, S. (1992). *Irrationality*. London: Constable and Company.
10. Mahoney, M. (1977). Publication prejudices: An experimental study of confirmatory bias in the peer review system. *Cognitive Therapy and Research, 1*, 161–175.
11. Brem, S., & Rips, L. (2000). Explanation and evidence in internal argument. *Cognitive Science, 24*, 573–604.
12. Kolata, G. (2008, September 30). Searching for clarity: A primer on medical studies. *The New York Times*, New York.
13. Goldacre, B. (2008). *Bad science*. Hammersmith UK: Fourth Estate.
14. Koen, B. (2003). *Discussion of the method: Conducting the engineers approach to problem solving*. New York, NY: Oxford University Press.
15. Jha, A. (2012, December 27). The F-word: Father of Higgs Boson calls out Richard Dawkins for 'Fundamentalism'. *The Guardian*, London.
16. Henry, R. (2012). Rep. Paul Broun's Service on House Science Committee Questioned after Comments on Evolution. *The Augusta Chronicle*, Augusta, GA.
17. Hall, S. (2011). Scientists on trial: At fault? *Nature, 477*, 264–269.
18. Hainey, M. (2012, December). All Eyez on Him. *GQ*.

3 Technology and Bioethics: What Can Scientists and Engineers Do and What Should They Do?

Nothing that you do in science is guaranteed to result in benefits for mankind. Any discovery, I believe, is morally neutral and it can be turned either to constructive ends or destructive ends. That's not the fault of science.

Arthur W. Galston

There is great potential for scientific and technological development to improve the quality of life and health. However, history has catalogued several instances of the misuse of science and technology which have prompted ethical and moral concerns about possible future abuses. The newest techniques of genetic manipulation have awe-inspiring power to control the growth and development of humans. Decisions made by physicians and patients who are confronting end of life are also replete with ethical questions and uncertainty. For example, should physicians assist patients who wish to commit suicide?

In this chapter, we will survey portions of the historical record to learn what lessons may be learned from the past and what safety measures have been put into place to protect the rights of the innocent or powerless. We will cover the rights and responsibilities of physicians, caregivers, and patients and see how the law has evolved to keep current with modern healthcare technologies. Specific cases and scenarios will be presented to illustrate realistic and problematic ethical dilemmas.

Finally, the introduction of several new drugs has made it possible to enhance the cognitive and athletic performance of human beings. Will this become the new "normal," or will society continue to condemn achievements made possible by artificial aids?

G.R. Baran et al., *Healthcare and Biomedical Technology in the 21st Century: An Introduction for Non-Science Majors*, DOI 10.1007/978-1-4614-8541-4_3,

3.1 Introduction

According to the US Centers for Disease Control and Prevention (CDC), someone who was born in 2006 can reasonably expect to live at least up to 78 years of age [1]. This is in a large part due to advances in the field of medicine, access to better healthcare, and general awareness of health-related issues. For example, physicians today have better tools to manage infections that were difficult to control only a few decades ago, and patients in a "coma" can be kept alive for long periods of time using ventilators and feeding tubes and successfully revived in some cases. Even with these advances, modern medicine does not have all the answers, and eventually there comes a point where physicians cannot help their patients anymore. The focus of care then shifts to allow the patient to die a dignified death, and many ethical, moral, cultural, and legal considerations come into play. This is often a very stressful time for the family of the dying patient, and conflicts can arise when opinions differ.

Ethical considerations have come to play an important role in assessing the new advances in biotechnology that have literally invaded our everyday lives. We now have the ability to genetically modify crops we grow for food, we can genetically engineer chickens to have more breast meat or cows to give more milk, we can clone animals, we can use drugs to enhance our memory and mental abilities, and we can fertilize human eggs in a dish and reinsert them into a woman's womb who can then give normal birth.

Many of these changes have been greeted with cheers; who can argue with the invention of wheat or corn species that are better able to resist drought or with the joy a childless couple greets news of pregnancy? Yet at the same time, many of these changes cause uneasiness; who are we to tamper with nature, after all? What are the long-term effects of changing the genetic makeup of plants we cultivate or the animals we breed? How should all this be regulated, and who should be in charge of making decisions?

3.2 A History of Bioethics

Physicians attempt to heal the wounds or illness of another person by using special talents or skills. In the USA, a Doctor of Medicine (M.D.) or a Doctor of Osteopathic Medicine (D.O.) degree is legally required to treat patients. In addition to these 4-year professional doctoral degrees, physicians are required to undergo rigorous additional residency training to specialize (e.g., internal medicine, general surgery, obstetrics, and gynecology) and pass licensing exams before they can practice their profession. Physicians are also required to participate in continuing medical education to remain up-to-date with advances in medicine.

In the modern world, scientifically grounded medical treatments are based on observation (origin and progression of disease), discovery (causes and influence), application (drugs and surgery), and evidence that a particular treatment is beneficial to the patient (evidence-based medicine). In preparation for practicing their profession, some physicians also take a *modern version* of the ancient Hippocratic

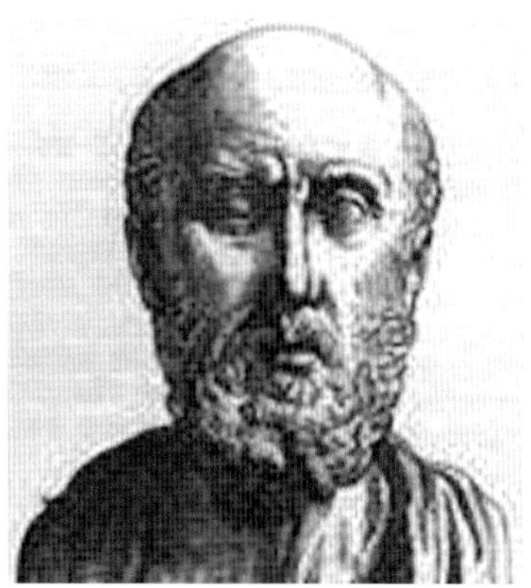

Fig. 3.1 Hippocrates of Kos, credited with compiling the first physicians' oath, promising that the caregiver shall do no harm

Oath, said to have been written approximately 2,400 years ago by Hippocrates of Cos (Fig. 3.1), swearing to practice medicine ethically. The most central tenet of the Hippocratic Oath is to "Do No Harm" to the patient.

The original oath has been modified in many instances to accommodate current medical practices and societal norms. For example, current laws and medical ethics in several states in the USA allow physicians to assist terminally ill patients to end their lives early (see "Physician-Assisted Suicide" discussed later in this chapter). Therefore, the modern versions of this oath vary slightly depending on a specific country's laws and medical practices.

The Hippocratic Oath was once administered to students graduating from medical schools, but has largely been replaced by The Declaration of Geneva, adopted by the World Medical Association. As currently amended, this declaration reads:

- I solemnly pledge to consecrate my life to the service of humanity;
- I will give to my teachers the respect and gratitude that is their due;
- I will practice my profession with conscience and dignity;
- The health of my patient will be my first consideration;
- I will respect the secrets that are confided in me, even after the patient has died;
- I will maintain by all the means in my power, the honor and the noble traditions of the medical profession;
- My colleagues will be my sisters and brothers;
- I will not permit considerations of age, disease or disability, creed, ethnic origin, gender, nationality, political affiliation, race, sexual orientation, social standing or any other factor to intervene between my duty and my patient;
- I will maintain the utmost respect for human life;
- I will not use my medical knowledge to violate human rights and civil liberties, even under threat;
- I make these promises solemnly, freely and upon my honor.

An additional Code of Medical Ethics for physicians has been adopted by the American Medical Association (https://www.ama-assn.org/ama/pub/physician-resources/medical-ethics/code-medical-ethics.page); it is considerably more extensive than the declaration above and covers many different situations, but its preamble reads as follows:

1. A physician shall be dedicated to providing competent medical care, with compassion and respect for human dignity and rights.
2. A physician shall uphold the standards of professionalism, be honest in all professional interactions, and strive to report physicians deficient in character or competence, or engaging in fraud or deception, to appropriate entities.
3. A physician shall respect the law and also recognize a responsibility to seek changes in those requirements which are contrary to the best interests of the patient.
4. A physician shall respect the rights of patients, colleagues, and other health professionals, and shall safeguard patient confidences and privacy within the constraints of the law.
5. A physician shall continue to study, apply, and advance scientific knowledge, maintain a commitment to medical education, make relevant information available to patients, colleagues, and the public, obtain consultation, and use the talents of other health professionals when indicated.
6. A physician shall, in the provision of appropriate patient care, except in emergencies, be free to choose whom to serve, with whom to associate, and the environment in which to provide medical care.
7. A physician shall recognize a responsibility to participate in activities contributing to the improvement of the community and the betterment of public health.
8. A physician shall, while caring for a patient, regard responsibility to the patient as paramount.
9. A physician shall support access to medical care for all people.

It is obvious that a concern for the patient's well-being is the number one priority in all these guidelines. We will see later, however, that the application of these principles is not always easy and the "right" decision is not always obvious. Many controversial cases arise that involve families, lawyers, the government, faith-based groups, and healthcare providers. Also, there have been abuses of human subjects in the name of "scientific research" that happened as recently as the twentieth century; we will discuss these in more detail later.

Even though physicians have an ethical and legal duty to treat patients, they may not be able to fulfill their duties for a variety of factors. These limitations may be due to economic issues (e.g., lack of medical insurance to pay for the treatment) or views of the patient (e.g., a patient may not wish to receive a particular treatment). And, many of the new treatment options being developed are very expensive, and the decision as to who should receive these treatments raises other ethical questions.

Because of the variety of complex situations brought about by technologic progress, a number of national and international organizations have been created to study these issues, and they generally focus on particular problems of interest to their membership. The United Nations Educational, Scientific, and Cultural Organization (UNESCO) has staffed an international bioethics committee with 36 independent members who work to ensure respect for human dignity and freedom. For example, this committee has issued declarations on the human genome and human rights, on human genetic data, and works to monitor doping activities in sports. The Vatican (Catholic Church) has also issued statements voicing its concerns about research on the human genome.

In the USA, the National Institutes of Health website lists the following organizations as being concerned with bioethics in a rapidly developing biotechnological setting: the American Society for Bioethics and Humanities, the American Society of Law, Medicine, and Ethics (which publishes The Journal of Law, Medicine, and Ethics and The American Journal of Law and Medicine), Public Responsibility in Medicine & Research, and The Society for Medical Decision Making. Many local groups and many large universities also have institutes or departments that focus on bioethics. Sometimes it seems that confronting difficult questions may be easier if a moral component is involved in addition to a scientific one. After all, for many of us the science and engineering behind these new possibilities is difficult to understand, and it is even harder to predict where it's all headed.

3.3 End of Life: The Integration of Technology, Law, Individual Rights, and Religious Belief

Starting in the mid-twentieth century, advances in medical technology have made it possible for patients with poor prognoses (patients who would otherwise die) to live longer on mechanical life support. For patients who are near death, it is now possible to maintain heart rhythm, blood circulation, to oxygenate the patient by means of a ventilator, to provide sustenance by means of a stomach tube, and to remove waste through a urinary catheter.

Due to the availability of these life-sustaining technologies, increasingly difficult decisions have to be made about when to stop medical treatment. These difficult decisions about prolonging medical treatment for seriously ill patients are often influenced not only by the medical options but also by personal, financial, legal, ethical, and moral considerations. For example, many people fear death and would like to delay it even when faced with late stages of terminal illness. In the past, patients on dialysis machines never considered stopping treatment even when the treatment was not working—sometimes the doctors had to decide. Fear of litigation also sometimes plays a role in forcing physicians and hospitals to continue life-sustaining treatments even if the patient has no chance of recovery. In modern societies difficult ethical and legal decisions often have to be made to decide who receives medical care, who pays for medical care, and at what point and by whom end-of-life decisions should be made. This section will deal with the ethics behind the current practices of modern medicine and research and describe some of the technologies that make prolonging life possible.

3.3.1 Technologies that Sustain/Prolong Life

Kidney disease is only one of the many debilitating illnesses that the aging population of the world is still struggling with. In the middle part of the twentieth century, the development of *kidney dialysis* machines gave rise to a debate over which

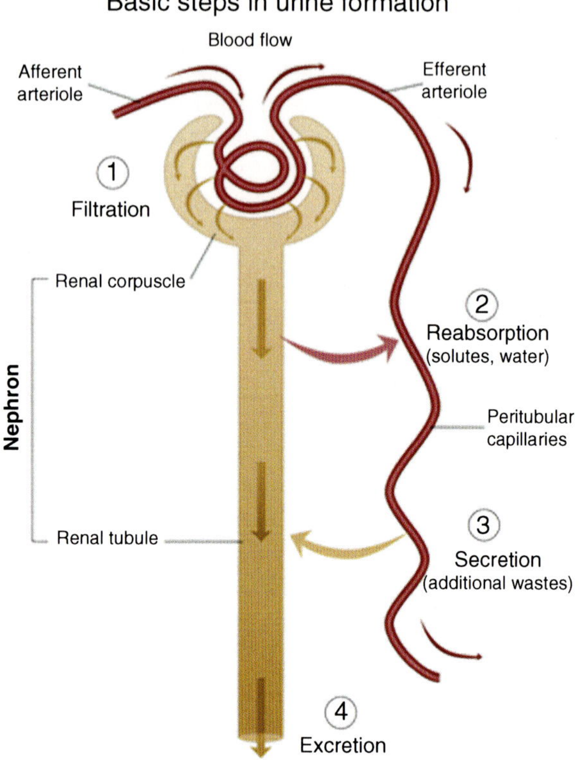

Fig. 3.2 The nephron, the basic functional unit of kidneys. The blood vessel drawn in red is the glomerulus, which is intertwined with the renal corpuscle; that's where the blood releases wastes and excess fluids into the urinary system. In addition, certain chemicals such as potassium, sodium, and phosphorus are also released into the renal corpuscle. However, because these substances are needed by the body, they are re-absorbed by the peritubular capillaries; the kidneys regulate the body's level of these important chemicals. The remaining wastes and excess fluid are excreted in the urine

end-stage renal disease (ESRD) patients should receive treatment and eventually gave birth to the field of modern bioethics.

Kidneys remove waste products and excess fluid from the body through urine. The basic functional unit of kidney is called the nephron (Fig. 3.2), and an average human kidney consists of about a million nephrons. Nephrons act as ultrafilters and process up to180 L of blood/day in an adult. Kidneys also regulate blood pressure, salts, vitamin D, and production of red blood cells (through the secretion of the hormone erythropoietin). Although people can live normal lives with only one kidney, once kidney function (the ability to filter blood) falls below 10–15 %, renal replacement therapy in the form of dialysis or kidney transplant is necessary.

Until the 1940s, kidney failure often meant an agonizing death over a period of approximately 6 weeks. As a short-term measure, Dr. Willem Kolff in 1943 developed a dialysis unit which used a semipermeable filtration membrane to separate low molecular weight waste products such as urea (the compound in urine with a strong smell, useful in excreting nitrogen from the body) from blood while retaining critical plasma proteins. Artificial dialysis can be used only as a short-term measure because it is a filtration device and cannot replace all kidney functions (e.g., vitamin D regulation).

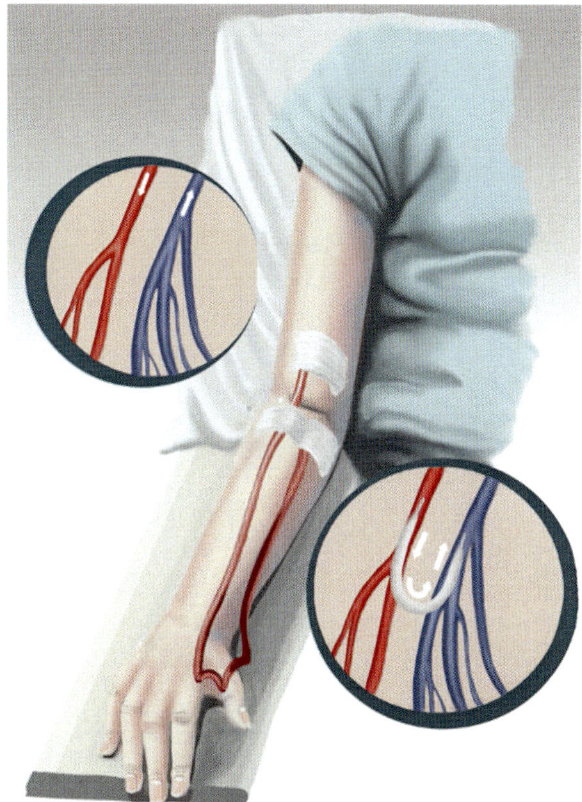

Fig. 3.3 Arteriovenous shunt used to improve blood access to dialysis machines. (http://www.cvtsa.com/MediaServer/MediaItems/MediaItem_209.jpg)

To perform dialysis, blood is usually removed from the patient, passed through an external dialysis unit, and the "purified" blood is returned safely to the patient. Removing blood from patients at regular intervals requires venous access, usually through a thick needle which is placed in the patient's vein to draw blood continuously. Maintaining a viable access to the vein is a challenge due to the possibility of thrombosis (clotting), infection, and/or weak veins. Dr. Belding H Scribner (1921–2003) solved the problem of vascular access by inventing the Scribner Shunt which minimized the possibility of thrombosis and infections. An arteriovenous shunt, or AV fistula, is a type of vascular access that establishes a direct connection between an artery and a vein (Fig. 3.3), thus allowing for adequate blood flow and leading to larger and stronger veins which makes repeated needle insertions easier.

Hemodialysis (Fig. 3.4) as a standard of care became available in 1960 after the invention of the Scribner Shunt. At that time, there were an estimated 10,000 patients who needed dialysis, but there were not enough of the expensive dialysis machines available to treat every patient. The first dialysis center, the Seattle Artificial Kidney Center, could handle up to 12 patients at any given time though normally 60 patients in the Seattle region needed dialysis. This posed a huge challenge and put the burden

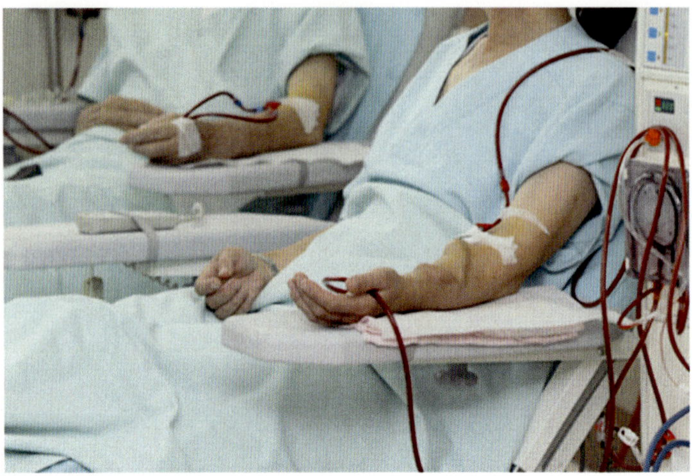

Fig. 3.4 A patient hooked up to a kidney dialysis machine for hemodialysis treatment

on physicians to decide who should benefit from the new option, because the denial of this treatment meant certain death for these patients.

Prior to this technology becoming available, doctors made decisions regarding the treatment of their patients with only some input from patients or their families. However, Scribner established an Admissions and Policy Committee to decide who would be accepted for this chronic dialysis treatment, thereby bringing societal norms and interactions into the treatment decision process. Scribner believed that in these situations, fair and ethical decisions could be reached by an independent group of citizens representing a broad array of interests, similar to the jury system used in the courts of law. The Admissions and Policy Committee used a number of objective and subjective criteria centered on "the social net worth of the patient" to arrive at its decisions. Other medical centers around the country also struggled with a similar dilemma and used similar criteria and various committees to select patients for treatment. This, for the first time, created a lively debate regarding the role of physician versus that of society in making healthcare decisions. This approach to rationing care was an imperfect solution but worked relatively well in dealing with difficult ethical issues arising from the development of a new technology. These committees were eventually dissolved when new treatment options such as neighborhood dialysis clinics and home dialysis allowed larger number of patients to be treated. In this case, a new ethical and legal framework necessitated by advances in technology (i.e., large, expensive dialysis machines) became unnecessary due to further advances in technology (i.e., smaller, cheaper, dialysis machines).

Even though the new treatment options increased the availability of dialysis treatment, many patients were not able to afford the high cost of dialysis treatment. This led to the establishment of a national health insurance program for treating all patients with ESRD in the USA in 1972. Currently, dialysis is considered a bridge solution to kidney transplant. However, at any given time there are not enough kidney donors, and approaches reminiscent of those employed by the Admissions and Policy Committee of the Seattle Artificial Kidney Center are now being used to decide which patients receive kidney transplants. In 2004, the number of ESRD patients reached 472,000 with an estimated total ESRD expenditures of $32 billion paid by the federal government.

Other life-support equipment that can be used to prolong life includes medical ventilators (machines designed to mechanically force air into and out of the lungs); neonatal incubators (small cribs for premature babies that provide warmth, clean filtered air, and may be fitted with a variety of sensors); heart–lung machines (devices that pump, clean, and oxygenate the patient's blood when the heart is incapacitated); left ventricular assist devices (implantable devices that help the natural heart to pump blood while the patient waits for a transplant); and feeding tubes (for patients who cannot swallow for any reason). One of the most difficult times for the family is to decide not only if these measures to prolong life should be deployed, but if there is no improvement, to decide when to discontinue these measures.

It is also important to remember that patients who have stayed in an ICU will show reduced mental capacity, muscular weakness, and high rates of depression. These consequences should be considered when deciding how long a person should remain in ICU care.

3.3.2 End-of-Life Case Study

Terry Schiavo, a woman in her 20s living in Florida, suffered a massive heart attack in 1990, was diagnosed with brain damage and was declared to be in a vegetative state after 2–3 months. For the next 8 years, her physicians attempted to return her to a state of awareness. Finally, her husband petitioned the courts in Florida to remove her feeding tube. He was opposed by Terry's parents, who believed that her condition was reversible and wanted her to be kept alive. In part because Terry did not have a living will, the legal scuffle continued in several state and federal courts even though CAT scans consistently showed severe atrophy of the brain. In the meanwhile, the US Congress and President George W. Bush passed a law making her case a federal rather than a state issue, but her husband prevailed in federal courts too. A number of religious and special interest groups also tried to intervene with various degrees of success. The feeding tube was finally removed in 2005 by the order of Pinellas–Pasco County Circuit Court, and Terry died several days later; the court order was issued after the judge discussed the case with Terry's family and friends and decided that Terry would not have wanted to live under such conditions. An autopsy revealed that her brain had in fact sustained severe and irrecoverable neurologic damage; modern technology was able to maintain this woman for 15 years at an exorbitant financial and emotional cost. This case is an illustration of the difficult decisions faced by patients and their families when they cannot process available information, or when there is a conflict between different family members. Even worse, this is an indication of how societal forces can often complicate these very personal difficult decisions.

In the Terri Schiavo case, the diagnosis was a "persistent vegetative state." This condition is characterized by a sleep–wake cycle even though the patient has no awareness of his or her surroundings. It is usually brought about by severe brain injury to the cerebral cortex but with preservation of the brainstem. While in this state, patients may have open eyes and even move or appear to display facial expressions, but in a non-purposeful manner. Neurologically damaged patients may also be diagnosed as being in a "minimally conscious state"; in this condition, they exhibit greater cerebral cortex activity and may respond to external stimuli that are emotionally relevant to them. Both conditions described are clinical diagnoses based on close clinical observation.

3.3.3 End-of-Life Planning and Care

In most modern societies, individuals, with the exception of children and mentally impaired, have the full authority to plan their own medical treatment. Therefore, the patient ultimately has the right to decide whether to accept or refuse a treatment option.

If the patient is unable to make decisions for himself/herself, as in the case of a comatose patient, decisions are often made in accordance with any advance directives left by the patient. An "advance directive" is described in the text box, and more information can be found here http://www.nlm.nih.gov/medlineplus/advancedirectives.html. The third layer of decision-making regarding medical care is moving from personal control to surrogate control (family, physicians, hospice, etc.). Finally, if the patient is not able to make his/her own healthcare decisions and has not left an advance directive, and if there is disagreement between various surrogates on how to proceed, the legal system through the courts and the executive/regulatory bodies will often make the final decision. In almost all cases, drawing up an advance directive and empowering trusted family members and friends will allow for these very personal decisions to be made according to the wishes of the patients and would prevent courts and/or executive/regulatory bodies from interfering in these often very difficult situations. The difficulties faced by the family of Terry Schiavo were in part due to the fact that she did not have any advance directives regarding her healthcare.

Advance directives are legal documents that allow you to spell out your decisions about end-of-life care ahead of time. They give you a way to tell your wishes to family, friends, and healthcare professionals and to avoid confusion later on.

A living will tells which treatments you want if you are dying or permanently unconscious. You can accept or refuse medical care. You might want to include instructions on:

- The use of dialysis and breathing machines
- If you want to be resuscitated if your breathing or heartbeat stops
- Tube feeding
- Organ or tissue donation

A durable power of attorney for healthcare is a document that names your healthcare proxy. Your proxy is someone you trust to make health decisions for you if you are unable to do so.

Source: the NIH, National Cancer Institute

An interesting counterpoint to end-of-life directives and the acceptance of death is the tendency of members of a generation who grew up in an age when technology conquered the moon, and new medical discoveries were being made every day, to simply refuse to believe that they are mortally ill. Many of us think that science is so powerful that doctors should be able to "fix" whatever is wrong with us. Who among us wants to hear that nothing more can be done, that it's now just a matter of time? After all, Dr. House (the fictional super diagnostician appearing on the television drama "House" now in reruns) hardly ever lost a patient, no matter what the unique assortment of symptoms his patients would exhibit. That attitude is frustrating to physicians, who don't quite know how to respond to terminally ill patients' demands to find a cure. That attitude may also be in part responsible for the high costs of end-of-life care. Baby boomers in particular are used to having it all and are persistent enough to scout out every possible lifesaving or life-prolonging measure discussed on the Internet. It is interesting to note on the other hand that physicians and nurses, who come into daily contact with the dying, are often less likely to wish aggressive treatment if they become terminally ill, demented, or in a persistent vegetative state and would decline aggressive care on the basis of age alone [2].

The American Medical Association (AMA) has developed a policy statement on end-of-life care, with a focus on providing the peace and dignity that people who are in their last phase of life hope to find [3]. This policy statement emphasizes that there should be opportunity for the patient and family to discuss various scenarios and preferences with physicians and to ensure that the patient's wishes are easily discoverable in time of need. Physical and mental suffering alike should be minimized to the degree possible. Patients must always believe that their physician is not abandoning them because they are dying, but will continue to provide the desired level of care. The burden to family, both financial and emotional, should be minimized. Resources such as hospice care, community support, or home care should be made available if possible, and family must be counseled on how to find the resources needed. Caregivers should also not cease their concerns for the family after the death of the patient, as the period of mourning and adjustment to the loss is one of intense emotions.

While progress in educating the public about end-of-life decisions has been made, only 25 % of Americans have a living will, and most have not had serious discussions with family member or friends on how they wish to die, e.g., in a hospice, at home, or in a hospital [4]. The majority of patients go to hospice 5–15 days before they die. Of course, it is impossible to predict the time of death exactly, and new technology makes this prediction even harder, because it is almost always possible to find a way to give the patient a few more hours or days before actual death. Nevertheless, physicians are often asked to make this prediction by family members trying to make decisions about hospice care. Rather than predicting the particular week or day of death, doctors ought to provide an estimate based on the trajectory of change in the health status of the patient.

In almost all cases, planning ahead makes sense for all concerned, as this allows the patient to die with dignity, and reduces the decision burden on family members. In cases where the patient is not able to make a decision for himself/herself, families often choose life-sustaining treatment for their loved ones sometimes even against patient's own wishes. Nevertheless, to be consistent with their oath "to be of benefit and do no harm," physicians are not obligated to provide medical care to terminally ill patients if the life-sustaining treatment is likely to provide more harm than good.

There is a growing public awareness of the need for advance end-of-life planning in order to help patients to decide ahead of time what kind of medical treatments they would or would not like to receive, who would make healthcare decisions on their behalf, and how long and to what extent they would like to be maintained on mechanical life support. A "living will" is a legal written document that can be drawn up by adults ahead of time to clearly spell out their wishes for end-of-life decisions.

One popular example of a living will is called "Five Wishes" (an example is found at http://www.agingwithdignity.org/forms/5wishes.pdf); this version includes not only the patient's wishes regarding medical treatment but also their psychological and religious needs and preferences.

In 2008, both houses of the US Congress formally recognized National Healthcare Decisions Day (S.Con.Res. 73 & H. Con.Res. 323), officially establishing the NHDD event as a national initiative to encourage every US resident to plan or start the conversation with family members about decisions relating to end of life and medical emergencies. In the United Kingdom, the Marie Curie Palliative Care Institute in Liverpool had formulated and promulgated the Liverpool Care Pathway for the Dying Patient, a systematic analysis of how best to incorporate hospice practice into other clinical setting. It is intended to improve the quality of life for the patient in the last days and hours of life and to involve and look after the surviving family as well.

Planning for end of life, which may come as a result of chronic illnesses or medical emergencies, starts with the acceptance that severe illness or death can happen at any stage in a human life. Older people can face end-of-life decisions as a result of chronic illnesses such as Alzheimer's, and younger people may face similar decisions when faced with emergencies such as accidents. However, without a proper directive, family members and physicians are left with difficult decisions if the patient is unable to make decisions about his/her medical care.

What do you think? Have your parents or grandparents ever discussed their end-of-life plans? At what point in time (if ever) would you feel comfortable bringing that up to them?

3.3.4 Death

Before the middle of the last century, someone was declared dead when he/she had no spontaneous activity of the lungs, heart, and brain. With advances in medical technology, it became possible to prolong heart and lung activity using mechanical devices even when there was very little or even no brain activity. These developments, therefore, changed our view of the definition of life and death and required a new ethical and legal framework for deciding when and under what conditions to stop medical care for severely ill or injured patients. In 1968, an ad hoc committee of the Harvard Medical School published a new set of criteria, widely adopted by others, that redefined death. Under these new guidelines, a patient can be considered dead if he/she is unreceptive and unresponsive (i.e., irreversible coma), cannot breathe without mechanical respirator, has no reflexes, and has a flat EEG for at least 24 h [5]. These new criteria represented a significant shift in bioethics of life and death as they effectively redefined life as consciousness.

However, the application of these criteria to comatose patients, for example, is much more complicated. In the case of "non-vegetative coma," defined by depressed consciousness, ability to respond to simple commands, and the possible presence of profound cognitive impairments, the patients can be considered to be alive. The use of these criteria becomes more controversial in the case of "vegetative coma" patients who are often unresponsive to stimulation but may be able to breathe without mechanical assistance and "eat" through feeding catheters (as was the case with Terry Schiavo). Similar issues complicate the decision-making process as to when and if to harvest the organs of brain-dead patients, for example. There are 16,000–35,000 Americans in a persistent vegetative coma at any given time in the USA. It costs between $40,000 and $100,000 per patient per year to care for these comatose patients. These cases are obviously driving up the cost of healthcare, but simply arguing that end-of-life care is driving the increasing costs of healthcare in the USA would be a mistake. It is not always easy to determine who will profit from additional care, and who will not, and what turn out to be the last days of life are often only apparent after death. There may not be a simple way to reduce these costs, especially under the current system of healthcare in the USA.

A third neurologic condition exhibited by some patients near the end of life is "brain death." In this condition, there usually has been severe damage to the cerebral cortex and the brainstem, no reflexes are present, and the patient is dependent on a ventilator to breath. An electroencephalogram (EEG) is flat after two readings obtained 24 h apart. At this point, the patient may be declared legally dead.

At some point, patients with serious illness are referred to hospice and/or palliative care facilities. There, the focus is on relieving pain or stress symptoms and not necessarily curing the underlying disease. Hospice or palliative care should not be confused with the nonexistent, so-called death panels (defined as a panel of bureaucrats who decides whether or not people with certain illnesses or age range can receive medical care). At the "death bed," science or medicine often plays a lesser role, while the societal laws and beliefs (e.g., religion) of the patient and family play a more prominent role.

At the end of life, palliative care often becomes a high priority in preserving the dignity of the individual. The first of the three particular symptoms that deserve attention is pain management, because pain is particularly feared by patients and their families. Almost all cancer patients experience pain, and pain is also present in other diseases. In most cases, modern medications, including narcotics, are capable of reducing this symptom, and there should be no stigma attached to requesting these medications. Another difficult symptom is dyspnea, or shortness of breath, affecting patients with lung diseases and congestive heart failure. There are few more terrifying feelings than not being able to breathe. The US Institute of Medicine has named improving care of dyspnea as one of five national priority areas for quality improvement. Finally, we need to understand that depression is also a cause of suffering. Dying patients are frightened, depressed, and anxious, particularly if they also suffer from dementia, because under those conditions they often cannot understand explanations of their condition and cannot understand where they are and why. This is particularly true of nursing home populations, where some patients are restrained, and many patients are confused and worried. Treatment for depression must be considered as a sensible and morally correct option in these cases.

It is a fact of life that death can potentially happen at any stage in life. Different cultures view death differently. In modern Western cultures, a "good death" is often associated with certain elements. They include an "aware" death—in which personal conflicts and unfinished business are resolved—pain-free death, open acknowledgment of the imminence of death, death as personal growth, and death at home, surrounded by family and friends. One's religious beliefs, or lack thereof, and their world view also often play an important role in determining how the person would want to live during the last days or hours.

3.4 Patients' Rights: Should They Be Told Everything?

We all would agree that a patient has certain rights that have to be protected, if for no other reason than the patient is vulnerable by virtue of needing treatment and at the same time is not as well informed as the healthcare professionals that are involved. Perhaps the first "right" a patient might be said to have is the right to information (Fig. 3.5). After all, the patient typically discloses a lot of personal data to the physician, and the physician has access to the results of various diagnostic tests the patient barely understands. The physician is relied on to explain the results and their significance. Clearly, all this takes time, and many of us have probably felt rushed during

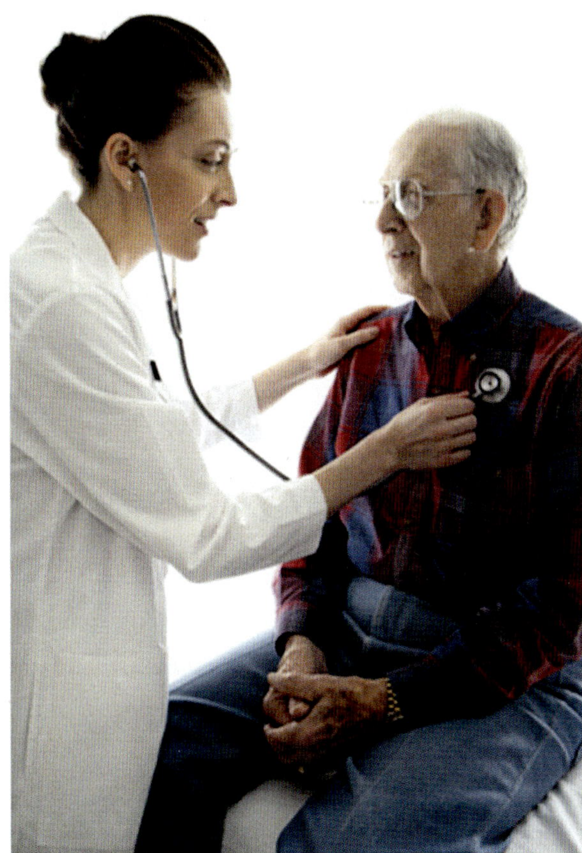

Fig. 3.5 A patient being informed of test results during a follow-up examination

our appointments with our doctor and would have appreciated to have had additional time with our physician after test results came back. It seems that about 15–20 min spent with a physician is the minimum for patient satisfaction, and physicians are also happier when they have the opportunity to spend time with their patients [6]. Many patients also would like to have a return visit scheduled for 2 days later so they could ask the questions they thought of after receiving the diagnosis!

Getting back to the question of the right to information, let's assume the physician learns that the patient has a disease for which there is no cure, is extremely painful, and has a long-time course before death. What is the obligation of the doctor in this scenario? Should the patient be fully informed of all the grisly details, or is it enough to give the patient the diagnosis and recommend interventional therapies? If the patient is told, it's possible that the depression that follows will torment the patient even while being in a relatively stable state of health!

The "correct" answer depends on the individual situation. If the patient asks the doctor directly about the disease and how it is expected to progress, the doctor has

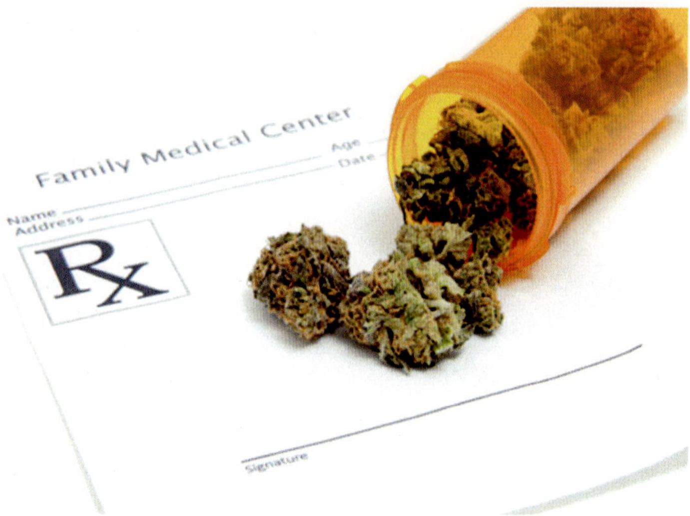

Fig. 3.6 Medical marijuana; prescriptions can be obtained in 17 states and the District of Columbia for relief of symptoms associated with chemotherapy, AIDS wasting syndrome, multiple sclerosis, spinal cord injury, and pain

an obligation to discuss the situation fully with the patient assuming that the patient is not a child or has diminished mental capacity. The real problem, of course, is that the doctor does not have a crystal ball and cannot predict with certainty how severe the disease symptoms will be, and how long the patient will suffer; that usually only becomes clear toward the end of the disease process. So, we can see that at least in some cases, the patient's right to know may not extend indefinitely, especially if there is doubt about a forecast.

If patients have the right to information, we must acknowledge that they also often get lots of misinformation from TV, Internet, magazines, gossip, etc. with which they or their family often confront their doctor, along with a demand for care that in the existing circumstances may be pointless. For example, a comatose patient suffering from liver cancer could conceivably profit from a liver transplant or being attached to a bioreactor that cleans and provides oxygen to the blood. If the physician informs the family, they may well decide to pursue this option, even though the physician's best expert opinion is that given the patient's overall condition, such treatment would be futile. In this case, the physician need not communicate the futile care options, even though this could have later malpractice implications [7].

What do you think: should physicians encourage patients to procure marijuana (Fig. 3.6) for medical uses in states where marijuana possession and/or use is illegal?

Physicians are people too and they do make mistakes. Do patients have the right to know every time a mistake is made? What if knowing about the mistake provides an avenue for a lawsuit by the patient for malpractice, even if no medical harm was done? Doctors are honor-bound to divulge mistakes to their patients if the mistake interfered with proper medical care. If not, it's more or less up to the doctor to decide whether to tell or not.

Patients also have the right to confidentiality. This is enshrined in the formal oaths and promises provided at the beginning of this chapter. Legally, patients acquired privacy protection in 1988 with the passage of the Uniform Health-Care Information Act which prohibited healthcare workers from providing any information to anyone without the patient's signed permission, restricted the power of a legal subpoena to acquire confidential information, and gave the patient full access to their medical records. Believe it or not, access to your own medical records was not certain before this law was passed! In 1996, the Health Information Portability and Accountability Act (HIPAA) was signed into US law, and it made health plans, healthcare clearinghouses, and healthcare providers legally responsible for keeping your information private. The US Office for Civil Rights implements and enforces healthcare privacy rights. Adhering to HIPAA sometimes becomes irritating, because every single time you see your doctor you have to sign yet another form; one wonders what happens to all those pieces of paper.

Are there some situations when patient confidentiality is not an absolute right? What if the patient is a psychiatric patient and discusses suicide or killing someone else with their physician? What if the physician discovers the patient has a communicable disease, a rare sort of flu virus infection, that is communicable to anyone with whom the patient comes into contact? If the patient is a minor and has been abused, should the physician notify someone in authority? In many such instances (e.g., a minor being abused), the physicians are obligated to ignore the confidentiality provision and seek help for such patients.

A particularly difficult decision for a physician occurs when a minor is ill, even in danger of dying, and the parents refuse to permit treatment because it runs counter to their religious beliefs. A Philadelphia couple, the Schaibles, was arrested in October 2009 for involuntary manslaughter in the death of their 2-year-old son who had died of pneumonia. When their son first became ill, the Schaibles prayed over him for 10 days rather than seeing a doctor, because their religion does not allow seeking medical care. When a physician is aware of such a situation, typically law enforcement is alerted and the child is placed under supervision of the court with or without the parents' approval. And although many of us would approve placing a sick child in a doctor's care because the child is not yet old enough to decide on their own, what about cases where parents refuse immunization for their children? We discussed this issue previously when we talked about bad or pseudoscience, but essentially it boils down to the fact that some parents believe (mistakenly) that, for example, the MMR vaccine (measles, mumps, and rubella) increases the possibility of the child becoming autistic. In this case, not only do the parents endanger their own child's health and safety, but that of other children as well by allowing their child to be the potential carrier of a dangerous disease. What should teachers, physicians, and day care center operators do? Not only the MMR vaccine is avoided, but also immunization against the flu, hepatitis A, chicken pox, polio, pneumonia, shingles, and whooping cough are resisted by some parents for religious reasons or because of erroneous information. At this time our society's only recourse in such cases is to educate parents and to isolate children and adults who are disease carriers.

What do you think? How many cases can you imagine where the law should have the right to protect a minor from "poor" healthcare decisions by their parents?

An interesting and tricky variation of the right to information which also involves the right to confidentiality occurs when a doctor or researcher discovers something unusual about the patient. For example, let's say the patient has an unusual resistance to bacterial infection; that could mean that there is something unusual about their immune system, which could be quite valuable to researchers developing treatments. The US Department of Commerce attempted to patent a cell line common to the Guaymi indigenous people in Panama, because it believed that the cells had some unusual antiviral properties. Even on the negative side there can be value: a patient with a certain type of cancer could become the source for cells of that cancer that are used by research labs to develop a cure. This happened in California in 1990, where a patient named John Moore diagnosed with hairy cell leukemia had his spleen removed on the advice of his doctor. The cancer that Moore had was developed into a cell line that was patented by Moore's doctor and commercialized by the University of California. Moore sued, but the state Supreme Court ruled that he had no right to his discarded cells or to profits made from them. The state of Oregon passed a law in 1999 called the Genetic Privacy Act, in which a person's genome (genetic information) was treated as personal property. The law was modified in 2001 to relax the individual's right to genetic information which is an indication that in the USA the courts generally rule against individual property rights to genetic material.

This topic (the ownership of cells or genetic material that has been discarded or manipulated) remains controversial. In Iceland in 1990, a company (deCODE) was granted the right to the genetic information of the entire population of Iceland, approximately 270,000 people. The company's interest in Iceland was based on the fact that the population was unusually homogeneous, which could allow careful studies of genetic profiles and identification of genes linked to specific diseases with the eventual goal of developing medicines for these diseases. The deCODE project ran into opposition from local groups, and in 2003 the Supreme Court of Iceland killed the project.

Companies like deCODE engage in an activity called "bioprospecting" (Fig. 3.7). In a parallel with the search for rare and valuable minerals, the goal is to search through large quantities of biologic material, both plant and animal, in hopes of identifying unusual compounds with bioactive properties. The search goes on in remote jungles and interrogates indigenous people who may have stumbled on miracle medicines unknown to Western science. Because the searches typically involve wealthy Western institutions carrying out research in poor countries, the United Nations Educational, Scientific and Cultural Organization (UNESCO) has issued several strongly worded declarations reaffirming the right of individuals to their own genetic material. It's not clear, however, what the legal implications of UNESCO policy are on actions by companies from the USA or other countries.

What do you think: is there a way to preserve the rights of the individual and yet pursue the development of novel medicines? If you were asked to donate cheek tissue cells as part of a clinical trial, would you agree? You know your DNA has a half-life of about 500 years, so that someone could make use of it a long time after you're gone.

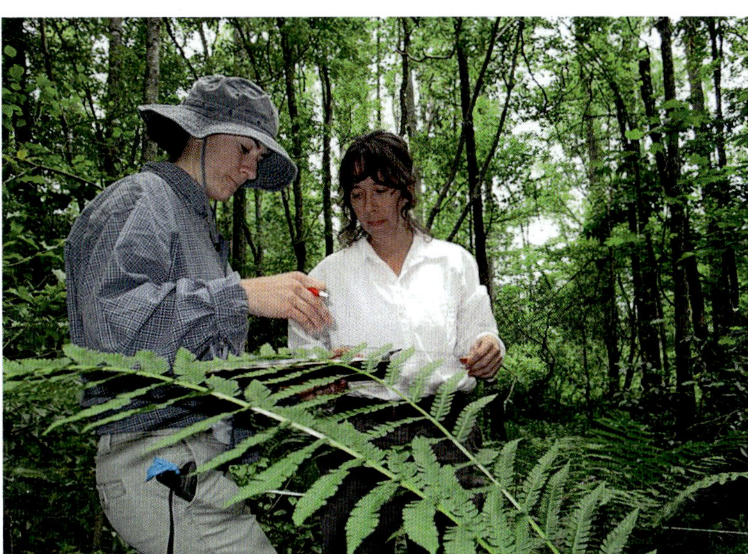

Fig. 3.7 Searching for rare plants to provide new medicines

3.5 Physicians' Dilemmas: Who Gets Treatment If Resources Are Limited?

Throughout medical history there have been many ethical challenges or questions regarding the issue of who receives a given treatment and who does not; in the end, who lives, who dies, and who decides. For example, in the 1800s, the surgeon-in-chief to Napoleon's Army gave treatment based on medical need but assigned higher priority to wounded members of the Imperial Guard (who were Napoleon's personal soldiers) over other wounded French conscripted soldiers.

There are occasions when physicians must personally confront many ethical and moral issues, even though their actions are guided by the applicable laws. The sacrifice of one life to save another is one such example. Such a case can arise with conjoined twins who share critical organs such as the heart or whose brains are linked. In a 2002 case in the UK, two conjoined female twins shared portions of the spine, but one twin was markedly weaker than the other, and doctors believed that unless they were separated, both would die. The parents, both devout Catholics, knew that the weaker twin would die as a result of the surgery and did not wish to proceed. However, the doctors went to court to get permission to operate; they won their case over the strong protests of the Church, and the operation ended with the preservation of the life of one twin. The ethical argument presented by the doctors and accepted by the court was that the weaker twin was already doomed and was literally sucking the life out of the healthier twin.

In November 2012, in a case in Dublin, an Asian woman went into premature labor in the 17th week of pregnancy. It soon became apparent that the pregnancy was difficult and that the fetus was in danger. The mother developed blood poisoning, and the father asked that the pregnancy be terminated. However, because Ireland is a Catholic country with strong anti-abortion laws, the hospital staff refused to

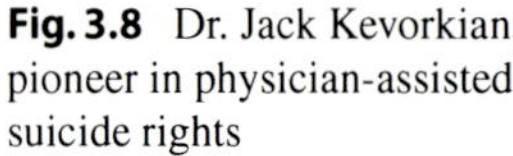

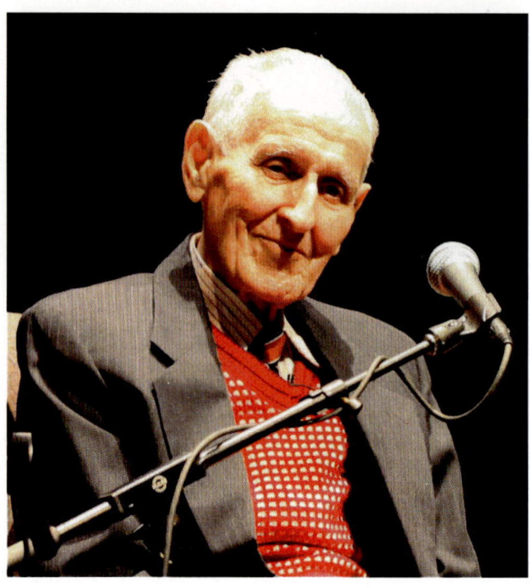

Fig. 3.8 Dr. Jack Kevorkian, pioneer in physician-assisted suicide rights

carry out the abortion, claiming they could hear a fetal heartbeat. Eventually, both the fetus and the mother died. Here, the issue was the strict legal bar to abortion, even though neither of the parents was Irish or Catholic.

Still another topic that arises on occasion is the debate about physician-assisted suicide. Despite significant advances in medicine, there are still many diseases and conditions for which no treatment exists. Furthermore, during the later stages of many of these diseases, patients often suffer from severe physical and psychological pain and discomfort, and a small but growing minority of these patients may request help to end their lives early. In several countries, physician-assisted suicide has been legalized in an attempt to hasten the death of terminally ill patients who are suffering from painful and uncomfortable conditions. In physician-assisted suicide cases, the patient normally has to make an enduring request to end his/her life and be subject to a battery of physical examinations to confirm the late stage of terminal illness and psychological examination to rule out psychological problems. Sometimes, a physician or other authorized healthcare workers may then administer drugs and/or other means to the patient to hasten his/her death; at other times the doctor provides a prescription for sedatives, and the patient will exceed the recommended dose privately. Physician and healthcare worker involvement in these procedures is completely voluntary and may in fact be prohibited by many medical professional codes [3].

Assisted suicide is currently legal in several countries, including Belgium, Luxembourg, the Netherlands, Switzerland, and three American states (Washington, Montana, and Oregon). The patient needs to meet certain medical criteria to be legally eligible for physician-assisted suicide. The person most often credited with raising the profile of this issue in the USA is Dr. Kevorkian, a.k.a. "Dr. Death" (Fig. 3.8), who has long maintained that physicians have the right to assist seriously ill patients who seek to die.

Physician-assisted suicide has gotten more attention since the state of Oregon passed the "Death with Dignity Act" in 1997, upheld by the US Supreme Court in 2006, and the states of Washington and Montana have also recently passed similar laws. This complex issue does not revolve simply around helping the patient to die, but rather helping the patient die versus letting the patient die without assistance.

Not surprisingly, much fierce debate occurs on this topic. Some religious groups vehemently oppose suicide and physician-assisted suicide, and many physicians also are opposed because of their fundamental vows to do all that is possible to preserve life. The decision is an intensely personal one, both for the patient and the doctor. Other arguments against permitting doctors to participate in PAS include the notion that pain control has evolved to the point that in many cases it is not necessary to die to alleviate pain, that assisting in suicide will lead eventually to accepting euthanasia, and that who knows how far we will go in accepting the notion that a doctor can assist in someone's death (Hitler is said to have killed 50,000 mentally incompetent individuals). However, experience in Oregon does not suggest that there will be an avalanche of cases; in the first 3 years after Oregon passed the law, 140 patients requesting physician-assisted suicide received medication, and of those only 91 died as a result [7].

3.6 Biotechnologies with Potential Ethical Issues: Frankenstein or Android?

Sometimes the introduction of new technologies brings up new ethical questions for discussion. For example, neurotechnologies typically involve the action of some magnetic or electrical stimulus on the neural system, typically the brain. They evoke fears of mind control and manipulation, and in fact they sometimes are capable of doing just that. These are powerful technologies that have the potential to cure some of the most resistant neurologic conditions, yet also could be used in less humanitarian ways.

3.6.1 Neurotechnology

Deep brain stimulation (DBS) involves implanting an electrode deep into the brain and connecting it with wires to an electric package containing a battery or a circuit that sends signals to the brain. This technology is used to treat Parkinson's disease, epilepsy, and stroke victims, but it can potentially be used to treat behaviors such as obsessive–compulsive disorder, obesity, and anorexia.

Transcranial magnetic stimulation (TMS) involves the application of a magnetic field to induce electrical currents in the brain. It is not as dramatic a procedure as electrode implantation, but it is also potentially capable of modifying behavior. A magnetic field is generated by a wire coil whose shape and placement near the

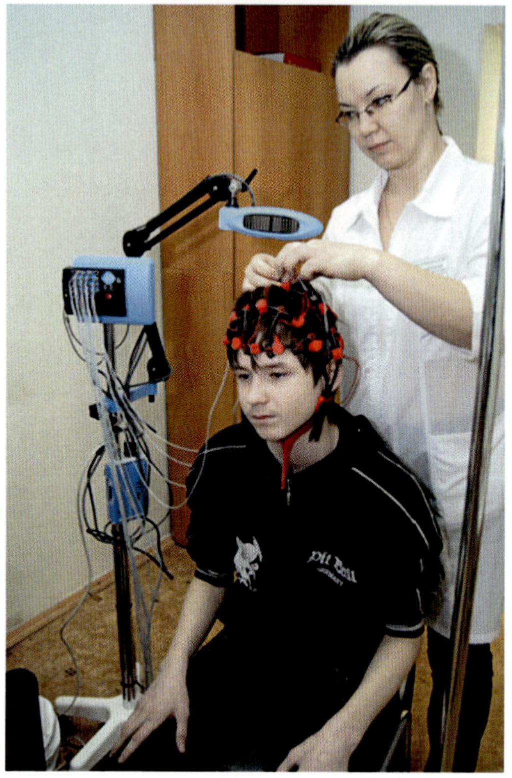

Fig. 3.9 A cap with electrodes which sense nerve impulses in the brain. The impulses can be relayed to a computer for the purpose of controlling electronic devices

head determines which part of the brain is being stimulated. This is based on the theory that some cells in the brain are not functioning properly, that they are over- or under-excitable, and that this leads to mental illness. A technique such as TMS could be used in psychiatric treatment, particularly for severe depressions or to strengthen functions such as attention and perception.

Brain–computer interfaces (BCIs, Fig. 3.9) connect the brain with a computer used to control devices enabling speech or locomotion and are therefore particularly useful for patients with disabilities. Of course it is possible to imagine any number of nonmedical uses, ranging from entertainment to enhancing war-fighting skills of soldiers.

3.6.2 Genetic Testing

The declaration by UNESCO, "Universal Declaration on Bioethics and Human Rights," adopted by acclamation in 2005 and which championed and proclaimed the rights of the individual, was issued because of concerns that large pharmaceutical companies would misuse the genetic data of humans. Some religious groups also wanted protection for persons unwilling, for reasons of conscience, to participate in certain types of genetic research, for example, cloning of humans, though there do not appear to be any serious plans on the part of anyone to actually clone people. Of course cloning of animals has been done for a number of years, typically for "good" causes. For example, researchers in Brazil have been gathering material from eight threatened species, including jaguars, in order to clone these animals for zoos [8]. The hope is that providing these cloned animals to the zoos will reduce the pressure on the wild population.

The Catholic Church also viewed as unacceptable that no specific reference was made to the rights of a human embryo. Its concern here was the use of prenatal genetic screening following a relatively common procedure, offered to women with a family history of genetic disorders and to some women over 30 years of age, known as amniocentesis. In this simple test, a needle is inserted into the cavity surrounding the fetus and a sample of the amniotic fluid is withdrawn. There are cells of the fetus floating in the fluid, and it is possible to examine the DNA of these cells for indication that the fetus will have down syndrome, Tay–Sachs disease, Duchenne muscular dystrophy, and sickle-cell anemia. Amniocentesis cannot be done before the 12th week of pregnancy; a procedure that could be performed earlier, chorionic villus sampling, relies on a tissue sample obtained by a catheter and guidance by ultrasound, but carries with it a 1–2 % risk of miscarriage. Several religious organizations were concerned that genetic information obtained at this time during pregnancy could lead to aborting a genetically challenged fetus.

There are similar tests that can be done earlier (preimplantation genetic diagnosis), on 3-day-old embryos produced by in vitro fertilization. Depending on the outcome of the test, the embryo can be discarded.

What do you think: should genetic testing be done to determine if a fetus will develop to be athletic or blond or free from genetic indicators of subsequent diseases such as breast or prostate cancer?

What do you think: would you be interested in learning about the genetic profile of your fiancé or fiancée before getting married? It could reveal the likelihood of them eventually developing specific cancers, heart disease, schizophrenia, Huntingdon's disease, or alcoholism.

What do you think: what would be the most important question(s) to ask if you are considering genetic testing?

3.6.3 Reproductive Biotechnologies

Approximately 10–15 % of couples in the USA are infertile (defined as those who have been unable to conceive children for 1 year). These would-be parents, who for various reasons do not wish to adopt, may pursue a variety of biotechnologies that assist them in conceiving a child. In about 30 % of infertility cases, the problem lies with the female; either they do not ovulate (hormonal malfunction, scarred ovaries,

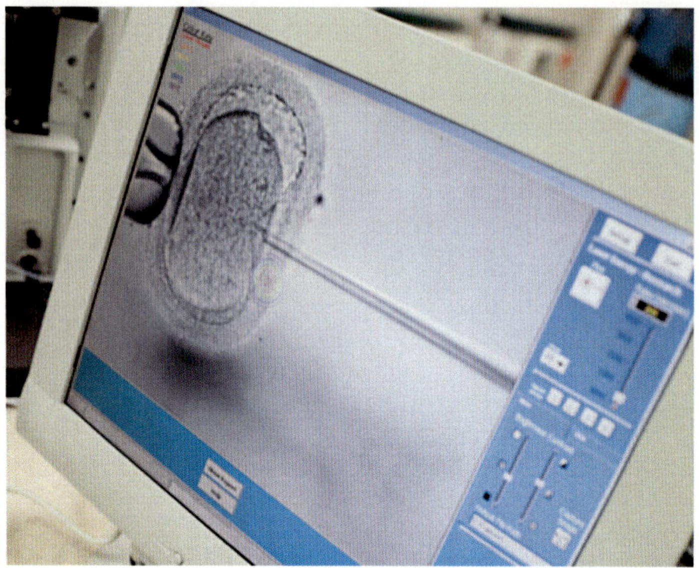

Fig. 3.10 Microscopic monitoring, displayed on a computer monitor, of sperm being inserted directly into an egg (artificial fertilization)

premature menopause), have poorly functioning fallopian tubes (infection, prior surgeries, abdominal diseases), suffer from endometriosis (an excessive growth of the lining of the uterus), or other factors are involved (lifestyle including drug and alcohol abuse, exposure to lead and other chemicals). Another 30 % of cases involve the male (low number of sperm or no sperm production). In the remaining cases, the cause of infertility may be a combination of those listed above or remain unknown.

Failure to ovulate is commonly addressed by prescribing hormonal treatments also known as "fertility drugs," which sometimes can cause multiple eggs to be released and could lead to multiple births.

Failure to conceive because of low sperm count can be addressed by a process called "in vitro fertilization," in which eggs are removed from the female and fertilized using sperm donated by the male partner, then reimplanted in the female 3–5 days later (Fig. 3.10).

During this procedure, several fertilized eggs may be reimplanted, and later, the embryos which do not appear to be developing normally are destroyed. Eggs that are not fertilized, or unused embryos, may be frozen and stored for later use. There are estimates that approximately a half-million fertilized embryos are currently being kept frozen (remember this when the topic of stem cell research comes up later). If the male partner cannot produce sperm or if a female has no male partner, it is possible to use sperm donated by an unknown donor that has been frozen and stored in what is called a "sperm bank." If successful, the procedure allows the female to have the baby in a more or less traditional way; typical success rates are less than 50 %.

What do you think: is it OK for a couple who are deaf to take advantage of in vitro fertilization and genetic testing to ensure that their child also be born deaf?

One of the trickier questions that have been raised by bioethicists concerns the possibility of creating "designer babies." Advertising has been spotted in Ivy League university newspapers offering $50,000 for the eggs of an athletic woman with no family medical problems and SAT scores above 1,400; a website auctions eggs from fashion models; a sperm bank advertises for male donors who are at least 6 ft tall, blond, have dimples, and an advanced college degree [9]!

If the female is unable to carry the fetus to full term because of her health, another option for the couple is to find a surrogate. A surrogate mother can be implanted with an egg from the female of the couple that has been fertilized with the sperm of the male of the couple, or a donated egg fertilized by the sperm of the male of the couple, or in some circumstances with a donated egg and donated sperm; this is called full surrogacy. Partial surrogacy occurs when the sperm of the male of the couple is used to fertilize the egg of the surrogate.

Many of the difficult issues concerning donor-conceived children arise after birth. For example, the donor in a successful birth may decide that he or she wants to have a role in the upbringing of the child. In later life, the parents may decide to tell the child it was conceived with the contribution of a donor and may not be able to tell the child much about the history of the donor. In the UK, donor-conceived children at the age of eighteen are legally entitled to find out the identity of the donor and make contact with him or her. Clearly, the parties involved in these cases may have conflicting interests; parents may not wish to have their child pursue the donor's identity, and the donor himself or herself may wish to remain anonymous. The roles of government and social and healthcare professionals are not clear in what are intensely personal matters.

In the USA, the laws concerning surrogacy are complex and vary from state to state [10]. Some states permit surrogacy contracts, while others prohibit them. There are many questions that can arise in a surrogacy case: what happens if the surrogate decides to keep the child; what happens if the surrogate demands additional payment; what happens if the surrogate wishes the child returned after a period of time; and what happens if the child is born disfigured or with a genetic impairment and is no longer wanted? For these reasons many surrogate cases end up in a court of law for a decision, and unfortunately it appears that the best interests of the child are not always the primary consideration during the court's deliberations. Sometimes baby brokers are also involved, taking a portion of the funds due the surrogate mother, and may also become participants in any legal action.

3.6.4 Organ and Tissue Transplantation

Even though biotechnology has progressed to the point that implants are available to replace tissues such as bone or tendon and skin may be grown in the laboratory for later use on burn victims, there remain medical needs that cannot be met at the present time. For example, there is currently no completely artificial heart or kidney or liver or lungs available. For patients needing those organs, transplants from human donors offer the best potential outcomes.

Unfortunately, there is a severe shortage of donated tissues and organs. The United Network for Organ Sharing (UNOS) is a private, nonprofit entity that manages the transplant system for the US government, and its website (UNOS.org) lists up-to-the-moment statistics related to transplant needs. For example, on November 15, 2012, there were 74,476 active transplant recipients on the waiting list for organs, and in the period from January 2012 to August 2012, only 9,504 donors. The Organ Procurement and Transplantation Network (www.OPTN.Transplant.HRSA.org) maintains a national patient waiting list in the USA and provides extremely detailed descriptions of the organ allocation policies stratified by donor and recipient age for life-sustaining organs such as kidneys, liver, pancreas, lung, and heart. We are now forced to ration organs similar to the way we used to ration kidney dialysis treatment in the 1960s.

The factors normally taken into account when matching donor and recipient include age, blood type, tissue type, medical urgency, waiting time, donor–recipient distance, the relative sizes of donor and recipient, and the type of organ. Patients on the waiting list can often track their positions on the list. If you had ever seen a news story featuring a grateful family member thanking the family of the donor, then it is likely that at the next opportunity you checked the organ donor question on your driver's license application, indicating you were willing to donate a needed organ in the event you had suffered a fatal accident. It is especially important to consider being a donor if you are a member of a minority, because minorities often favor certain blood types and may suffer from certain chronic conditions affecting the major organs, so the number of potential organ donors in minority groups is lower. Several states, including New York and Colorado, are considering organ donation as the default, meaning that you would have to purposely opt out of being an organ donor; if you did not, your organs would automatically be available for harvest upon your death.

If you make the decision to donate, you could potentially touch the lives of up to 50 people; very few other acts of kindness can have such a positive impact on the lives of so many people. There are some rumors circulating about organ donation that may put some people off, so the Mayo clinic has conveniently grouped them on its website www.mayoclinic.com/health/organ-donation/FL00077:

Fact: When you go to the hospital for treatment, doctors focus on saving your life, not somebody else's. You'll be seen by a doctor whose specialty most closely matches your particular emergency. The doctor in charge of your care has nothing to do with transplantation.

Fact: In fact, people who have agreed to organ donation are given more tests (at no charge to their families) to determine that they're truly dead than are those who haven't agreed to organ donation.

Fact: Organ donation is consistent with the beliefs of most religions. This includes Catholicism, Protestantism, Islam, and most branches of Judaism. If you're unsure of or uncomfortable with your faith's position on donation, ask a member of your clergy.

Fact: If you are under 18, you are too young to make this decision, but your parents can authorize it. You can express to your parents your wish to donate, and your parents can give their consent knowing that it's what you wanted. Children, too, are in need of organ transplants, and they usually need organs smaller than those an adult can provide.

Fact: Organ and tissue donation doesn't interfere with having an open-casket funeral. The donor's body is clothed for burial, so there are no visible signs of organ or tissue donation. For bone donation, a rod is inserted where bone is removed. With skin donation, a very thin layer of skin similar to a sunburn peel is taken from the donor's back. Because the donor is clothed and lying on his or her back in the casket, no one can see any difference.

Fact: There's no defined cutoff age for donating organs. Organs have been successfully transplanted from donors in their 70s and 80s. The decision to use your organs is based on strict medical criteria, not age. Don't disqualify yourself prematurely. Let the doctors decide at your time of death whether your organs and tissues are suitable for transplantation.

Fact: Very few medical conditions automatically disqualify you from donating organs. The decision to use an organ is based on strict medical criteria. It may turn out that certain organs are not suitable for transplantation, but other organs and tissues may be fine. Don't disqualify yourself prematurely. Only medical professionals at the time of your death can determine whether your organs are suitable for transplantation.

Fact: The rich and famous aren't given priority when it comes to allocating organs. It may seem that way because of the amount of publicity generated when celebrities receive a transplant, but they are treated no differently from anyone else. In fact, the United Network for Organ Sharing (UNOS), the organization responsible for maintaining the national organ transplant network, subjects all celebrity transplants to an internal audit to make sure the organ allocation was appropriate.

Fact: The organ donor's family is never charged for donating. The family is charged for the cost of all final efforts to save your life, and those costs are sometimes misinterpreted as costs related to organ donation. Costs for organ removal go to the transplant recipient.

Transplanting tissues, rather than whole organs, is more easily done, and tissues are more readily available; skin and bone are in greater supply than livers and kidneys. The most often performed tissue transplanted is the cornea, and the procedure is successful in 90–95 % of cases, permitting the recipient to once again be able to

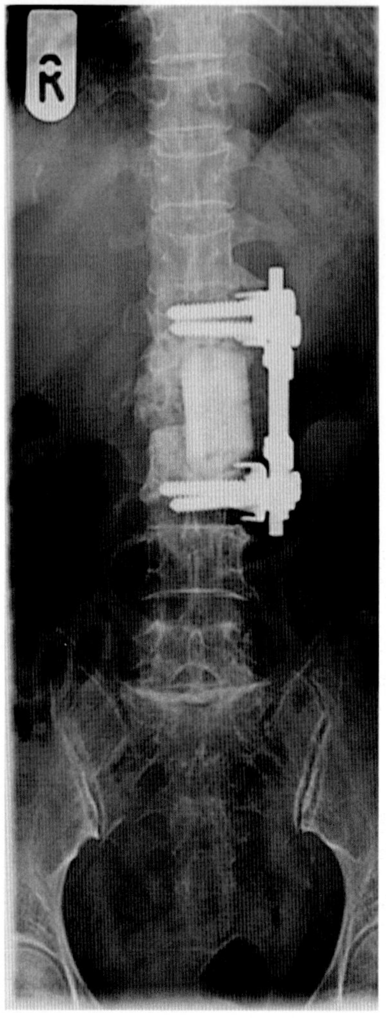

Fig. 3.11 A spinal fusion of two vertebrae, with a block of cadaver bone inserted to preserve intervertebral space and rods fixed with screws to stabilize the spine

see. Other transplanted tissues include skin, the bowel, bone, tendon, veins, and ligaments. Patients who rupture their anterior cruciate ligament (ACL) and require surgery to replace the torn ligament have the option of either receiving a ligament from a cadaver instead of ligament tissue being taken from another site on their body, e.g., the hamstring or the patellar tendon. Transplants of cadaver bone may be used in surgery of the spine, when a fusion of adjacent vertebrae is done to restore stability (Fig. 3.11). Veins are transplanted if the patient suffers from chronic deep vein thrombosis (blood clotting in leg veins) or in some cases of cardiac bypass surgery.

Potential ethical concerns do arise with transplants. For example, it is known that there is an active market in organ trafficking, with some 15,000–20,000 kidneys sold illegally worldwide each year (kidneys not apportioned by transparent methods), and even though the practice was once confined to the very poorest of countries, it has now spread into Europe [11]. Kidneys have asking prices as high as $32,000, and lungs are offered for sale at $250,000. Of course a donor can continue living with one kidney, but no one can live without lungs, so perhaps the lung donor was killed in the process? With 120,000 patients on dialysis in Europe in 2007, the demand is high, and where there is demand a supply will appear. This fact has given rise to the phenomenon of "transplant tourism," whereby wealthy potential recipients travel to the Philippines, Brazil, Pakistan, and China for cadaver organs. While there are stories recounting the extreme poverty and desperation of the donors, it must be remembered that organ trafficking is illegal, and in all cases, the donor receives the smallest portion of the payment with the broker getting the larger share. Just recently in March 2012, the government of China, conceding that it had relied on organs from executed criminals to augment its small supply of organs (voluntary donations are rare in China), announced plans to phase out organ harvesting from executed prisoners [12].

3.6.5 Stem Cells

Stem cells are precursor cells from which all other cells are derived; they have not yet differentiated (become different types of tissue, e.g., bone, muscle, skin). Because they have not yet "decided" what they will become someday, it is sometimes possible to encourage them to choose a specific direction or future. As stem cells divide, they become more and more specialized, eventually becoming characteristic of some specific tissue, so they need to be intercepted while they are still young.

Stem cells were first identified in mice embryos and then also in human embryos. The cells that are in the interior of a 3–5-day-old embryo called a "blastocyte" eventually produce cells for the entire human body. Research on human stem cells was originally conducted on human embryos left over from in vitro fertilization ("test tube baby") procedures, and it is the use of these types of stem cells that has provoked the most vehement opposition to stem cell research. In 2006, scientists developed a method to reprogram adult stem cells found in several body tissues (including fat cells) into embryo-like stem cells with the power to later differentiate (specialize and transform) into different types of tissue. This finding has relieved some pressure on stem cell research, but there are still interesting questions that remain. Jokes are going around suggesting that getting liposuction is a great way to harvest stem cells!

Embryonic stem cells may be immortal; they are often able to remain undifferentiated in laboratory conditions, while continuing to divide and making many (millions and millions) of copies of themselves. Embryonic stem cells can eventually grow into any kind of tissue (they are called "pluripotent"), but adult stem cells typically can only become one kind of tissue.

Although adult stem cells can sometimes be "tricked" into assuming some embryonic stem cell characteristics, scientists are still not certain if these adult cells that have been transformed into embryonic cells will remain potent and how they can be repeatedly encouraged to specialize. Because embryonic stem cells can be found in only one place (a human embryo), and many believe that destroying an embryo is immoral, other potential sources of stem cells continue to be investigated. For example, about 8 weeks postfertilization, embryonic stem cells can be obtained from an area called the gonadal ridge in a fetus. Not enough is yet known about these cells' ability to turn into any type of tissue, and the only available source is an aborted fetus, so there are some questions about using these cells too. Cord-blood stem cells (obtained from the umbilical cord at birth) are easily harvested with considerably fewer moral objections and are currently being studied to understand how they may differ from adult hematopoietic stem cells.

In 2012, there were 184 stem cell lines in the USA which may be used in NIH-funded research. This was not always the case; during the administration of President George W. Bush, the USA restricted stem cell research funded by federal grants to only 15 cell lines. Contrary to the hopes of opponents of stem cell research, this did not stop work by private foundations or in other countries around the world. Several states, such as New Jersey and California, passed legislation supporting stem cell research and budgeting funds to build stem cell research centers. Unfortunately, it was discovered in 2005 that many of the existing cell lines had been contaminated by DNA fragments found in the nutrients used in cell culture, when the embryonic stem cells were being grown and dividing. New stem cell lines are being developed.

Stem cells are central to the new concept of "regenerative medicine," where stem cells' ability to be programmed to develop into specific tissues will be harnessed to repair human bodies. Specifically, the hope is that neural tissues can be grown as a cure for Parkinson's disease (a goal of the Michael J. Fox Foundation), spinal cord injury (a goal of the Christopher Reeves Foundation), diseased heart tissue, bone marrow diseases, etc. If a way can be found to use adult stem cells, then presumably the patient could donate his/her own stem cells, have them cultured in a lab so that their quantities increase, and then use these stem cells to regenerate damaged tissue while avoiding any foreign body rejection reactions. If this technology were to become better understood and controlled, it could revolutionize the practice of medicine as we know it today.

The ethical questions surrounding embryonic stem cells emanate directly from the fact that an embryo has to be destroyed in order to obtain the cells. There are many who argue that the thousands of unused, frozen embryos will eventually be destroyed anyway and that using them in research that could benefit human life is ethically proper. A number of bioethicists have posed interesting questions about the use of embryos and drawn fine lines of distinction between specific stages of embryonic development [7].

For example, is it morally acceptable to use embryos that have been specifically donated for the purpose of serving as a stem cell source? In this scenario, a husband and wife could conceive and ask that the embryo be removed so that embryonic stem cells could be used to treat some disease in a member of the family. How about removing just a portion of the embryo, called a blastomere, during the earliest stages (day 3 after fertilization) of embryo development, because the remaining embryo will continue to develop (i.e., not be destroyed)? In both these cases, there is destruction of some or the whole of an embryo.

How about using an embryo that has died after thawing? After all, adult human organs are donated after death to needy patients. Here, however, the definition of death is tricky and specific guidelines need to be developed that would identify the "brain-death" equivalent for an embryo.

Many of the questions posed here could be answered once we decide when an embryo acquires "personhood," defined here as a condition that implies the right to life, the right to have that life protected, and the right to be treated with respect. The decision can be a personal one, but it is also likely that the federal government will eventually get involved, and as stem cell technology develops, laws will be passed that govern its applications. No doubt there will also be research and applications taking place in other countries that will not correspond to any laws passed in the USA, so get ready for a brave new world!

3.7 Human Enhancement: I Want to Be Better

Enhancing appearance, athletic performance, or mental capability is now within reach of anyone at any age who has the financial ability to pay. The word "enhancement" is interpreted to mean those procedures that are elective, i.e., not medically necessary, although the dividing line between sickness and enhancement is beginning to blur.

3.7.1 Enhancing Athletic Performance

That athletes take drugs to enhance their performance is no longer news, even though the long-term implications are not fully known, and the practice is mostly illegal and can result in the athlete being barred from the sport. Drugs banned at all times include anabolic steroids, beta-2 agonists, diuretics, and hormones such as human growth hormone (HGH), erythropoietin (EPO), insulin-like growth factor (IGF-1), human chorionic gonadotrophin (HCG), and adrenocorticotropic hormone (AVTH). Methods of performance enhancement that are banned at all times include blood doping, artificial oxygen carriers, tampering with samples, and gene doping. Substances banned in competition include stimulants such as amphetamine, ephedra, cocaine and narcotics, cannabinoids, and glucocorticosteroids. Lots of temptation is available to the motivated athlete!

Anabolic steroids are derivatives of the human hormone testosterone. Both synthetic and natural versions may be taken orally or by injection. Taking anabolic steroids will increase muscle bulk, strength, and muscle recovery time and reduce muscle breakdown after exercise. Sounds good, right? Of course taking steroids will decrease sex drive, increase irritability, cause acne, high blood pressure, raise cholesterol, cause liver disorders, and give rise to oversized mammary glands in men. For women, steroids will also lead to menstrual irregularities and beard growth. President George W. Bush signed the

Table 3.1 Some side effects of performance-enhancing drugs

	Performance-enhancing drug			
	Anabolic steroids	Human growth hormone	Erythropoietin	Androstenedione
Males	Prominent breasts, baldness, infertility, impotence			Acne, shrunken testicles, breast enlargement
Females	Voice changes, increased body hair, infrequent menstruation			Acne, voice changes, male pattern baldness
Males and females	Acne, liver abnormalities, elevated cholesterol, high blood pressure, depression, aggressive behavior	Fluid retention, diabetes, high blood pressure, muscle weakness	Increased risk of developing blood clots leading to death	

Anabolic Steroid Control Act in 2004, updating the list of illegal drugs to include these steroids; previously, they were sold over the counter as dietary aids.

Beta-2 agonists are dilators which cause the blood vessels to dilate, permitting easier blood flow. They are typically used by asthma sufferers who inhale the medication, and in that form there is no obvious enhancement of athletic performance. When taken orally or by injection, they may have effects similar to those of anabolic steroids. Side effects include heart palpitations, headaches, nervousness, and nausea.

Beta-blockers are drugs that weaken the effects of stress hormones. They have been taken by archers in competition to steady their arms and hands when aiming and shooting.

Diuretics remove excess water from the body and might be taken by athletes such as wrestlers, boxers, and jockeys seeking to meet a lower weight goal. They also help to get rid of traces of other drugs, because they lead to frequent urination. Side effects include dehydration, muscle cramps, and fatigue.

Human growth hormone, a $2 billion world market in 2008, is produced naturally by the pituitary gland in the human body and can be used for medical purposes such as increasing the growth of undersized children and in cases of kidney failure. It leads to increased muscle mass and a decrease in fat storage, but has many unpleasant side effects including high cholesterol, arthritis, impotence, abnormally excessive growth in height, and osteoporosis.

Erythropoietin is a hormone available as a prescription drug for treating anemia in the USA and stimulates bone marrow to make more red blood cells. Because these are the cells that carry oxygen, a high red blood cell count means that the muscle is able to receive more oxygen during endurance-type athletic events. Side effects include thickening of the blood, fever, nausea, anxiety, and headache.

Insulin-like growth factor is another hormone that plays an important role in the development of children, but its role with adults is unclear. Studies have not shown any effect on athletic performance, but some athletes believe it has steroid-like benefits.

Human chorionic gonadotrophin (HCG) is clinically used to stimulate ovulation in females. In male athletes, it is responsible for increasing the production of testosterone and epitestosterone, maintaining the ratio of the two within normal values and helping to evade detection of other prohibited substances. The side effects of HCG include development of large mammary glands in males, headaches, and depression.

Adrenocorticotropic hormone (AVTH) is used to increase the amount of androgen, converted later into testosterone. However, it also catalyzes the breakdown of muscle tissue, and so on balance it probably has an overall negative effect on performance.

It is important to remember that none of the hormones in Table 3.1 have been tested in FDA studies for enhancing performance, and that the doses, the timeframe, and the methods of taking these drugs by athletes can bear no resemblance to the way they are consumed by patients under medical care. It is a risky business to choose this type of human experimentation, and the experiences of one person may have little relevance to the potential effects on someone else. You may not achieve the celebrity status of athletes such as Lance Armstrong (cycling-EPO, testosterone, transfusions), Alex Rodriguez (baseball-steroids), or Bill Romanowski (football-steroids), but still have to live with the side effects.

Many people think that taking drugs to improve athletic performance should be allowed. They believe that the attitude of the world anti-doping community is based on flawed reasoning. If doping is illegal because the drugs are harmful and enhance performance, why not rule out drugs that are harmful but have no influence on performance (e.g., tobacco) or drugs that are not harmful but do influence performance (e.g., caffeine)? If use of drugs is contrary to the "spirit" of sports and fair competition, then why not address some of the other issues in the world of sports that do not exactly correspond to ethical treatment either, such as (over)training very young children to become gymnasts? And if a major concern is the health of an athlete, then why not test/evaluate the athlete's health status rather than their fluids for traces of drugs? This could end the game played by drug designers making substances that cannot be detected. An athlete's ability to improve endurance can be achieved either by taking EPO (with the understanding that taking EPO has many side effects) or by training at high altitudes; the latter strategy is presumably more expensive than simply taking a drug, so the ban on EPO would appear to discriminate against athletes from poor countries. We don't ban Kenyans or Ethiopians from the Olympic marathon simply because they were born into an environment that favored the ability to run long distances, so why ban athletes on EPO?

The most recent doping scandal involves Lance Armstrong, who was stripped of his seven wins in the Tour de France cycling race. This athlete had won more often than any other cyclist, was treated surgically for testicular cancer and came back to win again, established a foundation (Livestrong) that promoted fitness, and support to cancer patients, and yet when his old teammates testified to his use of blood doping and transfusions, his reputation was in tatters. Of course all of his achievements are still remarkable, and in the world of cycling, where typically ten cyclists per year are found to have taken banned substances, Armstrong was not unique.

Another focus of the sports fan is membership in the hall of fame of some particular sport. Athletes are voted in based on performance. So is it fair for an athlete who took banned substances to be eligible? What should happen to an athlete who has been voted in, and later his use of performance-enhancing drugs is discovered? These debates take place in every sports bar and pub during matches and are likely to never be resolved. In the 2012 baseball hall of fame ballot, there was no mention of formerly great players like Barry Bond, Roger Clemens, Mike Piazza, Sammy Sosa, and Mark McGwire, because the sports writers who vote on hall of fame membership will not even consider ex-players who were suspected of taking steroids [13].

In the end, many athletes are likely to do whatever they can (get away with) to win and to keep playing; they are known to disregard their health, not only by taking drugs, but by playing while injured, by not being truthful about their condition after suffering a concussion, and by playing recklessly (e.g., spear tackling in American football). Too much money, pride, and athletic ego are involved. Fans will have to decide for themselves how they feel about athletes who have been caught, and in the meantime, keep enjoying the arguments.

3.7.2 Cognitive Enhancement

Drugs can also be used to improve mental performance. The old routine used to consist of caffeine pills to stay awake, but even some scientists now admit to using stimulants like Adderall and Provigil to promote wakefulness [14]. Ritalin, normally prescribed for patients with attention deficit disorder, boosts neurotransmitters that help users stay focused and think more clearly, while Aricept, a drug developed for Alzheimer's patients, is used by some for memory enhancement. Other drugs are in clinical trials, and it is likely that at least some of them will be approved and become available. A typical precursor to Alzheimer's disease, and in many cases a normal outcome of the aging process, is memory loss. If that comes to be considered as an illness and given a formal diagnosis such as dementia or "mild cognitive impairment," then drugs may reasonably be prescribed for what was once viewed as normal. Does taking a memory-enhancing drug in this case constitute therapy or enhancement?

Beta-blockers are drugs prescribed for patients with high blood pressure; however, they also block the nervous system receptors activated in the "fight or flight" response known to many of us as causing rapid heartbeat and sweaty palms under stressful conditions. Studies have shown that beta-blockers can reduce stage fright and improve the performance of musicians and public speakers [9]. Is this medication a therapy or an enhancement?

Years ago, children and young adults who had few friends, stayed in their room, and spent all their time reading or playing video games were referred to as "shy"; it was always assumed they would probably grow out of that phase, particularly if they were going through physical changes to their body at the same time. Now, however, many parents worry: is my child OK? And a new diagnosis, "social anxiety" or "social phobia" joined the American Psychiatric Association's manual of mental disorders in 1987. In the late 1990s when GlaxoSmithKline received FDA approval for their drug Paxil as a treatment for social phobia and spent $92 million promoting this medication directly to consumers, the diagnosis became more frequently applied, and the drug was prescribed for treatment more often [9].

Several surveys have found that using drugs to improve one's ability to think does not carry the stigma associated with sport performance-enhancing drugs. Students taking these medications feel that they are taking the drug to improve their performance rather than to beat other students. The element of competition is directed inwardly, against one's self. The goal to be smarter is seen as being more righteous than just trying to bench press some extra weight.

Another factor in the different perceptions of sports versus cognitive enhancement seems to be the belief that the ability to become a better athlete is within reach for everyone—all you have to do is practice hard; to get bigger muscles, all you have to do is to lift more weight, do more repetitions. With intelligence, on the other hand, practicing is not believed to help; apparently you are born with a certain IQ and that's it, so raising your academic performance level using drugs is OK because that is the only way it can happen. And aren't drugs that make you smarter available to everyone? Fairness seems to matter to people; if everybody who wants to be "smarter" can just do it by getting a prescription and if being smarter doesn't hurt anybody, then what's the problem? Especially because it seems to be risk-free.

However, it seems that between 7 and 16 % of university students take these drugs, so it's hardly everyone who is getting "enhanced." And, the proportion of students taking them at elite (i.e., expensive) universities has been quoted to be 25 %. So if that is the case, then maybe it is not as fair as you think; the drugs are more likely to be taken by wealthy students than by those from lower-income backgrounds.

Is cognitive enhancement really risk-free? Amphetamines used to gain energy can cause psychosis and lead to addiction, and there are some good reasons why illegal drugs such as methamphetamine are so dangerous. Another question is do they really work, and here the answer is "yes," they do improve cognitive ability. The ability to focus improves, and the ability to recall facts at a later date improves. For some reason, the greatest improvements seem to be found with subjects who have less innate ability.

Now that these drugs are readily available, it may be pointless to debate if they should be used; they will be obtained by driven and competitive people, by those with connections or who know compliant doctors. Would any one of us object if going into a long surgery, our doctor was on medication to preserve or heighten alertness? Probably not. Indications are that enhancing mental ability through drugs will likely enter mainstream use within the next decade, particularly as more drugs become available. In an opinion piece written by eight prominent scientists and physicians in the prestigious scientific journal Nature, the argument is presented that humanity is always on a quest for innovation and improvement, and we continuously seek out ways of exercising and strengthening our brains [15]. The Internet, computers, and language are all tools that deliver high levels of information to us. The authors suggest that using drugs to improve cognition is similar (more sophisticated, but similar) to getting more exercise, sleep, and reading, all of which also benefit cognition. There may be subtle differences between the different methods of seeking enhancement, but these may not matter. There is little left in our lives that is truly "natural"; from the clothing we wear to the foods we eat, technology has intervened.

If it is true that the "genie is out of the bottle" with athletic and cognitive performance-enhancing drug biotechnology, then let's focus on issues that can be controlled. Let's find out how safe these drugs are when taken by different groups and for different lengths of time. What off-label uses ought to be strictly prohibited? Evidence-based approaches need to be brought to bear on these issues, because so much of the information available has been accumulated by word of mouth.

We should make sure that no one, including military or professional athletes, is ever forced to take these medications. Ways of ensuring fairness, for example, letting all students regardless of economic status have equal access to these medications, remain difficult to implement. There are existing laws that allow persons with diagnosed disabilities extra time for examinations; should these be extended to cover students without access to cognitive-enhancing drugs?

Many individuals and organizations are deeply interested and involved with these questions that are at the intersection of science, technology, ethics, and law. Additional topics to stimulate your interest may be found at the website of the President's Commission for the Study of Bioethical Issues (www.bioethics.gov) and the Hastings Center (www.thehastingscenter.org).

3.7.3 Enhancing the Ability to Work

The potential of using enhancement technologies to change the way people work is generally not fully appreciated. As the workforce ages in many developed countries, and in order to increase participation by those who might presently be excluded from work, medical technologies such as hearing aids, restoration of vision, improvement in mobility, and functioning of arms and legs could be made available to involve those with needed skills. Medication could be used to improve performance efficiency, motivate individuals, permit them to work in more extreme conditions, and enhance their potential to learn new skills needed for the workplace.

As most hearing losses occur in the cochlea, individuals suffer from an inability to understand speech in the presence of background noise. Implants have been available for approximately 40 years to correct this condition, and more commonly, hearing aids can be worn. Patients often complain about the discomfort associated with wearing hearing aids, and you may have noticed those with hearing aids always adjusting them. Electronic and audio technology for hearing aids is being developed that includes directional microphones, bilateral hearing aids (one on each ear). Also, research is being conducted on regenerating the hairs of the inner ear, as damage to these organs is often the case for cochlear impairment.

Visual enhancement is often needed by adults over 65 who suffer from age-related macular degeneration. Several technologies are being considered to improve vision for elderly adults. Retinal implants involve complex electronics that send a signal to the neurons leading from the retina; however, this particular technology is still in its infancy, and at this time is most useful for blind patients, as it permits them to see light and dark. Gene supplementation, another new therapeutic approach, has shown some limited success in animal models, but bright light is needed for vision and the means of delivering the genes remain problematic. Transplanting rod cell precursors has been shown to be effective in restoring vision in mice with degenerated photoreceptors, and it is conceivable that stem cells could be induced to differentiate into retinal cells.

We have all probably been asked at some point in our lives to help an elderly individual with a problem in arithmetic or a computer application. The British Academy of Medical Sciences in the UK reported that a 10 % improvement in memory could lead to marked improvement in scholastic standing; perhaps even the elderly could profit from medication for cognitive enhancement. However, even nonmedicinal intervention has been shown to help; using "brain training" software, researchers have achieved improvements in memory, processing speed, and reasoning ability in individuals over 65 years of age. Even video game playing may help, especially if the "winner" has to demonstrate that some learning has been achieved!

There is also evidence that the onset of dementia and Alzheimer's disease is currently diagnosed too late [16]. Improved diagnostic procedures could permit earlier interventions so that affected adults could lead more productive lives longer and potentially not require the same degree of care as they do now.

Many of the technologies described here are expensive, and it is not yet clear if the additional benefits will outweigh costs. There are also ethical and moral questions that will be debated; for example, is enhancing humans simply so they can work harder and longer a desirable and noble undertaking? Is it possible that society will take advantage of certain segments of the population more than others? What regulatory steps must take place to ensure the protection of individuals and maintain their freedom from being coerced by employers (e.g., the truck driver who is told to use medication in order to avoid sleep and deliver goods earlier)?

3.7.4 Enhancing Appearance

Cosmetic surgery continues to grow in popularity in the USA and around the world. In 2010, there were approximately 38,000 cosmetic surgery procedures carried out in the UK. Americans had nearly 14,000,000 procedures in 2011 and spent nearly $10.1 billion dollars on injections, surgeries, and implants. Can you guess what was the most frequently performed invasive procedure?

There were a little over 300,000 breast augmentations, 240,000 "nose jobs," 200,000 eyelid surgeries, and 200,000 liposuctions. In less invasive procedures, there were 5.7 million botox injections (this was the most popular procedure for both men and women, Fig. 3.12), 1.9 million soft tissue fillers, followed by chemical peels, and laser hair removal [17]. For teenagers aged 13–19, there were 79,000 cases of laser hair removal, 34,000 nose reshaping procedures, and 24,000 cases of laser skin resurfacing. 9,000 girls had breast implants. Recall that these statistics are for cosmetic surgery, not reconstructive surgery of the type that might follow an accident or mastectomies in breast cancer cases. In one sense, therefore, when comparing statistics across years, the total number of procedures is up by 5 % from 2010 and up by 87 % compared to the year 2000. And we all thought there was an economic recession!

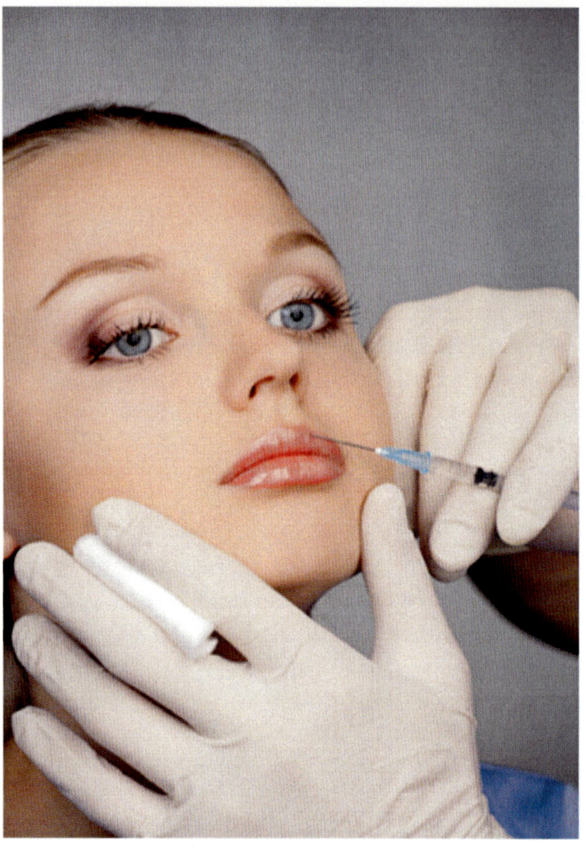

Fig. 3.12 Botox injection. The word "botox" is derived from botulinum toxin, an acute poison obtained from the bacterium *clostridium botulinum*. The toxin acts by blocking nerve impulses to muscles. Although injections of botox have been used to treat uncontrolled eye blinking, "lazy eye" syndrome, and other medical conditions, its cosmetic effect (first documented in 1989) is a result of muscle relaxation that reduces wrinkling

If all someone wants is to just look better, can there be any ethical issues involved? Actually, there may be quite a few. Let's consider the case of a young couple, in love, about to get married. They both like each others' appearance very much; both have thought about the beautiful children they'll have together, a product of the parents' good looks. What if, however, one (or both) had extensive cosmetic surgery? In that case, the other partner has no way of knowing what is in the gene pool. Imagine the surprise when the children are born and have huge crooked noses or grow extensive body hair? Accusations of "false advertising" might be made, and although there may not be any legal action, one or both of the partners will feel cheated and deceived.

How about the case of a young woman who is genetically predisposed to a breast size that is smaller than that of her friends? We are all aware of the dangers of body image problems sometimes leading to illnesses such as bulimia and anorexia, but as cosmetic surgery becomes more and more prevalent, society often encourages people to seek perfection. If many of your friends undergo surgery, then it may be likely that you will be expected to have these procedures too or else risk the chance of becoming unpopular. "Survival of the fittest has been replaced by survival of the fakest" according to Maureen Dowd in her book "Are Men Necessary." And yet, for all the complaining about how women's appearance is dictated by fashion magazines (with airbrushed photos), television, and the movies (with gauze filters and professional makeup applied), most women choose to go along. It is curious that we take pride in individualism and yet readily adopt fashion trends and body images that are thrust onto us by marketers; that young people undergo cosmetic surgery and orthodontic treatment to look better, yet fail to exercise sufficiently to maintain a healthy appearance; and that we make a virtue of being "sensitive" and not mocking people who are overweight, and yet obesity rates in the USA are skyrocketing.

While there can be disagreement about the use of procedures to enhance appearance, it is essentially a personal decision that adults are free to make. However, most people probably shudder at the thought of a parent encouraging a child to undergo cosmetic surgery, or who channels a child into an ultrahigh performance career, or who insists that the child be injected with human growth hormone so that they will grow to be taller than the norm. Children should have the right to decide for themselves once they reach a mature age.

What do you think: is it OK for someone to change the color of their hair in order to fit into or to challenge racial stereotypes? How about changing their skin color (lighten or darken) for the same purpose?

3.8 Summary

Many futurists believe that the growing reliance on computers and algorithms that make decisions far more quickly than humans (as an example, computers control some trading on the major stock exchanges and act when a predetermined set of criteria are met) will have unforeseen and dramatic influences on healthcare. It is entirely possible that students in college today will live to see these changes occur. If that is indeed in their future, then it becomes even more important to ensure that informed thought and consideration be given to ethical questions, such as those discussed in this chapter, before policies are in place and instructions to machines have been uploaded. Should we be concerned that decisions will be made by healthcare providers and communicated directly to life-sustaining devices? We will all be confronted with the issues discussed in this chapter, whether it be end-of-life planning or decisions or enhancing some aspect of ourselves with surgery or medication. The lines defining what is "ethical" and what is not are blurry. The Markkula Center for Applied Ethics has drafted a document that helps to guide ethical thinking [18], and it is summarized here. The authors make the point that for very difficult decisions, it is helpful to discuss and explore the problem with valued friends and colleagues, who may have unique insights and perspectives that would prove to be helpful. Finally, they present a multistep framework for ethical decision-making.

First, recognize if this decision could be damaging to someone and if more than a simple legal issue is involved. Next, get the facts to identify what is known and what is still to be discovered, identify stakeholders in the decision, and consult with them. Evaluate alternative options and ask which option will produce the most good and do the least harm, which best respects the rights of all stakeholders, which treats people equally or proportionally, and which has me act as the sort of person I want to be?

Then make the decision and evaluate it on the basis of which decision option best addresses the particular situation (e.g., perhaps you alone are involved, with no other stakeholders that would simplify your decision-making process), and think if you had to publically announce your decision, how would people you respect react?

Additional information related to bioethics with helpful links for more information may be found at www.biothics.com and at www.bioethics.od.nih.gov.

3.9 Foundational Concepts

- Throughout the centuries beginning with Hippocrates, physicians have codified rules of behavior for the treatment of patients; the fundamental concept is to do no harm.
- Many technologies such as kidney dialysis and heart-assist machines have the ability to prolong a patient's life. However, in cases where the patient is comatose or has other severe health problems, the decision to start or stop such lifesaving measures is enormously difficult for surviving family. Providing an advanced directory or living will does much to ease the family's concerns while honoring the wishes of the patient.
- Patients have the right to know their medical history and information and to control its distribution as enshrined in the HIPAA. The rights to genetic material, particularly when it could be used to develop new medications, are a topic of current interest and debate.
- Physicians face many difficult ethical decisions, including choices of whom to save in the case of separating conjoined twins and pleas for assisted suicide. The latter has become legal in several states in the USA.
- The development of new neurologic and gene-based technologies, as well as performance-enhancing drugs and reproductive technologies may usher in a "brave new world," where the potential for good is equaled by the potential for harm.
- The great shortage of human organs for transplant surgeries is sometimes alleviated by unethical and black-market suppliers. In the USA, there is a government-backed registry and system for assigning available organs to qualified recipients. All of us should consider becoming potential donors and should become familiar with the facts regarding organ donations.
- Human embryonic stem cells have the potential to transform into any tissue of the human body and are therefore a powerful and interesting source that could eventually relieve the shortage of transplantable organs. However, this technology has not yet been perfected.

References

1. National Center for Health Statistics. (2011). *Health, United States 2011*. Hyattsville, MD.
2. Gillick, M., Hesse, K., & Mazzapica, N. (1993). Medical technology at the end of life. What would physicians and nurses want for themselves? *Archives of Internal Medicine, 153*, 2542–2547.
3. American Medical Association. Retrieved from www.ama-assn.org/ama/pub/physician-resources/medical-ethics/about-ethics-group/ethics-resource-center/end-of-life-care
4. Callahan, D., & Lawler, P. (2012). *Ethics and health care: Rethinking end-of-life care*. The Heritage Foundation.
5. Ad Hoc Committee of the Harvard Medical School to Examine the Definition of Brain Death. (1968). A definition of irreversible coma. *Journal of the American Medical Association, 205*, 337–340.
6. Dugdale, D., Epstein, R., & Pantilat, S. (1999). Time and the patient physician relationship. *Journal of General Internal Medicine, 14*, S34–S40.
7. Budinger, T., & Budinger, M. (2006). *Ethics of emerging technologies*. Hoboken, NJ: John Wiley and Sons.
8. Watts, J. (2012, November 15). Brazilian scientists plan to clone endangered species to supply zoos. *The Guardian*, p.29. London.
9. Glazer, S. (2006). *Enhancement*. The Hastings Center. http://www.thehastingscenter.org/uploadedFiles/Publications/enhancement%20primer.pdf.
10. Spivack, C. (2010). The law of surrogate motherhood in the United States. *The American Journal of Comparative Law, 58*, 97–114.
11. Bilefsky, D. (2012, June 28). Black market for body parts spreads in Europe. *The New York Times*. New York.
12. Burkitt, L. (2012, March 22). China to stop harvesting inmate organs. *The Wall Street Journal*. New York.
13. Kepner, T. (2012, November 29). Hall of fame voters confront the steroid era and its questions. *The New York Times*. New York.
14. Carey, B. (2008, March 29). Brain enhancement is wrong, right? *The New York Times*. New York.
15. Greely, H., Sahakian, B., Harris, J., Kessler, R.C., Gazzaniga, M., Campbell, P., et al. (2008). Towards responsible use of cognitive-enhancing drugs by the healthy. *Nature, 456*, 702–705.
16. Drzezga, A. (2009). Diagnosis of Alzheimer's Disease with [18F]PET in mild and asymptomatic stages. *Behavioral Neurology, 21*, 101–115.
17. American Society of Plastic Surgeons. (2012). *2011 Plastic surgery statistics report*.
18. Velasquez, M., Moberg, D., Meyer, M.J., Shanks, T., McLean, M.R., DeCosse, D., et al. (2009). A framework for thinking ethically. Retrieved from http://www.scu.edu/ethics/practicing/decision/framework.html

Inventing, Evaluating, and Approving New Drugs and Devices

4

"Laughter is the best medicine."

Anonymous

Scientific discoveries and technological innovation are principal drivers of the world's economy. Development of new diagnostic procedures and treatments for disease only occurs in the presence of an incentive. The patent system preserves the right of inventors to profit from their discoveries and is an important component of technological progress. However, a patent does not ensure that a new drug or medical device is effective and does not protect consumers who are not equipped to evaluate the benefits of new healthcare-related products. For that reason, government agencies such as the Food and Drug Administration (FDA) in the USA are placed in charge of evaluating the effectiveness and safety of new biomedical technologies.

In this chapter, we will present a case study of a (fictional) drug and medical device as it progresses from an idea in a research lab to appearing on the market for purchase (the so-called bench to bedside journey). You will learn how ideas are developed, protected, and eventually turned into marketable and profitable products. Reasons why new drugs and medical devices carry such high costs will become apparent when you realize how much testing is needed before the FDA grants approval, and your appreciation for the work done by the FDA will increase markedly. You will also come to understand how human clinical trials are conducted, and how they play pivotal roles in the FDA approval process. Finally, you will learn where to go in search of unbiased and scientifically sound information about the effectiveness of various medical treatments.

G.R. Baran et al., *Healthcare and Biomedical Technology in the 21st Century: An Introduction for Non-Science Majors*, DOI 10.1007/978-1-4614-8541-4_4,

4.1 Introduction

At one time or another, we have all been helped by a drug or medication developed by the pharmaceutical industry. We, or someone close to us, have also likely benefited from a device developed and sold by the medical devices industry: a catheter, a digital thermometer, or an implant. When taking a medication or going through a surgery to implant a device in our body, did you ever ask yourself these questions?

- How was this drug developed?
- Who invented this device? Is it a first-generation device or a later, modified model?
- Is the drug safe?
- Will the device be effective?

Most of us probably assume that the medication or device is safe and effective, and the process by which the technology was developed does not particularly occupy our attention. It is unlikely that many of us actually attempt to learn about the drugs we are taking or if any problems with the drug have been reported.

It turns out that the development, evaluation, and regulation of drugs and medical devices is a huge business, involving doctors, patients, animals, the federal and local governments, lawyers, and technology companies. The size of the medical device market in the USA was approximately $106 billion in 2011, and $320 billion was spent on drugs that same year. The pharmaceutical (drug) industry employed 272,000 people in 2010 and spent $67 billion on research and development. These industries have a lot of clout with the government and will continue to play a significant role in the US and global economy as the population grows and healthcare's portion of the budget escalates.

Perhaps because we have trusting relationships with our pharmacist and with our doctor (and by extension the healthcare industry), we are often shaken and surprised when we hear news of breast implant failures, revision surgeries for metal hip implants, and food recalls. How can that happen? We are or will all be consumers of healthcare technology, so it's in our interest to learn where these technologies come from, who is in charge of making sure they are safe, and how do problems with drugs or devices get resolved.

4.1.1 Ideas for New Technologies

Ideas for new drugs or medical devices often come from clever and observant people: from scientists studying how diseases develop and progress, from doctors trying to help their patients, and on occasion even from patients themselves. Most often, ideas originate in a research lab, where a scientist or engineer is focusing on understanding the causes (mechanisms) of a particular disease or how to treat a particular symptom. Most scientists are not driven by the wish to develop a new product; however, sometimes an understanding of the mechanism suggests a treatment or cure. When such an inspiration strikes, the idea is carefully described in a laboratory notebook with the date noted and possibly discussed with other members of the research team to get their opinions. If the opinions are positive, the scientist who had the idea will usually conduct experiments to accumulate data that support the idea and to demonstrate the feasibility of an invention.

In order to illustrate how an idea progresses to the marketplace, let's imagine that a certain Professor Smart, who is employed by Bigname University and who maintains a bioengineering research laboratory, has had an idea for a novel method to deliver drugs to tumors. Although tumors have always been treated by drugs (chemotherapy), the drugs have always been delivered systemically (meaning that the patient's entire system is exposed to the drug). Professor Smart's new idea is to package the drug inside a special implant that would be surgically placed in the location of the tumor and slowly dispense antitumor medication at that site only, not throughout the entire body. At the same time, Professor Smart has had another idea, this one for a new drug that could be used to fight the tumor; instead of trying to poison the tumor, Professor Smart thinks that starving it by interfering with the ability of the cancer cells to process blood glucose will eventually cause the tumor to shrink and die.

So, there are two separate ideas: one for a device (the implant) and one for a drug. Professor Smart is excited about the potential for these two ideas and decides to plan some additional experiments. Sure enough, cancer cells grown in the laboratory show a response to the new drug. Professor Smart makes sure to tell her students and technicians to make careful and complete records in their laboratory notebooks and to date each experiment and each time the group discusses these two ideas. Professor Smart also mentions the experiments to a colleague, who agrees that the data strongly support the concepts, and urges Professor Smart to consider patenting the drug and the device.

4.1.2 The Patent Process

Professor Smart now sees the prospect not only of making a significant contribution to healthcare, but also of some financial gain to herself. She assigns a student to go online and to search for published literature or patents on any similar ideas. It turns out that there are no other papers or patents that describe such a drug-dispensing implant; there are patents that describe drugs that kill the tumor by preventing the growth of blood vessels, but none that interfere with processing of glucose. It seems that Professor Smart has two novel ideas.

As part of her employment-based responsibility to Bigname University, Professor Smart must go through the university's legal office for any patent-related activity. During the meeting with the university's lawyer and technology transfer officer (a person who seeks to commercialize inventions made at the university), the professor is asked to write two patent disclosures. These documents will be filed with the US Patent and Trademark Office (USPTO), and the filing date will be significant in determining who has the rights to the invention. The date could be important because other researchers are working on similar problems and may "beat" Professor Smart to the market. Filing a patent disclosure and a provisional patent application will protect her rights to the discovery for a year (in the USA) before a longer patent application must be filed. The date the provisional patent application is filed is important, because it determines priority rights to the invention. In other words, whoever filed first would be considered the holder/owner of the patent.

From a legal point of view, new ideas can be considered to be "intellectual property," and because they can result in new products that can be marketed for financial gain, the persons who come up with novel ideas usually want to protect their intellectual property with a patent. A patent is a right granted by the government to the inventor(s) to prevent other persons from making, using, selling, or importing the invention without first receiving a license (permission) from the inventor [1]. In the USA in most cases, a new patent is valid for 20 years from the date of its first submission to the US Patent and Trademark Office (USPTO). Each country has its own patent laws which often differ from those of the USA, and a patent filed in one country is only valid in that country. Therefore, Professor Smart probably has to file patent applications in Canada, Europe, South America, and a lot of other countries since her new treatment is likely to have a market outside the USA.

The professor and the university attorney meet often to discuss how the two patent applications should be written and what additional information might be needed to strengthen them. Finally, the applications are filed (sent) to the USPTO, where they are reviewed and evaluated by a patent examiner for three characteristics: is the invention novel, useful, and unobvious?

A utility patent may be granted for a process (how to make something), a machine (a new medical laser), an article of manufacture (a new tennis racket), composition of matter (a new kind of steel), or an improvement of any of the above. Design patents may also be obtained for a new shape of eyeglasses, for example; and finally, patents may be obtained for a novel plant or animal (e.g., a new transgenic mouse).

In the USA, for the invention to be novel, it must be new and not a reinterpretation of an existing invention; it must be different from what is called the "prior art." An idea that has been publicly described elsewhere (e.g., in a scientific journal) or produced before (e.g., already on the market) cannot be patented. Furthermore, an invention already patented cannot be patented again even by the same inventor. If there is any doubt in the mind of the patent examiner as to the novelty of the proposed invention, the USPTO will require that the patent application either be rewritten or reject the application. For an invention to be useful, it must have a useful purpose and work as it is described; theoretical descriptions of a time machine or perpetual motion machine, for example, would not be considered useful! Finally, the invention must be unobvious; someone skilled in the field of the invention would view the new idea as unexpected, even after having read all relevant publications, etc. Someone would not receive a patent simply by making an item already patented in a different size or a different color. If the USPTO denies a patent application or asks for revisions for any reason, the applicant can always appeal and provide additional evidence in support of the application, and of course, the application itself can be rewritten. This cycle of submission, review, and resubmission might be repeated

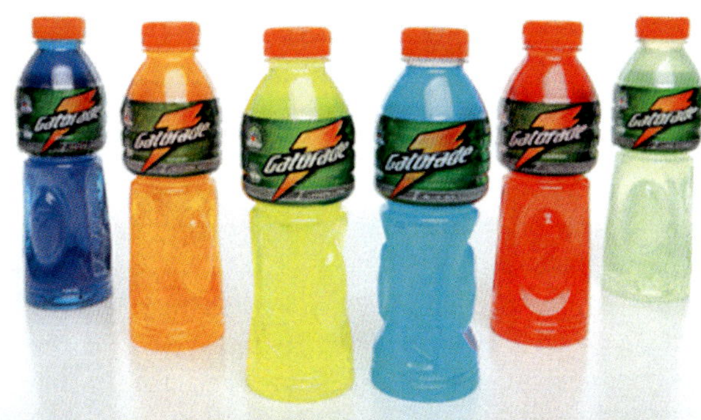

Fig. 4.1 Gatorade was developed and patented by a University of Florida professor in 1965

several times before a patent application is finally approved or rejected. The USPTO will publish the patent application 18 months after it has been submitted; after that time, the application is a matter of public record and available for anyone to see, even though the patent itself may not yet have been approved and granted. Large companies are always checking the website of the USPTO to discover what new patent applications are being evaluated so that they are aware of emerging technologies in their market sector and can potentially incorporate these new technologies in their product lines.

A large amount of work often goes into writing and developing a patent application because of the potential for large financial payoff. For example, a kidney specialist at the University of Florida received a patent for Gatorade in 1965 (Fig. 4.1); the University still receives some of the revenue from selling Gatorade even though the patent has expired (because of the settlement terms of a lawsuit over who owned the rights), which as of 2004 was worth $100M! Attorneys often try to write a patent application that is as broad as possible, so that it will cover as many different versions of the invention as possible. After the patent application is sent to the USPTO where it is reviewed, the invention can be sold or licensed, and the words "patent pending" will often be shown on the packaging of new products. Of course, this does not mean that the patent will be granted, only that it is being considered.

After about 2 years of waiting, Professor Smart gets the patents approved and frames the front pages of the patents to hang on her wall. In order to move forward, she schedules a meeting with the technology transfer officer to discuss ways of commercializing the inventions. A decision will need to be made: should the inventions be licensed to a larger biomedical company, or should the professor form a start-up company and try to market them on her own? In the meantime, her laboratory is working on identifying the most effective dose for the drug and for a method for miniaturizing the implant.

(A copy of a patent is provided in Appendix B for review; it is similar in structure to most all other patents).

Once a patent is granted and published and competitors learn about it, the invention or an imitation may be copied and sold, but if that happens, a "patent infringement" lawsuit will likely be filed by the inventor. In defense, a market competitor selling an imitation will likely challenge the validity of the patent in federal court, and there is the potential that the patent, even though it has been granted by the USPTO, will be reversed. During the court proceedings, the infringing party will typically argue that the patent is really invalid, because the invention was not truly novel or unobvious. You may have heard about several recent cases between the rival cell phone manufacturers Apple and HTC. As background, Apple had sued Samsung for infringing its patents on certain cell phone technology; it accused Samsung of copying the technology without paying Apple a license fee. Apple won that lawsuit (the two cell phones do look alike!) and then prepared to sue HTC. Once HTC saw that Apple won against Samsung, they decided there was a good chance they would lose too and decided to settle the lawsuit, paying Apple damages and avoiding an expensive legal fight.

Patents are valuable because they protect the holder of the patent for 14–20 years depending on the subject of the invention. When the patent nears its expiration time, the owner will typically try to apply for a new patent by, for example, changing the way a medication is administered (e.g., from a drug taken as a pill to a drug administered as a cream) and obtain a new period of patent protection. Because of a lack of new "blockbuster" drugs (like Viagra) receiving approval during the past few years, large drug makers are recycling many existing drugs for other diseases. For example, Rogaine was originally developed to treat high blood pressure, but is now being sold for hair growth. Viagra was originally meant for use against heart disease; Ibuprofen (e.g., Motrin™) was developed to treat hangovers and arthritis pain, but is now being suggested for protection against Parkinson's disease [2]. The advantage of recycling a drug is that the safety of the medication has already been established, so development costs are much lower. If a drug can be shown to be effective against another disease, a new patent will often be granted.

Other types of intellectual property include trade secrets (know-how) that a company does not want to disclose in a patent application, but prefers to keep private. Trade secrets (Fig. 4.2) are less easily protected, but the employees of technology companies are often required to sign noncompete contracts agreeing that if they leave their job, they cannot work for another employer in the same business for a certain period of time. The federal government does not regulate trade secrets, but individual states do.

4.1.3 To Market, to Market...

After considerable thought, Professor Smart decides to form a start-up company that will manufacture and market products resulting from her ideas. She recruits a business officer from her circle of friends outside the university and a product management leader who has experience with the biomedical product approval process.

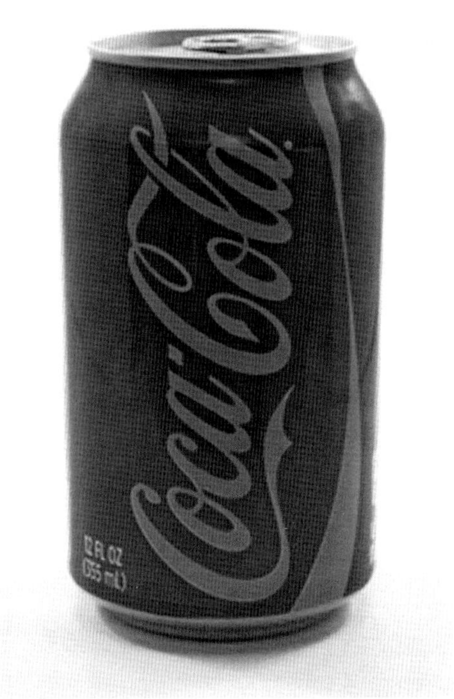

Fig. 4.2 The formula for the syrup in Coca-Cola is a trade secret and is not patented

They begin planning, knowing that they don't have the cash to make the products, to advertise, to hire salespeople, to develop a website, etc., all the things needed to bring the inventions to market. She starts to think of ways to raise money.

It's at this point that most technology-based small businesses fail. They enter the so-called valley of death, the zone between having demonstrated a successful idea and commercializing the idea. They need money either from "angel" investors (parents, family, personal credit cards), from government (Small Business Innovative Research grants), from banks (not likely), or from savvy rich investors (who are hard to convince and often want a big chunk of the business in return). Most of these funding sources will carefully consider how quickly and how likely they are to see a return on their investment. If the small business is credible and lucky, it will cross over the valley of death and be ready for a second or third round of venture capital funding, or possibly be bought out by a larger, well-established medical technology company, and the owners can retire. Large companies may find it easier to buy new technology than to develop it themselves, and this way they also eliminate a potential competitor.

(Portions of a Small Business Innovative Research Grant to the National Institutes of Health are found in Appendix A.)

Wall Street investors will consider the opportunity to invest very carefully. They know that the medical device industry grows in a pattern of "punctuated equilibration," meaning that sometimes there is rapid progress, and at other times, not much change occurs until someone comes up with a revolutionary new idea [3]. There are years where the only innovations that come up are "me-too" technologies representing evolutionary not revolutionary changes. It's the disruptive technologies that are the favorites of investors [4]. The company developing a disruptive technology is likely to grow quickly without any competition at least for a while, so investors are most likely to earn a good return.

Different issues come into play for the so-called orphan drug market. Rare diseases are defined as those that affect fewer than 200,000 patients; there are approximately 7,000 such diseases, with some 25,000,000 Americans affected [5]. Although the overall market for drugs to treat these diseases is large, the number of patients affected by any one disease is small. If it is considered that the typical costs of bringing a new drug is at least a billion dollars (costs of basic research, animal studies, human trials, legal, and marketing), then one can appreciate the disincentive for drug companies to address this market. Sadly, all the charity affairs and special events organized by sincerely motivated folks cannot possibly raise enough money to significantly address the goal of bringing a drug to market to combat diseases such as Huntingdon's disease, Burkitt lymphoma, amyloidosis, cystic fibrosis, familial hypercholesterolemia, Wilson's disease, glioma, multiple myeloma, phenylketonuria, and even snake venom poisoning [6].

This unfortunate state of affairs was addressed by the US Congress in 1983, when it passed the Orphan Drug Act. It established a new office in the FDA, the Office of Orphan Products Development (OOPD), which coordinates the development of incentives for drug and device companies to develop new products for diseases that the FDA has included in the Orphan Drug Designation program and the Humanitarian Use Device program (for treating or diagnosing a disease or condition affecting fewer than 4,000 individuals in the USA).

Incentives include an additional 7 years of patent protection, a 50 % tax credit for expenditures related to the clinical testing phase, and a waiver of FDA approval application fees. In addition, the OOPD offers two grant programs, funding clinical research testing safety and efficacy of products falling within the Orphan Drug or Device portfolio, and a Pediatric Device Consortia (PDC) Grants Program that as per the FDA website "provides funding to develop nonprofit consortia to facilitate pediatric medical device development."

The European Union has enacted similar legislation that includes some tropical diseases primarily found in developing countries.

4.2 Dealing with the Regulators

The professor knows that both of her inventions will have to be approved before they can be marketed and sold. There are several laws and regulations that will impact the work she needs to do over the next several years. The agency in charge of administering many of these regulations is the Food and Drug Administration (FDA).

4.2.1 The FDA

In 1906, the US Congress passed the Federal Food and Drugs Act, targeting misbranded or adulterated food and drugs being sold across state lines, to ensure that drugs met standards of purity. In 1912, the law was amended to prohibit manufacturers from labeling drugs with false claims. Nevertheless, it became obvious that still additional regulations were needed, and in 1938, Congress passed the Federal Food, Drug, and Cosmetic Act. This law required manufacturers to prove that drugs were safe before they could be sold, but not to prove that they were effective. For the first time, medical devices were included in the regulations.

In response to the thalidomide tragedy in Europe, which saw birth defects in children born to mothers who had taken this medication as a tranquilizer and antiemetic (to prevent morning sickness), Congress passed the Kefauver–Harris amendment in 1962, mandating that manufacturers conduct research to prove the drugs' efficacy. Laws often change in response to well-publicized adverse events; many women were injured as a result of using the "Dalkon Shield" intrauterine birth control device, and so in 1976, the Medical Device amendment was passed, which made it necessary for medical device manufacturers to register their products with the FDA and to conduct quality control evaluations before the device could be sold [7].

In 1986, a mechanical heart valve implant was withdrawn from the market because of premature failure of the device, and in 1990, a law was passed to institute postmarketing surveillance and reporting of failure events to the FDA. The primary responsibility for postmarketing surveillance and reporting of failure events is with the manufacturer of the device and not the clinicians or the hospitals treating the patient. Although the drug and medical device industry has seen ever more regulation, it should be clear that these laws have all been instituted with the health and safety of the consumer in mind.

The US Food and Drug Administration now has authority over a large variety of health-related products (Table 4.1), including (the information directly below was obtained at www.fda.gov):

No new drug or medical device may be sold in the USA unless it is approved for sale by the US Food and Drug Administration (FDA). A device is defined as an item that diagnoses, cures, lessens, treats, or prevents disease; that affects the structure or function of the body; and that does not achieve its effect through chemical action. A drug is defined as "articles intended for use in the diagnosis, cure, mitigation, treatment, or prevention of disease" and "articles (other than food) intended to affect the structure or any function of the body of man or other animals." As discussed in Chap. 10, it is becoming more difficult to distinguish between drugs and devices, for example, in targeted drug-delivery systems that employ a device (e.g., a polymer) to slowly release a drug (e.g., doxorubicin) for treating cancer.

This agency (Fig. 4.3) has the task of reviewing the safety of all food, drugs, medical devices, cosmetics, and other health-related products, although the US Department of Agriculture (USDA) regulates and inspects meat and poultry [8]. This is a huge responsibility, because these items account for about one-quarter of the US economy. All of the prescription drugs you have ever purchased and many

Table 4.1 Products within the US FDA's regulatory jurisdiction

Food	Biotechnology (genetically engineered plants and animals)
	Dietary supplements (safety only, not effectiveness)
	Food defense and emergency response help reduce the risk of tampering or other malicious, criminal, or terrorist actions on the food and cosmetic supply
	Food ingredients and packaging (ingredients and food contact substances)
	Food safety (information on seafood, fruits, vegetables, milk, canned foods, and infant formula) guidance, compliance, and regulatory information
	International activities (information on international outreach, exporting and importing into the USA, and trade agreements related to food safety)
	Labeling and nutrition
Drugs	Emergency preparedness (bioterrorism, drug preparedness, and natural disaster response)
	Drug approvals and databases (drug-related databases from FDA, information on drug approvals)
	Drug safety and availability (medication guides, drug shortages, drug safety communications)—development and approval process for drugs (conducting clinical trials, types of drug applications, forms and submissions requirements, labeling initiatives, drug and biologic approval reports)
	Guidance, compliance, and regulatory information (guidance for industry, warning letters, postmarket surveillance programs, rules and regulations)
	Science and research on drugs (research by FDA staff to evaluate and enhance the safety of drug products)
Devices	Products and medical procedures (approvals and clearances, home use, surgical, implants and prosthetics, in vitro diagnostics)
	Medical device safety (alerts and notices, recalls, report a problem, MedSun, emergency situations)
	Device advice (regulatory assistance, how to market a device, postmarket requirements, compliance, importing and exporting)
	Science and research on medical devices (chemistry and materials science, solid and fluid mechanics, imaging and applied mathematics, electrical and software engineering)
Vaccines, blood, and biologics	Allergens, blood and blood products, tissues and tissue products, cellular and gene therapy products, vaccines, transplantation of nonhuman tissues, industry guidance, safety and availability
Animal and veterinary topics	Animal feeds, animal drugs, salmonella, drug residues
Cosmetics	Cosmetic labeling, international activities
Radiation-emitting products	Medical imaging, mammography quality standards, radiation safety
Tobacco products	Labeling and marketing, tobacco and youth safety

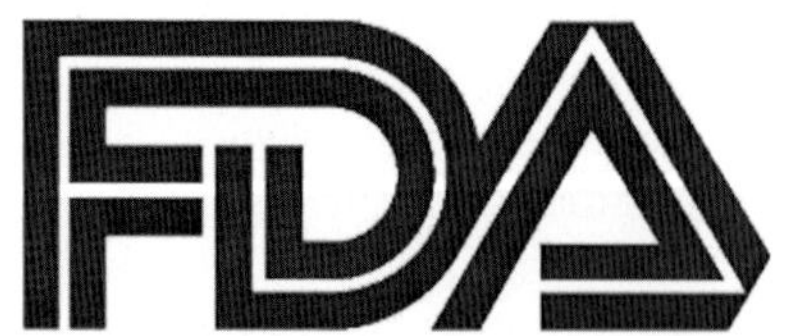

Fig. 4.3 The US Food and Drug Administration (FDA) regulates food, drug, and medical technologies marketed in the USA

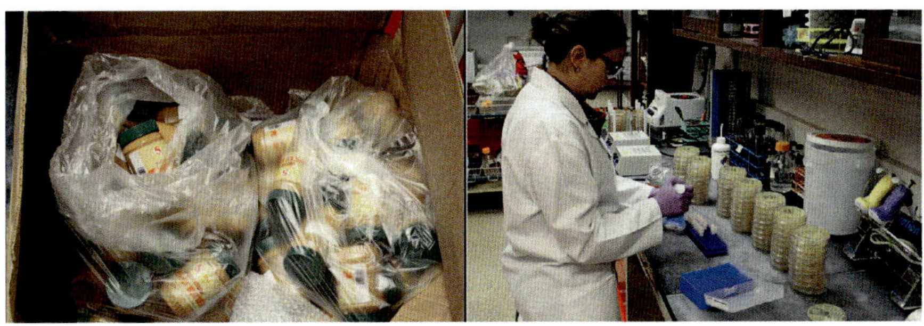

Fig. 4.4 (*Left*) Sunland peanut butter samples waiting for Salmonella testing and analysis. (*Right*) "October, 2012; FDA Sunland Microlab; Denver CO. Microbiologist Melissa Nucci prepping for "Bioplex," a method of determining the precise species of Salmonella present"

of the medical tools and devices you have seen your doctor use have been reviewed by some FDA committee and approved for sale. Though the public may not always be aware of all its actions, the FDA is constantly in the news when it approves a new drug or device, or mandates that a drug or device be withdrawn from the market, or issues an order to destroy contaminated food (Fig. 4.4).

The FDA is very busy; in the year 2000, it catalogued approximately 200,000 reports of harmful effects from drugs and received 70,000 consumer questions and 40,000 freedom of information requests. Each year it prevents hundreds of drugs, medical devices, and food products from reaching the marketplace because they are judged to be unsafe or harmful.

The FDA often hears from consumer groups who want the agency to be more vigilant and strict before approving new drugs or devices for sale and from the healthcare industry, who often wants the agency to speed up evaluations of drugs and devices and shorten the time needed before a drug or device is approved (and sold!). The FDA does its best to represent the consumer and to allow manufacturers to introduce new technologies, but sometimes it loses in Washington DC political power struggles. As an example, in the mid-1990s, the agency lost its power to regulate the effectiveness of herbal remedies and food supplements (Fig. 4.5); so, you should be aware that any reference to the FDA on food supplement product labels does *not* mean that the FDA has found these products to be safe or effective. And when a manufacturer claims to have registered with the FDA, that could mean only that a letter was sent to the agency, not that any FDA testing was necessarily conducted. Because the FDA does not regulate food supplements, no proof has to be provided that the supplements work as advertised. The manufacturers, and others who may financially benefit from promoting these supplements, are under no obligation to actually prove they are effective or even safe. The marketing of these products often relies on an indirect argument for their effectiveness rather than presentation of direct evidence of efficacy.

Let's take, for example, a popular supplement called CoQ10, often seen on the shelves of local drugstores. Its chemical name is ubiquinone, and it's been promoted as an energy pill. We all want to have more energy, right? Sounds like a winner.

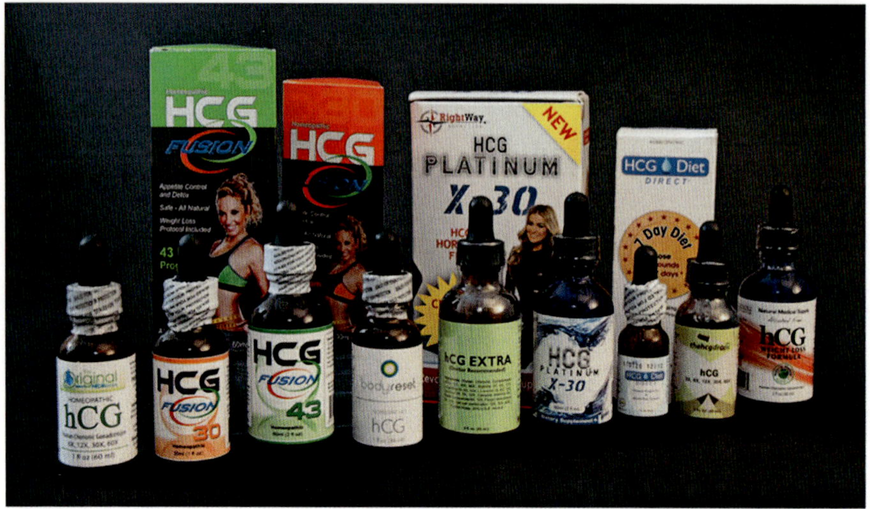

Fig. 4.5 Examples of dietary supplements not regulated by the FDA. "HCG Diet Products Are Illegal"; "These weight-loss products, sold online and in some retail stores, have been targeted by the U.S. Food and Drug Administration (FDA) and the Federal Trade Commission (FTC). FDA advises consumers who have purchased homeopathic (HCG) for weight loss to stop using it, throw it out, and stop following the dieting instructions."—FDA, Dec. 6, 2011, Updated 03/16/2013

Ubiquinone actually does play a role in the body's metabolism, being active in what's called the "oxidative pathway of adenosine triphosphate (ATP)." That much may be true; but has anyone demonstrated that activating this pathway will have anything to do at all with giving you more energy? No. Is being tired a disease? No. What is the best-known solution for being tired? Getting more sleep.

For a long time the FDA tried to regulate tobacco by classifying it as a drug; if it had been successful, cigarette manufacturers might have had to prove their product was safe. That didn't happen, because the US Congress had already taken on the role of labeling and monitoring tobacco products, thus in a way protecting the economies of tobacco-producing states. In 2009, the FDA was given new authority to regulate tobacco products and proposed that 50 % of a cigarette package had to be covered with a graphic anti-smoking image; an example is shown in Fig. 4.6. Cigarette manufacturers sued, claiming that forcing them to attach such images to packaging violated their right to free speech. As of November 7, 2012, the US Supreme Court had not decided the case.

What do you think: should government be involved in telling us or guiding us as to what to do (e.g., harsh tobacco warning labels), even if it is for our own good, or should it let us make up our own minds?

Because the FDA insists that manufacturers seeking to sell drugs in the USA prove the drugs are safe and effective, manufacturers are forced to conduct a variety of laboratory tests, animal experiments, and human clinical trials in order to provide

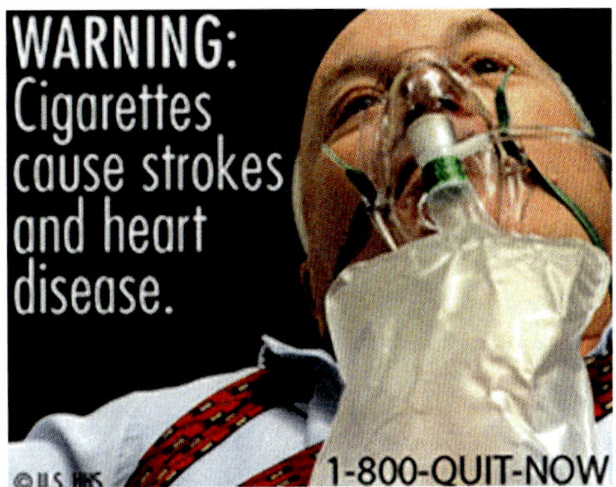

Fig. 4.6 One of the images proposed by the FDA to be used to cover 50 % of a cigarette package

that proof [7]. The data from these experiments provided by the company are reviewed by a panel of experts convened by the FDA, and if they are convinced, the drug is approved for sale. FDA actions are posted on its website (www.fda.gov), and lists of approved drugs as well as drugs taken off the market because of newly discovered health risks are found there too. (By the way, the website provides lots of consumer-friendly information about food, drugs, medical devices, recalls, and even cosmetics.)

During trips to your local pharmacy, you may have noticed that there is a class of products (cosmetics) that seems to make drug-like claims; the names of proteins and other organic molecules are included, and words that imply a healing effect are used. Because manufacturers of beauty products often liked to imply that these cosmetics have some medicinal effects, the FDA got involved. The agency defines cosmetics as "articles intended to be rubbed, poured, sprinkled, or sprayed on, introduced into, or otherwise applied to the human body…for cleansing, beautifying, promoting attractiveness, or altering the appearance." Among the products included are skin moisturizers, perfumes, lipsticks, fingernail polishes, eye and facial makeup preparations, cleansing shampoos, permanent waves, hair colors, and deodorants, as well as anything intended as a component of a cosmetic product.

Whether a substance is a drug or a cosmetic depends on its use. For example, the FDA would rule that an oil used as a fragrance is a cosmetic, but once the manufacturer claims it can be used in aromatherapy, it is classified as a drug. A massage oil is a cosmetic, but if someone claims that it relieves muscle pain, it is classified as a drug. This difference in classification is important to the manufacturer and to the consumer, because a drug must prove safety and efficacy, but a cosmetic does not. For the manufacturer, proving safety and efficacy is expensive because of all the testing involved; on the other hand, if the cosmetic meets the standard for a drug, it may be easily sold for a higher price than a beauty aid.

There are also differences between the approval process for prescription drugs versus over-the-counter (OTC) drugs; the latter must conform to a "monograph" (a set of rules or guidance) from the FDA, which lists compounds and chemicals that are generally safe and effective, having been in use for many years. Products that don't conform to published monographs (don't meet the GRASE "generally

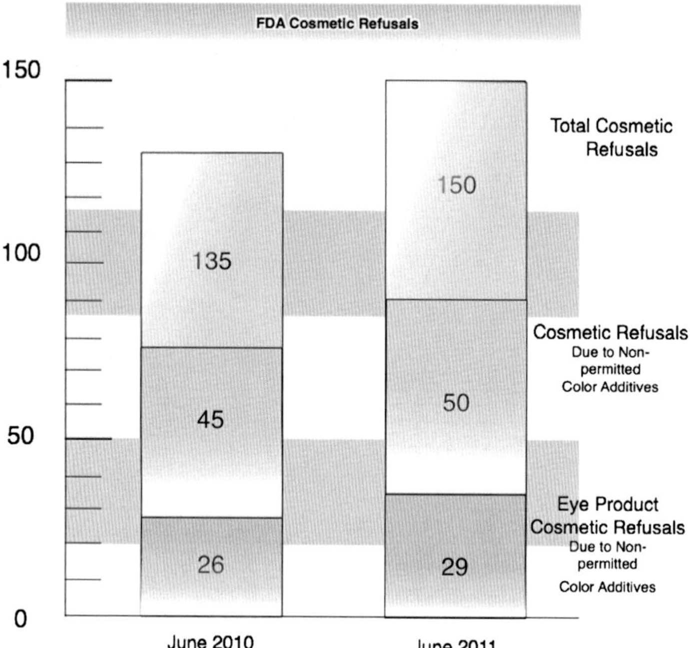

Fig. 4.7 The FDA will not permit sale or importation of cosmetics whose components do not correspond to those listed in its monographs. The above graph shows the number of cosmetic compounds not approved by FDA in 2010 and 2011

recognized as safe and effective" standards) are not permitted to be sold as OTC (Fig. 4.7). Examples of OTC drugs/cosmetics include acne medication, dandruff shampoos, and sunscreens.

4.2.2 Getting a Drug Approved

Professor Smart has two inventions, but drugs and devices follow different paths to achieve FDA approval. She has realized that it will not be possible to borrow sufficient funds to go through the 8–10-year drug approval process; she now establishes a subsidiary company that will attempt to find a buyer for the new drug. To make the sale more attractive, the professor's subsidiary begins to perform the preclinical studies on animals to assess safety and biologic activity. She hopes that these data, if they are convincing, will interest a large pharmaceutical company with deep pockets to take on the job of getting the drug approved.

And sure enough, after Professor Smart publishes the results of the animal studies, she is approached by a multinational company that wishes to license the drug patent and proceed with the studies needed for FDA approval. The professor and Bigname University are both delighted; they will be earning money for a long time,

	Preclinical Testing		Phase I	Phase II	Phase III		FDA		Phase IV
Years	3.5		1	2	3		2.5	12 total	
Test Population	Laboratory and animal studies	File IND at FDA	20 to 80 healthy vouluntеers	100 to 300 patient volunteers	1000 to 3000 patient volunteers	File NDA at FDA	Review process / approval		Additional post-marketing testing required by FDA
Purpose	Assess safety and biological activity		Determine safety and doasge	Evaluate effectiveness, look for side-effects	Verify effectivness, moniter adverse reactions from long-term use				
Success Rate	5,000 compounds evaluated			5 enter trials			1 approved		

Fig. 4.8 A representative timetable for the development and approval by the FDA of a new drug

but only if the studies go well. It's not enough to demonstrate the function of the drug in laboratory and animal studies; it has to be shown to work in humans too.

Here is where we learn why drugs cost so much money, and why a prescription plan is so important to have as a health benefit. First, only the patent holder or the licensee has the right to sell the drug; this monopoly allows the seller to set the price. Pfizer, the pharmaceutical company that developed Viagra, saw its profits go up by 38 % when Viagra was introduced to the market. Of course, Viagra costs about $25/pill in the USA which could explain this large jump in profits. As the patent rights to Viagra expire, the costs of the drug or its generic version will drop significantly.

But there are other reasons why prescription drugs are so expensive. Consider the drug approval process diagrammed in Fig. 4.8, which also includes the time spent on research. The company usually invests a lot of money in discovery and in the preclinical and clinical research stages, and remember that even after these studies are completed and paid for, the FDA can still deny approval. Manufacturers usually file for patents when they first start investigating a compound for medicinal purposes. However, on average it takes more than 12 years to bring a very small fraction of these compounds to market which means that even in the case of successfully approved drugs, the drug companies only have 8 years to recover their costs before the patent expires, at which time the generic versions of the drug can enter the market usually at a much lower price.

The large pharmaceutical company that licensed Professor Smart's drug patent must submit an Investigational New Drug (IND) application to the FDA. This application will discuss all the laboratory and animal data that was gathered by the professor and supplemented by additional work done at the company. If the application is approved, the company will begin with a Phase I trial on humans. This study will typically involve a small group of healthy individuals, and it will be used to establish the "pharmacodynamics" of the drug (how quickly it enters the bloodstream and then how quickly it is excreted), as well as safe dosage ranges. If successful, that study will be followed by a Phase II study, usually involving a slightly larger group of individuals (30–60), who have the disease targeted by the drug. This study is important as it provides some indication of the drug's efficacy (i.e., does it work in humans), further narrows down the dosage range, and identifies side effects.

Assuming the results are positive, the manufacturer moves on to a Phase III study; this will involve a still larger group (100–1,000) and will be primarily designed to evaluate efficacy. The professor's drug makes it through Phase III, and the licensee company submits to the FDA a New Drug Application (NDA), formally asking permission to begin marketing the drug. For the purposes of our story, the FDA grants permission, and the company begins to do all the necessary marketing steps: teaching the sales force about the new drug, taking out advertising in medical and even nonmedical magazines and newspapers, sending doctors samples, etc.

We end the story of Professor Smart's drug discovery here; now that the rights to the invention have been purchased by a large pharmaceutical company, it is they who will proceed with the FDA approval process we describe. All the issues related to animal and clinical trials that are yet to be discussed will come into play during the approval process. Eventually the marketing division will take over if/when FDA approval is obtained and salespersons will begin calling on individual doctors and hospitals convincing them to prescribe the new drug. Advertisements may appear in popular and medical journals highlighting study results. How a new drug is positioned in the market, how its price is established, and how its sales are controlled in foreign countries are all topics that would make for fascinating stories, but unfortunately lie outside the scope of this book.

4.2.3 Getting a Medical Device Approved: A Somewhat Different Process

The type of evaluation required by the FDA for medical devices depends on the impact the device can have on the life of the patient. The agency has identified as Class I various low-risk devices such as bedpans and tongue depressors, Class II includes medium-risk devices such as hearing aids and electrocardiogram machines, and Class III are high-risk devices such as pacemakers and catheters, devices that sustain or support life. Examples of other equipment regulated by the FDA include home health and consumer devices (blood glucose monitoring devices, pregnancy tests), surgery and life support devices (LASIK, liposuction), dental devices (X-ray machines, handpieces), general hospital devices and supplies (sterilizers, infusion pumps), implants and prosthetics (artificial hips and knees), cardiovascular devices (left ventricular assist devices, stents), and baby products with sudden infant death syndrome prevention claims (monitors, mattresses, positioners).

Recall that Professor Smart has still another patent on a device (an implant) that is surgically placed in the location of the tumor and slowly dispenses the anticancer medication. Before she proceeds with the approval process, she first must have an idea of the types of evaluations that are needed. The particular implant involved here is removable and is meant to be removed from time to time; it is classified as a Class II device. Had it been a permanent implant, it would have been classified as Class III and had to go through a process demonstrating that it was safe and effective. Only 2 % of medical devices submitted to the FDA are Class III.

Before any new Class I or Class II device is approved for sale, the manufacturer may submit what is called a 510k or "premarket notification" document to try to show that the device is substantially similar to one already approved and being marketed. If the FDA agrees with that claim, the device may be sold without additional evaluation. If the device is not similar to one already on the market or if it poses a significant risk of illness or injury (all Class III devices), the manufacturer must seek "premarket application" (PMA). In order to go through the PMA process, because the device is not approved yet for general sale or use, the manufacturer will need to obtain an IDE (investigational device exemption), permitting its use in controlled clinical trials. New devices will be approved if the studies show a "reasonable assurance" of safety and effectiveness, in contrast to the tougher requirement for drugs: "substantial evidence" of safety and effectiveness.

In the preclinical research stage, new technology is evaluated, so the company can show it is safe and effective by FDA standards. If a device is made in part or in whole from a newly developed or invented material (such as a new type of implant metal), the material must first pass a biocompatibility evaluation. There are many tests and analyses that are performed, but essentially the material must be shown to not irritate human tissues, to not release toxic chemicals, to not corrode or rust away in contact with bodily fluids, and to not cause cells to mutate into cancerous tissue. Most of these tests are performed "in vitro," meaning "in glass" as in a test tube or dish; that is, they are done in a laboratory and do not involve testing in animals. Human, animal, or bacterial cells initially serve as stand-ins for human tissue and are obtained from a biological supply company, then cultured in a sterile container together with the material to be tested, and nutrients are added to keep the cells alive. The activity of the cells is monitored, appropriate control samples are tested in parallel, and the behavior of the cells provides a first look at the potential biocompatibility of the material. If the cells die in the presence of material being tested, then the material is clearly not biocompatible. These tests are relatively inexpensive and can be repeated many times to enable screening of multiple variations of the material's composition. Various national and international organizations, such as the International Standards Organization (ISO), provide guidance as to how the tests are to be performed [9].

Fortunately for Professor Smart, the implant she invented is coated by a medical silicone material that is used frequently to coat other implants such as pacemakers, so there is no need to go through extensive biocompatibility evaluations. Also, it turns out that there is already an FDA-approved implant on the market that dispenses medication, though it is used in the mouth for treatment of persistent oral yeast infections.

The professor is therefore able to submit a convincing 510(k) arguing for substantial equivalence and begins to sell the product through her start-up. The initial steps are difficult, and she enlists the help and support of experienced medical device executives who are placed on the board of directors and negotiates with local city and state government to receive tax benefits in return for employing local workers to fabricate the device. Professor Smart decides that she is not quite qualified to be the company president and hires an experienced businessperson who in return for a sizeable stock option is willing to work for a reduced salary. This enables the professor to return to her lab to conduct more research and to pursue her first love: teaching undergraduates!

We don't know how this story ends; is Professor Smart's company bought out by a larger device manufacturer? Does she sell her ownership share and retire? Does she move fabrication and assembly offshore to a less expensive labor market? What do you think?

In this section, the topics of animal testing and human clinical trials were introduced without much detail in order not to distract the reader from the description of the FDA approval process. We will now look at these two topics in depth.

4.3 Use of Animals in Biomedical Research

If a new drug, material, or device is found to do no harm in vitro (in the lab), it is then subjected to testing in animals; this may involve animal surgery or dissection (vivisection) and possibly the death of the animal. The use of animals in research is controversial, as experimenting on animals is believed by some to be unnecessary and cruel; the writer Mark Twain was a very vocal anti-vivisectionist in the late nineteenth century. Those opposed to animal testing often argue that results obtained through animal experimentation can't be applied to humans and cite the example of the drug thalidomide, which was found to be safe in animal trials, yet when taken by humans led to many thousands of children born with birth defects. Of course, thalidomide was intended as a sedative for pregnant women, so it's possible that the animals that were administered with thalidomide in the study were not observed to see if their offspring were deformed, but only to see if the drug sedated them. Other examples of discrepancies in results from animal versus human tests include penicillin which kills cats and guinea pigs but not humans; arsenic which is not poisonous to rats, mice, or sheep, yet kills humans; and morphine, which is a sedative for humans but a stimulant for cats, goats, and horses. The philosophical argument is made that if harm to animals is done, then we must be certain that some good will come of it; at this stage of drug evaluation (animal testing), the benefit is not certain, only probable [10].

There is no doubt that experiments conducted on a living creature need to be strongly justified, and before permission is granted by a review committee (Institutional Animal Care and Use Committee, IACUC) located at the university or hospital where the testing is done, the scientist must have a good argument that the testing is necessary, that the specific animal used exhibits a response similar to that of a human, that only the minimum number of animals needed will be tested, that the animals will be maintained in an appropriate environment under the supervision of a veterinarian, and that any procedures including the possible sacrifice

Table 4.2 Three principles of humane animal use

Reduction: minimize number of animals used
– Don't conduct unnecessary animal experiments
– Use the least number of animals without sacrificing the quality of research
Replacement: use "lowest" species in the evolutionary ladder
– Rodents preferable to dogs and cats
– Primates require overwhelming justification
– Are computer models/cell culture experiments a reasonable alternative?
Refinement: minimize pain and suffering
– Use of analgesia and anesthesia even if animal shows no signs of pain
– Strict and humane euthanasia when necessary

(euthanasia) of the animal be conducted without pain (Table 4.2). The US government first passed a law (The Animal Welfare Act) that included guidelines for animal testing in 1966; the law was revised in 1985 and 1992, and the National Institutes of Health as well as the Department of Agriculture have also provided guidance for committees reviewing proposals that include experimentation with animals in its Institutional Animal Care and Use Committee Guidebook. All US government funding agencies such as the National Science Foundation and the National Institutes of Health, as well as many private agencies that fund medical research, support research that will reduce reliance on animals in evaluation of new drugs and devices.

You may be interested to learn of some benefits to mankind that came about as the result of experiments performed on animals: these include asthma inhalers (tested on dogs and guinea pigs), meningitis vaccine (developed using mice and rabbits), leukemia chemotherapy treatments, and heart and kidney transplants plus antirejection medication (developed using dogs and pigs). Drugs and devices need to be tested in a biological system in order to optimize device design or the exact composition of a new drug before experimenting on humans. Animal studies permit retrieval and analysis of devices after they have been in the animal, and the devices can be wired to provide real-time data while they are being used; that can't happen with human trials. Well-controlled animal studies also allow the isolation of a single variable (e.g., diet, degree of exercise), which would not be possible in a human study. In addition, drugs developed in animal studies are often used for treating pets and other animals.

As will be discussed later in Chap. 12, because our knowledge of molecular biology and genetics has progressed, it is now possible to develop "transgenic" and other genetically modified animals for experimentation. If we know that a certain disease has a genetic component, it may now be possible to modify and breed laboratory animals so that they will possess the gene predisposing them to some disease. For example, mice have been genetically engineered to develop Alzheimer's disease, making it possible for scientists to study the effects of various drugs on the progression of that disease. Other animal models have been developed for study of Parkinson's disease, alcohol and drug abuse, and various cancers. Mice have been bred to have no hair, making them easily observed for skin irritation and skin cancer research. A company in Cambridge UK called Kymab, breeds mice which contain human DNA; about 0.1 % of the mouse's genome is human. As a result, the company can use these mice to make antibodies that can work with humans. Mice are first inoculated with antigen (a bacterium virus, toxin, abnormal protein, or cancer cells). The mice then begin to make antibodies to the antigen, and some months afterwards, the spleens of the mice are removed. Special cells called B-cells are identified in the spleen and taken to be grown in a laboratory, where they replicate and make many additional copies of themselves. All the B-cells are able to make the antibody, which can be extracted from the cells and used to make drugs for humans.

An additional ethical consideration for developing or cloning such animals is that they are to be used for studies of disease mechanism and cures, not as pets. Nevertheless, genetic engineering techniques have been used to create, for example, new pet dog breeds that are hypoallergenic.

What do you think: is it OK to breed pigs and immobilize them so that they become obese and use them to study the effects of fat-modifying drugs?

As stated earlier, the use of animals in research is governed by a number of laws and regulations, and as a result, the purchase and care cost of animals used in research is usually extremely high. The use of animals in pet and food industries is far less regulated despite the fact that a much larger number of animals are used in these industries. In almost all countries today, animals are treated as property and as such are not legally regarded as "persons" [11]. However, almost all modern societies have stringent laws and regulations that require their citizens to treat animals humanely and with care.

4.4 Use of Humans in Research

"Principal 6: The degree of risk to be taken should never exceed that determined by the humanitarian importance of the problem to be solved by the experiment" [12].

Assuming that animal testing has been conducted and the material, device, or drug has shown some effectiveness, the next step in the clinical evaluation process is usually a human trial. There are some differences between the trials for drugs and those needed for devices. Drugs require more than one clinical trial, but a single clinical trial may be sufficient for a new device. The reason for this difference is that the clinical outcome of a drug trial is determined by the interaction between the patient and the drug, while the outcome of a device trial is determined also by the skill of the physician intermediary. Any device will typically perform better and better as physicians advance along the learning curve for the surgery needed to implant the device (e.g., artificial hip or cardiac pacemaker), and improvements are made as the device is evaluated. Another characteristic of a device trial that contrasts with a drug study is that neither the physician nor the patient can be "blinded" to the device, i.e., it is difficult if not impossible to study the placebo effect in device trials.

Although the use of animals for evaluating new drugs and devices often provokes strong feelings and even opposition, experimenting with humans poses much greater ethical and moral challenges. The twentieth century saw horrific crimes committed by the Nazis on concentration camp inmates who were subjected to often bizarre experiments; that practice resulted in the Nuremberg Code, a list of ten principles that guide medical investigations involving humans, and shown below.

1. The voluntary consent of the human subject is absolutely essential.

   This requires that the person involved should have legal capacity to give consent; should be so situated as to be able to exercise free power of choice, without the intervention of any element of force, fraud, deceit, duress, over-reaching, or other ulterior form of constraint or coercion; and should have sufficient knowledge and comprehension of the elements of the subject matter involved, as to enable him to make an understanding and enlightened decision. This latter element requires that, before the acceptance of an affirmative decision by the experimental subject, there should be made known to him the nature, duration, and purpose of the experiment; the method and means by which it is to be conducted; all inconveniences and hazards reasonably to be expected; and the effects upon his health or person, which may possibly come from his participation in the experiment. This requirement for voluntary consent of course presents a challenge in cases such as testing of drugs specifically targeted for children, who are not considered mature enough to give consent, or testing interventions for people in coma, who cannot give consent.

   The duty and responsibility for ascertaining the quality of the consent rests upon each individual who initiates, directs or engages in the experiment. It is a personal duty and responsibility which may not be delegated to another with impunity.
2. The experiment should be such as to yield fruitful results for the good of society, unprocurable by other methods or means of study, and not random and unnecessary in nature.
3. The experiment should be so designed and based on the results of animal experimentation and a knowledge of the natural history of the disease or other problem under study, that the anticipated results will justify the performance of the experiment.
4. The experiment should be so conducted as to avoid all unnecessary physical and mental suffering and injury. People cannot be used simply as a means to an end (e.g., developing a new drug) disregarding risks to human test subjects.
5. No experiment should be conducted, where there is an a priori reason to believe that death or disabling injury will occur, except, perhaps, in those experiments where the experimental physicians also serve as subjects.
6. The degree of risk to be taken should never exceed that determined by the humanitarian importance of the problem to be solved by the experiment.
7. Proper preparations should be made and adequate facilities provided to protect the experimental subject against even remote possibilities of injury, disability, or death.
8. The experiment should be conducted only by scientifically qualified persons. The highest degree of skill and care should be required through all stages of the experiment of those who conduct or engage in the experiment.

9. During the course of the experiment, the human subject should be at liberty to bring the experiment to an end, if he has reached the physical or mental state, where continuation of the experiment seemed to him to be impossible. Extra protections should be provided to those with diminished autonomy (e.g., prisoners, cognitively Impaired).
10. During the course of the experiment, the scientist in charge must be prepared to terminate the experiment at any stage, if he has probable cause to believe, in the exercise of the good faith, superior skill, and careful judgment required of him, that a continuation of the experiment is likely to result in injury, disability, or death to the experimental subject.

In 1964, the Declaration of Helsinki was first published by the World Medical Association, which provided a distinction between therapeutic and nontherapeutic research, and protected the rights of patients needing medical care who are also recruited for medical research. The declaration has been amended six times, most recently in 2008. Other policies developed by the World Medical Association (www.wma.net) and adopted by the United Nations include "Guidelines for Physicians Concerning Torture and other Cruel, Inhuman or Degrading Treatment or Punishment in Relation to Detention and Imprisonment," treatment of hunger strikers, and prison medicine.

We don't have to go to Nazi Germany for evidence of mistreatment of human subjects in medical studies; the year 1972 saw the exposure of the infamous Tuskegee syphilis study. In the course of this clinical trial, which had been conducted since 1932 under the auspices of the US Public Health Service, 399 poor African-American sharecroppers in Alabama who had contracted syphilis were followed by doctors of the Tuskegee Institute and provided with free medical care and food. However, they were never told they had syphilis, and even though it was known that penicillin was a cure for syphilis, they were never treated. This wasn't necessarily a racial issue; some of the doctors and nurses monitoring the patients were also African-American. It wasn't until 1997 that President Clinton on behalf of the US government apologized to the survivors of this study.

Human clinical trials are important because they are the gold standard that helps to establish the safety and efficacy of new drugs and devices. All research that involves human subjects in the USA must conform to standards of the Department of Health and Human Services as outlined in the 1979 version of the Belmont Report, written and developed after the details of the Tuskegee syphilis study became known [10]. The FDA, which has oversight over research on drugs or devices, has issued guidance most recently in 1998 for clinical investigators and committees reviewing studies with human participants. All research with human subjects that is paid for by the US government must be approved by an Institutional Review Board (IRB) at the institution where the clinical trial will be held. The IRB committee has rules that state who should be included as members of this committee, and the Belmont report provides guidelines for its work. The IRB will review the protocol (study plan) as well as the informed consent form that all patients involved in the study will have to sign. The protocol should identify well-defined end points, the number of subjects that the device must be tested on, the characteristics of the patients (e.g., age, gender, weight, medical condition), how many sites will sponsor the trial, and how long the trial will take. The IRB has to also consider, for example, if the consent form is easily understood by the proposed patient population; that's why it's called the "informed" consent form. There are three categories of IRB review process: full (e.g., testing a new implant), expedited (e.g., amendments to existing protocols), and exempt (e.g., retrospective chart analysis of patients in a hospital—no risks to patients).

(An example of an informed consent form for a clinical trial is found in Appendix C.)

IRBs may encounter difficulties deciding if a device is a "significant" or a "non-significant" risk. This is an important finding for the manufacturer, because a non-significant risk determination means that the trial can proceed without informing the FDA. A determination that the device is a significant risk will mean that the manufacturer will have to obtain an IDE from the FDA before the trial begins.

As a result of government regulations, clinical trials involving human subjects typically progress along fairly well-documented paths. In a Phase III trial, for example, an experimental drug will be administered to half of the participating patients, with the other half receiving either a placebo or, if one exists, the standard treatment for their particular disease. The doctors and patients in clinical trials are usually "blinded" as to whether a given patient is being treated with the drug or with a sugar pill to remove biases that may arise as, for example, when a doctor may be eager to show positive results for a drug that he may have helped develop.

There is actually some controversy about when a placebo should be used as a control. Most experts generally agree that a placebo is appropriate for evaluating what are called "first-generation" drugs, or drugs that have been developed to fill a gap in available medications, and also when there is little or no evidence that some existing therapy is effective. However, in evaluating "second generation" drugs, or those that are modifications of existing and successful medications, many experts believe that the control should not be a placebo, but rather the existing standard treatment. In other words, the trial should be conducted to determine if the new medication is more effective than what is currently available; isn't that the information that you and your doctor would find to be most interesting and useful? Drug manufacturers, on the other hand, would rather use a placebo control in all cases, because it is easier to prove effectiveness compared to a placebo than to prove a better result over an existing treatment. Also, the manufacturers point out that the FDA's function is only to determine if a drug is safe and effective, not if it is "better" than an existing drug. The decision over whether a placebo or the standard treatment should be used as a control is made by the Institutional Review Board (IRB). Perhaps you can see how important the role of the IRB is in protecting the rights of patients and of ensuring that the study produces information of importance not only to the manufacturer but also to the consumer. Sometimes, manufacturers complain that IRBs are "tougher" in the USA than in other countries and end up conducting their clinical trials in other countries with friendlier IRB's even though the intended market is primarily the USA. There are no international agreements for informed consent, so manufacturers often have much more flexibility as to what they may tell persons participating in these studies in other countries. At the present time, more than 50 % of drug clinical trials are done outside the USA.

What do you think: should clinical trials be conducted using poor people in foreign countries as subjects? They do get paid, but they are not likely to afford taking the medication ever again if needed.

By the way, do you realize how truly powerful the placebo effect is? Our mind really can affect the way our bodies react. For example, it has been shown that patients who believe that they are receiving medication, but in fact are receiving two sugar pills, feel better than patients who receive only one sugar pill and that when a placebo is administered by an injection (i.e., getting a shot), it is more effective than when it is given as an oral medication.

We are all susceptible to the placebo effect. A study that involved medical students found that the color of the pill influenced their belief as to its effectiveness; students who took pink sugar pills were more alert than students who took blue sugar pills [13]! Pills for hyperactivity are usually green, and pills for depression are usually yellow; why do you think Viagra is blue?

The more elaborate the ritual in taking the drug, the greater its perceived benefit. Patients routinely say that brand name drugs are more effective than generic medications, even though the ingredients are identical. The fancier the packaging, the better we think the medication will work. We also believe what we are told: if your doctor is upbeat and optimistic, chances are you will feel better sooner than if he is down and pessimistic. In a study involving hotel maids (i.e., ladies who clean hotel rooms), one group was told that the work they do is very beneficial to their health because it provides them with exercise. The other group was not told this information. Four weeks later, the group that had been told their job was good for them reported feeling better, with lower weight and body fat than the other group even though both reported doing the same amount of work [14].

Keep the placebo effect in mind when you read about miracle cures.

Which patients in a clinical trial receive the drug, and which receive the placebo or standard treatment, should be determined randomly. A well-designed study will have an elaborate randomization plan that goes beyond simply alternating between groups as patients are recruited. In what is called a "double-blind" study, designed to reduce the chance of bias to a minimum, the patient will receive a medication identified by a code, and neither the patient nor the physician will know if the medication is the new drug or a placebo. Only at the end of the trial, 6 or 12 months later, will the key to the codes be unsealed, and the meaning of the codes revealed.

A particularly problematic aspect of the placebo effect is that patients will do better while being in a trial just because they are in the trial and get attention!

The clinical trial processes described earlier (Phase I, II, III) are interventional; they rely on an experiment where an independent variable (the drug and its dose) is manipulated, and the effect on the dependent variable (some measure of health) is noted. Other types of interventional trials also exist; some involve large populations where a relatively benign treatment is evaluated versus a placebo. For example, in the 1940s several limited studies had found that an elevated fluorine content in drinking water seemed to reduce the prevalence of tooth decay in children. Based on this preliminary data, it was decided to conduct a large-scale trial which began in 1945, with the population (28,000 children 4–16 years old) of the town of Grand Rapids, Michigan, receiving fluoridated water and the population (77,000 children 4–16 years old) in the neighboring town of Muskegon, Michigan, acting as a control (no fluoridation). No placebo was used because the investigators were certain that the placebo effect could not influence tooth decay. The rate of tooth decay in these children was followed for 15 years, and it was found that decay decreased by 48–63 % (depending on age bracket) in children from Grand Rapids. The results of this large group interventional study provided the foundation for water fluoridation in many cities of the USA.

Other clinical trials are characterized as observational. In this type of study, a large free-living population is observed for many years to search for relationships between lifestyle and the risk of some chronic disease or between genetic factors (heredity) and the risk of some chronic disease. These trials don't prove cause and effect, but provide useful associations. For example, the association between lung cancer and smoking cigarettes was found in this type of study.

Would you like to be a human "guinea pig"? Someday you might be offered the

What do you think: what are some examples of population groups well-suited to study the role of heredity in determining health and others appropriate for the study of the effect of lifestyle on health?

opportunity to participate in a clinical trial; advertisements can be frequently heard on the radio posted by researchers looking for participants. You might also have the chance to be part of a clinical trial (and want to be included) if you have an illness for which there is no effective standard treatment or if the medications/procedures you need are expensive and are not covered by your insurance; in a clinical trial for a drug, there is usually no cost to the patient. Remember that some diseases are rare, and the drugs used to treat them can cost thousands of dollars/month because the drug company has only a small population of patients it relies on to redeem its costs of developing the drug.

If you choose to participate in a trial, what questions should you ask? First, take your time and read the informed consent form carefully; it must explain the purpose of the study, the foreseeable risks, potential benefits, appropriate alternative procedures, the extent of confidentiality, any compensation (especially for risky procedures), whom to contact with any questions, and a statement that participation is voluntary. Ask questions if you don't understand something about the trial. Other topics that should be covered in the consent form include unforeseeable risks to the patient, circumstances under which your participation in the study may be terminated, any additional costs resulting from participating in the study, and any consequences if you choose to withdraw from the study [15]. It is also worthwhile to ask if you will be able to participate in any future clinical trials for your condition if you participate in the one being considered. Sometimes, your participation in one trial will knock you out of consideration for other trials, especially if you did not respond well to the drug being investigated.

4.5 Postmarket Surveillance: How Do Products Perform Years After They Have Been Sold?

New medical devices undergo considerable development and evaluation by a manufacturer before they are submitted for FDA approval and then again during the approval process. After they are approved and sold to doctors and hospitals, manufacturers continue to modify the devices as they see fit to improve them, but these minor changes do not require that the newest device version be reevaluated; the manufacturer will claim "substantial equivalence" of the new device to the older, approved model. A criticism of this regulation is that manufacturers use this strategy to avoid going through the approval process from the very beginning, even for Class III devices [16].

As a safety measure and just in case a problem was not detected in the PMA process or under the claim of "substantial equivalence," the FDA mandates that manufacturers continue to monitor the performance of drugs and devices after approval [17]. They are required to investigate complaints, keep records, and submit individual reports about device malfunction, deaths, or injuries. Devices whose failures could have serious adverse consequences (e.g., permanent implants or life-sustaining devices used outside a healthcare facility) must be tracked by the manufacturer, usually by serial number. If the FDA decides a device or drug poses an unacceptable risk to patients, it may suggest that the manufacturer issue a voluntary recall, though the FDA is also empowered to mandate a legally binding recall if the manufacturer refuses to act on their own. Other sanctions that may be applied by the FDA include a warning letter, a citation (warning that the company will be prosecuted if violations are not corrected), prosecution (criminal action filed by the FDA), and seizure (the FDA removes the products from the market).

Devices are imperfect and inevitably some patients will develop long-term complications. One way in which manufacturers and regulators can learn from their mistakes is to actively promote a device retrieval system [18]. In this scenario, implants and other devices that are removed from a patient would be sent to a centralized laboratory facility where they would be systematically examined, the cause of failure (if any) identified, and improvements could then be made to the next generation of devices.

4.6 Room for Improvement: What Can Be Done to Increase Reliability and Utility of Clinical Trials?

There is much room for improvement in how clinical trials are planned and reported. There is a concern, for example, that manufacturers selectively choose to reveal only positive not negative or inconclusive study outcomes [19]. Let's pretend that ten different trials were conducted, and four of them showed no effect of the drug. The manufacturer is not very likely to publish the results of those four trials and has no obligation to do so. And yet, not including information from all studies can give a very misleading impression to patients and to doctors. Drug manufacturers should register all studies of new treatments, so that the doctor and even the patient can learn about all clinical trials that were conducted on a particular drug or device, including those that might have shown there to be no effects.

Drug studies paid for by drug companies are also more likely to show that the drug is safe and effective, and 70 % of all drug trials reported in the scientific literature are funded by manufacturers. Furthermore, if a drug trial is conducted in several locations (i.e., a multicenter trial), it is likely that each center will publish their findings in a separate scientific paper. So, even though only one clinical trial is held, the large number of publications that come out implies that many different studies have been conducted. The FDA is often shown early results from these studies, which may not be indicative of long-term use.

A sensational recent case involved the drug Vioxx. This drug was developed to treat arthritis, and its claim to fame was that unlike other arthritis medications, it did not cause stomach irritation. So, a trial was conducted, and the authors reported that in fact Vioxx was much better at not causing stomach distress. What the published reports did not say was that there were several deaths due to heart attacks in the patient group that had been taking Vioxx. That was not reported because it occurred a few months after the study had "officially" ended, and the authors decided that the data were not pertinent to the primary focus of the study. When this news got out, Vioxx was taken off the market, and the New England Journal of Medicine, a very prestigious publication where the results of the study had been first announced, wrote a scathing editorial "expressing concern" with the way the news of the deaths had first been concealed [20].

Another flaw in the current system is that the results provided to FDA regulators are secret and not disclosed to a wider scientific audience. So, the FDA often makes decisions without the benefit of scrutiny by a large number of experts. Still another significant problem is that for many major diseases, no one knows what is the best treatment, simply because it is in nobody's financial interest to actually find out; that's the case for the so-called orphan drugs, which are medications used for rare diseases [12]. If the potential pool of patients that need the drug is small, companies are more inclined to spend their time and money on drugs that will be prescribed for large patient pools with the potential for greater profits.

From a consumer's point of view, some aspects of placebo-controlled trials fall short of the ideal. For example, don't you want to know how a new medication compares against one that's already approved, which drug actually works best in head-to-head competition? Of course you do. And yet, companies don't want to provide that information, preferring to use the easier placebo control. When pharmaceutical companies do run comparison trials, there are many ways they can game the outcome. For example, they can compare their drug against a competitor's drug that is administered at a very low (ineffective) dose, or administer the competitor's drug at a very high dose (causing major side effects), or provide the competitor's drug in the wrong way (orally rather than by injection). And, unless you are familiar with the way these drugs are intended to be used, you can't really spot if there was any cheating involved.

A minor problem that arises with clinical trials is the practice of over-recruiting patients, because device manufacturers are allowed to recover device costs from patients, and the clinicians conducting the trial are allowed to charge the patient (or the insurer) for procedures or services associated with the device. In other words, if the trial has more patients, the clinician and the manufacturer earn more money. Drug manufacturers, on the other hand, are not permitted to charge for treatment in a clinical trial.

What can you do as a consumer to find out what's best for you? There is a relatively new way of thinking about the practice of medicine, called "evidence-based medicine." According to those who practice it, only sophisticated analysis of many different clinical studies will identify what is the best course of treatment. Of course most of us cannot do these analyses, but fortunately there is an organization called the Cochrane Collaboration, an international network of people working to help us make informed decisions about healthcare (www.cochrane.org), which publishes reviews (some 5,000 so far) of treatments for prevention, treatment, and rehabilitation. Examples include reviews discussing cranberries for urinary tract infections, fish oil for preventing dementia, exercise for depression, and the list goes on and on. You can see that these reports cover topics that are not too difficult to understand, and the Cochrane people have no incentive to mislead anybody. Best of all, the information is available online, and it's all free. You owe it to yourself to browse their collection. And for anybody who's interested, there is another group called the Campbell Collaboration (campbellcollaboration.org) that conducts similar reviews summarizing research reports of social policies.

4.7 Manufacturer–Consumer–FDA Relations

There will likely always be tension between manufacturers seeking to speed up the introduction of their product into the marketplace and consumer groups who want to ensure safety and certainty that the medication or device will function as advertised. Consumers also want rapid introduction of new treatments because they are thought to be improvements over what is currently available. The suggestion by manufacturers that the FDA budget should be increased so that the agency can expand its workforce as a strategy to speed up the review process will most likely benefit manufacturers and consumers alike. On the other hand, many consumers, and possibly some representatives of the legal system, don't fully understand the complexity of the interactions between the human body and drugs, devices, and materials. For example, bodily fluids will leach (dissolve) out some components of polymers (plastics) implanted in the human body. It's not possible to exactly simulate such behavior, i.e., years of service in the human body, in a laboratory setting, or in a short clinical trial. Therefore, it is also impossible to know for sure which components are leached out and what happens with them once they are freely available inside the body.

What do you think: if you were a patient needing an implant that would be in your body for decades, how much time would you be willing to wait until testing was completed in a laboratory?

The FDA's concern for safety and efficacy extends to the labeling *and* advertising of prescription drugs and devices. Labels must include adequate directions for use and warnings against harmful use, and there should be no false or misleading statements. Advertising materials must contain the name of the drug, its ingredients, and a summary of side effects, contraindications, and effectiveness. This information is found in the small print when drugs are advertised directly to consumers in the pages of newspapers and popular magazines or on television. Did you know that the advertising budgets for direct-to-consumer drug advertising is climbing at much higher rates than for advertising targeted at physicians?

Although drug companies eventually lose patent protection for their products, they may maintain a marketing advantage after patent expiration if they can successfully argue that generic forms of the drugs are not truly similar to the brand name medication. Currently, some of the most profitable drugs are made not in chemical factories, but in living cells; examples include the arthritis drug Humira™ and cancer drugs Herceptin™, Avastin™, and Rituxan™. Manufacturers claim that unless the generics are made with the identical cell line used by the original drug developer, they are not truly identical and are called "biosimilars" and should be subjected to the same FDA approval process as the original drug [21]. These arguments are being made in state legislatures and the courts, and the way they will eventually be resolved will have great implications for healthcare costs.

Information found on the Internet poses a challenge for drug and device manufacturers [22]. Often, drug company-sponsored links on search engine sites don't contain all the FDA-mandated information, even though the links themselves may lead to pages where the required information is posted. Does the consumer typically follow these links? If not, then he is left with an incomplete understanding of what the drug does. Furthermore, the Internet contains much information provided by third parties about drugs. The manufacturers can't reasonably be held responsible and liable for such incorrect postings by third parties.

The drug and medical device industry is also involved in considerable litigation, possibly because the industry is seen as having "deep pockets," i.e., lots of money, and because drug or device failures have such significant, human-interest consequences. Since the early 1990s, there has been continuing mass litigation brought against the health industry. Law suits have been filed concerning breast implants, pedicle screws (a screw used in spine surgery), the Norplant birth control device, several diet drugs (the "fen-fens"), a pain medication for arthritis sufferers (Vioxx), an antidiabetes drug (Rezulin), a drug for gastrointestinal ailments (Propulsid), a statin designed to lower cholesterol and prevent heart disease (Baycol), and, most recently, metal-on-metal artificial hip implants (the articular hip replacement) [23]. Manufacturers have lost enormous sums of money and consequently are always searching for ways to lower their exposure if they lose court cases. One way is to employ the so-called learned intermediary strategy, which boils down to shifting part of the blame onto the physician, who is, after all, responsible for prescribing the medication and its dosage and duration [24]. Another is to lobby the US Congress to pass laws limiting exposure; in 2011, the medical device industry spent approximately $33 million on lobbyists. At the same time, the industry is pushing for accelerated reviews by the FDA, pointing out that many medical device companies are often small and can't afford to wait through a lengthy review. In counterpoint, groups like Public Citizen provide evidence that in 2011, for example, the FDA issued 50 Class I recalls and 1,151 Class II recalls. In a report issued in February 2012, the organization listed several recommendations on policies that would strengthen the enforcement powers of the FDA and also increase the burden of reporting and proof on the manufacturers [16].

Although smoother approval processes and less burdensome reporting requirements are "good for business," it is wise to recall that some 50 years ago, the FDA stood firmly against the approval of the drug thalidomide, intended for pregnant women who suffered from morning sickness. Dr. Frances Kelsey at the FDA refused to approve this drug, even though it had been approved for use in Canada and 20 other countries. She demanded additional tests. Only later was it found that the drug was responsible for horrific birth defects, and it was pulled out from the international market. Dr. Kelsey received the distinguished federal civilian service from President John F. Kennedy for her stand, and the US Congress was moved to pass legislation in 1962 that outlined the steps drug manufacturers had to take to prove safety and effectiveness. Interestingly, thalidomide is available for use again, but not as a sedative, but rather as a treatment of leprosy and some cancers.

A complicated reality is the "off-label" use of drugs or devices. This happens when a drug or device is used in a way that's not specified in the FDA-approved labeling for the drug or device. After all, once a drug is approved, there is nothing stopping your doctor for prescribing it for any condition whatsoever. The argument for such use is that new medical developments and discoveries are sometimes made by physicians treating patients, and they could find that a drug or device is useful in an application not originally intended or approved. The FDA is aware of off-label use and permits it in certain situations, because it is not in the position of practicing medicine; that is the role of the doctor. Off-label use is also allowed with certain populations, e.g., late-stage cancer patients who have little to lose by trying new therapies and for infants and children, because few medications have been specifically FDA approved for children. The problem of course is that few health insurance companies will pay for off-label use of cancer-fighting drugs, because they argue there is no proof the drug works. Common examples of off-label drug use include using antihistamines as sleep aids rather than for allergies and asthma medications for bad coughs, and you can imagine the variety of uses for Viagra. You should be careful, however; if a drug is used off-label for a different population than the one it was first intended for, the company has no obligation to divulge any information it might have about side effects for that population. For example, if a drug was approved for treating depression in adults and is prescribed off-label for teenagers, the manufacturer doesn't have to tell anybody what it knows about the effect(s) of that antidepressant on teenagers.

What do you think: why are there few FDA-approved drugs for infants and children? Should and could this be corrected?

At the conclusion of this chapter, we would like to illustrate an interaction between medical device manufacturers, consumers, and the legal system. The story of breast implants includes all these elements. The story also contains an example of a dilemma confronting manufacturers and patients: how is it possible to predict the long-term effects of new medications, materials, or devices, when it is not realistically feasible to conduct clinical trials for the length of time that a patient would be exposed to the new drug or device? In other words, both manufacturers and patients have an interest in new products being introduced; and yet, no manufacturer is able to evaluate a new product for the 10, 20, or more years that the product would be in service. Preliminary laboratory, animal, and human testing can yield an absence of evidence of harm, but that is not quite the same thing as evidence of absence of harm.

4.8 Case History: Silicone Breast Implants

The first silicone breast implants were developed in the 1960s, and the first woman received them in 1962 (Fig. 4.9). In 1976, the FDA published the Medical Devices Amendment and was given the authority to review the safety and effectiveness of new devices. However, silicone breast implants had been on the market for so long that they were "grandfathered" in and didn't have to go through the extensive FDA testing that had just become mandatory. Just 1 year later, in 1977, the first lawsuit against Dow Corning, a manufacturer of medical silicone, was won by a woman who claimed her ruptured implants caused pain and suffering, and in the 1980s the Public Citizen Health Research Group sent out a warning saying that silicone breast implants cause cancer.

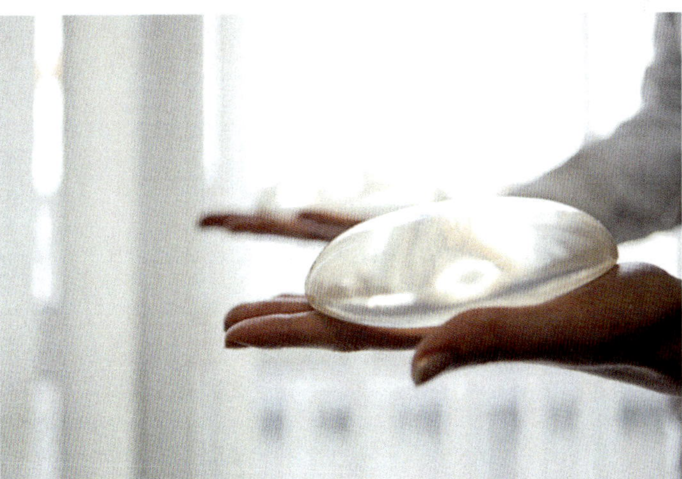

Fig. 4.9 Silicone-gel-filled breast implants

In 1982, responding to many complaints, the FDA proposed that silicone breast implants should be classified as Class II devices, and their safety should be proved. In 1984 Dow Corning lost another court case, and in 1988 the FDA classified implants as Class III devices, further upgrading their perceived potential danger. Silicone breast implants became the focus of popular TV news programs and congressional hearings. In 1991 Dow Corning submitted the results of 329 studies to the FDA, but the FDA ruled that the studies were inconclusive and requested additional data. By that time there were 137 lawsuits filed, and several internal documents were found in the Dow Corning files which damaged its legal position. In 1992, several manufacturers voluntarily withdrew silicone breast implants from the market, but that year marked the filing of the first class action lawsuit (a group of people joined together and filed a lawsuit on behalf of all breast implant patients). In that same year Dow Corning and Bristol–Myers Squibb quit the breast implant business, as there were now over 3,000 lawsuits, and multimillion dollar awards were being made to the women winning some of these cases.

In 1994, the class action lawsuit was settled, but manufacturers continued to claim that there was no scientific evidence linking silicone breast implants to autoimmune disease. Interestingly, a Mayo clinic study published that year also did not find any such evidence. Nevertheless, Dow Corning, which was facing 20,000 lawsuits, filed for Chapter 11 bankruptcy in 1995 (a form of bankruptcy that allows the organization to continue in business while under the supervision of the court).

In 1996 a federal judge in Oregon ruled that lawyers may no longer present evidence that silicone breast implants cause disease because there is no scientific evidence backing up that claim. Manufacturers started to win lawsuits, although Dow Corning chose to settle the class action lawsuit, paying out $3.2 billion. In 1999, the Institute of Medicine released a report that although silicone breast implants may be responsible for scarring and tissue hardening, they do not cause any major disease. Silicone implants are now available for women who have had breast cancer surgery.

At this time, silicone-filled breast implants are approved by the FDA, though it is noted that they are not lifetime devices and are likely to require surgical removal at some point.

What do you think: is there a winner and a loser in this story? What effect, if any, do these events have on healthcare technology and patients needing breast implants in the USA?

4.9 Summary

The regulatory process for drugs and medical devices has evolved for over 100 years, and as we have seen, it often changes in response to bad publicity or when a widespread adverse event occurs. It is at those times that the Congress develops the political will to pass another law or amendment. Although legitimate criticism may be leveled at aspects of this regulatory system, it's likely that because it is a product of compromise between the sometimes competing demands of consumers and manufacturers, future improvements will be incremental. The FDA will likely be confronted by more and more sophisticated treatment modalities, including many emerging technologies such as genetic engineering, and it is probable that additional questions will arise about how best to regulate drug–device combinations.

The rather broad description of ways in which the clinical trial process could be improved should not reduce our confidence in the "system." It has protected the American consumer well, particularly when compared to many other countries.

4.10 Foundational Concepts

- The patent process is designed to provide inventors with financial incentives to invent; the patent provides the inventor with exclusive rights to market the invention for 14–20 years. Obtaining a patent requires careful record-keeping to preserve the "first to invent" claim, and the invention must be novel, useful, and not obvious.
- Inventors often have difficulty finding funding to perfect and to market their invention. Health-related inventions (drugs or devices) have the extra burden of having to be proved to be safe and effective in a manner acceptable to the US Food and Drug Administration (FDA). The FDA has regulatory authority over drugs, medical devices, some food products, vaccines, blood, biological, animal feeds and drugs, cosmetic labeling, medical imaging devices which emit radiation, and tobacco labeling.
- The FDA does not regulate herbal remedies or food supplements; therefore, those substances do not have to be proved safe and effective.
- The approval process for new drugs includes preclinical testing in the laboratory or using animals, followed by Phase I, II, and III clinical trials using human subjects. Human trials are first reviewed by an Institutional Review Board convened at the institution where the trial is to take place and must include adequate protection for the human subjects including informed consent. The principles of sound experimental design (e.g., control groups, double-blind studies) must be followed.
- Proposed animal studies must also be reviewed and found to be humane without untoward suffering. The use of animals at this time is essential, although research is ongoing to find alternative ways to evaluate new drugs and devices.
- The approval process for new medical devices depends on a finding that the device is essentially similar to an existing device in use. If so, the manufacturer is free to market the device. If not, the manufacturer must provide data from controlled studies to the FDA in order to obtain marketing approval.
- Drug companies pay for drug trials, and so it is possible that negative results are never known because they are suppressed. No one else has the resources to conduct such trials.
- The Cochrane Collaboration publishes an analysis of treatments for various diseases and conditions and bases its findings and recommendations on an objective analysis of the results of all published and controlled human trials that have assessed a particular drug or treatment.

- There is a tension between the FDA, manufacturers, and consumers. The manufacturers want as rapid a path to market as possible, while consumers want a guarantee of safety and effectiveness. Both groups blame the FDA for shortcomings in the approval system.

References

1. Moazzam, M., & Bednarek, M. (2006). Intellectual property protection for medical devices. In K. Becker & J. Whyte (Eds.), *Clinical evaluation of medical devices* (pp. 117–139). Totowa, NJ: Humana Press.
2. Kollewe, J. (2012, November 28). Drug recycling is big pharma's bright hope. *The Guardian*, London.
3. Galeon, A. (2006). Wall Street's perspective on medical device evaluation. In K. Becker & J. Whyte (Eds.), *Clinical evaluation of medical devices* (pp. 187–196). Totowa, NJ: Humana Press.
4. Christensen, C. (1997). *The innovator's dilemma*. Boston, MA: Harvard University Press.
5. Winegarden, W. (2012). *A primer on the orphan drug market: Addressing the needs of patients with rare diseases*. San Francisco, CA: Pacific Research Institute.
6. Pipes, S. (2012, October 29). To cure rare diseases, unleash orphan drug innovations. *Forbes*. http://www.forbes.com/sites/sallypipes/2012/10/29/to-cure-rare-diseases-unleash-orphan-drug-innovations/
7. Sweet, B., Schwemm, A., & Parsons, D. (2011). Review of the processes for FDA oversight for drugs, medical devices, and combination products. *Journal of Managed Care Pharmacy, 17*, 40–50.
8. Harris, G. (2008, September 30). What's behind an F.D.A. stamp? *The New York Times*, New York.
9. International Standard Organization. (2003). ISO-10993 biological evaluation of medical devices Part I. Evaluation and testing. http://www.fda.gov/MedicalDevices/DeviceRegulationandGuidance/GuidanceDocuments/ucm080735.htm.
10. Budinger, T., & Budinger, M. (2006). *Ethics of emerging technologies*. Hoboken, NJ: John Wiley and Sons.
11. Miller, G. (2011). Animal rights. The rise of animal law. *Science, 332*, 28–31.
12. The Nuremberg Commission. (1949). *Trials of war criminals before the Nuremberg Military Tribunals under Control Council Law No. 10* (pp. 181–182). Washington, DC: The US Government Printing Office.
13. Blackwell, B., Bloomfield, S., & Buncher, C. (1972). Demonstration to medical students of placebo responses and non-drug factors. *Lancet, 299*(7763), 1279–1282.
14. Crum, A., & Langer, E. (2007). Mindset matters: Exercise and the placebo effect. *Psychological Science, 18*, 165–171.
15. Kracov, D., & Dwyer, L. (2006). Regulatory requirements for clinical studies of medical devices and diagnostics. In K. Becker & J. Whyte (Eds.), *Clinical evaluation of medical devices* (pp. 21–58). Totowa, NJ: Humana Press.
16. Mouzoon, N., & Garome, M. (2012). Substantially unsafe: Medical devices pose great threat to patients; safeguards must be strengthened, not weakened. *Public Citizen*.
17. Onel, S. (2006). Postmarket requirements for significant risk devices. In K. Becker & J. Whyte (Eds.), *Clinical evaluation of medical devices* (pp. 81–97). Totowa, NJ: Humana Press.
18. Schoen, F. (2006). Role of device retrieval and analysis in the evaluation of substitute heart valves. In K. Becker & J. Whyte (Eds.), *Clinical evaluation of medical devices* (pp. 305–329). Totowa, NJ: Humana Press.
19. Goldacre, B. (2012). *Bad pharma: How drug companies mislead doctors and harm patients*. Hammersmith, UK: Fourth Estate.

20. Curfman, G., Morrissey, S., & Drazen, J. (2005). Expression of concern: Bombardier et al. "Comparison of Upper Gastrointestinal Toxicity of Rofecoxib and Naproxen in Patients with Rheumatoid Arthritis". N. Engl. J Med 2000;343: 1520–1528. *New England Journal of Medicine, 353*, 2813–2814.
21. Pollack, A. (2013, January 28). Biotech firms, billions at risk, lobby states to limit generics. *The New York Times*, New York.
22. Sampson, K., & Spector-Bagdady, K. (2010). The regulation of prescription drug and restricted medical device advertising. *Engage, 11*, 4–8.
23. Meier, B., & Roberts, J. (2011, August 22). Hip complaints surge, even as the dangers are studied. *The New York Times*, New York.
24. Thornton, R. (2002). Defending claims related to prescribing drugs or using medical devices. *Baylor University Medical Center Proceedings, 15*, 102–104.

A Visit to the Physician: Diagnoses and Enabling Technologies

5

"Any sufficiently advanced technology is indistinguishable from magic."

Arthur C. Clarke

Many folks regard an appointment with a physician with fear and trepidation; after all, something is wrong, and it's likely that by the time the appointment is made, the patient is in some discomfort. The memory of other, earlier appointments, when diagnostic tests were ordered and the results came back with an indecipherable or incomplete explanation, only contributes to the patient's anxiety.

In this chapter, we plan to demystify much of what happens in the doctor's office by explaining why certain tests are important, and what they can contribute to an understanding of your state of health. The technology underlying many tests and diagnostic imaging procedures will be discussed so that you will appreciate the reasons why tests are conducted in specific ways.

5.1 Introduction

What a terrible thing it is to have symptoms of disease and yet not know what exactly is wrong, is the matter "serious," how long the symptoms might last, and what can be done to relieve them. Although the Internet provides a lot of information and many opportunities for "self-diagnosis," more than likely searches of medical sites will only contribute to more worry. Obtaining an accurate diagnosis is critical to prescribing proper treatment, and the medical profession can now take advantage of many tools developed by biochemists and engineers that are essential in the management of a patient who is ill. Unfortunately, there is still much that is unknown about the functioning of the human body, and although the cause of a disease may be identified, the best treatment may elude the healthcare provider. Not all patients progress

G.R. Baran et al., *Healthcare and Biomedical Technology in the 21st Century: An Introduction for Non-Science Majors*, DOI 10.1007/978-1-4614-8541-4_5,

in their disease at the same rate, nor do all medications have the same effects on all patients. When the diagnosis suggests a serious or life-changing sickness, it makes sense to seek other opinions and to become an informed and active patient.

5.2 Home or Self-Diagnosis

Most folks avoid making an appointment to see a physician for as long as possible. There are many reasons to put off making the phone call; it's often difficult to make an appointment at a convenient time, there is usually a co-payment involved, the appointment will take a long time, travel may be required, etc. If the complaint is minor, a home diagnosis will sometimes suffice.

Most homes have one or two diagnostic devices on hand, namely, a thermometer and a blood pressure measuring instrument (the technical name is "sphygmomanometer") with a cuff that is fitted around the arm, a battery-powered air pump that inflates the cuff, and a mechanical or electrical gauge to read out blood pressure. An elevated body temperature is often the hallmark of a disease or infection, while an elevated or depressed blood pressure is also a sign that professional care may be needed. In this way, these home diagnostic aids do not provide a diagnosis, but rather validate the decision to seek help.

The normal core body temperature for humans is close to 37 °C or 98.6 °F, and the aim when measuring temperature is to get as close to the core reading as possible. Thermometers can be placed sublingually (under the tongue), and that location provides a good measure of the core temperature; however, this is not a practical monitoring method, because the individual will find it uncomfortable to keep the thermometer in the mouth, and if nasal congestion accompanies a fever, there is a tendency toward mouth breathing, which lowers the temperature reading. It's also possible to measure temperature under the arm (axillary temperature), but it's important to be consistent and be able to find the same location when positioning the thermometer. Thermometers placed into the rectum also provide readings of core temperature, but are often uncomfortable for the individual and cannot be used without assistance. The tympanic membrane of the ear provides another site where the temperature may be measured, and a local drugstore will usually stock electronic thermometers with a package of protective covers for the tip that may be used in the ear.

The probe thermometer (Fig. 5.1) often seen at a hospital or a physician's office has a long tip that contains a device called a "thermistor," which is based upon a material whose electrical resistance changes with temperature [1]. The thermometer passes an electric current provided by a battery through the thermistor and measures its resistance to current flow. Once it has been calibrated, it can easily and quickly read body temperature. Probe thermometers are usually placed sublingually. The sensory portion of a tympanic thermometer (Fig. 5.1) does not come into direct contact with the inner ear; rather, the tip contains a device called a "thermopile," which is capable of measuring the infrared radiation given off by the tympanic membrane inside the ear. It is important to place the tip of the thermometer far enough into the ear canal to obtain a reliable reading.

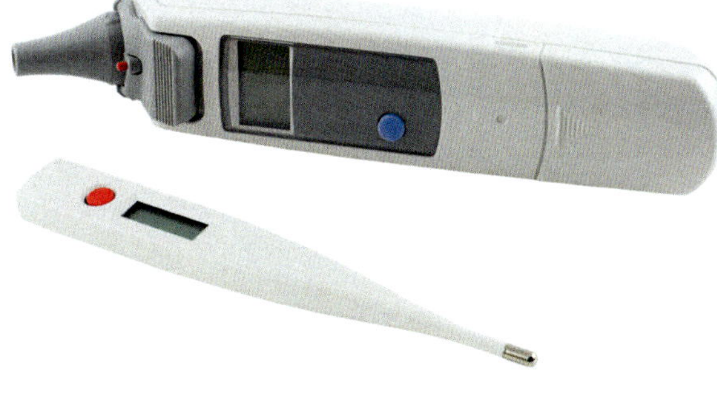

Fig. 5.1 A tympanic thermometer (*upper*) and a probe thermometer (*lower*)

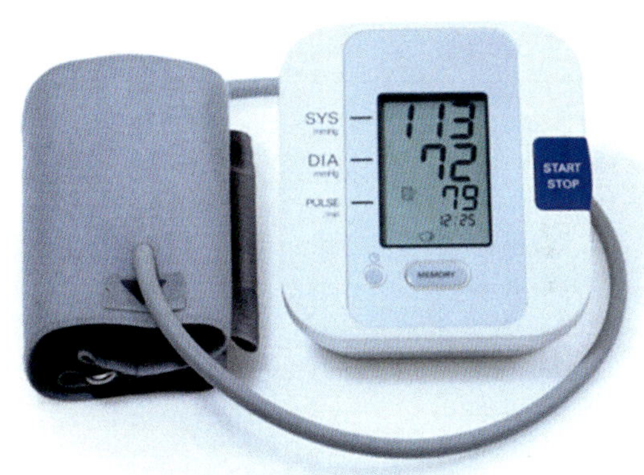

Fig. 5.2 A sphygmomanometer (blood pressure measuring device) suitable for home use

Blood pressure monitoring devices used at home or at a physician's office measure the "systolic" pressure (the highest pressure coinciding when the chambers of the heart called the ventricles have contracted to send blood through the body) and the "diastolic" pressure (the lowest, coinciding when the ventricles are filling with blood) in the brachial artery (found in the upper arm). When the device is turned on and air is pumped into the cuff, it increases pressure on the arm and forces the brachial artery to close. If the physician or assistant uses a stethoscope while a blood pressure measurement is taken, they are listening to the sound of the artery opening and closing. A device often used at home (Fig. 5.2) does not rely on sound, but the pneumatic tube within the cuff also senses the pressure fluctuations in the artery. The home user is usually better off with devices that automatically provide systolic and diastolic readings on an electronic dial rather than trying to interpret dial gauge-type instruments.

One other test conducted within the privacy of the home has proven to be popular: the home pregnancy test. The FDA claims that one-third of all American women have used such a test at some point in their lives [2]. The first version appeared in 1977 and was quite complex, with various components that had to be assembled at the time of use. The initial one-step test was introduced in 1988. Home pregnancy tests rely on the device to sample female urine for the presence of the hormone "human chorionic gonadotropin," or hCG, which is secreted by the placenta soon

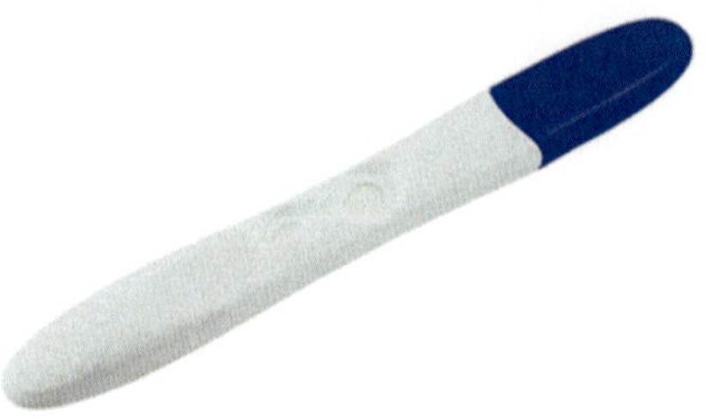

Fig. 5.3 A home pregnancy test device

after fertilization of an egg. The urine wets a compressed fiber strip that has been coated with an antibody molecule that binds to hCG; when the binding occurs, a further sequence of chemical steps occurs causing a color change. The earliest this test can be reliably used is 6 days after fertilization, because the placenta takes time to form. Note too that fertilization does not always occur at intercourse; it may occur later, so that waiting longer (2 weeks) increases test reliability even more. For some 10 % of women, the egg does not implant until after the first day of a missed period; it is also reasonable, therefore, to wait until the first missed period to use the test. Although the FDA participates in premarket review of these tests, it only assures consumers that today's tests perform as well as the tests that were available in 1976. Of course, they may perform better, but the consumer cannot know that. The tests are capable of providing false negatives and false positives; a more reliable test performed at a physician's office is indicated when certainty is desired (Fig. 5.3).

5.3 The Beginning of a Visit to the Doctor

What happens when a patient visits a physician for a checkup or with a complaint? We all remember from our own experiences that the sequence of events begins with an administrator or receptionist requesting that us to fill out forms providing personal information: address, date of birth, insurer, list of medications, and specific complaint if any. The patient will also be asked to sign and date a HIPAA document; this document will be signed and dated every single time the patient visits a doctor, even if he or she had been seen previously as a patient by the same doctor. These documents are to protect the patient's privacy; no one has the right to see those medical records without the patient's express and written permission, and because the patient's history will be updated during each visit, a new form will need to be signed, usually to allow the office to send information to the insurance company. The Health Information Portability and Accountability Act was adopted in 1996, and the www.HHS.gov/ocr/privacy/ website provides this explanation:

> The Office for Civil Rights enforces the HIPAA Privacy Rule, which protects the privacy of individually identifiable health information; the HIPAA Security Rule, which sets national standards for the security of electronic protected health information; and the confidentiality provisions of the Patient Safety Rule, which protect identifiable information being used to analyze patient safety events and improve patient safety.

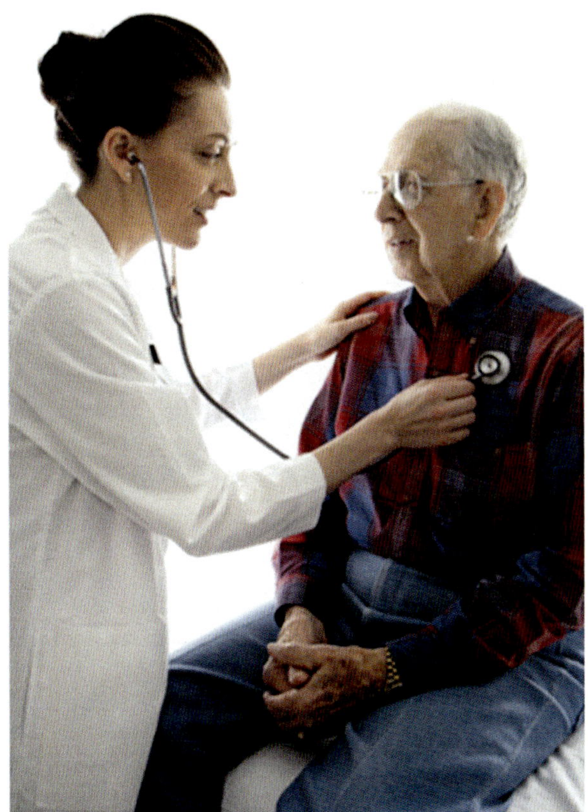

Fig. 5.4 A physician performing auscultation or listening to the patient's breathing and heartbeat using a stethoscope

After filling out paperwork, the patient is typically taken back to get weighed, has their blood pressure taken, and temperature and pulse and blood oxygen level are often measured. Eventually, the patient is seen by the physician who will begin by asking about any symptoms or concerns, and a physical exam is conducted.

The exam is a critical and fundamental component of diagnosis. The various actions of the doctor, even though they may seem very "low-tech," provide important information that lets the doctor zero in on what might be wrong and what follow-up tests (if any) should be ordered. During the physical exam, the doctor will perform an inspection, palpation, percussion, and auscultation (Fig. 5.4).

During the inspection, the physician examines different parts of the body, searching for clues that could suggest a health problem. For example, the condition of the eyes could reveal an overactive thyroid gland, while a growth on the eyelid could indicate a high cholesterol level. Large or prominent neck veins are symptomatic of heart failure to the physician. If the tongue or nail beds are bluish, low blood oxygen content could be responsible; a pale appearance could indicate low blood hemoglobin.

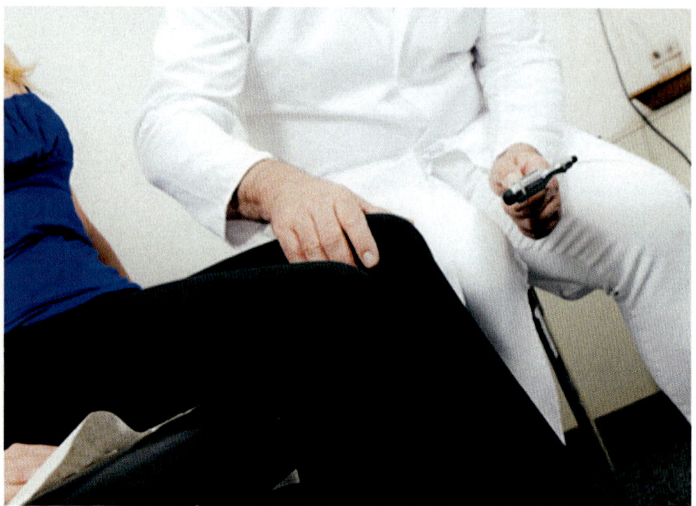

Fig. 5.5 Testing reflexes as part of a physical exam focusing on neurologic issues

Next, the doctor proceeds with palpation, a very hands-on examination involving the application of pressure to the legs and feet to check for excess fluid accumulation or swelling and to the belly, which could reveal liver enlargement or an active ulcer. The physician places one hand on the patient and taps it with the index finger of the other hand in a procedure called "percussion." The physician will be able to feel differences in the way tissues vibrate in response to the tapping, and these could hint at enlargement of the heart or liver. Tapping can also suggest fluid buildup in the chest or stomach.

Finally, auscultation (listening through a stethoscope as shown in Fig. 5.4) helps the physician to determine if heart disease should be suspected either due to the presence of a heart murmur caused by turbulent flow through the heart valves or turbulent flow through the arteries of the neck or legs caused by cholesterol plaques interfering with blood flow. Listening to the lungs can help diagnose pneumonia, asthma, or bronchitis.

A physical exam can be more extensive during a regular checkup or if a specific complaint is presented. For example, opening the mouth and saying "aaaah…" displays the mouth and tonsils and the condition of the gums and teeth, which provides a general indication of health. A neurologic exam will examine balance (e.g., standing on one foot, walking while placing one foot directly in front of the other), reflexes (hitting the joints with a rubber hammer (Fig. 5.5) to evaluate nerve conduction), and pricking fingers and toes with a pin to ascertain if there has been any sensory loss (e.g., diabetic patients commonly lose sensation in their feet). Finding loss of sensation in certain areas will permit the physician or neurologist to identify which nerve may be injured. A discovery of sensory loss will in many cases be followed up with vibration and temperature sensation testing using a tuning fork. These techniques may not appear to be highly sophisticated, but if performed by a skilled diagnostician will provide information which will determine if additional tests are needed.

There are, however, some cautionary comments now being expressed about routine physical exams [3]. As technology has become more and more prevalent in healthcare and as the financial pressure to see more patients throughout the day impacts the amount of time that physicians spend on the physical exam with each patient, there are concerns that the skills of young physicians related to this exam are becoming deficient [4]. Furthermore, some of the diagnoses made as a result of the physical exam may not have rigorous underpinnings. Because of these concerns, the American Medical Association has gathered reviews of relevant publications, entitled "The Rational Clinical Diagnosis," which can serve as a primer for physicians seeking more certainty in their diagnosis [5].

A second consequence of the increasing availability of technology and the pressures on physicians to reduce time spent on individual patients is the expanding reliance on laboratory tests and diagnostic imaging. In the case of patients with health insurance, there may also be a financial incentive for physicians and hospitals to order tests routinely. In fact, however, many of these tests may be unnecessary, and many are duplicated, particularly when a patient goes for a second opinion. The American Board of Internal Medicine Foundation recently joined forces with a number of national professional healthcare organizations representing other medical specialty areas and pharmaceutical trade groups to inaugurate a project called "Choosing Wisely," joining with Consumer Reports to publish lists of diagnostic tests and procedures that are routinely ordered but which provide little if any value. According to a recent Institute of Medicine report, these types of tests may be partially responsible for the approximately $750 billion (30 % of health spending in 2009) spent unnecessarily on needless administrative costs, fraud, and unnecessary services [6].

5.4 Beyond the Physical Exam: Blood Tests

Let's assume that the patient has been feeling ill, fatigued, has difficulty sleeping, and from time to time suffers dizziness. During the appointment, the patient will go through the administrative ritual described earlier, discuss symptoms with the physician, who will usually order blood tests. Many of us have undergone this procedure, during which a phlebotomist, a person trained in taking blood, inserts a needle into an arm vein (Fig. 5.6) and draws blood collected into tubes with colored caps. The color of the cap corresponds to a specific analysis or analyses the blood will be subjected to, and the inside or bottom of the tube will be coated with chemicals to preserve some essential characteristic of the blood or to prevent degradation of the blood component of interest to your physician. A partial vacuum inside the tube helps to draw the blood out of the vein and into the tube. The number of tubes filled depends on the number of analyses the physician has ordered.

The blood is sent to a laboratory for analysis, and a full report is prepared and sent to the physician within approximately 2 weeks, though a partial report can be ready in

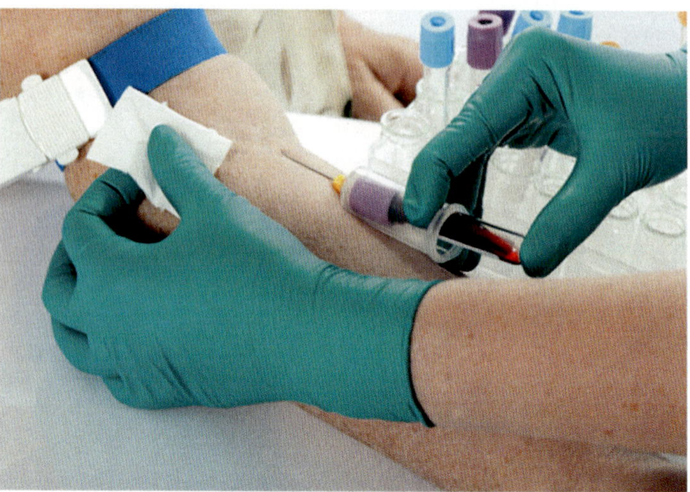

Fig. 5.6 A phlebotomist drawing blood for analysis

a matter of hours. Blood contains many different cells and chemicals (Fig. 5.7), and conceivably, they can all be analyzed for a clue to the patient's condition. During a follow-up visit, the physician will discuss test results with the patient, who should ask for a printout of those results to take home, unless they are available online; these results will be useful when seeking a second opinion. There are a number of common tests that are done, and the specific "numbers" will be quoted alongside the reference or "normal" range. Any abnormal results will be identified.

The most common blood test ordered is a "Chem 7" which surveys the amount of seven substances found in blood plasma, the liquid component of the blood, in contrast to blood cells, which are solid blood components. Blood urea nitrogen (BUN) measures kidney function, with a high level possibly indicating poor function. Carbon dioxide (CO_2) is a measure of how well the lungs and kidneys are managing the amount of bicarbonate in the body. High creatinine levels, produced during muscle breakdown, are associated with kidney problems. Excessive amounts of glucose, a sugar, could indicate the presence of diabetes. Serum chloride plays a role in maintaining the acidity of the blood, and an imbalance could indicate over hydration or dehydration, poor kidney function, or other endocrine gland issues. Serum potassium deviations from normal could be responsible for decreased heart and muscle function. Finally, serum sodium levels are measured to determine if the patient is properly hydrated or has endocrine (hormonal) disorders.

The second most common test is the CBC or complete blood count. The WBC or white blood count is the number of white blood cells; an elevated level may be an indication of infection, while low levels may be a sign of bone marrow disease or an enlarged spleen. Hemoglobin (Hgb) is the concentration of this oxygen carrying protein in red blood cells, and hematocrit (Hct) is the volume of the blood occupied by red blood cells. Low levels may be an indication of anemia, which can be caused by a number of diseases as well as dietary factors. The mean corpuscular volume or

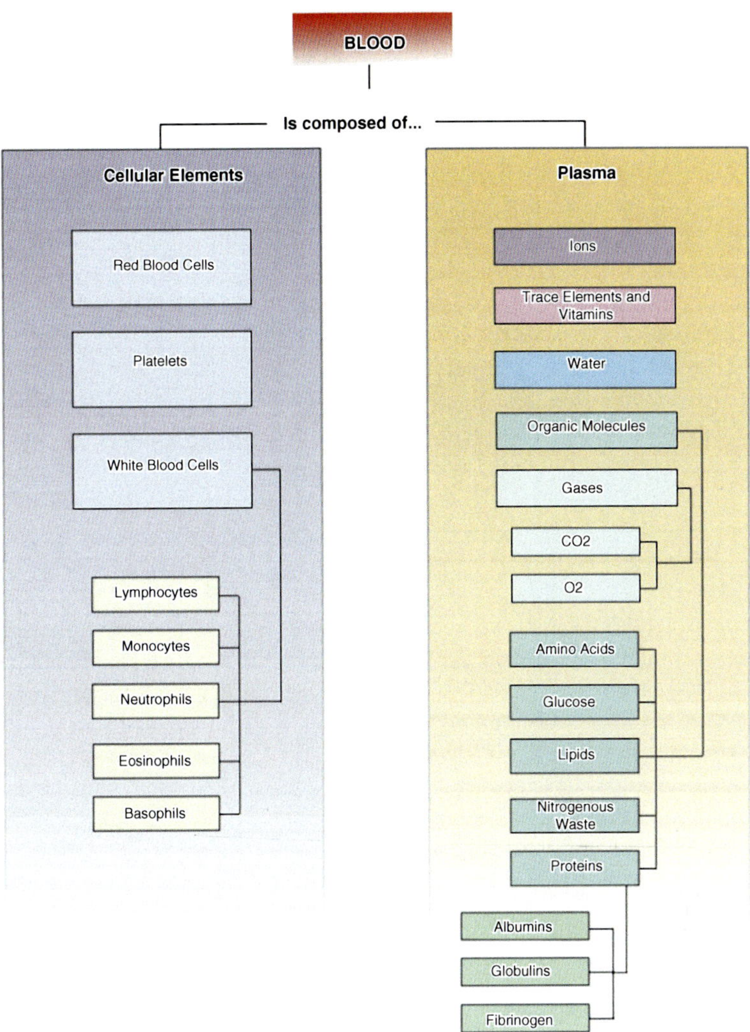

Fig. 5.7 Chemicals and cell types found in blood

MCV helps to determine if anemia is caused by an iron deficiency, whereas high values are associated with deficiencies of vitamin B12 or folate. Finally, the platelet count (PLT) provides an indication of how many of these clotting cells are in the blood. A high value can be associated with bleeding or cigarette smoking, while a low value can result from blood loss, infections, or bone marrow failure.

Other substances may be measured if the physician believes it to be necessary. There are several general groups:

(a) Enzymes such as alkaline phosphatase are important for enabling chemical activity in the cells throughout the body, and injuries to cells cause enzymes to be released. Alcoholism and other diseases can give rise to high enzyme levels.

(b) Albumin and globulin are proteins found in the blood, and their levels are a general indicator of health. Globulin is associated with the immune system, so changes in the amount of globulin could be associated with a variety of ailments, including bone marrow disease.
(c) Elevated blood fats (cholesterols and triglycerides) are associated with increased risk of heart disease. LDL cholesterol is the "bad" cholesterol associated with deposits on the insides of arteries, while HDL cholesterol is the "good" variant because it helps to remove LDL cholesterol deposits. C reactive protein is a cardiac disease risk factor, as are homocysteine and lipoprotein, so if the physician suspects the patient is a candidate for heart disease, these compounds will be measured.
(d) The level of various hormones, including those associated with the thyroid gland, insulin, estrogen (estradiol), and testosterone may be measured to aid in the diagnosis of thyroid disease, diabetes, pregnancy or menopausal issues, and reduced testicular function respectively.

5.5 Heart Function

If a patient mentions symptoms such as shortness of breath or chest pains during exercise or if there were instances observed during the physical examination when the heart was beating irregularly, the patient may be scheduled for an ECG (also EKG), short for electrocardiogram. This is a relatively simple and short diagnostic test. Essentially, the patient lies down on an examination table and is asked to unbutton their shirt and provide access to the lower portions of the leg. Then, the nurse or technician will attach up to 12 electrodes to different sites on the body. These electrodes are provided with a sticky coating so that they adhere to the skin; it may be necessary to clean the skin with rubbing alcohol or even shave the skin to ensure good skin–electrode contact.

The electrodes are distributed in such a way as to surround the heart at different angles. Six are attached to the skin on the chest and are placed at specific locations on the rib cage. The additional electrodes or leads are placed on the arms and legs. When the ECG monitoring machine is turned on, the leads communicate the electrical activity occurring in the heart, and the familiar shape of the heart pulse is recorded, with the curve consisting of five waves labeled P, Q, R, S, and T (the letters don't really stand for anything) as shown in Fig. 5.8.

Analyzing the size and shape of these waves provides information about the relative health of the heart (Fig. 5.9). For example, the wave pattern during supraventricular tachycardia (excessively rapid beating of the heart) looks like the one shown in Fig. 5.10.

ECG monitoring can be performed while the patient is resting, in which case the test takes no longer than a minute, or it can be performed as part of a stress test, where data are taken from time to time at specified intervals. If a patient complains of an irregular heartbeat that occurs only from time to time, a small heart monitor may be attached to the patient and then worn over a period of a day or longer.

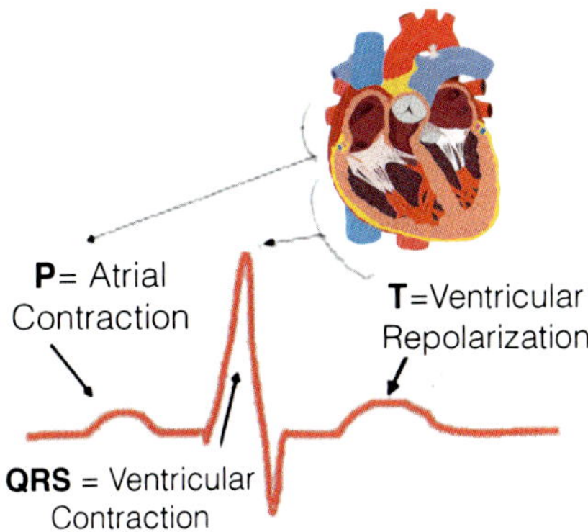

Fig. 5.8 An electrocardiogram (ECG) tracing in normal subjects has a "PQRST" waveform with each portion of the wave resulting from electrical activity of different parts of the heart

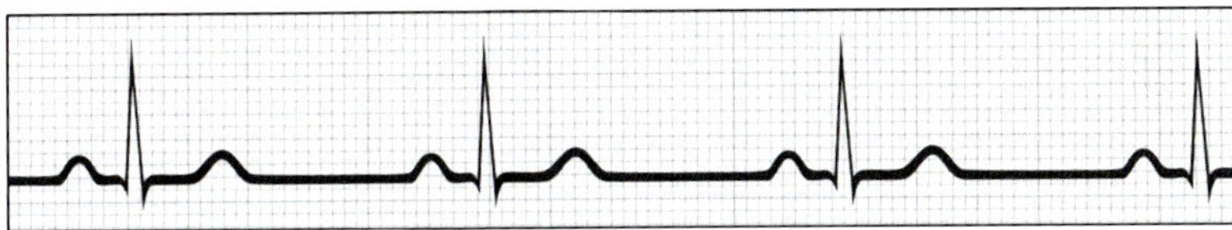

Fig. 5.9 An electrocardiogram (ECG) tracing showing the typical "PQRST" waveform in a normal (healthy heart) patient

If the ECG done in the physician's office is inconclusive (the test does last only a short time), a cardiac stress test may be ordered. Some heart problems become more apparent when the heart is stressed, for example, during exercise, and begins to beat rapidly. If the patient has arthritis and cannot run, the stress test is conducted using medication to make the heart beat quickly. If no arthritis or similar medical problems exist, the patient is asked to exercise on a stationary bike or a treadmill, and ECG monitoring is performed before, during, and after exercise. Stress testing evaluates the possibility of coronary heart disease often caused by reduced blood flow to the heart; the reduction in flow is usually a consequence of plaque or blood clots in the arteries that have narrowed the artery. If heart disease is in its initial stages, the disease may only manifest itself during the exercise encountered during a stress test.

Additional analyses carried out during stress tests may include monitoring blood pressure and requiring the patient to breathe into a tube so that oxygen consumption and carbon dioxide output may be monitored. In addition, an echocardiogram may be obtained; this test uses ultrasound to image the heart in real time while it is beating. In this test, the patient lies down, and a gel is rubbed on the chest, with the technician moving a transducer (a device that emits ultrasonic signals and also records the reflected sound waves) over the area of the heart (we will discuss how an echocardiogram is obtained a bit later in this chapter). The images collected during the echocardiogram can indicate areas of poor blood flow, dead heart muscle, and if the heart valves are operating properly. It's important for the physician to know the

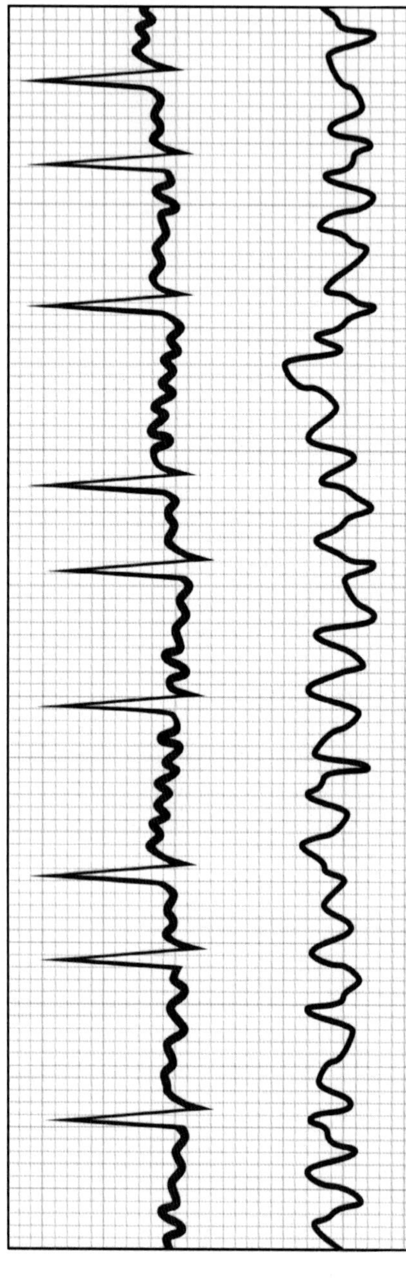

Fig. 5.10 Electrocardiogram (ECG) tracing of a subject experiencing atrial fibrillation (*top tracing*) and another subject experiencing ventricular fibrillation (*lower tracing*). Note the relative regularity of the waveforms and the absence of the typical "PQRST" waveform as shown in Fig. 5.9

ejection fraction (how much blood the left ventricle pumps out with each contraction). If that fraction is low, near 30–40 %, meaning that only 30–40 % of the blood is pumped out of the left ventricle during each beat, the physician may suspect heart failure. Symptoms of heart failure include shortness of breath, fatigue, and swelling in the feet and ankles.

5.6 Gender-Specific Diagnostic Tests

Certain diagnostic tests are gender specific. Middle-aged men or men describing problems with urination will usually have their prostate gland examined by a physician who will insert a gloved and lubricated finger into the rectum. The physician will move the finger around, probing to identify the lobes and groove of a normal prostate gland, which is 2–4 cm long and triangular in shape. Deviations from normal shape and feel will alert the physician to order additional tests. One such blood test that may be ordered measures the amount of protein called the prostate-specific antigen (PSA); elevated levels indicate potential prostate disease. These examinations and tests are performed to determine if the patient is at risk of developing prostate cancer, and a pattern of continuously elevating PSA is sometimes grounds for a biopsy. However, in May 2012, the US Preventive Services Task Force published a recommendation against PSA testing on the grounds that the benefits may be small and potential harm (e.g., through exploratory surgery and biopsies) may be substantial.

Common screening and diagnostic tests for women include a clinical breast exam (a physical exam of the breast and underarms to feel for lumps), the mammogram (an X-ray of the breast to screen for breast cancer), and a pap test (a swab of cells from the cervix or opening of the uterus) to screen for cervical cancer. The frequency with which these tests are performed depends on family history, the patient's age, and other relevant general health characteristics.

5.7 So Many Tests...

When we become ill, we want to have the certainty of a correct diagnosis so that the best treatment possible can be prescribed. Unfortunately, the complexity of our bodies sometimes precludes a rapid diagnosis. In times when the diagnosis is elusive, it is natural to want more and more testing, even though tests can yield contradictory results and provide even more anxiety. What is the wise and responsible course of action for us to follow as healthcare consumers [7]? To begin, we as patients should be better informed about our health and our healthcare choices. For example, if a patient is generally healthy and not exhibiting particular symptoms, then more testing often provides little benefit while contributing to the overall burden on the healthcare system. Most of us are concerned about tests that miss the presence of some dangerous disease, that provide the so-called false negative. However, the opposite is also true: false-positive results (indicating the presence of a disease where there is none) will lead to stress and unnecessary and potentially dangerous follow-up tests, including surgical intervention.

It is important to remember that there are no perfect diagnostic tests. Each test has associated with it a particular sensitivity (which can be thought of as related to the percentage of people with a particular disease who are correctly identified as having that disease) and a particular specificity (which can be thought of as related to the number of people who are healthy and are identified as such). Unfortunately, tests usually do not have both a high sensitivity and a high specificity. Those that are highly sensitive tend to give higher rates of false positives; tests that are highly specific usually sacrifice some sensitivity and tend to give higher false negative results. Knowing this, physicians will prescribe a highly sensitive test for a screening examination (to identify everyone having the disease even if some who are healthy are also misdiagnosed) and follow that up with a test that is highly specific (to confirm a diagnosis and eliminate the false positives). So, a highly sensitive test that yields a negative result will correctly identify a healthy patient, while a highly specific test that yields a positive result will correctly identify a patient who is ill.

Knowing the sensitivity and specificity of a diagnostic test permits us to define a positive predictive value and a negative predictive value for that test. Let's assume that we are testing a group of 100 people, and of that group, 20 test positive for the presence of the flu. We also know from other tests and evaluations that of that group of 20 positives, only 15 actually have the flu. We can calculate the positive predictive value of the test we used by dividing the number of people with the flu who tested positive (15) by the total number of people who tested positive (20), or 15/20 or 75 %. We can therefore say that a person who tested positive has a 75 % chance of actually having the flu.

In this same group of people, we know that of the 80 that tested negative, 5 actually have the flu. The negative predictive value is calculated as the number of healthy people who tested negative (75) divided by the number of people who tested negative (80), or 75/80 or 93.75 %. We can say that a person with a negative test result has a 93.75 % chance of not having the flu or has only a 6.25 % chance of actually having the flu.

In practice, the diagnostic value of a test is improved if it is limited to those patients who are likely to have the disease. Test results are more meaningful if they are applied after careful consideration of the patient's history and indications from the clinical examination [8].

Being better informed also means knowing what are the recommended tests and test frequencies for persons with our characteristics of age, family history, gender, ethnicity, and lifestyle. For example, while the United States Preventive Services Task Force recommends a cholesterol screening every 5 years, that recommendation is not relevant for a middle-aged obese patient who should be tested more frequently. Similarly, tests for the prostate-specific antigen test for men, breast cancer screening for women, and colonoscopy for diagnosing colon cancer are probably useful for a subset of the population and not for all who undergo a checkup.

The websites http://consumerhealthchoices.org and http://choosingwisely.org provide an entry to various topics related to medical tests, hospitals, and other public health issues.

5.8 Medical Imaging

Diagnostic imaging is a central component of modern medicine, and advances in imaging technologies have vastly improved the accuracy of medical diagnoses and treatment options. Humans are highly visual creatures, i.e., we heavily rely on our sense of vision to gather information from our environment, and the acquisition and analysis of images play a major role in our day-to-day activities. Many animals, on the other hand, sometimes utilize other senses to gather information from their surroundings. For example, bats and dolphins depend on sound waves to navigate their environment, fish have pressure sensors that provide information about their surroundings, snakes can detect infrared radiation from prey, dogs use scents to identify other creatures, and some birds can detect magnetic fields to guide them in their annual migrations [9, 10].

An image is defined as a physical likeness or representation of a thing. Even though humans have a well-developed vision system, we can only see down to a certain size or detect only parts of the electromagnetic spectrum (Fig. 5.11). For example, we cannot see objects that are smaller than 1 μm (e.g., microbes) or see through our skin with naked eyes.

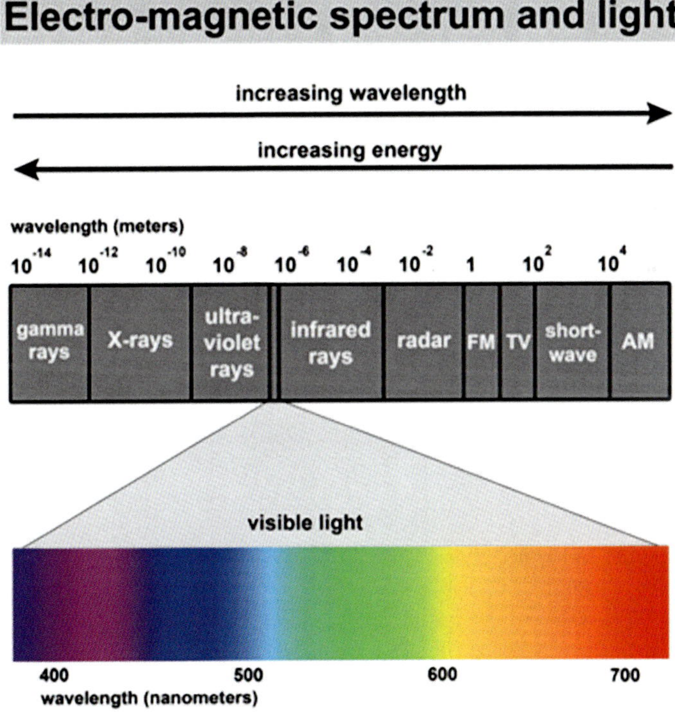

Fig. 5.11 Wavelengths of different types of radiation in the electromagnetic spectrum

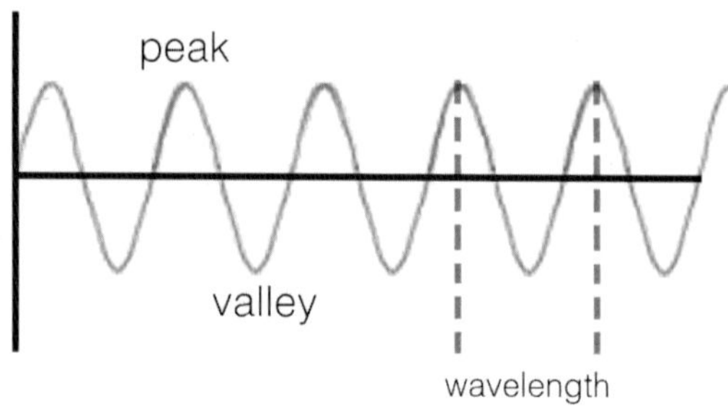

Fig. 5.12 A graphic representation of a wave

With advances in imaging technology, it's now possible to detect the entire band of the electromagnetic spectrum. Different systems use certain ranges of that spectrum (e.g., visible light, X-rays, gamma rays) to create images. Physicians use their knowledge of medicine and advanced imaging technologies to diagnose a disease or injury. Radiology is the field of medicine that relies heavily on imaging techniques. There are two major radiological subspecialties: diagnostic radiology and interventional radiology. Diagnostic radiology deals with the detection and diagnosis of a disease or injury using various imaging technologies, while interventional radiology combines these imaging technologies with other surgical techniques to treat diseases and correct tissue abnormalities.

We will first review the basic principles of imaging and discuss several imaging modalities. A central theme will be that the same fundamental physical processes that allow us to see our picture in a mirror can also be used to generate an X-ray image of our bones.

5.8.1 Imaging Basics

A basic understanding of waves and their properties is required to grasp all modern imaging techniques. Waves are defined as signals that have repeating patterns. From sunlight to water ripples on a pond, we are surrounded by waves. Light and sound are also transmitted by waves. Visible light belongs to a family of waves called "electromagnetic" waves, while sound is transmitted by pressure waves. Electromagnetic waves are different from sound waves in that they can travel through a vacuum whereas sound waves cannot. Any wave (Fig. 5.12) can be described by the following characteristics:

1. *Frequency*: Number of times an event (e.g., peak/valley) occurs in a specific period of time. Frequency is usually expressed in cycles per second or hertz (Hz).
2. *Wavelength*: The distance between two adjacent peaks. Wavelength is usually expressed in meters or nanometers.

For a given wave, frequency (f) and wavelength (λ) are related by wave velocity (v):

$$f = v / \lambda.$$

Table 5.1 Examples of the system of prefixes

Prefix	Scientific notation	Example
Kilo (K)	$1,000 = 10^3$	Kilogram (kg)
Mega (M)	$1,000,000 = 10^6$	Megawatt (Mw)
Giga (G)	$1,000,000,000 = 10^9$	Gigabyte (gb)
Milli (m)	$1/1,000 = 10^{-3}$	Millimeter (mm)
Micro (μ)	$1/1,000,000 = 10^{-6}$	Microliter (μl)
Nano (n)	$1/1,000,000,000 = 10^{-9}$	Nanometer (nm)

Wave velocity (ν) usually has a unit of meter/second and changes with the properties of material conducting the wave. Because many scientific disciplines in general and imaging systems, in particular, often deal with both very large and very small numbers, scientific notations are generally used to denote various quantities. Examples of some prefixes that are used to denote large or small numbers are presented in Table 5.1.

As the name suggests, electromagnetic waves are created when electrical and magnetic fields combine and/or interact with each other to produce waves. Human eyes, cameras, radios, televisions, cell phones, and microwave ovens all use electromagnetic waves to operate. For example, our eyes detect visible electromagnetic (light) waves, radios detect radio waves, and microwave ovens use microwaves to operate.

All forms of electromagnetic radiation have the dual property that they travel as waves and carry energy in a stream of particles called photons. All electromagnetic radiation travels at the same speed, i.e., 3×10^8 m/s (the speed of light). Photons are assumed to have no mass or electric charge, but photons of different electromagnetic waves carry different energy levels. Electromagnetic waves with lower wavelengths have higher-energy photons; photons of radio waves or visible light, for example, carry less energy compared to photons of X-rays or gamma rays. This is why visible light cannot penetrate tissues, whereas X-rays or gamma rays can.

Sound is produced when molecules or objects vibrate at various frequencies and travel in all directions by molecule-to-molecule interactions. Sound is a mechanical wave and unlike electromagnetic waves needs molecules of matter to travel. For this reason, sound cannot travel through a vacuum. Human ears can detect sound frequencies between approximately 12 and 20,000 Hz (20 kHz). However, an individual's frequency detection capabilities depend upon many factors, including age. Certain high-frequency sound waves (e.g., ultrasound) are used in medical imaging.

Attenuation (absorption) of various forms of radiation by dense matter (e.g., the human body) can be described by an expression similar to the Beer–Lambert law:

$$I = I_0 \exp^{(-\mu x)}$$

where I is the transmitted radiation intensity, I_0 is the incident (initial) radiation intensity, μ is the mass absorption attenuation coefficient (cm^{-1}) which depends on the properties of the material, and x is the thickness of the material (cm).

Reflection of visible light from various objects in our immediate environment enables us to see and is the most familiar imaging modality for most people. During a doctor's examination, the physician's eye uses visual light to create images of the patient which are later processed in the physician's brain. Visual images captured by cameras or microscopes are used in many disciplines of medicine. Examples include skin photographs (dermatology), arthroscopic images (orthopedics), endoscopic images (gastroenterology, minimally invasive surgery), and microscopic images (pathology). As you will hopefully see in the discussions below, the same physical principles that allow you to see a picture on the wall of your house also allow us to image a broken bone in an intact body.

5.8.2 X-Ray Imaging

Before 1895, physicians had no way of looking into a patient's internal organs without making an incision. This changed overnight when a German physicist named Wilhelm Conrad Röntgen found "a new kind of rays" on November 8, 1895. These "mysterious rays" were later called Röntgen rays, or X-rays. X-rays have the seemingly extraordinary ability to pass through many substances that are quite opaque to light. Röntgen immediately realized that these rays have immense applications in the field of medicine and communicated his discovery to the Physico-Medical Society of Würzburg, Germany. Within a few months after the discovery, physicians all over the world were using X-rays in their practices. Röntgen was awarded the first Nobel Prize in physics in 1901 for his discovery of X-rays.

There is of course nothing magical about X-rays except that compared with visible light, X-rays have highly energetic photons and a shorter wavelength. X-ray's photons are produced when high-energy electrons (negatively charged particles) are emitted from a high-temperature cathode and strike a target (anode) made of tungsten or another metal. The amount of energy acquired by these electrons depends upon the voltage applied between the cathode and anode [11]. A simple X-ray generation setup is shown in Fig. 5.13.

X-ray photons are highly energetic and are, therefore, more penetrating than visible light. Like light rays, X-rays also have different attenuation coefficients for different materials (Table 5.2). Attenuation of X-rays in solids takes place by absorption and scattering of the X-ray beam and can be described by the Beer–Lambert law.

X-ray attenuation is proportional to the density of a material and so is significantly higher in bones as compared with another tissue; therefore, bones appear lighter on X-ray images as compared to muscle. X-rays are particularly well suited for imaging broken bones. Most metals have even higher attenuation coefficients for X-rays than bone, and for this reason, lead is used to protect humans from the harmful effects of X-ray ionizing radiation.

The most common radiological imaging procedure is the production of still images of various tissues and organs (film X-Ray). In this procedure, X-rays are passed through a patient's body, and the transmitted X-rays are captured using a photographic film; like photography, however, X-ray films are increasingly giving

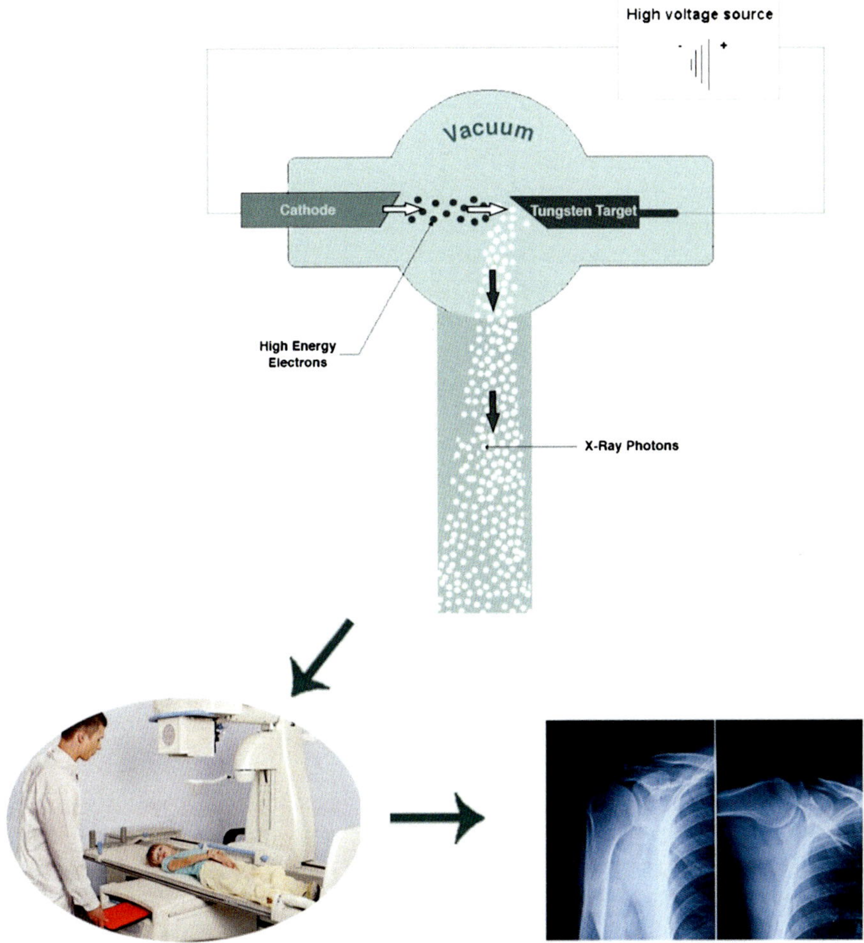

Fig. 5.13 Schematic of a simple X-ray generation device (*top*), a picture of an X-ray machine (*bottom left*), and typical images produced by an X-ray machine (*bottom right*)

Table 5.2 Attenuation coefficients of different materials for X-rays

Material	Attenuation coefficient
Air	−1,000
Fat	−100 to −40
Water	0
Spinal fluid	0–20
Brain white matter	20–35
Brain gray matter	30–40
Blood clot	55–75
Calcification	>150
Bone	1,000
Metallic foreign body	>1,000

way to digital imaging systems. Some frequent uses of film X-rays include chest X-rays to diagnose tuberculosis progression and to detect bone fractures.

Low-dose X-ray imaging is often used to detect breast diseases in both male and female patients. Even though mammography is used for the early detection and diagnosis of breast cancer lesions, it can also be used for other purposes, such as imaging breast implants. In the case of X-ray mammography to detect cancer, radiologists look for abnormal masses and microcalcifications, or calcium deposits, in a radiographic image. Abnormal masses and calcium deposits are easy to detect using X-rays, because they are much denser and have higher attenuation coefficients for X-rays than the surrounding normal soft tissues. Even though calcifications are extremely common in breasts, it is the subtle changes in morphology and distribution of breast calcifications that characterize an underlying disease [12].

Bone mineral density (BMD) measurement remains the best method for accessing the risk of bone fractures [13]. It is well accepted that the amount of mineral is the main determinant of mechanical properties in bone. Bone mineral density or bone mass can be measured noninvasively by using X-ray absorptiometry, which is based on the principle that bone attenuates or absorbs ionizing radiation. In this technique, two X-ray beams with different energy levels are used to image a patient's bone. BMD measured by using DEXA, defined as the ratio of bone mineral content divided by the two-dimensional projected bone area, is then used to diagnose the existence and progression of degenerating diseases such as osteoporosis.

5.8.3 Nuclear Imaging

Radioactive isotopes, such as carbon-11 and nitrogen-13, naturally emit radiation that can penetrate tissue. These isotopes, also referred to as radionuclides, may accumulate to a greater extent and/or faster in some types of tissue (e.g., tumors). Once taken up by the tumor, the isotope undergoes decay, releasing a positron (a particle with a positive charge) which then meets an electron (a particle with a negative charge). This encounter creates mutual destruction, which is detected by specialized detectors known as scintillators, which record the release of energy, and processed by computers, which ultimately re-create an image of the tissue. This image can then be used to diagnose various pathologies. Growing medical applications of radionuclide imaging range from detection of tumors to assessing cardiac function.

Radionuclide scanning is done by injecting a tiny amount of radioactive isotope into a vein. Because different radionuclides tend to collect in different types of tissue, the radionuclide used for each patient varies with the particular diagnosis being sought. For example, scanning for bone cancer other than multiple myeloma utilizes technetium phosphate. Scans detect physiologic changes in bone in contrast to the morphologic changes seen by traditional X-rays. The increased uptake of radionuclide by the bone in some area is typically due to the increased activity of bone cells called osteoblasts associated with the formation of new bone caused by infection, tumor, fracture, or synovitis (inflammation of the synovial membrane which covers joints such as hips and knees).

Scanning for infections and some malignant tumors may be carried out using gallium citrate radionuclide, but this agent also congregates in fracture areas and in locations of inflammatory arthritis. Still other radionuclides include indium-111 and technetium-99, which are used to label white blood cells that eventually assemble in areas of infection or inflammation.

A more sophisticated variant of radionuclide imaging is single-photon emission computed tomography. In this technique, a gamma-ray camera is rotated around the patient's body and records one-dimensional projections of radioactivity. A computer processes many such images and develops a two-dimensional image of the cross-sectional distribution of the radionuclide in the body.

Perhaps the latest (and most expensive) form of imaging technology is positron emission tomography, or the PET scan. For the test, the patient is injected with a short-lived nuclide such as fluorine 18, which is incorporated into a radioactive version of the blood sugar glucose. After the patient rests for about an hour, the radioactive tracer distributes itself within the body; it travels to wherever glucose is needed to provide energy, and because tumors use glucose in a different way than normal tissue does, the tumor will contain a different amount of the radioactive glucose than the normal tissue near the tumor. As the radionuclide decays, it gives off a positron (hence the name of the technique). The positron travels an extremely short distance in the body before it encounters an electron, and the two particles annihilate each other. This annihilation is accompanied by the emission of two gamma rays, which travel along a line in exactly opposite directions. A detector outside the patient's body senses these rays and is able to determine the location where the annihilation occurred. Many such detection events occur during the time the test requires, and once a computer analyzes the data, an image can be constructed locating the tumor in the body.

PET scans are often administered at the same time as a CT or MRI, and this hybrid technique provides both anatomic and metabolic information. It is possible to know what the structure is and what it is doing biochemically at the same time. This is a great advantage over just knowing what the organ or tissue of interest looks like. Common uses of PET include determining how far a cancer has spread, how well the cancer is responding to treatment, planning brain surgery if the patient's epilepsy does not respond to treatment, helping to diagnose dementia and Parkinson's disease, and because it is effective in tracking blood flow around the heart, can help the surgeon decide if the patient could benefit from heart surgery.

An attractive aspect of PET is that it utilizes a short-lived radionuclide, so the patient absorbs only a small amount of radiation. Unfortunately, the radionuclide has to be made on site, i.e., at the hospital or clinic, and the facility has to invest in a cyclotron to prepare the radionuclide. Not all hospitals are able to afford these costs.

5.8.4 Imaging with CAT Scanners

Computed axial tomography systems, or CAT scanners, use computers to combine multiple two-dimensional X-ray images to produce a three-dimensional image of an object. CAT was invented in 1972 by Godfrey Hounsfield of EMI Laboratories in

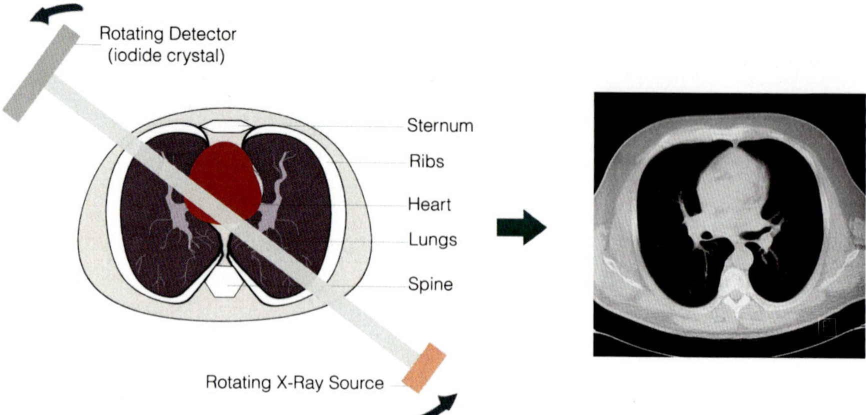

Fig. 5.14 Simple schematic of a CT imaging device

England and Allan Cormack of Tufts University in the USA. Both were later awarded the Nobel Prize in Physiology or Medicine in 1979 for their invention. The first clinical scanners appeared in 1974 and were almost exclusively used for scanning the head, with later scanners in 1980s incorporating the whole body. Currently, the CAT scan is the imaging modality of choice to assess bone, heart, and the lungs. Its ease of use, high-quality and high-resolution images, and relatively low morbidity (pain and discomfort) to the patient make it an outstanding diagnostic tool for the physician. The word tomography comes from two Greek words "tomos" which means "cut" or "section" and "graphein" which means "to write" or "to draw."

Computed tomography (CT) scanning uses a computer to mathematically reconstruct thin slices of cross-sectional imaging of the human body from multiple two-dimensional X-ray images. In a CT gantry, a collimator is used to focus narrow beams of X-rays from the X-ray tube which are then used to generate multiple images from various directions (Fig. 5.14).

A narrow beam of X-ray originates on one side of the patient and passes through the body. Some X-rays are absorbed, while others scatter and are ultimately detected by a sensitive detector on the other side of the patient. This process is then repeated in order to obtain multiple two-dimensional images as the X-ray generator rotates circumferentially around the patient in a 360° fashion. As the beam passes through different types of tissue, different attenuation values (depending on material density) known as Hounsfield units (HU) are assigned. For example, the HU for water is 0, while a beam through air is given an HU of −1,000 and that of cortical bone is more than +400 HU. The multiple two-dimensional X-ray images are then processed by a computer using a mathematical algorithm to produce three-dimensional voxels (volume elements, analogous to pixels on a TV monitor).

The current generation of CT scanners can acquire an image in approximately 4–5 s. This rapid time permits the acquisition of less-blurry images, as the patient can be asked to stop breathing during the scan. New systems coming online will acquire images in milliseconds.

Table 5.3 Comparison of low radiation exposures during various imaging procedures

X-ray procedure	BRET (days)	Effective dose equivalent (mrem)
Dental	2	1–2
Chest	6	1–5
Skull	20	10–20
Pelvis	65	70–140
Lumbar spine	130	130–270
Head CT	300	200–400
Barium enema	390	510–880

5.8.5 Health Concerns with X-Rays

An important property of X-ray is its ability to ionize atoms, which can cause significant damage to cells and DNA. The biological hazards of X-rays were soon realized after their discovery, when Thomas Edison's chief assistant, Clarence M. Dally, died of cancer in 1904. Dally's hand cancer was due to X-ray overexposure.

Data accumulated over the years have shown that ionizing radiation (X-rays, gamma rays, UV light) can cause skin burns, radiation sickness, genetic mutations, sterility, and cancer. Radiation dosage in mammals is measured in terms of "rem" or "Röntgen equivalent for mammals/man." If a mammal or human being is exposed to 25–100 rem of ionizing radiation, harmful changes in blood composition and the immune system may occur. Survival is unlikely if a radiation exposure occurs in the range of 1,000 rem [14]. This type of high radiation exposure can occur during nuclear fallout.

In a clinical setting, patients, and especially healthcare workers, normally receive low levels of radiation (in units of millirems) during various radiological procedures. However, the long-term risks of such low levels of radiation exposure are not well understood. Humans who are exposed to radiation from imaging devices are continuously monitored for cumulative radiation exposure using radiation dosimeters (badges). All living systems, including humans, are exposed to a background level of radiation from cosmic and other natural sources on a daily basis. In the USA, a person is exposed to an average background radiation level of 1 millirem, or 1 Background Radiation Equivalent Time (BRET), per day. For comparison purposes, exposure to other sources of radiation, Effective Dose Equivalent (EDE), is usually expressed in terms of multiples of Background Radiation Equivalent Time (BRET) (Table 5.3). For example, a typical dental X-ray exposes the patient to the equivalent of two extra BRETs of radiation.

Because CT imaging relies on generating three-dimensional images from a large number of two-dimensional X-ray images, it generally delivers relatively large doses of radiation (Table 5.3) to the patient. The more detailed the scan, the higher the dose of radiation and therefore, unnecessary whole-body scans should be avoided. Radiation received from CT scans accounts for close to 50 % of all radiation patients receive from diagnostic studies.

Table 5.4 Speed of sound waves through different media

Medium	Speed (m/s)
Air	343
Fat tissue	1,450
Water	1,520
Muscle	1,580
Bone	3,800
Aluminum	5,000

5.8.6 Ultrasound Imaging

Ultrasound imaging, also called ultrasound scanning or sonography, uses high-frequency sound waves to create images. Sound waves with a frequency of more than 20,000 Hz (cycles/s) or 20 kHz are usually defined as ultrasound. In medical imaging, however, sound frequencies in the order of 1–15 MHz are usually used. Humans cannot hear ultrasound, though animals such as echolocating bats, porpoises, dolphins, and whales are adept at "seeing" in the dark using ultrasound. Dogs are also able to detect high-frequency sounds which are inaudible to humans, which make them especially suitable for hunting as they can hear the sounds created by prey.

During the 1790s, Lazzaro Spallanzani (1729–1799) an Italian priest and physiologist, in his search to explain the ability of bats to navigate and fly in darkness, conjectured that non-audible sounds may exist in nature [15]. He found that covering the bat's ear with hot wax impaired its ability to navigate in darkness. The presence of non-audible sounds remained a scientific mystery until 1938, when Donald R. Griffin and Robert Galambos used sonic detectors to record ultrasound noises produced by bats [16]. Karl Dussik, a neurologist at the University of Vienna, was the first to report the use of ultrasound for medical diagnostic purposes in a paper that was published in 1942 [17].

In a way similar to audible sound waves, ultrasound is a pressure wave that cannot travel through a vacuum and can only be transmitted through a medium, and its velocity depends upon the medium through which it travels (Table 5.4). In the table below, you will note that ultrasound travels through water and animal tissue at nearly the same velocity. This is due to the fact that tissues have a high water content. You will also notice from the table that ultrasound travels more quickly through denser materials (e.g., metal) and more slowly through materials that are easily compressible (e.g., air).

An echo is defined as the repetition of a sound caused by its reflection from neighboring matter. Hard surfaces like mountains or walls can reflect sound waves better than softer surfaces such as rubber or fabrics. Similarly, ultrasound waves are reflected differently by different tissues throughout the body, and they are partially reflected from the interface where two different materials meet. An echo can be used to measure distances and is used extensively in naval warfare (sonar) as well as medical imaging. Knowing the speed of sound in a certain medium, one can measure the distance from any object that reflected the sound waves, and knowing the location of the interface allows the device to create an anatomic image of the tissue or organ. For example, if you were to hear an echo 10 s after shouting "hello" near a mountain range, you could estimate the distance to the mountain range in the following manner:

$$\text{Distance travelled} = \text{Speed of sound}(\text{in air}) \times \text{time} = 343\ \text{m/s} \times 10\ \text{s} = 3{,}430\ \text{m}.$$

For calculating the distance of the mountain range from the listener, one should divide the total distance traveled by half. In other words, it took 5 s for the sound to travel from you to the mountain and another 5 s for the reflected sound wave to travel back. In this case, the distance from the mountain range is 1,715 m.

Similar to X-rays, ultrasound is attenuated differently by different materials. In the body, ultrasound attenuation and reflection depend upon the type of tissue and its pathological state.

Production of high-frequency sound waves was made possible by the discovery of piezoelectric materials. In 1880–1881, Pierre and Jacques Curie first demonstrated that some materials (e.g., quartz, bone, and ceramics) generate an electric potential in response to an applied mechanical stress. These materials also deform when an electric potential is applied to them. Depending on the applied electric field, these materials can produce ultrasound (due to rapid repeated contraction and expansion) at different frequencies. The critical component of an ultrasound imaging system is the transducer, a device made from one or several piezoelectric crystals, which is coupled with the body using a gel. In order to produce the image, the transducer is moved across the body while in continuous contact with the gel.

A simple setup used to produce an ultrasound image is shown in Fig. 5.15. A piezoelectric transducer emits ultrasound waves. As the waves travel through tissue, they are reflected (echo) differently by different tissue interfaces. The reflected sound pattern is picked up by a receiver which converts them back to electrical signals. These electrical signals are then processed by a computer to produce the image of the tissue structure. Liquids/fluids are very good conductors of sound/ultrasound and cause low ultrasonic attenuation. That makes ultrasound a good imaging modality for fluid-filled structures such as a fetus in the amniotic sac and the heart which contains blood. Ultrasound is significantly attenuated through air or bone and, therefore, is not effective for imaging parts of the body that either contain gas (e.g., thoracic cavity or lungs) or that are obscured by bone (e.g., an adult brain). The spatial resolution of ultrasound, or the smallest detail that can be seen, is approximately 1 mm.

Ultrasound may also be used to evaluate other soft tissues such as cysts and tendons to diagnose plantar fasciitis and tendinitis and is employed to provide guidance when injections are to be given to highly localized bodies such as calcific deposits.

A property of the sound wave, the Doppler effect, can be used to measure dynamic characteristics of living tissue. The Doppler effect, or Doppler shift, was first described by the Austrian physicist Christian Doppler in 1842 and describes the change in frequency of a wave moving relative to an observer. The change in the frequency, or pitch, in the siren of an emergency vehicle when it first approaches and then passes is an illustration of the Doppler effect. The frequency detected by the observer is higher than the emitted frequency during the approach, identical with the emitted frequency at the instant of passing, and lower while receding from the observer. The velocity of the passing object increases with the magnitude of the difference between emitted frequency and that detected by the observer. Therefore,

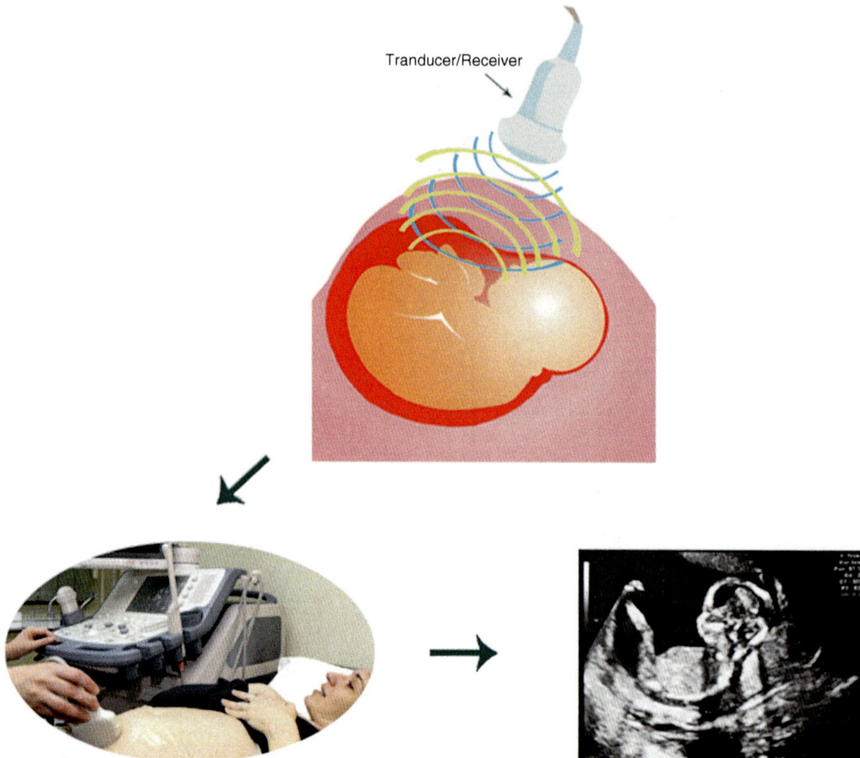

Fig. 5.15 An ultrasound transducer produces high-frequency sound waves (illustrated in *blue* in the *top panel*) which are reflected differently by different tissue (illustrated in *yellow* in the *top panel*). These reflections are then collected by the ultrasound receiver and mapped out as an ultrasound image (*bottom right panel*)

the Doppler effect can be used to measure the velocity and direction of moving objects by targeting a sound wave at the moving object and measuring the frequency of the reflected sound wave.

The Doppler effect has applications ranging from creating special effects in the entertainment industry to predicting weather patterns in meteorology. Doppler ultrasound systems can also be used to measure the velocity and direction of movement for many tissue and body fluids in the body. For example, Doppler echocardiography is widely used to measure movements of cardiac muscle, heart valves, and blood in the heart to diagnose and detect various pathologies during a stress test. Similarly, Doppler ultrasound can be used to measure blood flow in a fetal heart to determine if the fetus is growing at a normal rate.

Ultrasound imaging systems are relatively safe to use because they do not produce any ionizing radiation. Ultrasound imaging devices are portable, require no radiation shielding, and are cheaper compared to other medical imaging devices (e.g., CT or MRI).

5.8.7 Magnetic Resonance Imaging

The concept of magnetic resonance was discovered by two American scientists, Felix Bloch and Edward Purcell, who received the Nobel Prize for their discovery in 1952. Magnetic resonance has been used extensively to analyze the structure of molecules since the 1940s. However, clinical applications of magnetic resonance became possible in the early 1970s when the first magnetic resonance imaging (MRI) system was developed by Paul C. Lauterbur and Sir Peter Mansfield, who later also received the Nobel Prize in 2003 for this important contribution.

Many materials in nature can be magnetized in the presence of a magnetic field. Some materials, such as iron, can be easily magnetized in a weak magnetic field, but other materials, such as hydrogen, can only be magnetized in the presence of very large magnetic fields. Magnetic resonance imaging (MRI) relies on the inherent magnetic properties of hydrogen atoms in water molecules within the body. To understand how MRI works, one needs to remember that the human body is largely composed of water. Each water molecule is made of two hydrogen atoms and one oxygen atom. MRI utilizes a powerful magnetic field to bring together the protons of the hydrogen atoms in the body in line with the field. Modern MRI systems use superconductors to create a magnetic field with strength up to 10 T (Tesla). For comparison purposes, the earth's magnetic field has a strength of 30–60 μT.

Individual hydrogen nuclei (protons) have magnetic properties as the result of their spin. Normally, hydrogen atoms are randomly oriented so the sum of all the spins gives a null net magnetization. However, within a large external magnetic field, the nuclear spins align with the external field. Most of the spins align with the field (parallel), but some align against the field (antiparallel). It is slightly easier to be aligned with the magnetic field (parallel) because the aligned position is at a lower energy state. About ten out of every one million hydrogen atoms are aligned opposite (antiparallel) to the magnetic field. Thus, in the presence of a large external magnetic field, there is a slight net magnetization in the tissue in line with the magnetic field. It is these unmatched atoms that are essential in producing the MR image (Fig. 5.16).

When a person is placed in an MRI system, they become slightly magnetized! To obtain an MR image, a large external magnetic field is used to align the hydrogen atoms of the tissue of interest. A very short pulse of energy, in the form of radio frequency (RF) waves, is then directed into the body using a radio transmitter which knocks some of these hydrogen atoms out of alignment (Fig. 5.17). When the radio transmitter is turned off, the hydrogen atoms shift back into their aligned position through a process of "relaxation." This relaxation process releases energy in the form of another radio wave, which can be detected using a sensitive radio receiver using a phenomenon known as resonance. Two systems may exchange energy when they both oscillate at what is referred to as the "resonance frequency." Magnetic resonance corresponds to the energetic interaction between spins of the hydrogen atom and electromagnetic radio frequency (RF).

The signal received by the radio receiver is then analyzed by a computer to determine the amount and configuration of water in different parts of the tissue being imaged. Because the body is composed of more than 60 % water and the water in

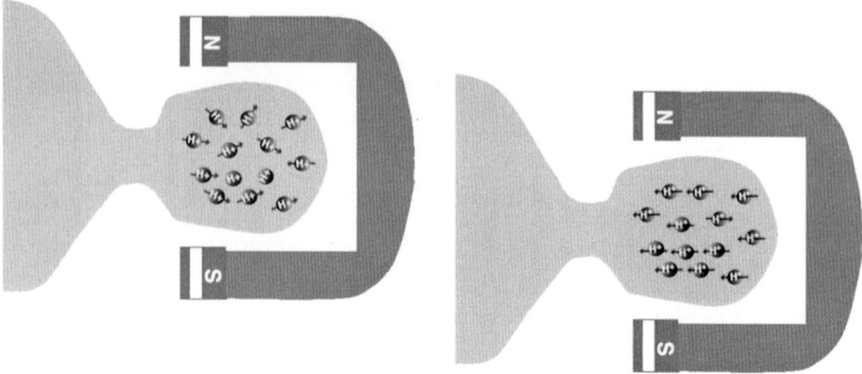

Fig. 5.16 Hydrogen protons in living tissue such as brain are aligned randomly (*left panel*) in the absence of an external magnetic field. However, these protons are mostly aligned with the magnetic field (*right panel*) in the presence of a strong external magnetic field

different parts of the body is bound differently to various tissues, MRI provides information about almost all tissue types and can be used to differentiate between tissues of very similar density. Similar to CAT scans, a computer uses several different two-dimensional MR images taken from different directions to generate a three-dimensional image of the tissue. These images can then be used to detect disease states such as cancerous tumors in which the protons are realigned differently than in normal tissue. The MRI signal obtained from a tissue is sensitive to a number of parameters, including hydrogen density, relaxation times (the so-called T1 and T2 signals), and blood flow within the tissue. By analyzing these signals and comparing them to existing calibrations, a map of different tissues can be generated, which can then be used for diagnostic purposes.

At this time there are no major studies indicating that MRI may be unsafe to patients or fetuses. However, MRI is contraindicated in patients with implants that have metallic and/or electronic components because the strong magnetic field may cause the movement of metallic implants and/or disrupt electronic systems. These include patients with implanted pacemakers, insulin pumps, aneurysm clips, and skin staples. It should be noted that one reason why titanium metal is often used for implants is that it is safe to use in magnetic fields. Similarly, MRI is not recommended for those patients with bullets, shrapnel, or metallic implants in their bodies. MRI may even be counter indicated in patients with tattoos as magnetic ink particles are often used in tattoos.

5.8.8 MRI Versus CT Scan

A CT scan may be preferable over an MRI because of its lower cost, easier access, faster imaging, thinner slices of imaging, better imaging of bone, and no contraindication to metal implants. MRI may be preferable over CT scans for greater

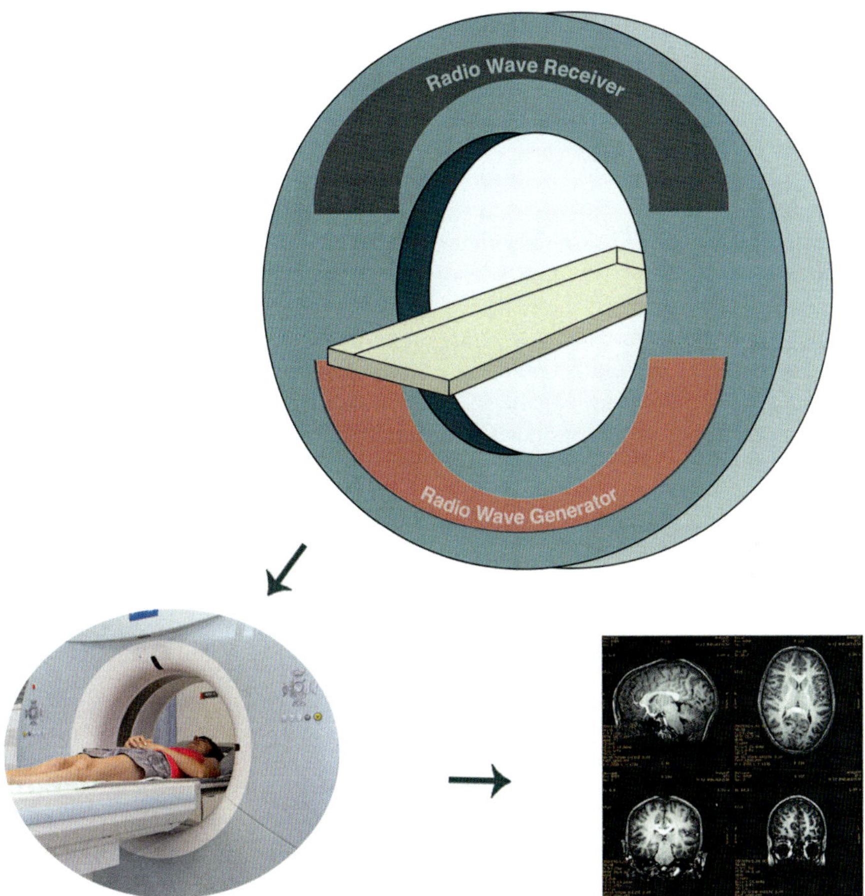

Fig. 5.17 A simplified illustration (*top*) and a picture of (*bottom left*) an MRI machine with an MR image of the human brain (*bottom right*)

resolution of soft tissues and higher sensitivity in detecting many disease processes. MRI is often more expensive and requires subjects to remain still for relatively long periods of time in a tightly confined space, but has better resolution (<1 mm). Because of this high resolution, MRI is commonly used to diagnose many conditions, including changes in bone marrow, diagnosis of bone tumors, sports injuries, and damage to tendons, ligaments, and cartilage. As noted earlier in this chapter, X-ray attenuation of most soft tissues is similar, and hence X-ray imaging is often unlikely to provide much useful information about soft tissue. However, MRI plays a vital role in diagnosing various pathologies associated with soft tissue, including herniated discs in the spine and injury to the brain. Furthermore, use of contrast agents can help resolve differences between scarring and recurrent injury.

5.8.9 Contrast Agents

If a compound with a high X-ray attenuation coefficient is injected intravascularly (into a blood vessel) in a patient before taking the image, the level of contrast between vasculature and surrounding tissue is increased significantly. Contrast agents enable the radiologist to distinguish between tissues which look similar in X-ray images and may also help differentiate between normal and diseased tissue.

Typically, contrast agents in the form of nanoparticles are injected into the body, and if they are passively targeted, they will interact with a tissue or organ because of the physiology or abnormality of the tissue. For example, because tumors have poorly formed vascular systems, nanoparticles may selectively penetrate and accumulate in tumors. The liver contrast agent Feridex is taken up by healthy liver and spleen tissues, but not by cancerous tissues, and thereby provides a discriminatory image for these organs.

Actively targeted contrast agents have been treated with a surface agent that is designed to preferentially bind to a specific protein in a tissue of interest, and therefore, these particles will aggregate at the site where those tissues are located.

Compounds with high X-ray attenuation coefficients can be used to detect blockage of small vessels in applications such as angiography. Iodine-based intravenous (IV) contrast agents can be used to enhance contrast between vessels and their surrounding tissue, especially in the brain. For example, in healthy subjects, the so-called blood–brain barrier keeps harmful substances from entering the brain parenchyma (the nervous tissue in the brain). However, in disease states such as brain tumors, strokes, and infections, CT imaging can be used to detect when IV-injected iodine crosses the blood–brain barrier and enters the brain parenchyma. In MRI, water can be used to visualize the stomach or bowel. However, most often the element gadolinium is used to enhance vascular tissues, the brain, tumors, and infected sites. Many contrast agents have undesirable side effects. For example, gadolinium can be toxic to kidneys, especially in patients with preexisting kidney failure. Several examples of contrast agents used in various imaging modalities are listed in Table 5.5.

Technological issues related to nanoparticle contrast agents include size; nanoparticles that are too small (<5 nm) are rapidly cleared from circulation by the kidneys. Particles that are too large are also rapidly cleared from circulation, although they typically yield high signal strength in the image. The issue of circulation time requires optimization: it must be long enough to permit the particles to accumulate in the region of interest and allow image capture, yet not too long, as the particles do need to be eventually cleared from the body. The surface characteristics of nanoparticles also play a role in determining circulation time.

Continuing new advancements in MRI are anticipated. For example, a kind of MRI called functional MRI (FMRI) is already available. It turns out that the hemoglobin present in red blood cells and which enables oxygen transport to tissues is diamagnetic when oxygenated, but paramagnetic after giving up its oxygen burden. This small difference in magnetic properties means that the blood provides a slightly different MRI signal depending on its oxygenation state. Because blood oxygenation depends on neural activity, this imaging method provides a window into brain function. Although FMRI does not provide a direct measure of mental activity, it

Table 5.5 Examples of contrast agents

Agent	Route of administration	Modality	Tissue
Fluorescein sodium [14]	Eye drops	Optical	Ocular diseases
Barium	Oral	CAT/X-ray	Gastrointestinal tract
Iodine	Intravenous	CAT/X-ray	Thyroid
Air liposomes	Intravenous	Ultrasound	Heart
Gadolinium	Intravenous	MRI	Rectal conditions

nevertheless does provide a more objective measure than behavioral observations by psychologists, and simultaneous measurements by EEG can provide complementary information. Potential future applications of FMRI include use as a lie detector!

5.9 Getting Small: Micro- and Nanotechnology

Many of the sophisticated imaging devices we have just reviewed depend on sophisticated electronic circuitry and dedicated computers in order to function. MRI machines use powerful electromagnets that must be cooled by liquid helium and liquid nitrogen. Many of the chemical analyses done routinely and rapidly in medical laboratories to provide a diagnosis based on blood chemistry also depend on electronic components and automated chemical equipment with prepared and self-dispensed reagents. The characteristic all these technologies have in common is miniaturization and, where possible, automation. In this section, we will discuss some of the ways in which devices can be made smaller, as well as the effects that size has on the behavior of matter. Believe it or not, portable phones once looked like this (Fig. 5.18).

One reason that they don't look like that anymore is that there has been a revolution in the manufacturing of miniature electronic circuits (called "integrated circuits") used in many devices, and practically all modern technology utilizes some form of an electronic circuit. Gordon Moore, the co-founder of the Intel Corporation, predicted in 1965 that the number of components such as transistors in integrated circuits of the same size will double every year. His prediction has proven to be accurate to this day; in 1971, a typical integrated circuit contained 2,300 transistors, but in 2011, they contained over one billion. As the number of components grows, much more capability can be packed into the same amount of space.

5.9.1 How Microelectronic Devices Are Made

The special techniques used to manufacture ever-smaller circuits often rely on a type of printing method called lithography. In this technique, the surface (the substrate, often made of elemental silicon) on which features are to be printed is first coated by a layer of photoresist (a polymer that can be dissolved by special solvents after it has been exposed to light). Then, a beam of light (for coarse features) or electrons (for fine

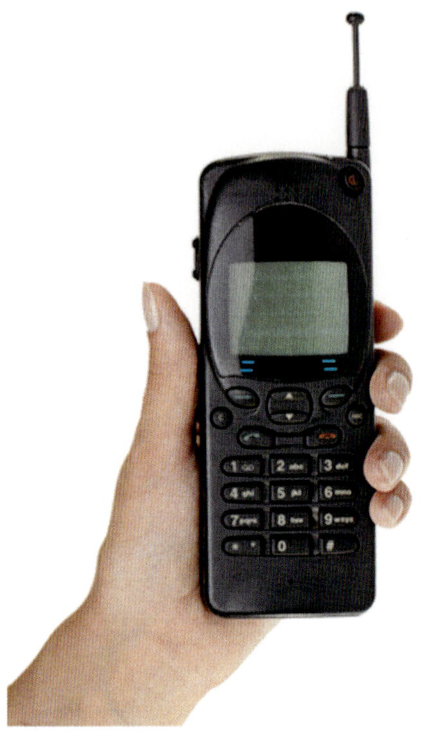

Fig. 5.18 An old portable phone

and small features) is passed through a mask so that only portions of the photoresist are exposed to the radiation. The entire substrate is dipped in a solution that dissolves away the exposed photoresist, leaving sections of the original surface uncovered in a pattern onto which thin layers of the materials needed to make transistors can be deposited. The deposition can be carried out in different ways, depending on what is being deposited: a metal or a gas that turns the silicon substrate surface into silicon dioxide. Sequencing different masks, each with a different pattern, and repetition of the exposure and dissolving processes yield complex designs. Today, rather than manufacturing individual electronic components such as transistors and connecting them together to form an electronic circuit, lithography and vapor deposition processes are used to deposit thin coatings of the materials needed for many transistors directly onto a circuit board and at the same time connect them together (Fig. 5.19).

This technique enables a manufacturer to manufacture circuits looking like the one in Fig. 5.20, which contains hundreds of components too small to be seen with the naked eye.

The lithography process can be used to make a variety of complex shapes on a variety of substrates, including ceramics, and hard and soft polymers. Lithography technology has now been linked with advances in surface science and surface chemistry and a better understanding of microfluidics (the science of how fluids behave in very narrow channels and tubes), allowing the development of devices such as biosensors and the "lab-on-a-chip."

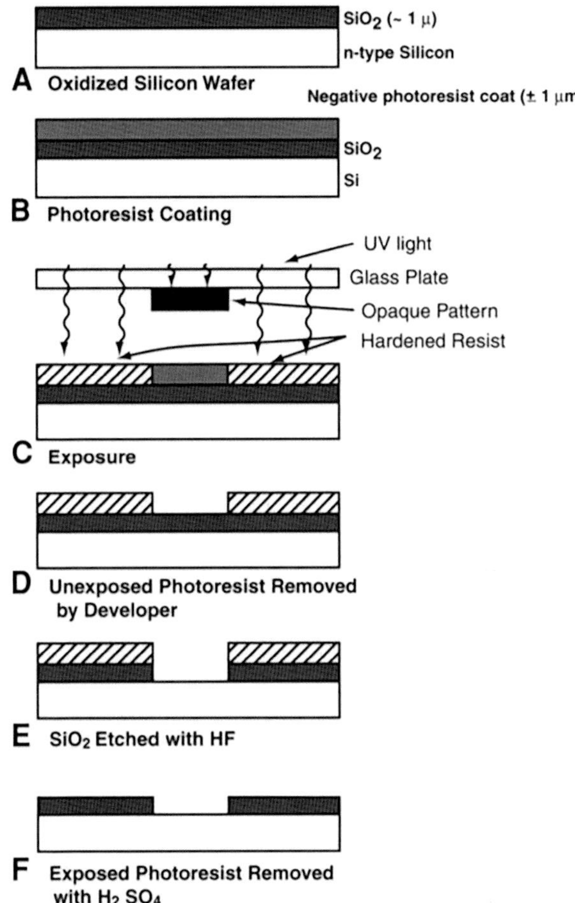

Fig. 5.19 Schematic illustration of photolithography. Copyright Humana Press

5.9.2 Biosensors

Biosensors are devices that may be used to analyze components in fluids such as blood or saliva, the presence of toxic gases in the atmosphere, or the presence of specific compounds in drinking water. The substance of interest that is being analyzed is called the "analyte."

For a biosensor to function, a receptor is needed, which is the component that will "receive" or bind with the analyte. If it is to be a useful receptor, it must be quite specific and only permits the molecule of interest to bond. For example, if we were interested in knowing the concentration of lead in drinking water, a receptor that only binds to lead is essential. In the case illustrated in Fig. 5.21, the receptor only senses the round molecules, not the hexagonal ones. In practice, these receptors are quite complicated (and molecules do not come in a color or in a neat geometric shape).

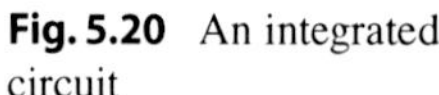

Fig. 5.20 An integrated circuit

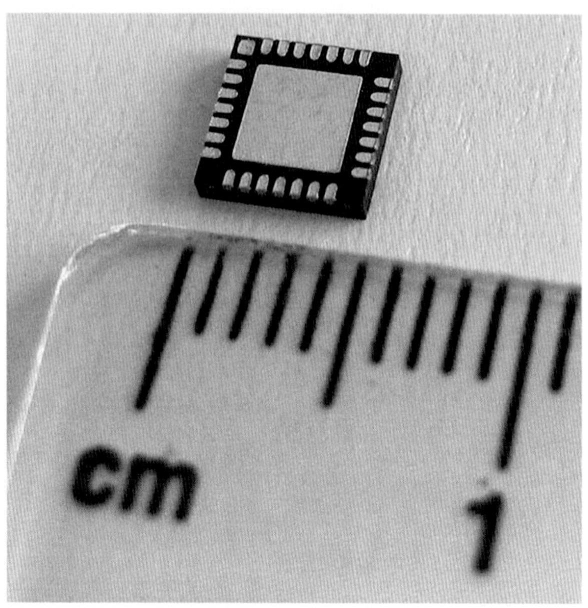

After a receptor is identified, a "transducer" must be designed and made. The transducer is the component that recognizes the binding event and sends out some sort of signal. For example, in a glucometer (Fig. 5.22; a device used by diabetics to measure their blood sugar level), the patient is required to prick their finger to bring up a drop of blood. The blood is then conducted into a test strip, which contains a micro-sized electrode and is coated with an enzyme called glucose oxidase. When the sugar in the blood encounters the enzyme, a reaction occurs, which also causes a small electrical current to flow; the current is the signal.

Finally, a readout component is necessary. This is typically an electronic circuit that would recognize the signal from the transducer and indicate something about its intensity or magnitude in a way that an observer could understand. For example, in the case of the glucometer, a small meter converts the intensity of the electric current into the blood glucose concentration, and that number is displayed for the patient to see.

Just as with the glucometer, many biosensor transducers rely on a change in electrical property when the binding event occurs to provide a signal; however, changes in mass (weight) or temperature can also provide signals. Transducer technology is mature and available in many applications. Design of a new receptor often presents a challenge because of the need for "specificity," or certainty that only the compound or molecule of interest is being detected. Receptors often rely on sophisticated chemical conditioning of the receptor surface, and receptors for large numbers of proteins and chemicals found in the human body have been identified.

Dramatic developments in biosensors are forecasted as miniaturization methods make them smaller and smaller, and therefore, more portable. As one example, sensors can be made small enough to be incorporated into a cell phone and could then be used to sniff out toxic gases and place a call to a safety responder! Having such

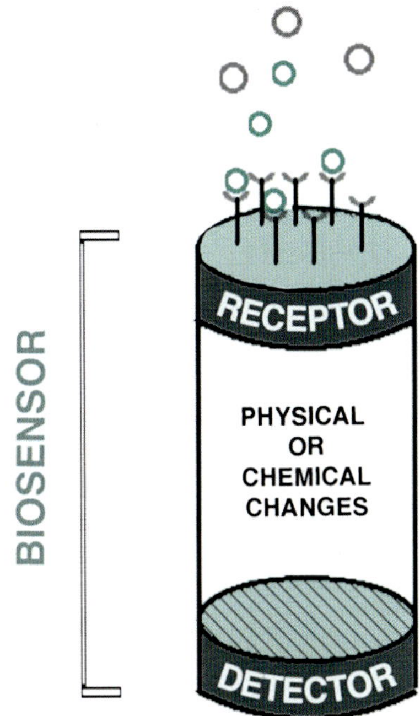

Fig. 5.21 Schematic of a biosensor

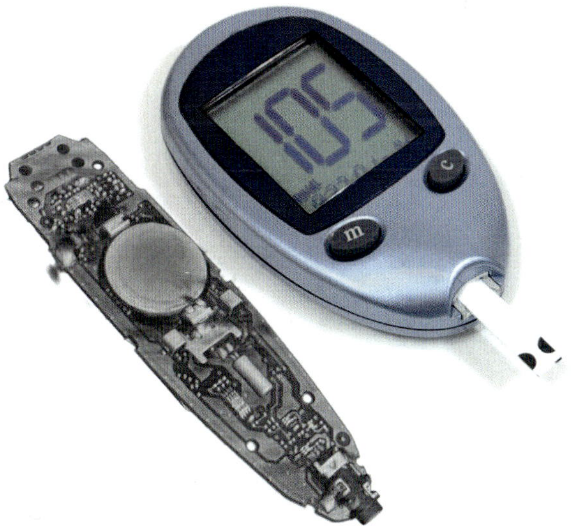

Fig. 5.22 A glucometer for measuring blood glucose level

sensors present in cell phones could serve as a "crowdsourcing" method for detecting dangerous compounds in the environment or even measuring air pollution.

A lab-on-a-chip (LOC) is a miniaturized chemical analysis laboratory. These devices may only be a few centimeters in size, but they pack a lot of power and capability into a very small space. They can be used to detect and quantify pollutants in water or air and even to perform DNA sequencing. The development of LOC took off in the mid-1990s when the US government became interested in using these devices for early warning of biological and chemical warfare attack. Today, however, the LOC are seen as potentially vital components in the effort to improve global health. They function as "point-of-care" devices, meaning that they may be used at remote locations and in circumstances where elaborate and complex full-size biochemical laboratory facilities are impractical or impossible.

LOC devices depend on an additional micromachined support structure, often made from a polymer, which contains many small tubes and channels such as those seen in Fig. 5.23.

These devices may be stand-alone devices or components of much larger systems such as medical imaging machines; they may operate within or outside a living organism and either contain their own power systems or be connected to an external power source.

The LOC is activated when the analyte-containing fluid flows through an opening in the micromachined support platform. The fluid winds its way through all the channels, and along the way it interacts with biosensor receptor components placed at strategic locations. Movement of the fluid through the narrow tubes is made possible by capillary forces (the same forces that are responsible for water flowing up a narrow vertical glass tube), and the study of fluid in narrow channels is called "microfluidics." Some devices are much more complex than what is shown in Fig. 5.23 and contain many fluid channels, with electrodes placed at several locations to monitor chemical reactions.

The small size of these devices immediately confers significant advantages. The devices are portable, meaning that the patient is not required to travel to a clinic or hospital. The devices are not costly, meaning that large numbers can be dispatched to areas where there are emergencies. Perhaps best of all, certainly from a patient's point of view, only a very small amount of fluid is needed—a pinprick of blood. The devices are often intended for single use only and then discarded.

5.9.3 Nanotechnology; Getting Smaller Still

The concept of nanoscience and its applications in nanotechnology got its push from Richard Feynman, a Nobel Prize winner in physics, who gave a lecture in 1959 at the California Institute of Technology titled "There's Plenty of Room at the Bottom" (you can read this lecture here [19]). In the lecture, he foresaw developments in computer chips, tiny machines, and other strange physical phenomena that are size dependent. In order to appreciate the wide range of applications of nanotechnology, please visit the website of the Nanotech Project group,

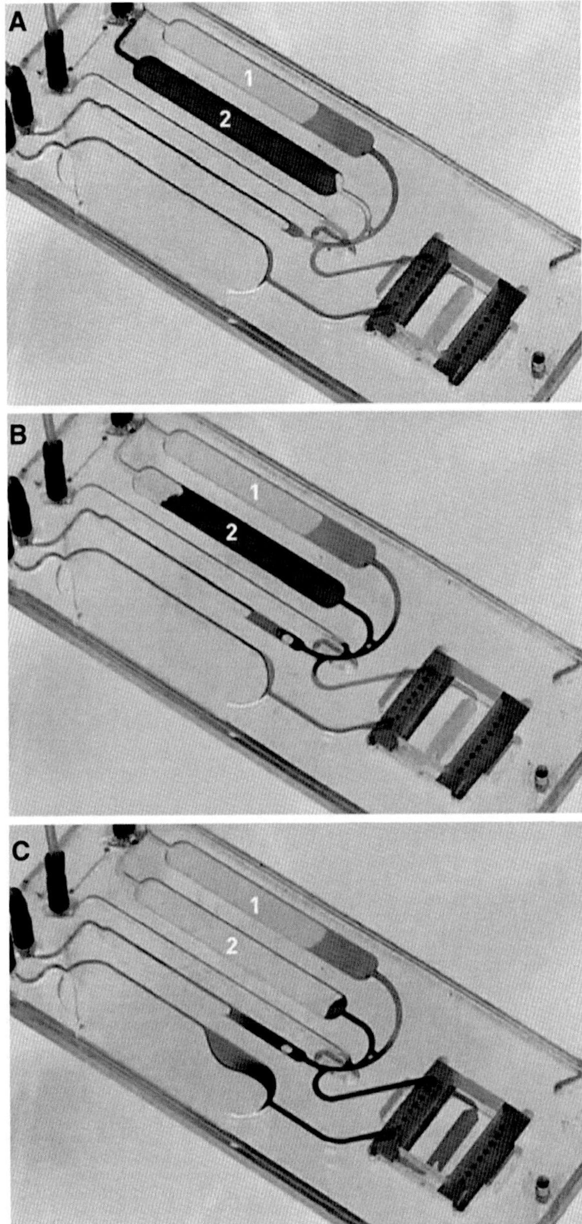

Fig. 5.23 Photograph of a lab-on-a-chip machined in clear polymer. The small channels permit fluid which are housed in reservoirs to flow in a sequence designed to permit fluid analysis. In the sequence shown here, liquids are delivered from reservoirs 1 and 2 to sensing chambers, or they may first be mixed prior to entering the sensing chamber. Eventually, they will occupy a waste chamber. Copyrighted by Springer-Verlag USA

which lists a number of actual, present-day applications at www.nanotechproject.org; they include coatings for television displays, ultrawide-angle camera lenses, and cosmetics containing nanoparticle moisturizers that deliver their contents into small wrinkles and pores.

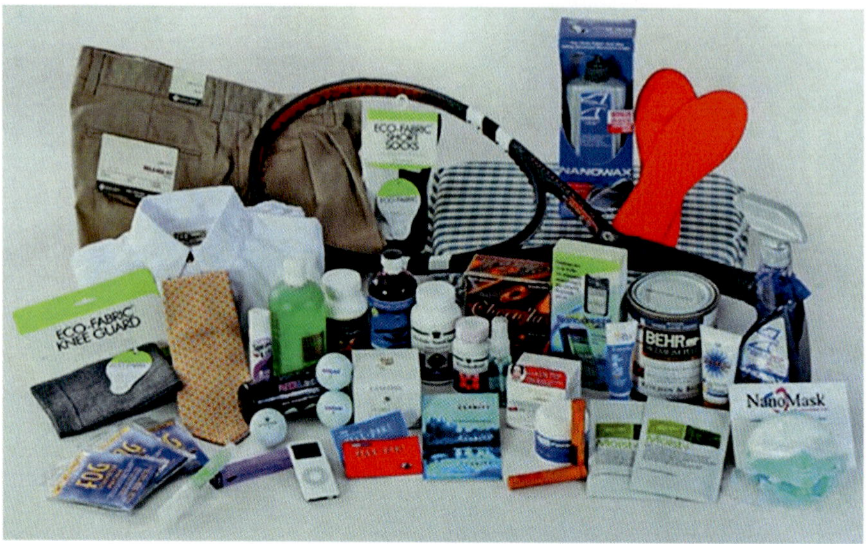

Fig. 5.24 Examples of products affected and enhanced by the presence of nanomaterials. Nanoparticles are added to paint, to structural materials such as tennis racket frames, and to fabrics to provide them with stain resistance. Copyrighted by Springer-Verlag Berlin Heidelberg

Nanotechnology is any technology that uses components that are very small, with dimensions measured in nanometers, and whose effectiveness depends significantly on the small size of the component. A common misconception about nanotechnology is that all things miniaturized are nanotechnological. Not true; a nanotechnological device has to depend on some critical component being 1–100 nm in size and behaving differently because it is small. Many products are affected by nanotechnology and nanomaterials (Fig. 5.24).

Nanotechnology has also captured the public's imagination, with the result that many futuristic technologies are predicted, including some that will impact healthcare (Fig. 5.25).

Recall how small a nanometer is—10^{-9} m, a billionth of a meter. If an average human hair is approximately 50 μm thick, it is 50,000 nm thick. Anything that small is impressive if it actually manages to perform a desirable function.

A comparison of various structures and their sizes might make the concept of nanotechnology easier to understand. A typical nanoparticle could be 26 nm in diameter (26×10^{-9} m), a marble is 26 mm (26×10^{-3} m) in diameter, and the earth is 2,600 km ($2{,}600 \times 10^{3}$ m) in diameter. The average fingernail grows approximately 1 nm/s, flu virus particles are about 75–100 nm wide, and scientists have created carbon nanotubes, which are 1,000 times thinner than a human hair but 200 times stronger than steel.

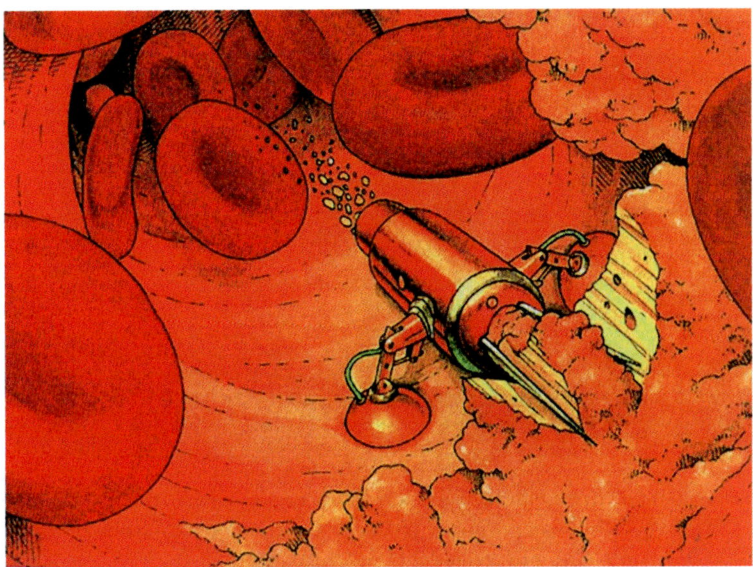

Fig. 5.25 An artist's rendering of a nanorobot cleaning up an artery by removing cholesterol plaque. Copyrighted by Springer-Verlag Berlin Heidelberg

5.9.4 Matter at the Nanoscale

Scientists have found that matter at the smallest scale has properties that are often far different than the properties of that same matter in bulk. These different properties enable novel applications. For example, the element gold on a macroscale is yellow and shiny, but on the nanoscale, when gold nanoparticles are dispersed in water, they display a reddish color. Another example is the compound titanium dioxide, which in a powdered form is used as a white pigment in paint; however, when the powder particles are nanosized, the titanium dioxide is transparent. Still another example is aluminum, the metal element used to make aluminum foil; when the aluminum is a nanosized powder, it is spontaneously explosive as it comes into contact with air.

As we see from these examples, the optical as well as chemical reactivity properties of a material change depending on its size. You can appreciate the effects of size from personal experience; powdered sugar will dissolve much more quickly in water than a lump of solid sugar crystal weighing the same amount. That's because the powdered sugar has a much greater surface area, and it is more reactive because more sugar molecules are exposed to water in powdered sugar than in a lump of sugar crystal (Fig. 5.26).

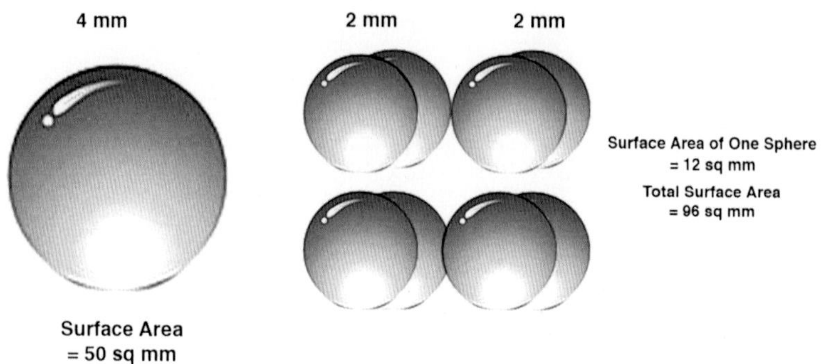

Fig. 5.26 Schematic illustration of effect of size on surface area. The eight spheres, with smaller diameters that add up to the diameter of the larger sphere have twice the surface area of the large sphere

Nanoparticulate matter becomes even more useful when it is "functionalized" (given a coating with a compound or molecules that can react or bind to other substances of interest). The compound or molecule used as the coating is called a "ligand." The ligand is often used as a trigger or an activation switch, because when it binds to another molecule, a small local chemical reaction occurs that may result in a color change, a small electrical signal, or a change to the shape of the bound molecule. By varying the ligand or by changing the type of chemical coating the nanoparticles, it is possible to provide particles with "specificity," or the ability to bind only to a cell that displays the molecule (e.g., protein) of interest. In this way, scientists can use functionalization strategies to force nanoparticles to bind only to certain tumor cells, or selected regions of a cell, or to some other tissues of interest. For example, Fig. 5.27 is a drawing of a nanoparticle coated with targeting molecules that enable the particle to adhere to cells exhibiting that molecule's target on their surface. Once the particle binds, the drug it is also carrying can be dispensed exactly at the site where it is needed. The small size of these particles (they are 100–1,000 times smaller than the cell they target) ensures that many nanoparticles have the chance to interact with the cell of interest.

Gold nanoparticles are also useful as heat-absorbing agents. When they aggregate on a tumor, surgeons can shine a laser onto the general area where the tumor is located. The laser beam wavelength is chosen to ensure that it can penetrate skin and body tissues for a short distance. As the gold nanoparticles are irradiated, they heat up, and essentially "cook" the tumor, resulting in tumor control.

Quantum dots are small (20–50 nm) crystals of inorganic compounds that emit visible light when irradiated by ultraviolet light. They are extremely bright, and as with other nanoparticles, the color they emit is dependent on their size. It is therefore possible to synthesize a series of quantum dots in various controlled sizes, and they will emit visible light in a range of colors. The dots could then be coated with a thin (1–2 nm) antibody ligand. If various-sized quantum dots, each size coated with antibodies to a different specific protein found on the surface of a tumor cell are placed in circulation, it is likely that the dots will bind through the antibody to

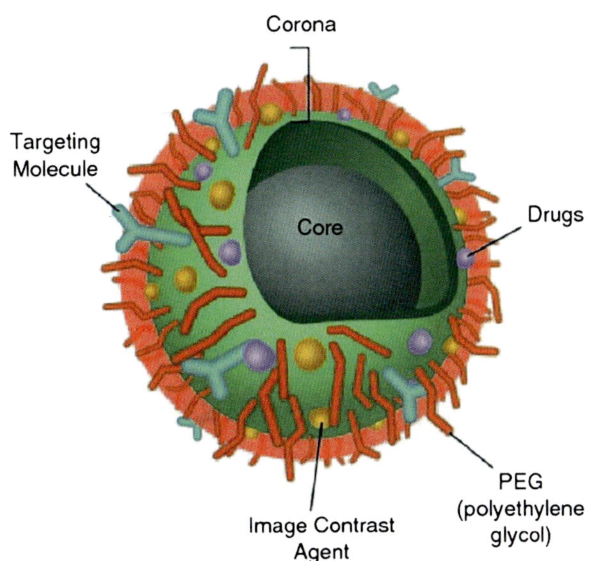

Fig. 5.27 A multifunctional, therapeutic nanoparticle. It has been coated with PEG to make it hydrophilic, with a targeting molecule to ensure it preferentially binds to a cell of interest, with a drug that is designed to treat the diseased cell, and with an image contrast agent to enable the particle to be visualized. Copyrighted by Springer-Verlag Berlin Heidelberg

the site where the proteins are located. Subsequent irradiation by ultraviolet light will reveal where quantum dots have congregated and help to locate the tumor.

Quantum dots are so small that they can be used to tag certain components inside cells. In Fig. 5.28, quantum dots were coated with folic acid. A type of throat cancer cell expresses many receptors for folic acid on its surface. Therefore, folic-acid-covered quantum dots will adhere to throat cancer cells, indicating the presence of these cells.

5.9.5 Hybridizing Imaging with Other Technologies

An even more exotic use of nanoparticles is their enlistment into nanorobotic systems that can be used for therapeutic and diagnostic applications. We will discuss targeted drug delivery methods in a later chapter, but this application is mentioned here because of its relationship to imaging. Nanoparticles can be useful for therapeutic applications because they can travel everywhere in the human body; the narrowest portions of the blood vasculature (blood vessels) can only be penetrated by objects between 30 and 300 nm in size. It has proven possible to construct "nanobots" that consist of magnetic nanoparticles functionalized with specific ligands and which carry drugs. These nanobots may be guided into the proper site using the magnetic forces generated by an MRI; once they are in place (e.g., example at a diseased tissue site), a second signal from the MRI causes them to release the drug [20]. Although the technology still has some way to go before it is widely implemented, it may fulfill the fantasies of many science fiction writers who had speculated about the future of tiny machines that could circulate through our bloodstream rooting out disease (see the movie "Fantastic Voyage" and Fig. 5.25).

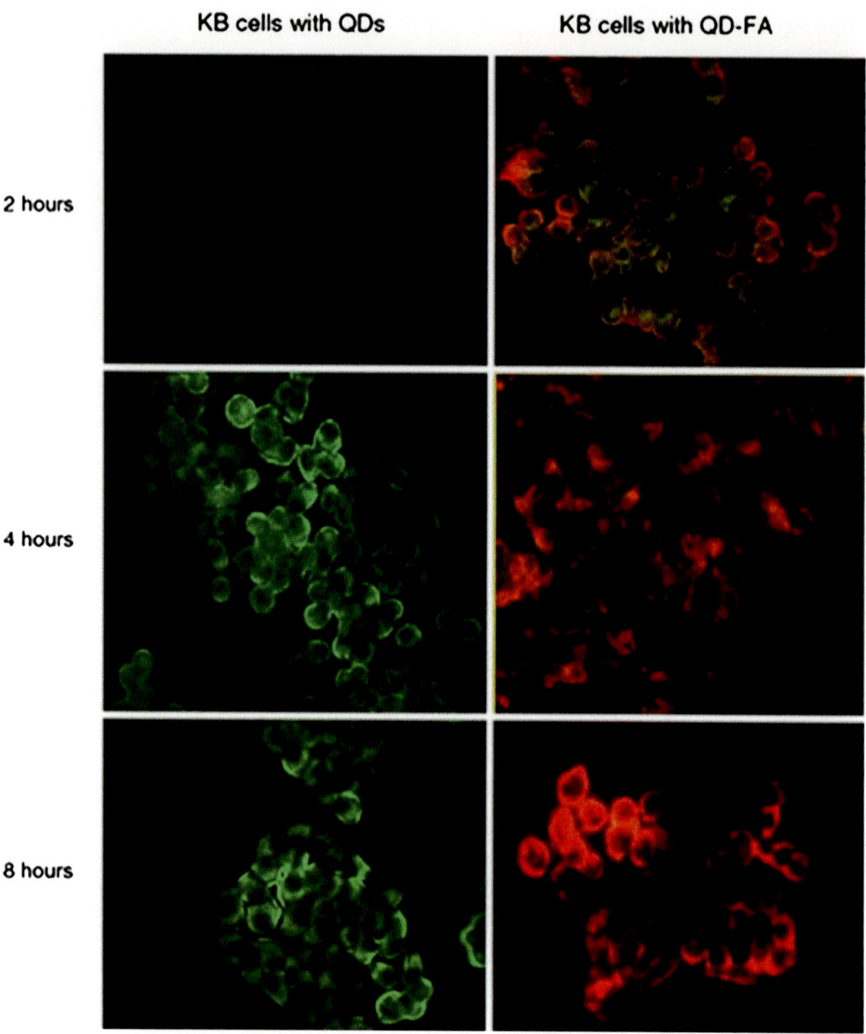

Fig. 5.28 Micrographs of cells incubated with quantum dots coated with folic acid. Human throat cancer cells have an abundance of folic acid receptors. On the *left*, an image of cells alone; on the *right*, an image of the cells labeled with the folic acid-coated quantum dots. Copyrighted by Springer-Verlag

The hybridization of imaging and therapy giving rise to a powerful symbiotic technological relationship actually had its start in 1895, when only 8 days after Roentgen's paper, a surgeon used the new X-Ray technology to help in removing a sewing needle from a woman's hand [21]. In 1908, two scientists reported the invention of the "stereotactic frame," a contraption that could be fitted onto the patient's head, and by aligning the frame with certain anatomical markers such as the ear canals, they could assign coordinates to various portions of a human brain to guide them in neurosurgery [22].

Similar frames are still used today. In various types of surgery, image-guided interventions that take advantage of computers usually follow a sequence of steps beginning with preoperative imaging, superimposing the image onto the patient's anatomy, and tracking the surgical instruments to place them within the image [23]. The software innovations that make image-guided surgical interventions possible are custom developed, but their parallels are found in other applications too, such as the entertainment and electronic gaming industries. For example, virtual reality and three-dimensional rendering algorithms are used not only for training surgeons in new procedures, but by surgical systems to integrate data from CT or MRI (i.e., technologies that can peer inside a patient) with visual microscopic data, so that the surgeon can actually "see" the relationship of bones and ligaments to the location of the instruments and be less likely to cause any accidental harm [23].

Image-guided or facilitated surgical interventions occur in several specialties of medicine. In neurosurgery, surgeons use imaging during craniotomies for brain tumor removal, and imaging has been used to guide placement of electrodes or ablation probes in the treatment of patients with Parkinson's disease or epilepsy [24]. In the case of Parkinson's patients, although it is difficult to visualize many of the deepest portions of the brain, databases have been developed from prior surgical experiences cataloguing the positions where electrodes had been placed in other patients and yielded some reduction of the typical Parkinson's tremor symptoms. For tumor surgeries, the image registration becomes complicated (as in the cases of other surgeries where a change of pressure occurs), as the brain tissue shifts position when the skull is opened. Development of "surgical suite-friendly" MRI systems that permit ready access to the patient is in progress, as MRI is not associated with the radiation danger posed by CT systems to the surgeon and operating room personnel.

In spine surgery, accurate placement of "pedicle" screws (these hold the metal rods that are used to straighten the spine or to support a degenerated spine segment) during insertion into the vertebrae is essential to avoid impingement into the spinal canal where the spinal cord is located and to ensure proper screw angulation. Commercial image-assisted surgical systems for this purpose are available from companies such as Medtronic, Inc. In the next chapter, we will discuss implants used for hip or knee replacement and the importance of proper alignment of these implants for proper distribution of forces during walking, but here it is just worth mentioning that surgical planning that relies on imaging is already used in many operating rooms [25].

Patients suffering from arrhythmia (irregular heartbeat) are often implanted with a pacemaker; however, it is necessary for the cardiac surgeon to ablate (destroy using extreme cold or a radio frequency discharge) the portions of the heart that are responsible for the arrhythmia so that they do not compete with the pacemaker. Catheters (thin tubes that are passed inside blood vessels to the surgical site; they typically include a miniature camera for visualization, as well as miniature surgical instruments at their tip) are available that can both map the heart, the locations of the targeted heart tissue, and perform the ablation too. Another application in cardiac interventions is found in bypass surgery. Here, the traditional procedure has been to open the patient's chest and separate the ribs in order to obtain a full view of the

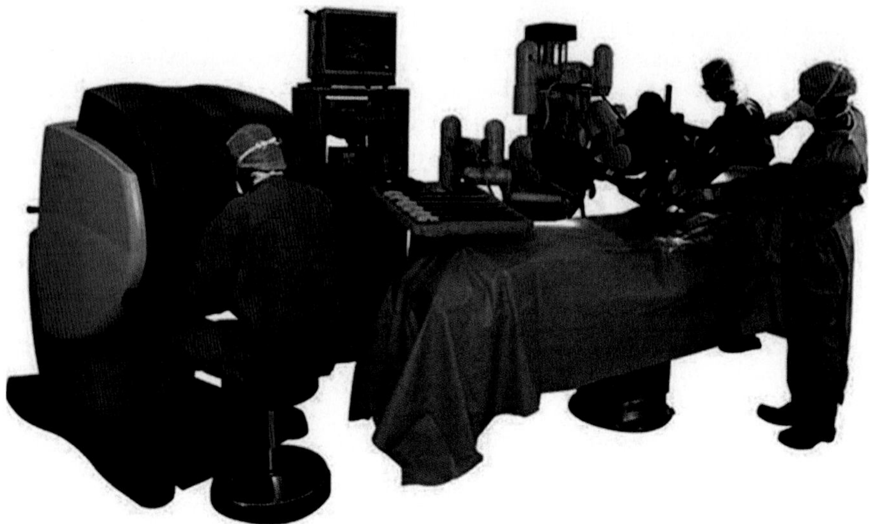

Fig. 5.29 The operating room setup for cardiac surgery using the da Vinci™ Robot. Copyrighted by Springer Science + Business Media B.V.

heart and access the blood vessels needing bypass. The surgery is followed by a long convalescence, and many healthy tissues are traumatized because of the need for observation and access. More recently, endoscopic heart surgery has been seen as a realistic alternative to traditional open-heart surgery, as it is accompanied by less trauma and shortens patient recovery time. The da Vinci robotic surgery system which relies on strong imaging capability has been used for this purpose (Fig. 5.29).

Lung and abdominal surgeries have proven difficult for image-guided system assistance for the same reason that brain surgery involving opening the skull: the soft organs shift position once the cavity (chest or skull) is opened and the pressure on the organs changes. However, bronchoscopy, the examination of the lung airways by a camera potentially followed by biopsy of suspicious lesions, and lung biopsy, using a needle that enters through the skin on the chest, have both been enhanced by development of imaging and positioning systems and software.

Finally, in a continued quest to minimize the collateral damage to healthy tissues during surgery and to reduce patient recovery times, a new surgical approach has been recently proposed, the so-called NOTES, an acronym for Natural Orifice Transluminal Endoscopic Surgery [26]. In this methodology, the surgeon enters the patient's body through one of the natural orifices: the mouth, rectum, or vagina using an endoscope (essentially a complex catheter which includes a camera and surgical instruments). The potential for wound infections, hernias caused by a misplaced cut, and postoperative pain is reduced. The need for software and imaging guidance is great because the flexible endoscope traverses, making many turns, and it is vital to know what the relationship of the tip is to nearby organs. When viewing an image, the surgeon needs to know which direction to follow! In any case, while the challenges are great, the potential advantages of still-less-invasive surgical practices are high.

5.10 Summary

Obtaining a correct diagnosis is the fervent wish of any individual who is ill. The only way to prescribe a proper and potentially effective treatment is to utilize the skills and experience of a physician during the examination to guide the remaining diagnostic tests' procedures. Advances in chemistry and biochemistry have provided analytical methods for determining the presence and amount of chemicals in the blood that can provide an indication of health or sickness, and engineering innovations have given us imaging techniques that can see at macroscopic, microscopic, and molecular levels. A fusion of imaging and surgical practice has occurred, which promises to result in less trauma and potentially better outcomes to the patient.

5.11 Foundational Concepts

- Blood chemistry analyses provide a good indication of a patient's health. Although visits to a physician are needed in cases of poor health or ailment, routine visits for a "checkup" may not be necessary for individuals in generally good health.
- A physical exam consists of inspection, palpation, percussion, and auscultation. The results of this exam may prompt the physician to order other tests, including an EKG which provides an indication of the health of the heart by measuring the frequency and relative intensities of the heartbeat.
- No diagnostic test is 100 % accurate; each has a certain specificity and sensitivity, which define the positive predictive value and the negative predictive value of that test. That's why additional and different tests are ordered if the potential for a serious disease is uncovered.
- Electromagnetic radiation covers a wide spectrum of frequencies and energies. Visible light is only a small portion of that spectrum, and higher-energy radiation such as X-rays can be used to probe the interior of bulk matter. As X-rays pass through an object, they are absorbed to a degree that depends on the matter itself. The differential absorption is responsible for being able to discriminate between different tissues on a standard X-ray print.
- Differentiation between various tissues by the emission of gamma radiation by nuclides is possible because different tissues take up nuclides to varying degrees.
- The Doppler effect is responsible for the ability of ultrasound imaging to measure the speed of blood flow in a beating heart. The high water content in human tissue enables the function of diagnostic MRI.
- The miniaturization of electronic devices is made possible by a technique called photolithography. The development of biosensors and the lab-on-a-chip was made possible by techniques of surface functionalization and the science of microfluidics.

References

1. Street, L. (2012). *Introduction to biomedical engineering technology* (2nd ed.). Boca Raton, FL: CRC Press.
2. Kennedy, P. (2012, July 27). Who made that home pregnancy test? *The New York Times*, New York.
3. Laine, C. (2002). The annual physical examination: Needless ritual or necessary routine? *Annals of Internal Medicine, 136*, 701–703.
4. Dunnington, G., Reisner, E., Witzke, D., & Fulginiti, J. et al. (1992). Teaching and evaluation of physical examination skills on the surgical clerkship. *Teaching and Learning in Medicine, 4*, 110–114.
5. Simel, D., Rennie, D., The American Medical Association (Eds.). (2009). *The rational clinical examination: Evidence based clinical diagnosis*. McGraw-Hill: New York.
6. Smith, M., Saunders, R., Stickhardt, L., & McGinnnis, M. The Institute Of Medicine, et al. (Eds.). (2012). *Best care at lower cost: The path to continuously learning health care in America*. The National Academies Press: Washington, DC.
7. Rosenthal, E. (2012, June 2). *Let's (Not) Get Physicals. The New York Times*. The New York Times Company: New York.
8. Akobeng, A. (2007). Understanding diagnostic tests 1: Sensitivity, specificity, and predictive values. *Acta Paediatrica, 96*, 338–341.
9. Reading, A. (2006). The biological nature of meaningful information. *Biological Theory, 1*, 243–249.
10. Barth, F. G. (2003). 1. Sensors and sensing: A biologist's view. Sensors and sensing in biology and engineering (p. 3). Springer, Vienna.
11. McCollough, C. H. (1997). The AAPM/RSNA physics tutorial for residents. X-ray production. *Radiographics, 17*, 967–984.
12. Sickles, E. A. (1986). Breast calcifications: Mammographic evaluation. *Radiology, 160*, 289–293.
13. Faulkner, K. G. (2000). Bone matters: Are density increases necessary to reduce fracture risk? *Journal of Bone and Mineral Research, 15*, 183–187.
14. Brown, M. H. (1962). Effect of ionizing radiation on immunity. *Canadian Medical Association Journal, 87*, 1183.
15. Van Tiggelen, R., & Pouders, E. (2003). Ultrasound and computed tomography: Spin-offs of the world wars. *Journal Belge de Radiologie—Belgisch Tijdschrift voor Radiologi, 86*, 235–241.
16. Kane, D., Grassi, W., Sturrock, R., & Balint, P.V. et al. (2004). A brief history of musculoskeletal ultrasound: 'From Bats and ships to babies and Hips'. *Rheumatology, 43*, 931–933.
17. Dussik, K. T. (1942). Ueber die möglichkeit, hochfrequente mechanische schwingungen als diagnostisches hilfsmittel zu verwerten. *Zeitschrift für die Gesamte Neurologie und Psychiatrie, 174*, 153–168.
18. Licha, K. (2002). Contrast agents for optical imaging. *Topics in Current Chemistry, 222*, 1–30.
19. Feynman, R. (1959). *There's plenty of room at the bottom*. www.zyvex.com/nanotech/feynman.html.
20. Vartholomeos, P., Fruchard, M., Ferreira, A., & Mavroidis, C. et al. (2011). MRI-guided nanorobotic systems for therapeutic and diagnostic applications. *Annual Review of Biomedical Engineering, 13*, 157–184.
21. Burrows, E. (1986). *Pioneers and early years: History of British radiology*. Alderney, UK: Colophon.
22. Horsely, V., & Clark, R. (1908). The structure and function of the cerebellum examined by a new method. *Brain, 31*, 45–124.
23. Cleary, K., & Peters, T. (2010). Image-guided interventions: Technology review and clinical applications. *Annual Review of Biomedical Engineering, 12*, 119–142.
24. Guo, T., Finnis, K.W., Parrent, A.G., & Peters, T.M. et al. (2006). Visualization and navigation system development and application for stereotactic deep-brain neurosurgeries. *Computer Aided Surgery, 11*, 231–239.
25. Jaramaz, B., DiGioia, A.M. 3rd, Blackwell, M., & Nikou, C. et al. (1998). Computer assisted measurement of cup placement in total hip replacement. *Clinical Orthopedics and Related Research, 354*, 70–81.
26. Coughlin, G., Samavedi, S., Palmer, K.J., & Patel, V.R. et al. (2009). Role of image-guidance systems during NOTES. *Journal of Endourology, 23*, 803–812.

Properties of the Host (The Human Body)

6

"The cell, over the billions of years of her life, has covered the earth many times with her substance, found ways to control herself and her environment, and ensure her survival."

Albert Claude

It will be much easier to follow the discussion in later chapters on the subjects of implants and other biomedical technologies if an appreciation of certain anatomic and physiologic characteristics of the human body has been obtained. In this chapter, we will describe and discuss the building blocks of the human body, and certain diseases such as arthritis which affect the structure and performance of the body. You should be better able to understand why implants are designed in certain ways so that they can be used to rehabilitate normal function.

6.1 Introduction

Man-made materials have been used for centuries to replace tissues of the human body. Egyptian mummies were found with gold taking the place of their missing teeth, and ivory was used in the nineteenth century to replace teeth and bones [1]. Development of prosthetic body parts goes back to at least 800 BC, the date associated with a discovered pair of two artificial big toes found on the feet of an Egyptian mummy. A bronze and wooden leg dated to 300 BC was unearthed in a Roman burial ground in southern Italy.

There is a wide range of implants available today, some to replace hard tissues such as teeth and bones others that replace soft tissues like skin or blood vessels. Implants can be made from synthetic materials, from materials derived from natural sources, and even from other animals. We will begin exploring this topic by first discussing how the systems of the human body, particularly the immune system,

G.R. Baran et al., *Healthcare and Biomedical Technology in the 21st Century: An Introduction for Non-Science Majors*, DOI 10.1007/978-1-4614-8541-4_6,

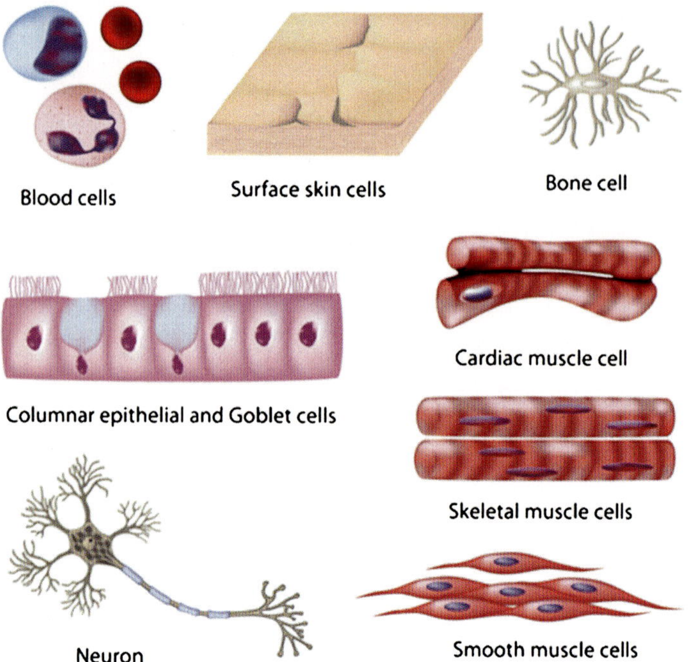

Fig. 6.1 Picture of various cell types

affect implant material selection and design. Then, in Chap. 7, we will move on to introduce concepts related to the properties of the materials used to make implants, how properties can be modified, and how materials and implants are standardized to enable reliable implant performance. Finally, in Chap. 8, we will discuss applications of materials and implants in specific clinical cases.

6.2 Cells: The Basic Building Blocks of Tissues in the Body

There are approximately 10^{13} cells comprised of about 200 different types of cells in humans. They are discrete structures, having shapes that vary by type of cell (Fig. 6.1), and their sizes range widely. Red blood cells are approximately 8 μm in diameter; certain neurons may be over a meter in length but only 10 μm thick, while muscle cells are approximately 100 μm in diameter and about a millimeter long, and skin cells are about 10 μm in length.

The border enclosing the cell is called the cell or plasma membrane, and it serves to keep the various subunits of the cell's structure isolated from the external environment (Fig. 6.2). Although the membrane appears to be solid, it is, in fact, porous, and many unseen substances such as proteins extend from within the cell, through the membrane, and out to the exterior. These proteins often serve as receptors, or sensors, that tell the cell what is going on outside. The cell is given shape by other, internal proteins arranged

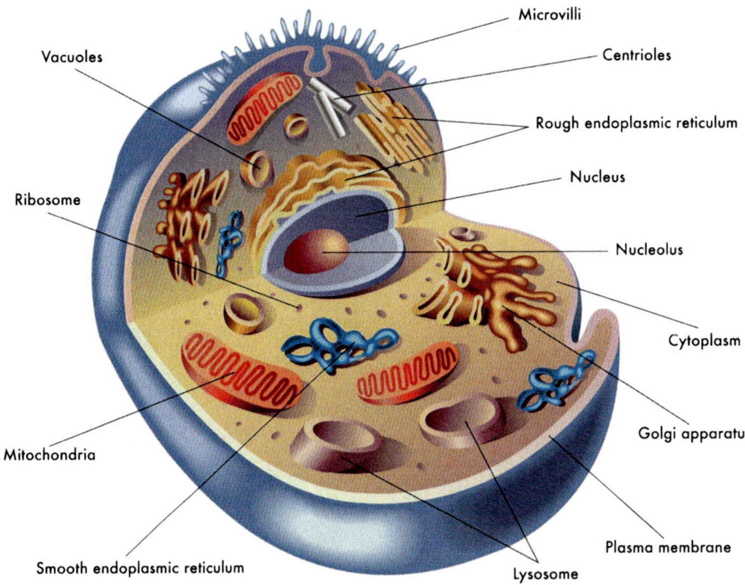

Fig. 6.2 The components of a cell

in the shapes of microfibrils, filaments, and microtubules, ranging in size from about 6 to 25 nm in diameter. Think of these as tubes that form a type of scaffold for the cell; in contrast to a building scaffold, however, these tubes are able to realign and change position within the cell, allowing the cell to change its shape and to move.

Cells are derived from parent cells by the process of cell division. A mature cell will divide, and both daughter cells will have a full complement of all the necessary parts of a cell's machinery, including genetic information (except for red blood cells, which do not have a nucleus). This process of division results in cell proliferation. Some cells (stem cells) begin life uncommitted; they have not yet assumed a specific shape or function. The process by which they do so is called "differentiation"; think of this as the way the cells become "different" or specialized and turn into bone, muscle, skin, blood, or nerve cells. The trigger for differentiation may be internal (provided by the DNA in the cell) or external. External influences that cause differentiation can be chemical (substances released by other nearby cells or introduced artificially into the environment; these are usually called growth factors) or mechanical. Cells sense mechanical signals such as stresses when they are in a portion of the body that carries a load (e.g., cartilage) or when they are in a part of the body where fluid flow occurs (e.g., endothelial cells lining the walls of blood vessels). Even though the stimulus may be mechanical in origin, it is converted into biochemical or bioelectrical signals within the cell in a process called mechanotransduction.

A cell can be thought of as a micro-sized factory that is in active communication with its environment, constantly processing signals and synthesizing proteins. Many cell types are capable of attaching and adhering to surfaces through receptor–ligand interactions (ligands and receptors were introduced in Chap. 5), in which the cell extrudes a portion of the cell membrane like a foot and forms multiple adhesion points. In this process, the cell shape changes (flattens), and cells conform to the shape of the surface. For example, cells that attach to a grooved surface will try to fit into the grooves and adopt a long, thin shape. If cells receive an appropriate biochemical signal, they will move either toward or away from that signal in a process called chemotaxis; cells can migrate from one location to another.

The interactions of cells with materials used to construct medical devices determine if the device will be tolerated by the body (be biocompatible) or if the body will attack the device using elements of its immune system. We now have the technology to analyze how an individual cell responds to the presence of implanted materials, and the knowledge gained in those experiments is used to design better and more bioactive implants and devices.

6.2.1 Cell–Surface Interactions

Whenever a material or device, for example, a splinter, a catheter, or a hip implant, is inserted into the body, what is it that the blood, skin, or muscle cells encounter? It is the surface of the device that the blood and cells respond to, not to what lies underneath. This important insight empowers scientists and engineers to design devices using bioactive materials best suited for the operation and performance of the devices; advances in surface modification chemistry permit designers to optimize the surface for desirable biochemical interaction with blood, bone, skin cells (fibroblasts), bacteria, and nerve cells. Material surfaces can also be modified to improve their physical characteristics, such as lubricity, which makes insertion of cardiovascular and urinary catheters less painful for the patient.

Insertion of a permanent implant or temporary device entails the simultaneous formation of a wound. As with any wound, the insertion site is flooded with blood and with fluids spilling out of cells that have been cut or damaged. Within minutes, the surface of the implant or device is covered with components of blood or intracellular fluids, among the most important of which are proteins. This is similar to what happens when one inserts a knife or a fork into a piece of meat or an egg while eating; the utensil is immediately contaminated and covered with protein from the meat or the egg. Proteins are complex molecules that fold in a particular shape, called a "conformation," and the specific conformation adopted by a protein depends on its environment at any given time. You can easily appreciate that the conformation of a protein floating freely inside a cell or in blood plasma can be quite different from the conformation of the protein when it is adsorbed to the surface of an implant. The conformation of the protein on the surface is determined by chemical characteristics of the surface, and engineers and scientists can try to modify the chemical composition of the implant surface in order to affect the protein's conformation. As an example, in Fig. 6.3, a protein called fibronectin has settled onto the surface of an implant, and its conformation has changed so that a group of amino acids called RGD (arginine–glycine–aspartic acid) is presented for interaction with a cell's transmembrane

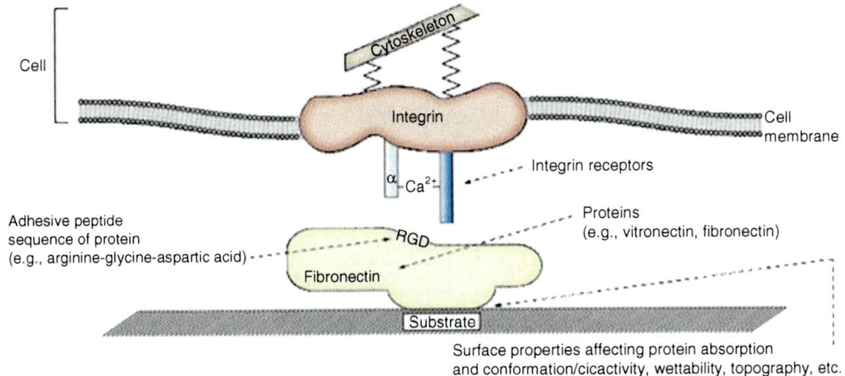

Fig. 6.3 An implant surface with adherent fibronectin. Copyrighted by Springer Science + Business Media, LLC

protein called an integrin receptor. The binding between the RGD group and the integrin is the event that "tells" the cell that an implant is in the immediate vicinity.

Each human tissue cell has hundreds of different receptors; for example, the neurons in your nose which sense odors have over a thousand different receptors. A protein adsorbed on an implant surface is likely to have a specific conformation characteristic of the material that implant is made from, and therefore some reactive group will be exposed that is dependent on the properties of the implant surface.

If cell receptors are proteins, then it follows that they also have a specific conformation. The way receptors preserve specificity (react to only a very limited number of stimuli) is to ensure that the only successful interaction occurs with a molecule (ligand) whose conformation is compatible with the receptor's conformation. So, if the receptor conformation resembles a jigsaw puzzle piece, then the only activator is another puzzle piece with a conformation that allows the stimulating substance (the ligand) to fit into (bind to) the receptor. When the ligand docks or binds with the receptor, the receptor changes its conformation again. This change in conformation is communicated to the interior of the cell, triggering internal biochemical reactions.

Sometimes, the binding event can be used to prevent the cell from performing certain functions. This is one strategy followed by pharmaceutical companies when designing new drugs. If it is known, for example, that a particular virus attaches to certain receptors on the cell surface (Fig. 6.4), then interfering with the attachment/binding could prevent the virus from gaining entry into the cell, a necessary step for the virus to multiply and spread. The particular drug molecule that binds to the receptors preferred by the virus would then be considered as a preventive medication.

The trick is in knowing which ligands bind to which receptors and what are the implications of the binding event. With that knowledge, for example, the designer of a bone implant could modify the implant surface to attract proteins that in their new conformation would enable the adhesion of osteoblasts that make bone, anchoring the implant. Alternatively, the designer could modify the implant surface in such a way as to render it non-fouling such that no proteins or bacteria could adhere to the surface.

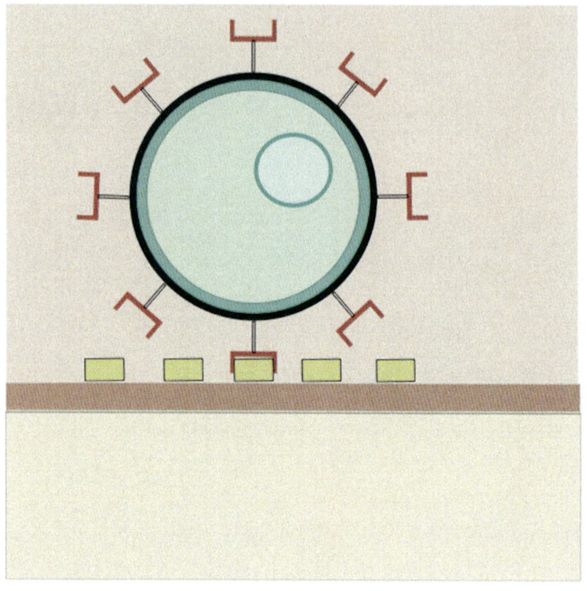

Fig. 6.4 A virus covered with proteins (*red*) that bind to specific receptors on the cell surface (*yellow*)

6.2.2 The Defensive Systems of the Human Body

The human body utilizes cell–surface interactions to react to implants and any other foreign body that penetrates the skin. The body is equipped with a complex and sophisticated defensive and healing mechanism. This system employs various methods to protect tissues and detect and destroy harmful pathogens (infectious microorganisms), while the wound healing mechanism is geared toward minimizing damage caused by injury, eliminating any microbes or foreign material left behind at the site of injury, and replacing damaged tissues with healthy new tissue.

Examples of the first line of defense for the body are the skin, the digestive system, the respiratory system, ears, eyes, and the urinary tract. Skin acts as a physical barrier that also regulates body temperature and excretes some metabolic waste products through the sweat glands. The digestive system uses a low pH in the stomach to destroy some microorganisms found in food, and the alkaline pH in the intestines, bile salts, lysozyme (an enzyme that breaks down bacterial cell walls), presence of harmless stomach bacteria, and the peristaltic action (movement to excrete) of the intestine all discourage harmful colonization of microbes. The respiratory system takes advantage of fine nose hairs, baffles of the nares (nasal membranes), the mucosal surfaces of the trachea, and ciliated (covered with fine hairs) epithelium of the lower respiratory tract to entrap inhaled microorganisms. The respiratory tract is also colonized by harmless bacteria and cells that secrete substances which can neutralize many harmful pathogens.

These tissues and organs employ defense mechanisms that are nonspecific (they don't depend on the exact nature of the foreign substance involved) and are designed to prevent harmful pathogens (microbes/viruses that cause diseases) from colonizing.

Interestingly, many of these nonspecific defense systems work in conjunction with harmless bacteria that have themselves already colonized these tissues and which secrete antimicrobial or acidic substances that inhibit harmful pathogens. For example, the vagina is colonized by lactic acid bacteria (vaginal flora) that keep the vaginal lining acidic, an environment that is hostile to many harmful pathogens.

The second line of defense includes cellular defense mechanisms, also known as the immune system. The immune system is the body's natural defense in combating (infectious) organisms. Usually, it effectively protects the body from pathogens such as parasites, bacteria, and many viruses. However, even with a fully functional immune system, many bacterial or viral infections will require treatment with powerful antibiotics or antiviral drugs. The success of the immune system depends on its ability to discriminate between foreign (nonself) and host (self) cells. The immune system will recognize xenografts (tissues from animals), sometimes allografts (from other humans), and many microorganisms (harmful versus harmless bacteria) as foreign. In some cases, the immune system may mistakenly recognize the body's own cells as foreign and attack them (autoimmune diseases). Other functions of the immune system include scavenging dead, dying, or abnormal (cancerous) body cells.

If a harmful pathogen successfully enters a tissue, the immune system will try to disable or destroy it. The immune system consists of a network of various cells, tissues, or organs positioned throughout the body. The cells as a group are called leucocytes (white blood cells, so-called because when blood is centrifuged, they settle as a white layer between the red blood cells in the bottom and the clear plasma at the top of the specimen container). There are many different types of leucocytes, including monocytes, macrophages, and lymphocytes. Both red and white blood cells are formed in the bone marrow, and some of the white blood cells travel to the thymus (an organ located partly in the neck and chest) for maturation. Those cells are called T-cells (thymus cells). Human immunodeficiency viruses (HIV) are shown to infect T-cells primarily. T-cells play a major role in the rejection of transplanted allografts, organs, or xenografts. Other white blood cells mature in the bone marrow itself and then travel to lymph nodes found throughout the body, including the armpit and stomach or spleen.

The cells of the immune system can recognize pathogens or foreign bodies (through ligand–receptor binding events as has been previously described) and use many different mechanisms to destroy the invaders. Macrophages can engulf dying cells and pathogens. Other immune cells such as natural killer cells secrete proteins that can lyse bacteria (puncture the cell wall), killing them in the process. Medical devices made from synthetic materials (e.g., polymers, metals, composites) are not attacked by the immune system in the same way that microbes or other allografts or xenografts are attacked. Sometimes, the immune system does not "see" the implants because within seconds of implantation, the implants are coated with the patient's own proteins. These proteins, undergoing a change in conformation, might then signal other cells (macrophages, foreign body giant cells) in the body to attack the implant. Finally, a fibrous tissue is usually formed around the implant (encapsulation) [2, 3]. The presence of such tissue may be advantageous in some implants and detrimental in other. Examples of situations where fibrous tissue formation is not desirable include tissue around blood vessel stents or implantable sensors.

6.2.3 Other Implant–Host Interactions

Biocompatibility is the ability of a medical device or implant to perform its intended function with an appropriate tissue response. Any implantable device that comes into contact with tissue or blood should satisfy two criteria: biofunctionality and biosafety. Biofunctionality means the implant should function as intended without eliciting any undesirable responses. A simple example is the ability of a suture to hold injured tissues together until the tissue is completely healed. Biosafety means that after implantation the medical device should not release any toxic products or degradation by-products that might cause death, chronic inflammation, diseases, or cancer. For example, the human body is a very harsh environment and can cause metallic implants to corrode (dissolve). The consequences of corrosion include weakening of the implant and the release of corrosion by-products that can be toxic to the surrounding local tissue or to the body as a whole. Another example is the release of acidic by-products by biodegradable sutures, which causes chronic inflammation and pain. The nature of the body's response to an implant will determine if the implant will function properly and as intended. The outcome depends on many factors, including the type of tissue, the biocompatibility of the medical device, and the length of time the implant will be in contact with live tissue. The following are some examples of deleterious local or systemic responses to implants.

- Many of the biomaterial implants used in orthopedics, cardiovascular surgery, etc. contain metals, including nickel. Nickel is primarily responsible for contact dermatitis (an itchy rash and inflammation) and is found in furniture, coins, earrings, and other jewelry for body piercings. As much as 10–15 % of the world's population is allergic to nickel and may be diagnosed using skin patch testing. Interestingly, many patients allergic to nickel usually do not develop metal allergy symptoms to orthopedic or cardiovascular implants, although they can develop reactions to dental appliances such as partial dentures that contain nickel. This may be due to the differences in the way skin tissue and other internal tissues react to implants. There is also a major controversy about the use of mercury-containing (amalgam) fillings in dentistry, though there has been no peer-reviewed evidence presented that the mercury in fillings causes problems to the dental patient.
- Pyrogens are fever- and inflammation-causing agents, usually derived from bacterial cell walls. Implants must be free of any microbial contamination, and this can usually be achieved by various sterilization techniques. However, the remnants of dead microbes and microbial components alone may induce an inflammatory immune response such as fever. Before a medical device can be introduced in a market, agencies such as the FDA require pyrogenicity study results for device approvals. These studies can be conducted in animals or using state-of-the-art blood or cell culture pyrogen tests. In a rabbit model, a sterilized medical device is washed in sterile saline. The wash saline is then injected into rabbits, and the rabbits are monitored for a rise in rectal temperature.
- Some medical devices are designed to be in contact with vascular structures or blood. They can be grouped into short-term extracorporeal devices (kidney dialysis units or heart lung machines) or long-term in situ implants (heart valves, heart pumps, or stents). Improperly designed implants can cause local (e.g., clot-

ting, calcification) or systemic (small blood clots called emboli) reactions leading to stroke, myocardial infarction, pulmonary embolism, damaged blood proteins and eventual implant failure or death. Blood–medical device interactions are very complex and depend on many factors, including the surface roughness of the implant (a rough surface promotes faster blood coagulation), surface wettability, or surface charge (negative surfaces delay clot formation). Each blood-contacting device design needs to be tested extensively for unforeseeable failure mechanisms using in vitro testing and animal models.

- There has always been a concern that biomaterials may cause tumor growth. However, tumor occurrence at implant sites is very rare. There are two types of tumors: (1) benign (pathological and clinical behavior is relatively innocent) or (2) malignant/cancerous (deadly). Humans don't get foreign body tumors nearly as often as rodents do; therefore, animal models used to test tumorigenesis need to be carefully selected. However, there is a possibility that other patient or environmental factors may initiate a foreign body tumor.
- All load-bearing orthopedic implants wear and release small particles (wear debris) into the immediate environment. The human body's innate foreign body response to the particles is to recruit specialized cells called macrophages to the area where particles have been released in order to scavenge them. The macrophages engulf the particles in a process called "phagocytosis," and each macrophage is capable of consuming many particles, depending, of course, on the particle size. As a side effect of phagocytosis, macrophages will release biochemical substances called cytokines which cause local inflammation. Another, more pernicious side effect of cytokine release, is that the bone in the immediate area begins to resorb (disappear). The cytokine triggers the activity of a cell called an "osteoclast," whose normal function is to break down bone as it participates in bone remodeling (i.e., bone resorption and bone deposition). Because the bone begins to disappear, the implant loses some of the stability provided by the bone; as a result, the implant begins to move slightly, and the movement further loosens the implant. Eventually, the patient cannot tolerate the pain and discomfort, and the implant has to be replaced. Now that bone has been lost, the replacement implant must be much larger. Because this process occurs to some degree with almost all implants, it is generally believed that implants have a certain lifetime, approximately 15 years, and will need replacement thereafter.

Even though animal models can provide preliminary information or design criteria about various biomedical device interactions, many times biomedical devices behave very differently when implanted in humans. Therefore, it is best to study the effect or behavior of implants in humans. This can be done ethically by studying implants that have failed and been extracted or retrieved from patients after their death.

6.2.4 The Wound Healing Response

The wound healing process can be divided into four phases: hemostasis, the inflammatory phase, the proliferative phase, and the remodeling phase [4]. Immediately after injury, chemicals are released by the platelets (a component of blood) to constrict blood vessels around the site of the injury. Constriction of blood vessels prevents further blood loss. The platelets also coagulate, forming a blood clot that plugs the injury site and prevent further blood loss. This stage (hemostasis) is followed by the inflammatory phase which is marked by swelling, production of heat, and the population of the injury site by white blood cells to destroy and clear any microbes. The proliferative and the remodeling phases are a complex series of events that include the formation of new blood vessels, reconnection of neural structures, and collagen formation by fibroblasts The culmination of these phases is the replacement of skin structures with scar tissue and subsequent formation of normal tissues. Wound healing is affected by a number of factors, including medications, infections, and the patient's nutritional/physiologic status.

6.3 Bone

Many of the implants we are most familiar with are either anchored to or replace bone, the tissue that forms a scaffold for the human body. As we consider how to design relevant implants, an understanding of the structure and properties of bone becomes essential.

The human skeleton is composed of 206 bones, though this number could be higher because of the presence of accessory bones (e.g., extra toe bones) in the limbs. Bones play a major role in load bearing, locomotion, eating, and protection of vital organs (e.g., skull protects the brain, ribs protect the heart and the lungs) and serve as a mineral reservoir. Muscles, ligaments, cartilage, and tendons attach to bones, and they are essential for force creation and transfer.

6.3.1 Bone Structure

Bone is a composite made up of 65 % mineral (mainly hydroxyapatite) and 35 % organic matrix (organic materials contain the element carbon; in bone, collagen and other non-collagenous proteins bone cells are organic). The inorganic (non-carbon containing) mineral component contributes to bone strength, while the organic matrix (the adhesive phase that binds the mineral phase and holds it together) is responsible for toughness (i.e., crack resistance). The mechanical properties of bone depend on the anatomic location and function of a particular bone. These properties can be fine-tuned according to loading requirements by changing the ratio of inorganic/organic components and water content [5]. Many examples can be found in nature where the proportions of these three components are varied to obtain the desired mechanical property. The mineral content is also related to bony function: tooth enamel—97 % mineral (strong), ossicles of the middle ear—90 % mineral (stiff), long bone—65 % mineral (strong and resistant to fracture), and antler—30 % mineral (fracture resistant). Even though the quantity of different components plays a role, there is also evidence that the quality of the organic components affects bone performance.

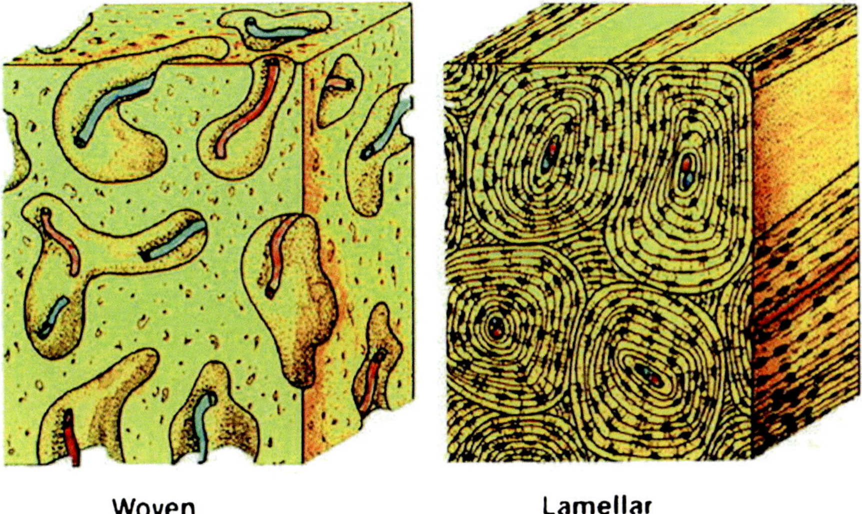

Fig. 6.5 Structure of woven and lamellar bone. Copyrighted by Humana Press, a part of Springer Science + Business Media, LLC

The microscopic structure of bone is such that small crystals of hydroxyapatite with the formula $Ca_{10}(PO4)_6(OH)_2$, shaped like minute plates, surround the collagen fibers. These crystals nucleate (start to grow) at specific places along the collagen molecule; in this way, the protein acts as a template for mineralization.

The bones in children are less mineralized than in adults, i.e., contain less hydroxyapatite, and more organic matter. A less mineralized bone will be more flexible (and less brittle) and thus be able to absorb more energy. This property helps children to avoid fractures during frequent falls. It is interesting to note that elderly adults lose bone mineral content in the context of osteoporosis. Although osteoporotic bones have low mineral content just as children's bones do, they are at greater risk of fracture because the quality of the organic component has degraded too.

If we consider bone structure at a level more coarse than the molecular level, then bone may be classified as either woven or lamellar (Fig. 6.5). Woven bone is formed quickly, as in a fetus and during fracture repair. Lamellar bone grows more slowly, and is better organized, and can form hollow cylinders that house blood vessels [6]. Woven and lamellar bone can coexist forming a fibrolamellar bone.

Moving up still another level in the hierarchical structure of bone, bone is organized as spongy (also known as trabecular or cancellous bone) and compact (also known as cortical) bone (Fig. 6.6). An adult human skeleton consists of 80 % cortical bone and 20 % cancellous bone. Cortical bone forms the outer wall of all bones, and trabecular bone is found in the inner parts of bones.

Cancellous bone has obvious porosity, and the individual small plates of bone called "trabeculae" (Fig. 6.7) are arranged in a way so as to provide reinforcement

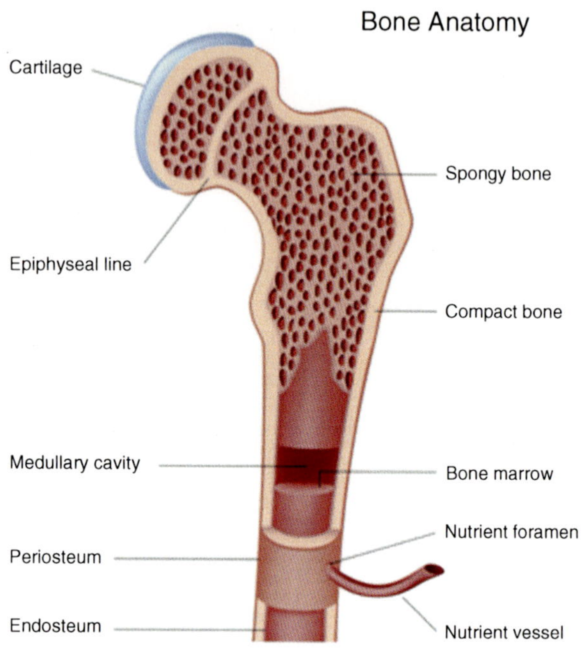

Fig. 6.6 Cross section of a long bone, showing spongy (cancellous) bone and compact (cortical) bone

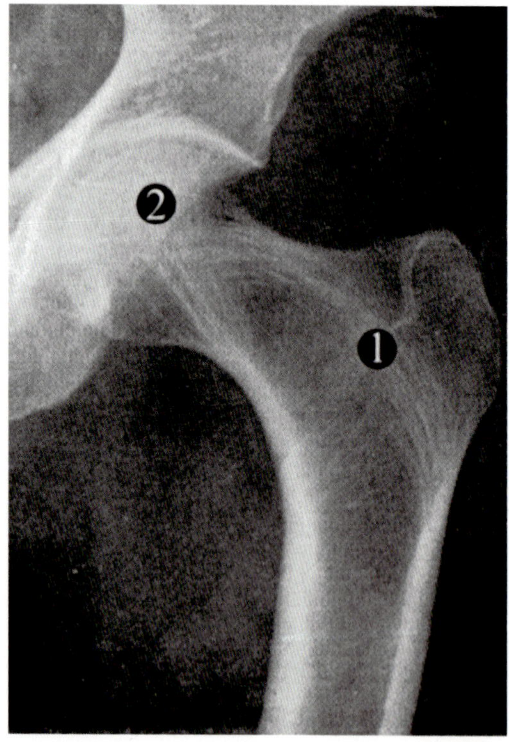

Fig. 6.7 Radiograph of a human femur and acetabulum, showing the two principal patterns of arrangement of trabeculae along lines of stress. Copyright by Rudman, KE; Aspden, RM; Meakin, JR. BioMedical Engineering OnLine *Vol.* 5 *Issue* 1. *DOI*: 10.1186/1475-925X-5-12 *Published*: 2006–12–01. Creative Commons Attribution License

along the principal stress directions. Certain weight-bearing skeletal sites benefit from the presence of large amounts of cancellous bone. For example, the vertebral bodies and the calcaneus (heel bone) consist primarily of cancellous bone surrounded by a thin cortical shell. Cancellous bone offers some advantages in these skeletal sites. First, it tolerates great deformation (think of a sponge) when compared to cortical bone, thereby accommodating flexion, rotation (in the case of spine), and high-impact loading (in the case of the calcaneus). Second, the porous network makes the material lighter [7].

Microscopically, compact (cortical) bone is nonporous and consists of many units called osteons making up the Haversian system. The porosity in cancellous bone is typically filled with marrow. The (red) marrow found at the ends of long bones and in flat bones is responsible for producing red blood cells, platelets, and most white blood cells. Marrow found in the medullary canal is a type called yellow marrow and consists primarily of fat cells. The body may convert yellow marrow to red marrow if needed.

6.3.2 Bone Activity

Bone is a living tissue and has several different types of active cells. The outer covering of bone is called the periosteum and is composed of bone-lining cells and a sheet of collagen, while the inner surface of bones is called the endosteum, also composed of bone-lining cells. These cells give rise to osteoblasts, cells that are involved in the formation of new bone by laying down the collagen fiber that is later mineralized. Osteocytes are cells that are found inside the body of the bone. Finally, osteoclasts are cells that destroy bone by dissolving it and passing the debris through their own body into the space outside the bone. Bone tissue is in a constant state of remodeling, i.e., portions of our bone are being destroyed by osteoclasts and at the same time osteoblasts are laying down new bone. These two types of cells communicate with each other and maintain bone homeostasis (the equilibrium between bone density and mineral availability in the body). A breakdown in these communications causes diseases such as osteoporosis.

Because osteoblasts and osteoclasts are able to remodel bone in response to external loads, bone has the wonderful ability to appear where it is needed. The practical design of bones was appreciated even by Galileo, but it was Wolff, publishing in 1892, who codified what is now known as Wolff's law: bone reshapes itself in response to external forces. Many later observations by other scientists have added to this initial finding, and we now know that bone remodels in response to flexure, that repetitive loads cause remodeling (not static loads), and that bone is added to the concave surface that is formed during bending [8]. Because bone remodeling is the product of cell activity, there must be a way that osteoblasts and osteoclasts sense loads. The prevalent theory today is that because bone is piezoelectric (it accumulates an electric charge in response to pressure), osteoblasts are responding to electric fields when they begin to lay down new bone. Interestingly, it is thought that the electric charge forms in the collagen, rather than in the hydroxyapatite crystals. This response, i.e., of new bone formation in response to electricity, demonstrated on rabbit bone in 1953, was the basis for development of various electronic devices currently used to accelerate bone formation in difficult to heal bone fractures [9]. Because of this finding, additional research has been done showing that application of ultrasound can also accelerate bone healing and shock waves (similar to those used to fracture kidney stones) can also accelerate bone healing. There are several devices currently being marketed that provide low-amplitude (intensity) ultrasonic stimulation. In some, ultrasound is delivered via a small transducer that is placed on the skin near the fracture site (Exogen™), while in others (Marodyne LivMD™), low-intensity vibration is produced by a pad on which the patient stands for a short period of time (approximately 15 min) daily. An increase in muscle mass and bone mineral density is claimed after regular use of the low-intensity vibration devices.

It's interesting that repetitive (dynamic) loading of long bones is what triggers bone remodeling. This is of course not the case in dental orthodontic treatment, where it is the application of a static, long-term load that causes tooth movement. The jaw bone is resorbed where it is subjected to pressure by the tooth which is seeking to change its position, and new bone is deposited behind the moving tooth. It should be remembered, however, that the forces used in orthodontic movement are much lower than those applied to long bones and the tooth socket is lined with a periodontal ligament, a complex tissue which itself responds to load by altering its blood vessel network and whose cells release a variety of biochemicals thought to affect osteoclast activity. Also, while the load delivered by the orthodontic appliance is static, there are some dynamic forces in play while the patient is chewing.

In any event, the fact that bone cells respond to load is responsible for the loss of bone mass experienced by astronauts who have spent an extended period under zero-gravity conditions, e.g., while at the international space station. Where there is no gravity, there is no weight-induced loading of bones, and therefore, no need for them. Under normal conditions too, exercise workouts which involve some weight lifting will help to maintain bone mass. The need for bone to be loaded in order to keep from being resorbed is a crucial consideration when choosing materials for implants that will be used together with bone, as we will discuss later.

6.3.3 Bone Degradation and Fracture

As with any other load-bearing structure, the most obvious mechanical requirement for bone is to avoid fracture (Fig. 6.8). Healthy bones do not develop spontaneous fractures during voluntary physical activities of life [10]. The consequences of bone failure are tragic in humans and animals.

Bones fail when a force exerted against the bone in any direction is stronger than the bone can structurally withstand. Fractures in healthy individuals frequently occur as the result of trauma: during sporting activities, automobile accidents, and falls in children (where fractures take the form of green stick fractures, torus or buckle fractures, characteristic of less mineralized bone). Adults with severe bone

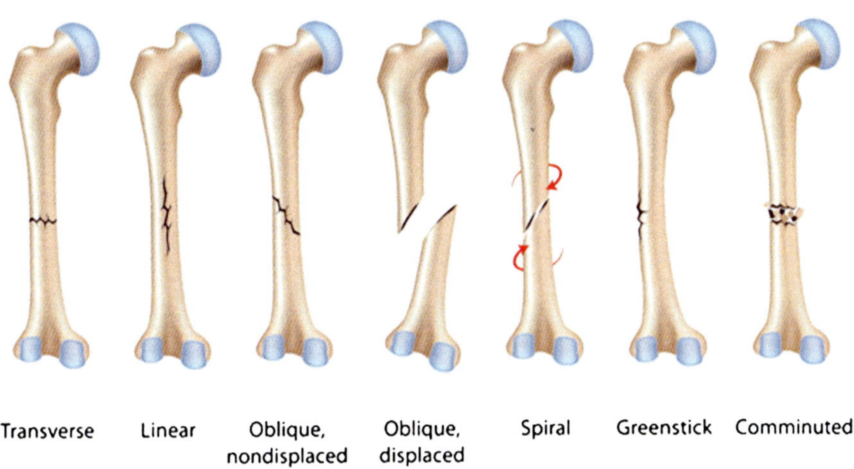

Fig. 6.8 Different types of bone fractures

mineral loss (such as characteristic of osteoporosis) are prone to traumatic, as well as nontraumatic fractures (those due to voluntary muscle forces stronger than the bone can structurally withstand). Most osteoporosis-related fractures occur in the hip, spine, or near the wrist joint [11]. Bones also fail when they are subjected to new, strenuous, and repetitive stresses (e.g., fatigue fractures). Fractures of this type usually happen when an individual's relatively sedentary lifestyle suddenly changes to a more active lifestyle as in the case of new military recruits.

There are three major factors that interact in a number of ways to cause fracture: the bone, the patient, and the magnitude and direction of force/load. Here we will focus on the bone and the patient.

A growing body of evidence indicates that factors other than bone mineral density, such as bone geometry, microarchitecture, molecular structure of inorganic and organic bone components [12], and bone remodeling [13], equally contribute to bone fragility. There are also many patient-related factors that increase the risk of fractures, such as age, gender, drug treatment [14, 15], systemic diseases, vision problems, gait instability, or nervous disorders.

All individuals lose bone strength with advancing age. This occurs primarily as the result of bone mineral loss, but other reasons include deterioration of bone collagen quality [16] and change in bone microarchitecture (Fig. 6.9). Osteoporosis is a systemic disease characterized by reduced bone mass and deteriorated bone microarchitecture. The elderly are more susceptible to bone fractures regardless of gender, mainly due to osteoporotic changes in their bones. Sadly, hip fractures are often the "beginning of the end" for these patients; the mortality risk for women doubles in the year following a hip fracture. Because of the severe effects of mineral

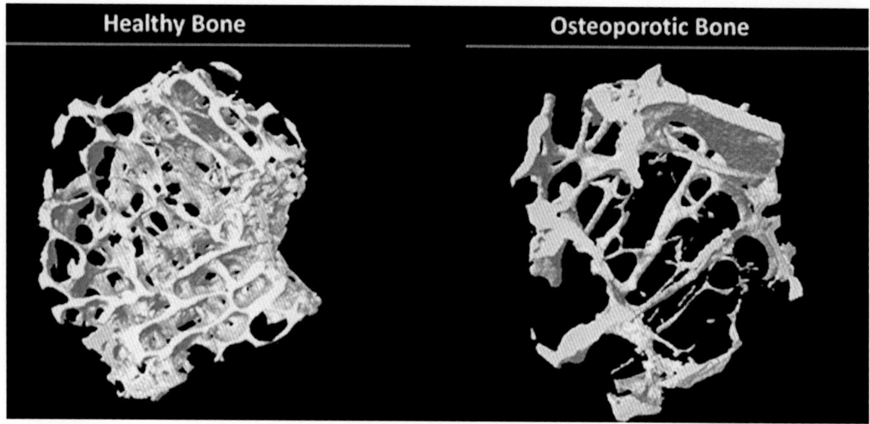

Fig. 6.9 High-resolution photographs of normal healthy bone (*left*) and osteoporotic bone (*right*). Copyright Springer Science+Business Media New York

loss, it is wise to maximize the amount of calcium in the diet where possible. Recalling that men and women reach peak bone mass between the ages of 25 and 30 and start to lose bone mass after that age, it makes sense not only to ensure that there is plenty of calcium in the diet during youth, but also to avoid lifestyle choices that reduce bone mineral density, such as smoking and excess soda consumption.

There are gender differences in bone size, rate of bone loss, and bone loss pattern. Males have larger skeletons compared to females [7]. For example, vertebral bodies are wider and taller in men than in women. The onset of puberty plays a major role in determining the size of the skeleton, and for females, estrogen produced after puberty limits the diameter of the bone by inhibiting periosteal bone formation.

The size of the skeleton plays an important role in fracture. For example, in long bones larger cross sections have greater strength in bending and torque (twisting) than smaller cross sections with equal amounts of bone. Thus, their smaller bone size makes women more vulnerable to fractures than men. It is also not surprising to observe that long bones usually become wider (periosteal bone formation) and thinner in older adults. In this way bones can maintain their strength despite having lesser bone mineral density.

By age 50, the risk of sustaining a fracture is three times greater for women than for men [17]. The main trigger for this is menopause. Postmenopausal bone loss is mainly caused by estrogen deficiency. Although men also develop osteoporosis, the pattern of cancellous bone loss is different in men and women. In men, bone loss occurs mainly through a reduction in bone formation and trabecular thinning. Cancellous bone loss in women is primarily the result of a complete removal of some trabeculae, leaving those that remain more widely separated and less well connected. The loss of trabecular connectivity is almost irreversible and leads to permanent alteration in trabecular bone microarchitecture, and because connectivity is a more significant component of bone strength than thinning, bone strength is better preserved in men than in women.

Strategies for preventing bone fracture focus on strengthening bone and preventing falls or other traumas. In children, optimal mineralization of the skeleton can be achieved by making sure their diet contains adequate calcium and that they participate in bone-loading exercise [18]. In adults, osteoporosis can be treated with antiresorptive agents (e.g., bisphosphonates, estrogen) or anabolic agents (e.g., parathyroid hormone, fluoride, prostaglandin E). The majority of the pharmacological treatments now available for osteoporosis work by inhibiting bone resorption. It should be noted that the drug treatments have side effects, and therefore it is important to prevent bone loss before the first fracture, particularly in women, and to maintain bone strength before the first fracture, because bone loss is largely irreversible (e.g., loss of trabecular connectivity) by the time the first fracture occurs. The best way to prevent bone loss during old age is to participate in physical activity and maintain a proper diet [19].

Microcracks develop over time in loaded bone. In youth, an individual can deal with these "wear and tear" problems by activating osteoclasts to remove old bone, by relying on osteoblasts to put down new bone, and by performing dynamic exercises, since these seem to have beneficial effects across the age spectrum and across multiple skeletal sites. As a person ages, however, there is (1) a tendency to exercise less, and (2) hormonal and physiologic processes combine to create a negative bone balance. This is especially problematic in cancellous bone regions and increases the likelihood of hip fracture, spinal collapse, and wrist fractures following a fall. Remedies to the hip fracture epidemic are likely to involve multiple approaches, including but not limited to osteoclast inhibitors, osteoblast activators, and appropriate exercise regimens. Altered lifestyles (e.g., wearing padded undergarments) and perhaps modified living arrangements (such as stiff but collapsible bathroom flooring) may also benefit particularly high-risk individuals [18].

To briefly recapitulate, bone fracture is due to a variety of reasons, including osteoporosis, and is often the reason an implant is needed. However, the most common causes for hip and knee replacements are not, strictly speaking, bone diseases. Arthritis, which often attacks the articular cartilage (cartilage found in articulating joints where two or more bones are in moving contact), is the most frequent cause for joint replacement.

6.4 Diseases of the Joints: Arthritis

Arthritis is defined as an inflammation of the joints. Although there are approximately 100 different types of arthritis including gout, lupus, and scleroderma, the most common forms requiring joint replacement because of a deterioration of cartilage are rheumatoid arthritis and osteoarthritis.

The cause of rheumatoid arthritis (RA) is not known, but it is an autoimmune disease in which the body's immune system mistakenly attacks its own tissue. Manifestations of this form of arthritis are found in joints such as knees, fingers, ankles, and wrists on both sides of the body equally, accompanied by swelling and inflammation that can cause severe deformation of the joint (Fig. 6.10).

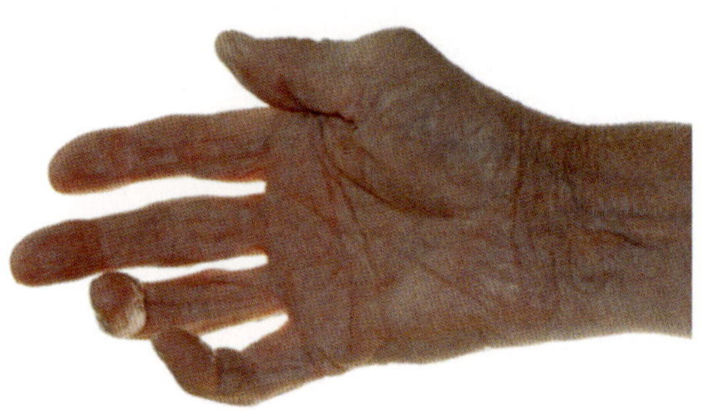

Fig. 6.10 Severely deformed hand and finger joints due to rheumatoid arthritis

Other symptoms include morning stiffness in the joints that lasts over an hour, pain, and a loss in the range of motion. There is no cure for RA; common aids include anti-inflammatory drugs, physical therapy, exercise, and other medications. If the joints become severely disfigured and if there is a loss of mobility, surgery with joint replacement may be recommended.

Osteoarthritis (OA), as shown in Fig. 6.11, is a different disease, whose cause is relatively well understood. It is characterized by morning aches, pains, and stiffness, a cracking noise when joints are moved (e.g., while kneeling), and inflammation. Because the cause is the wear and tear of the cartilage, there may come a time when the cartilage has worn away enabling bone-to-bone contact. At that point, the pain may become severe enough to limit movement and mobility. Palliative measures that reduce pain and discomfort include anti-inflammatory medication, physical therapy, exercise to strengthen the muscles of the joint, and injections of hyaluronic acid-based lubricants such as Synvisc™ or Hyalgan™. Injections into the knee joint may provide relief for up to 3 months; in Europe, these treatments are also approved for shoulder and ankle osteoarthritis. Because hyaluronic acid is obtained from the combs of roosters, patients allergic to poultry products should not be given injections of hyaluronic acid. Eventually, surgery to replace the joint may be required. Being overweight and out of condition are known to bring on osteoarthritis, as greater loads are placed on the joints (particularly the knees) and the muscles are unable to adequately control movement. Although both men and women suffer from osteoarthritis, above age 55 more women than men are diagnosed with OA.

6.5 Summary

All medical devices, both permanent and temporary, encounter the immune system of the body whenever they are used in contact with human fluids or tissues. The aim of the biomedical engineer is to design devices that are well tolerated, so that they may function without provoking fibrous tissue encapsulation. In order to rationally

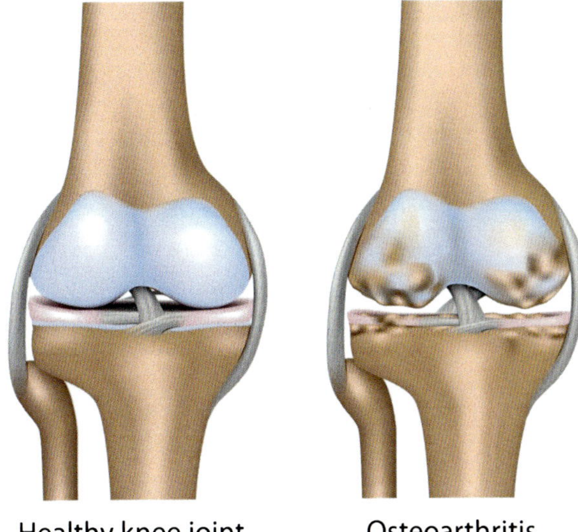

Fig. 6.11 Diagram of an osteoarthritic knee, with extensive cartilage destruction

design such devices, the engineer must appreciate and understand the surface interactions between materials and the cells of the body.

The skeleton serves as a scaffolding system in the body. Bones change with age, becoming weaker, and the bearing surfaces in joints, typically cartilage on cartilage, can degrade as the result of wear and tear or arthritis.

6.6 Foundational Concepts

- The approximately 200 different kinds of cells found in the human body are the building blocks for tissues and organs. Cells vary in size and shape and, in addition to carrying genetic material in the nucleus, are equipped with many sensory features that protrude beyond the cell membrane and inform the cell about its environment.
- Stem cells are undifferentiated, meaning that they have not yet been transformed into muscle, skin, bone cells, etc. Differentiation is caused by environmental cues.
- Changes in a cell's environment cause a cascade of biochemical reactions which can alter the cell's shape, cause the cell to move, trigger the release of signaling molecules to recruit other cells that are part of the immune system, or provoke local reactions in the neighboring tissue such as swelling.
- Cells can sense the shape (conformation) of a protein adsorbed on the surface of an implant and, in doing so, can trigger a foreign body response.
- The body's defenses respond to intrusion by foreign substances, both natural (as, e.g., bacteria) and synthetic (metallic implants). A number of different cells such as macrophages or killer cells participate in attempting to inactivate, isolate, or remove the foreign substance. Sometimes a change in shape and size of a

material can trigger a defensive response; solid materials may be tolerated, but small particles of the same material from an implant will often result in a response that will include inflammation and bone resorption.

– Bones lose mineral content with age and become weaker. Osteoporosis is an age-related disease that affects females more significantly than males. Cartilage, present in load-bearing joints, can wear away with time or because of osteoarthritis. In severe instances, replacement with an artificial joint may be required if the patient is to remain mobile.

References

1. Cerruti, M., & Sahai, N. (2006). Silicate biomaterials for orthopedic and dental implants. *Reviews in Minerology and Geochemistry, 64*, 283–313.
2. Anderson, J. (2001). Biological responses to materials. *Annual Reviews in Materials Research, 31*, 81–110.
3. Anderson, J., Rodriguez, A., & Chang, D. (2008). Foreign body reaction to biomaterials. *Seminars in Immunology, 20*, 86–100.
4. Kirsner, R., & Eaglstein, W. (1993). The wound healing process. *Dermatologic Clinics of North America, 11*, 629–640.
5. Currey, J. (1999). The design of mineralised hard tissue for their mechanical function. *Journal of Experimental Biology, 202*, 3285–3294.
6. Currey, J. (2002). *Bones. Structure and mechanics*. Princeton, NJ: Princeton University Press.
7. Seeman, E. (2003). The structural and biomechanical basis of the gain and loss of bone strength in women and men. *Endocrinology and Metabolism Clinics of North America, 32*, 25–38.
8. Park, J., & Lakes, R. (2007). *Biomaterials. An introduction* (3rd ed.). New York, NY: Springer.
9. Galkowski, V., Petrisor, B., Drew, B., & Dick, D. (2009). Bone stimulation for fracture healing: What's all the fuss? *Indian Journal of Orthopedics, 43*, 117–120.
10. Frost, H. (2001). From Wolff's law to the Utah paradigm: Insights about bone physiology and its clinical applications. *Anatomical Record, 262*, 398–419.
11. Melton, L., 3rd. (2000). Who has osteoporosis? A conflict between clinical and public health perspectives. *Journal of Bone and Mineral Research, 15*, 2309–2314.
12. Oxlund, H., Mosekilde, L., & Ortoft, G. (1996). Reduced concentration of collagen reducible cross links in human trabecular bone with respect to age and osteoporosis. *Bone, 19*, 479–848.
13. Heaney, R. (2003). Is the paradigm shifting? *Bone, 33*, 457–465.
14. Gage, B.F., Birman-Deych, E., Radford, M.J., Nilasena, D.S. & Binder, E.F. et al. (2006). Risk of osteoporotic fracture in elderly patients taking warfarin: Results from the national registry of atrial fibrillation 2. *Archives of Internal Medicine, 166*, 241–246.
15. Hubbard, R., Tattersfield, A., Smith, C., West, J., Smeeth, L. & Fletcher, A. et al. (2002). Inhaled corticosteroids and hip fracture: A population based case-control study. *American Journal of Respiratory and Critical Care Medicine, 166*, 1563–1566.
16. Zioupos, P., Currey, J., & Hamer, A. (1999). The role of collagen in the declining mechanical properties of aging human cortical bone. *Journal of Biomedical Materials Research, 45*, 108–116.
17. Chevalley, T., Hoffmayer, P., Bonjour, J.P. & Rizzoli, R. et al. (2002). An osteoporosis clinical pathway for the medical management of patients with low trauma fracture. *Osteoporosis International, 13*, 450–455.
18. Boot, A.M., de Ridder, M.A.J., Pols, H.A.P., Krenning, E.P. & de Muinck Keizer-Schrama, S.M.P.F. (1997). Bone mineral density in children and adolescents: Relation to puberty, calcium intake, and physical activity. *Journal of Clinical Endocrinology and Metabolism, 82*, 57–62.
19. Beshgetoor, D., Nichols, J., & Rego, I. (2000). Effect of training mode and calcium intake on bone mineral density in female master cyclists, runners, and non-athletes. *Intenational Journal of Sport Nutrition and Exercise Metabolism, 13*, 290–301.

Properties and Behavior of Materials and Some Design Considerations Too

7

"Mathematics (and materials science, our considered addition), rightly viewed, possesses not only truth, but supreme beauty."

Bertrand Russell

It is not always immediately appreciated that the human body and whatever devices are used to treat its diseases are made from materials. And therefore, a study and an understanding of the behavior and characteristics of materials can provide insights into failures of the body's tissues, as well as clues regarding the desirable properties of materials used for tissue replacement.

In this chapter, we will provide an introduction into materials science and engineering, explaining why materials behave as they do and how material properties may be characterized in a way to facilitate communication between engineers and physicians. It is likely that you have not been exposed to this content before in any health- or biology-related courses, so why are we introducing it now? Because we believe that it is helpful to learn about materials and how they are described and characterized before learning about implants made from those materials. We hope that you will gain a new appreciation for how implants are designed and how material properties are involved in implant performance.

7.1 Introduction

Where do the materials used for implants come from? In some cases, the patient is the source; for example, in the case of a bony nonunion (a situation when the ends of a broken bone are too far apart to grow together and heal), a small sample of bone can be obtained from the iliac crest (the edge of the hip bone) and implanted in the space between the two fractured ends. The implant will act as a seed to assist new

G.R. Baran et al., *Healthcare and Biomedical Technology in the 21st Century: An Introduction for Non-Science Majors*, DOI 10.1007/978-1-4614-8541-4_7,

bone growth. An implant that is obtained from the same organism that is also the recipient of the implant is called an "autograft."

However, a patient cannot always provide an adequate amount of implant material. There may be many broken bones, or much of the skin lost as the result of a burn, and what if the patient requires a new heart? Materials like bone can be obtained from other human donors, often cadavers; and because there are no artificial complete heart replacements, the only option is for a heart transplant from another human. An implant obtained from another organism that is of the same species is called an "allograft."

Although there are opportunities to obtain cadaver bone and to treat it with powerful chemicals so that it will not provoke a strong foreign body response by the recipient of the implant, the availability of complex and organized tissue structures such as heart valves from human donors is almost nonexistent. In these cases, pig heart valves can be used instead; the valves are similar in size and in function and have been shown to work in humans. Implants from species other than the recipient's are called "xenografts."

We have already discussed in the chapter on medical ethics how difficult it is to obtain donated organs for transplant, and earlier too (Chap. 6) we wrote about the foreign body response. Patients who undergo organ or tissue transplants need to be placed on immunosuppressive medication for their entire lives, and as a result, they run the risk of not being able to easily fend off common infections. Because at the present time there are few alternatives, there is a need to use implants made primarily of synthetic materials to replace or repair diseased or injured tissues or organs. The questions are which materials to use and how to design the implant so that it functions as needed and has an adequate lifetime that justifies the surgical procedure needed to insert the implant.

Selection of a particular material for an implant or prosthesis involves a consideration of material mechanical, physical, chemical, and biologic properties, as well as product-specific requirements such as ease or economy of processing and even appearance. In this chapter we will discuss synthetic and natural materials used in healthcare biotechnology and learn why different materials possess such a variation in properties and behavior.

7.2 Types of Synthetic Materials

There are essentially three classes of materials: metals, ceramics, and polymers. In order for any of them to be used in the body, they have to meet a stringent set of requirements. First, they should be "biocompatible," meaning that they cause no tissue reactions. However, it is just as important that the body does not significantly change desirable physical or chemical properties of the implant material and that any degradation of the material does not lead to the release of chemicals or particles that could be harmful to the body. The mechanical properties, such as strength and hardness, are also significant, but the exact requirements vary with the specific implant location and application. For example, an implant that replaces a portion of a large bone such as the femur must be able to carry some of the body's weight, while an implant that replaces a portion of the middle ear need not be chosen on the basis of its weight-carrying ability. Finally, implant materials must be able to be fabricated into specific shapes, their surfaces must lend themselves to be polished, and they must be sterilizable [1].

Metals include materials such as steel and copper, ceramics include materials such as glass and porcelain, and polymers (perhaps an unfamiliar word at this point) include materials such as Plexiglass, Teflon, and silk. Polymers are commonly called "plastics," but the word polymer is preferred, because it more accurately describes the molecular structure of these materials. The word "plastics" is used in everyday language because many polymers can be easily shaped and molded, i.e., they are "plastic" in a way similar to plasticine or modeling clay.

These three classes of materials are made using different processes, possess quite different properties, and yet one can find examples of all three classes being used in the manufacture of medical implants and medical devices. The challenge for the engineer designing a medical device is to determine which material is best suited for any given application; and in order to do that, a way to describe the design and material property requirements must be found and used. After all, it does little good to state that a "strong" material is needed without specifying what exactly is meant by the word "strong." There could be no possibility of unambiguous communication between the designer and the eventual client (e.g., hospital, surgeon) unless a common language was used. In the next few sections of this chapter, we will first discuss some fundamental aspects of the three classes of materials, then introduce the terminology used to describe material properties, and provide examples of specific materials and their biomedical applications.

7.2.1 Metals

In considering which synthetic materials are most often used to replace missing or diseased tissues, it would be apparent that metals are most frequently used for load-bearing implants such as artificial hips and knees. Metals are ubiquitous in contemporary life and are among the oldest synthetic materials "domesticated" by man. Today, they are used for orthopedic implants, surgical staples and wires, bone screws, dental implants, artificial heart valve components, stents, etc. Metals are used either in their pure, elemental state (e.g., titanium) or combined with other metals and nonmetals in an alloy (e.g., stainless steel). We all have a kind of "gut" feeling about the properties of metals, and the way in which metals behave can be readily explained by the way in which metal atoms are assembled.

A pure metal contains only one kind of atom. In metals, the atoms are arranged in a regular and orderly arrangement as shown in Fig. 7.1. Of course this is only a two-dimensional view, and in reality the atoms are arranged in three dimensions.

The atoms have a neutral charge; the importance of this will become apparent later. This orderly arrangement is called a "crystalline" structure as opposed to a disordered arrangement which would be called an "amorphous" structure. Crystalline used here

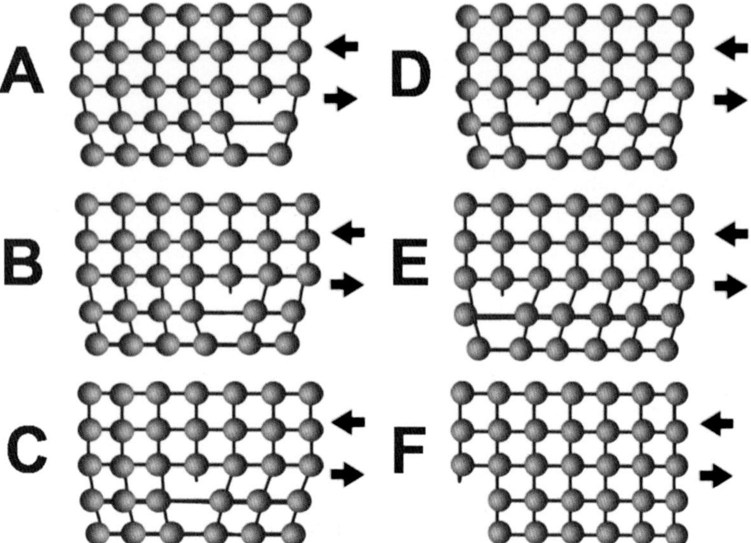

Fig. 7.1 Idealized depiction of metal atoms with a dislocation showing how metals are able to deform. In drawing **a**, note the dislocation (the line of atoms second from the *right*). In succeeding drawings **b** through **e**, the application of a shear force causes the dislocation to move from right to left. Eventually, in **f**, it has left the shape of the atoms permanently changed. This process mimics plastic or permanent deformation in metals. Note too that each movement was made easier by the presence of the dislocation, as the atoms had vacant space to move into

does not mean the sparkling glass used to make vases or costume jewelry, but rather the orderly arrangement of atoms. In metals, the exact type of arrangement can be different in different elements. Because it is extremely unlikely that a perfect crystal would form when liquid metal cools and freezes, imperfections are known to exist, but these can be beneficial. In Fig. 7.1, for example, there is a missing row of atoms shown; this is called a "dislocation" in metallurgy. If we were to apply a shear force to this grouping of atoms, then the dislocation will travel from the right to the left. In the end (drawing f), the crystal has undergone a translational movement, i.e., a permanent change in its shape. The phenomenon of dislocation movement is called "slip."

Imagine this going on literally in millions of locations in a piece of metal, such as, for example, in a piece of wire that's being bent or a sheet of metal forged into the shape of an automobile body. If there were no dislocation imperfections and the crystal structure were to be perfect, it would require a great deal more force to deform the wire. The ability to shape metals is critical for the manufacture of countless metallic goods, so it may be said that dislocations make metalworking possible.

If we consider the structure of metal alloy (not a pure metal), where there is a mixture of different atoms of different sizes, it is possible to speculate on the effect that alloying will have on the deformation potential of metals. In essence, an alloy is made by dissolving one or more metallic elements in another metallic element. In Fig. 7.2, an idealized structure of several types of alloys is shown.

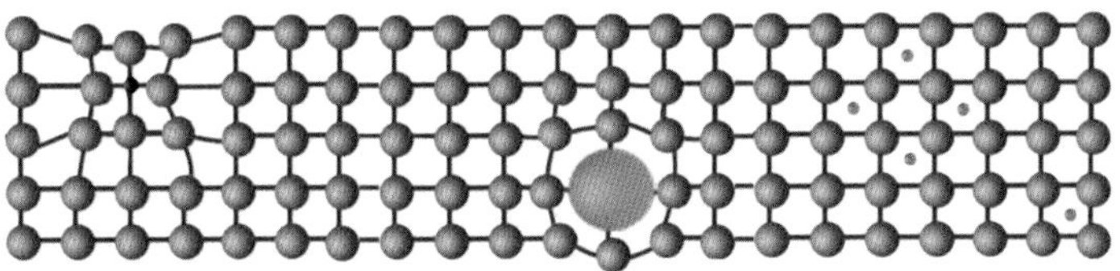

Fig. 7.2 Idealized depiction of substitutional and interstitial alloys. The substitutional alloy is shown on the *left*, where a small atom has replaced (substituted) one of the larger gray atoms, and in the *middle*, where a large green atom has replaced (substituted) for one of the gray atoms. The interstitial alloy is shown on the *right*, where small green atoms have found their way into the spaces (interstices) between atoms of the parent metal

The result of the additions of elements has also had the effect of somewhat distorting the regularity of the crystal structure; it remains ordered, but there are indications of strain, shown by the distorted drawings of "bonds" between the atoms of the host element. If you imagine that a force is applied to the structure, it may be easily understood that the presence of the foreign alloying elements makes any dislocation movement more difficult, and therefore more force is required to deform the alloy. If deformation is more difficult to achieve, we have in essence strengthened the original host metal! This is one reason why alloying is done: to achieve solid solution strengthening.

In addition to the application of force, another way to shape metals is by casting them, i.e., heating them to a high temperature so that they melt then pouring the liquid metal into a mold. This is a process invented thousands of years ago and is usually the first step after refining metal ore. Casting can be an efficient way to fabricate a complex piece to near-final shape, and a technique called the "lost wax" process has been used for centuries to fabricate jewelry and statues. In this method, a wax pattern of the desired object is made then covered with a clay and sand mixture that is allowed to harden. The assembly is heated until the wax melts and runs out (the lost wax), then molten metal is poured into the mold. When metals solidify from a melt, they form grains that are visible under a microscope (Figs. 7.3 and 7.4).

Grains are found in both pure metals and in alloys. Grains form grain boundaries where they meet (the dark lines in Fig. 7.3d). In Fig. 7.4, separate grains are easily visible. The boundaries are a direct result of the misalignment in crystal structure from one grain to its neighbor, and one could imagine that a dislocation in one grain could not easily move through a grain boundary into another grain. This insight reveals a second way to strengthen metals: the smaller the metal grains, the higher the grain boundary content in a given area of metal and the shorter the distance that a dislocation may travel before being stopped at a grain boundary. Once a dislocation cannot move, further deformation of the metal becomes difficult; grain refinement (decreasing grain size) is therefore an effective strengthening mechanism. Grain boundaries are also the locations where impurities segregate during freezing. These grain boundaries therefore will have a different composition than the grain itself, and this disparity in composition has consequences for the corrosion behavior of the metal.

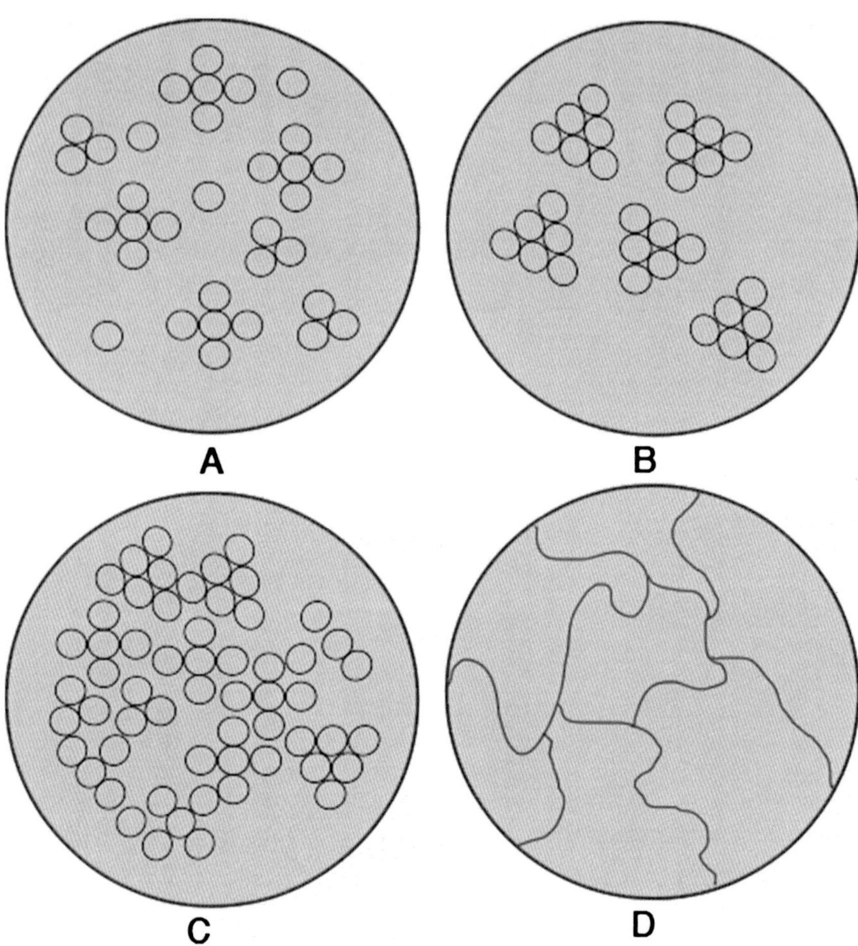

Fig. 7.3 Diagram of the formation of grains from a melt showing how the crystal structure in each grain is aligned differently than in the neighboring grains

In metals, therefore, their "malleability," or the ease or degree to which they may be permanently deformed, is a function of dislocation density, grain size, and the inherent interatomic forces. Any process that hinders dislocation movement will have the effect of strengthening a metal, and conversely, any process that enables dislocation movement will weaken a metal. For example, the sequence of events in a blacksmith shop or in some other metalworking operation is typically to first heat the metal (an increased temperature will provide vibrational energy to atoms and make dislocation movement easier), deform the metal (dislocations undergo slip and become trapped at grain boundaries, or they interfere with each other and deformation becomes increasingly difficult), then reheat the metal (increase in temperature will help release pinned dislocations and can enable grain growth) prior to further attempts at deforming the metal.

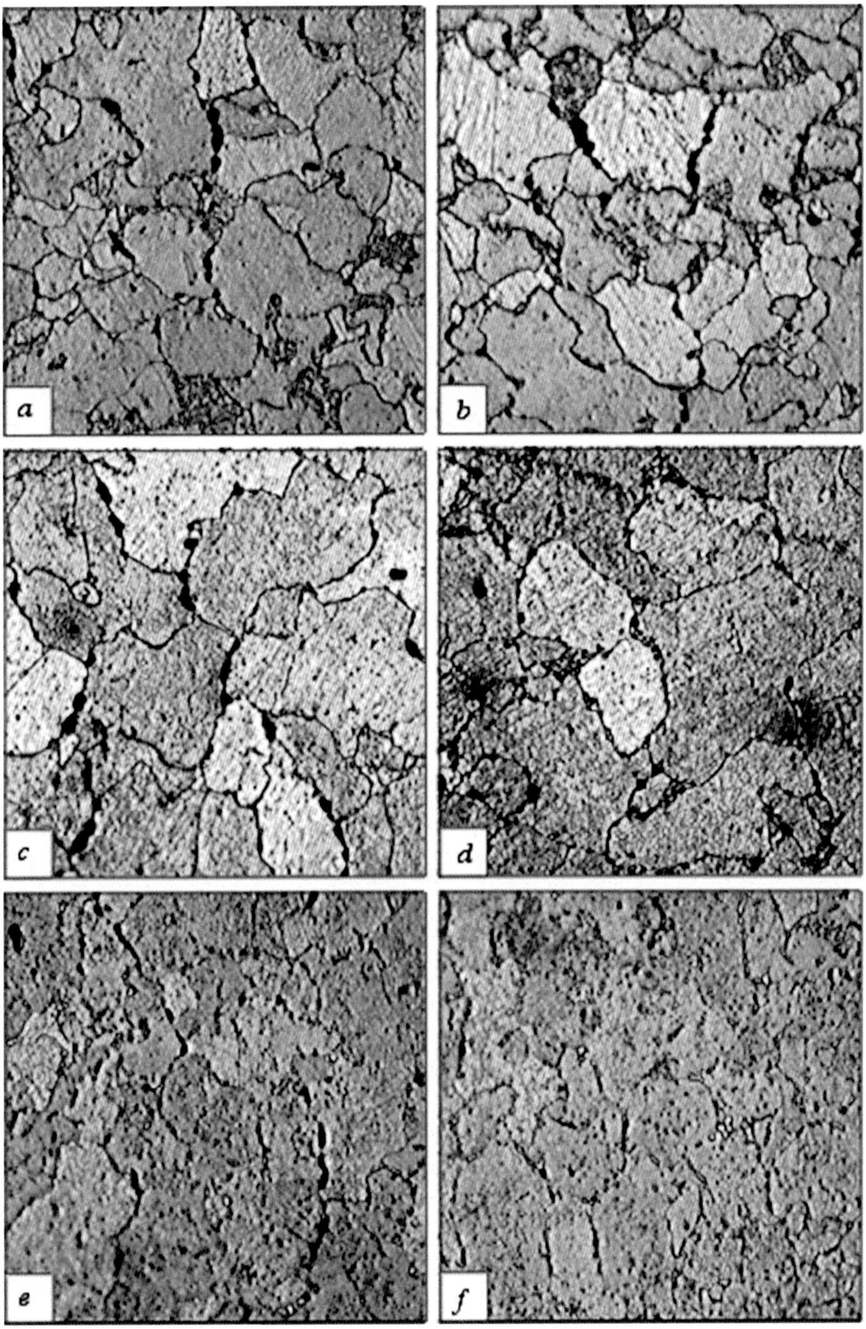

Fig. 7.4 Microscope images of metal grains of various sizes. Copyright Springer Science + Business Media New York

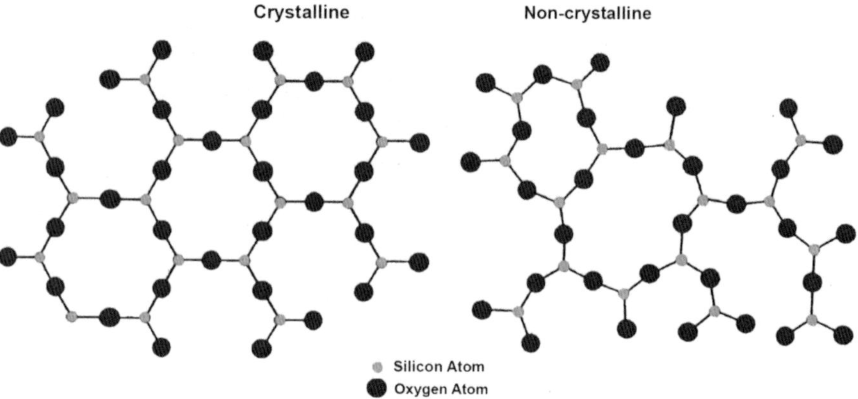

Fig. 7.5 A depiction of the structure of silica (SiO_2) in two forms: crystalline (quartz) and non-crystalline or amorphous (fused silica)

7.2.2 Ceramics and Glasses

Examples of ceramic materials include brick, cement, glass, all the precious and semiprecious stones such as rubies and amethysts, and computer memory materials, a wide range indeed. They behave quite differently than metals, and just as the structure of metals is responsible for their characteristics, so too is the rather different structure of ceramic materials responsible for their properties.

Ceramics and glasses are usually composed of oxides, which are chemical compounds consisting of a metal or the element silicon and the element oxygen. In contrast to metals, which are composed of atoms in a neutral state, ceramics consist of ions, which are atoms that have lost or gained electrons. Ions therefore have a charge associated with them; an atom that loses a single electron will become an ion with a single (excess) positive charge, while an atom that gains a single electron will become an ion with a single (excess) negative charge. As in many cases, opposites attract; with ions of opposite charge, the attraction is quite strong. However, unlike metals which almost always are crystalline, ceramics may be crystalline or amorphous; this difference in structure has important consequences for the physical properties of ceramics.

To understand more about ceramic structure, we can look at an idealized depiction of the ionic distribution in silica, the most common mineral on earth (Fig. 7.5). The chemical formula for silica, also known as silicon dioxide, is SiO_2. Silica is found on every beach in the world and is the main component of glass.

In this figure, the crystalline form of silica on the left (commonly called quartz) is regular and orderly; the structure possesses long-range order. The noncrystalline or amorphous form of silica on the right is not regular; the structure is distorted, and the angles of the lines drawn to represent ionic bonds are all slightly different as well.

The crystalline form of silica is obtained when molten silica is allowed to cool very slowly until it becomes solid, as the slow cooling process permits all the ions to assume well-ordered positions. The noncrystalline form on the right is commonly

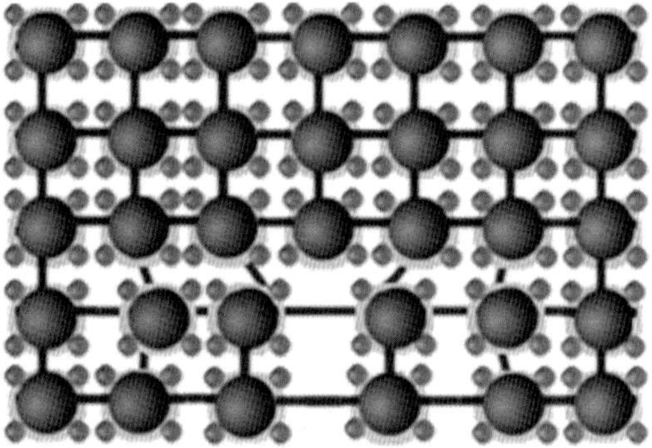

Fig. 7.6 Depiction of a dislocation in a crystalline ceramic structure. A row of missing unit cells (groups of positive and negative ions) is responsible

called fused silica and is obtained when molten silica is cooled more quickly and the ions do not have time to assume well-ordered positions.

In ionic materials, the dislocation situation is somewhat more complex than in metals; the structure is required to maintain an overall charge balance, so that if a negatively charged ion is missing, a positively charged ion must be missing too. That makes the appearance of dislocations in ionic crystals such as ceramics rather more complex than in metals, as entire assemblies of linked positive and negative ions (called unit cells) must be missing for the dislocation to be actually present (Fig. 7.6).

In this structure, it is apparent that in order for movement or deformation to occur, one row or plane of ions must slide past another row of ions. If this is to occur in a row containing both positive and negative ions, then it is inevitable that at some point the negative ions in one row will approach the negative ions in the neighboring row and the positive ions in one row will approach the positive ions in the neighboring row. Because both groups of ions have similar charges, the negative ions will repel each other, and the positive ions will repel each other, in effect making it more difficult for movement or slip to occur. It is the like-charge repulsion which makes ceramics and ionic materials so resistant to plastic or permanent deformation.

If the regularity of the structure is partially responsible for hindering slip in ionic crystals, then perhaps a change in structure will enable deformation. A change from a crystalline to an amorphous structure, as shown in Fig. 7.5, provides for relatively greater interionic distances, and with the additional vibrational energy provided by higher temperatures, the fused silica will flow. Still another example of structure–property relationships is provided by common clay. This naturally occurring mineral is a complex mixture of many oxides arranged in a complex pattern as shown in Fig. 7.7.

The groups of tetrahedra based on silicon, aluminum, iron, or magnesium are arranged in sheets; when water is present, it finds its way between these sheets. It is this structural feature that provides damp clays with their slippery feel.

The way that metals and ceramics or glasses deal with flaws, however, is quite different. For example, a scratch on the surface of a piece of glass is a flaw, a crack waiting to grow. Automobile windows that are chipped by flying gravel require repair because if none is performed, the chip will grow in size until the window

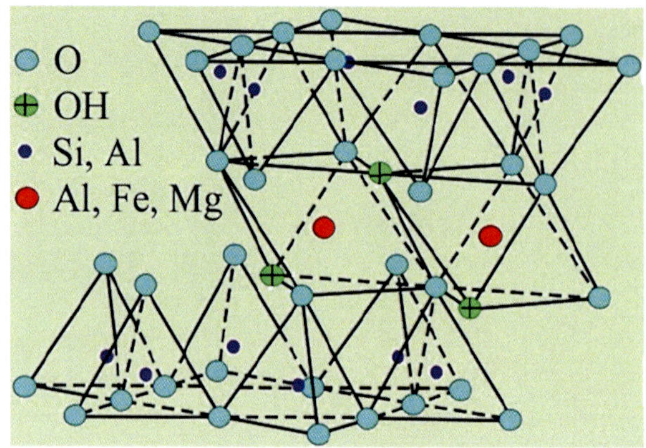

Fig. 7.7 The structure of common clay. Copyright Springer Science+Business Media B.V.

breaks; a scratch on a pane of glass is sufficient to behave as the source of the crack that follows when the pane is stressed. On the other hand, metal surfaces contain many scratches or flaws without any obvious harm to their mechanical properties.

The intrinsic flaws (scratches, bubbles) present in glasses and ceramics are called Griffith flaws. Griffith proposed a novel explanation for the strength of glass in 1921, following the observation that although the theoretical strength of glass (calculated using the strength of interionic bonds) was quite high, on the order of 1,000,000 lb/in^2 or more, the measured strength was considerably lower. He formulated an equation for the strength of glass as follows:

$$\sigma_f = \left(\sqrt{2E\gamma / \pi}\right) / \sqrt{a},$$

where σ_f is the fracture strength, E is Young's modulus (a measure of stiffness), γ is the surface energy of the material, and "a" is the length of the flaw. In essence, this equation predicts that the failure strength of a material is inversely proportional to the square of the flaw size; the larger the crack, the weaker the material. This prediction has been verified in many experimental studies of glasses. However, the equation fails for metals and other materials that are capable of plastic deformation. That's because the magnitude of stress concentration at the crack tip assumed by Griffith does not occur in those materials, because they dissipate stress by deforming at the crack tip, thereby blunting the crack. A consequence of this finding is that the strength of glasses and ceramics is strongly dependent on the way they are prepared. A ceramic or glass body containing small flaws such as bubbles or surface scratches will be stronger than the same body containing large flaws. Also, any techniques, such as surface polishing, that reduce the size of the flaw will serve to strengthen the component.

While metals are made by refining from ores and subsequent melting, casting, and machining or plastic-forming operations, ceramics and glasses are shaped using other techniques. Ceramic materials possess melting temperatures that are too high for practical casting; hardly any mold could be made to contain them. Instead, ceramic bodies are prepared either from powders of naturally occurring oxide

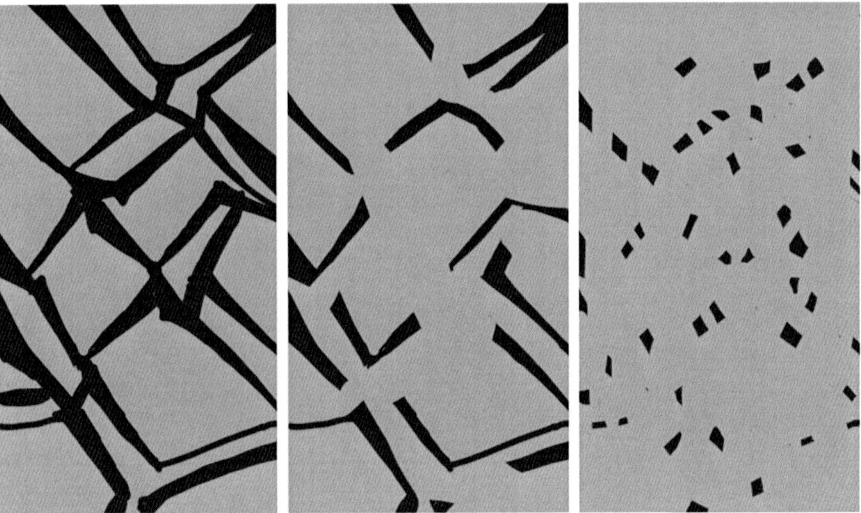

Fig. 7.8 Idealized illustration of the sintering process

minerals or from oxides converted from pure non-oxide compounds, blending the oxides together in the proper proportions, then forming the powders into a useful final shape in a process called sintering. The finely powdered ceramics are first either compacted under pressure in a mold or, with fluid added to form a "slip," poured into a mold. After the slip has dried, both the pressure-molded and the slip-formed components have adequate strength to be handled and are then heated for a period of some hours or days (the time depends on the specific ceramic) to allow the process of sintering to occur, illustrated in Fig. 7.8.

During sintering, the particles begin to fuse together at points of contact. With time, the contact areas become larger, and eventually the particles become one large mass. Often, air is entrapped, resulting in residual pores (which then become Griffith flaws). Usually, the particles do not undergo melting.

Glasses, in contrast to crystalline ceramic materials, have historically been prepared by melting together the various minerals and components in a large crucible then pouring the viscous melt into molds to form a finished item or into water where the glass breaks up and is eventually ground into a finer powder called a "frit." Frit can be also be used in molding processes. Today, there are chemical synthetic methods relying on "sol-gel" techniques that produce complex glasses and ceramics which could not be made using melting methods.

7.2.3 Pyrolytic Carbon

Pyrolytic carbons are a unique class of materials. Although they consist almost entirely of carbon (C) and would normally be treated as an organic material, their method of manufacture and their mechanical properties are ceramic-like. This form of carbon is entirely man-made, and its structure is unlike any of the naturally occurring forms of carbon including graphite or diamond. Pyrolytic carbon is only available as a coating and was originally developed to coat pellets of radioactive elements for use in nuclear reactors. It was discovered that this material also has outstanding compatibility with blood; it does not support clotting and also appears to not fatigue; its mechanical properties do not deteriorate with use. Now, almost every artificial heart valve has components that are coated with pyrolytic carbon. Anticlotting drugs still need to be taken by patients with artificial heart valves, but pyrolytic carbon is superior to other synthetic materials in this application.

The process for manufacturing carbon-coated components begins with a "preform." This is a substrate shaped in the form of the final product but somewhat smaller (because the coating will add to the final size). The preform is made of a material which can withstand high temperatures; metals such as tantalum, rhenium–molybdenum alloy, or graphite may be used. The preform is cleaned and placed in a "fluidized bed reactor," a metal vessel that contains small ceramic particles. An inert gas such as nitrogen flows from underneath the bed of particles, suspending them. The preform is also present in the reactor, which is heated to temperatures above 1,000 °C, and a hydrocarbon gas such as ethane (C_2H_6) is allowed to flow into the reactor chamber. Because no oxygen is present, the hydrocarbon gas does not burn, but dissociates into atoms of carbon and hydrogen, and the free carbon atoms coat the preform and the ceramic particles. After a suitably thick (a few hundreds of microns) coating is formed, the piece is taken out, machined if necessary to final dimensions, and highly polished using diamond paste. During assembly of heart valves, care must be taken because pyrolytic carbon is quite brittle, and excessive bending of the disc will cause cracks to form.

7.2.4 Polymers

Polymer materials are used more frequently as medical device components than any other class of material. These organic (carbon-containing) substances occur in nature but can also be synthesized in the laboratory. The word "polymer" comes from two Greek words, the first being the prefix "poly" meaning many and the second "meros," meaning parts. Accordingly, polymers are composed of many parts connected together. A useful way to imagine what the structure of polymers looks like is to think of them as a chain of individual units connected together (Fig. 7.9).

In a piece of ultrahigh molecular weight polyethylene (UHMWPE), there are millions of molecules existing together in chains, all tangled together. It's possible to think of them resembling a bowl of spaghetti. Of course, it's not necessary that each chain remains as a simple strand. It's possible to synthesize chains with other configurations (Fig. 7.10). Here, in addition to a simple linear polymer, are idealized renderings of other polymer configurations.

In order to learn about the phenomenon of cross-linking, it may be useful to reconsider the bowl of spaghetti noodles, imagining them after they have cooled and rested for several hours. Any attempt to pick out an individual strand will be

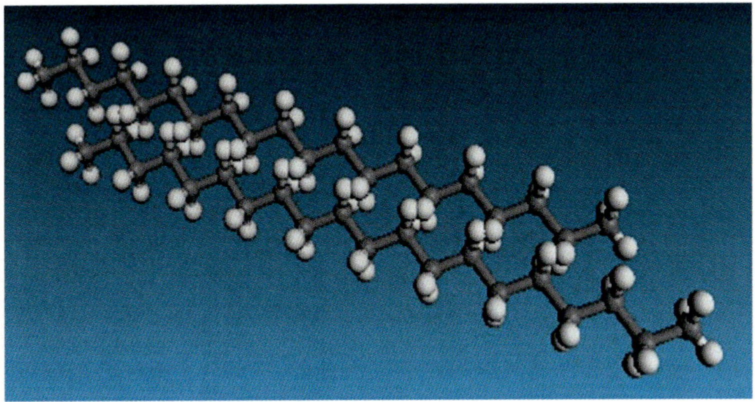

Fig. 7.9 A depiction of a simple polymer chain of poly(ethylene). It is composed from mers of ethylene. In this illustration, the carbon atoms are *dark spheres*, and the hydrogen atoms are the *light-colored spheres*. An ethylene mer consists of two carbon atoms, each bonded to two hydrogen atoms. In the real world, the chain can contain 200,000 individual ethylene units forming a single molecule of ultrahigh molecular weight polyethylene (UHMWPE), the material used as a liner in artificial hips and knees (and the bottom of snow skis and snowboards). The number of monomers in a polymer molecule is termed the "degree of polymerization." Copyrighted by Springer Science+Business Media, LLC

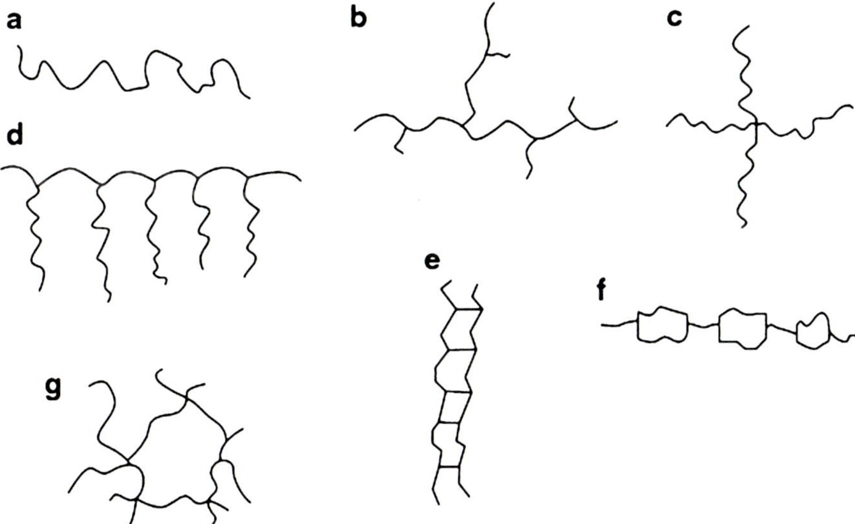

Fig. 7.10 Representations of polymer chain structures. (**a**) Linear polymer, (**b**) branched polymer, (**c**) star-shaped polymer, (**d**) comb shaped polymer, (**e**) ladder polymer, (**f**) semiladder polymer, and (**g**) network structure. Copyright Springer Science+Business Media LLC

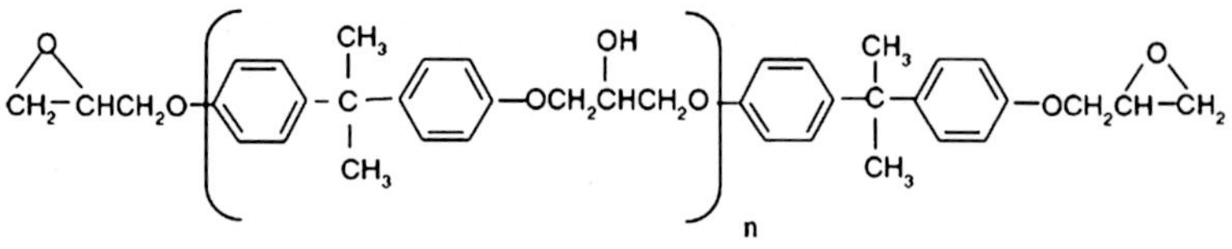

Fig. 7.11 Structure of an epoxy resin. Copyright Springer Science + Business Media B.V.

fruitless, as the spaghetti strands have become connected (glued) to each other. This is simulated in drawing "e" in Fig. 7.10 above, which depicts two polymer chains connected to each other by "cross-links." The two chains cannot move individually; a load applied to one strand is shared by the other. If many polymer chains are cross-linked in this way, it is readily understood that a cross-linked polymer is stronger than a simple linear polymer, even though their compositions may be identical.

The power of cross-linking was discovered accidentally by Charles Goodyear in approximately 1840. At that time, there was a great deal of interest in natural rubber, as it was thought that many useful articles could be made from it, including life preservers and shoes. Unfortunately, pieces made from natural rubber deteriorated with time; they would rot and were unable to withstand raised temperatures. In addition, the natural rubber was sticky and difficult to work with. Goodyear, who had had a roller-coaster history in business, decided it would be worthwhile to experiment with natural rubber in hopes of making it more useful. He worked in an old factory building he bought and pursued a strategy of adding various dry powdered chemicals, one after the other, to the sticky rubber. One story about his discovery has it that one day, he went to the local store to brag about his latest mixture, which included sulfur powder. The news was greeted with laughter, and Goodyear became so angry that he threw the piece of rubber he had brought. It accidentally landed on top of a hot stove, and after Goodyear managed to retrieve it, he noticed that the properties of the rubber had changed; it was no longer sticky. Continued experimentation led to the vulcanization process, which consisted of mixing sulfur powder with natural rubber and heating. The durable material which resulted was soon in use in the USA and in England. Forty years later, two brothers from Ohio founded a tire company and named it after the inventor of the vulcanization process.

Of course, most polymers are not as simple as poly(ethylene). In fact, most have complex structures. Just for comparison, Fig. 7.11 depicts the structure of an epoxy resin material, similar to that found in epoxy cements. The six-sided rings are representations of structures with carbon atoms at each corner. Also, polymers can have more than one type of repeat unit (mer); these are called "copolymers," as shown in Fig. 7.12. In these representations, A and B denote mers with two different compositions. The figure shows that the monomers may be distributed randomly, in a block arrangement, or as a graft copolymer.

The reactions that result in the bonding of individual monomer units together are called "polymerization" reactions. There are two common reactions, "addition" and "condensation."

Addition polymerization reactions are simpler; they also involve catalysts and accelerators, but no by-product is given off. The end of the polymer chain is activated, and additional units are added on with the active site continually migrating to

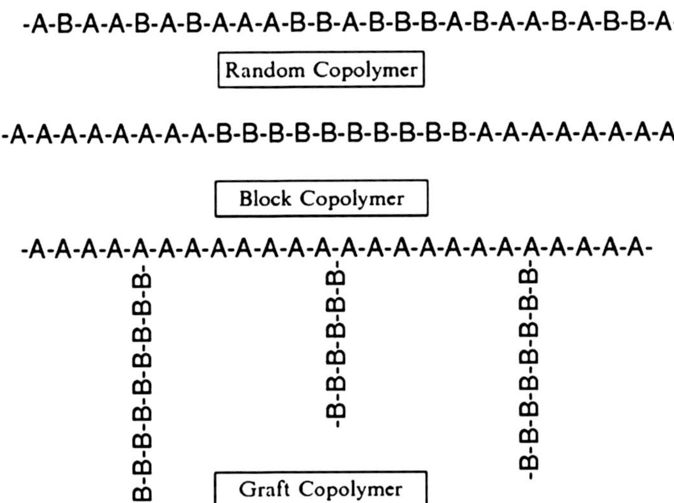

Fig. 7.12 Representations of various kinds of copolymers. Copyright Springer Science + Business Media B.V.

the end of the chain. Examples of addition polymerizing materials are synthetic rubbers, polystyrene (Styrofoam), polytetrafluoroethylene (Teflon), polymethyl methacrylate (Plexiglass), and polyvinylidene chloride (Saran wrap).

Polymers react to heat in different ways. Thermosetting polymers keep their shape once they are polymerized; heating them will only degrade them. Thermoplastic polymers can change their shape because they soften and flow when heated. The explanation for the difference in behavior lies in their structures. Thermoset polymers have undergone some cross-linking, so that their shape is permanent; reheating will not permit reshaping. Thermoset polymers cannot be recycled, but are generally less expensive than thermoplastic polymers.

Because of their long chains, polymers are difficult to crystallize, and the basic structural component of an ordered region is not an atom or ion, but rather a chain. In Fig. 7.13, a crystalline polymer is visualized; in some areas, the chains are aligned to form a type of crystal, but the ordered regions are bounded by disordered regions. Whereas crystalline structures in metals and ceramics are obtained by slow cooling from a melt allowing atoms or ions to occupy preferred locations, in polymers the ordered structures are most often obtained by mechanical methods. Forcing a polymer through a narrow opening like a nozzle orients the polymer chains in the direction of flow. In general, amorphous polymers are transparent, while crystalline polymers are opaque.

Polymer components are fabricated in ways that depend on whether they are thermoplastic or thermosetting. Thermoplastic polymers are prepared in a chemical plant, and during their synthesis and polymerization, additives such as colors, mechanical property modifiers, antioxidants, reinforcing fillers or opacifiers, lubricants, and mold release agents are added. Ultraviolet light stabilizers will be added to articles that are meant for outdoor use; polymers degrade in the presence of UV

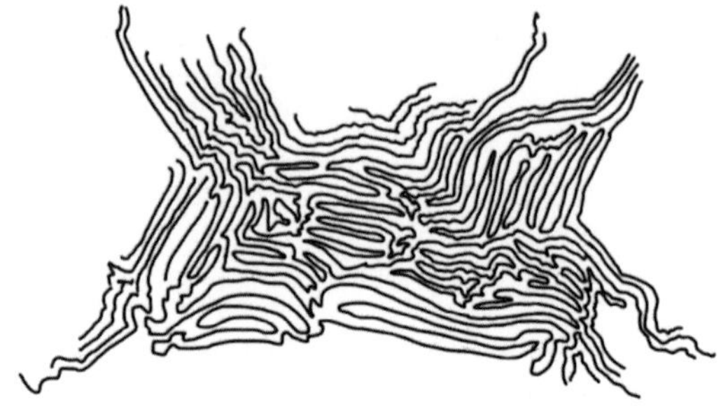

Fig. 7.13 Representation of a crystalline polymer. The polymer chains are folded together, and in some areas, they form a somewhat regular and ordered structure

light, and the stabilizers absorb UV. The product leaving the plant is in the form of granules; these granules are used by fabricators who heat and inject or force them into molds that provide a final shape. Gas may be bubbled through the polymer in order to produce porosity. After cooling, the finished article is removed, although fibers may also be drawn from thermoplastic polymers by forcing the molten mass through a small diameter nozzle; the fibers can later be used to weave cloth. Thermosetting polymers are usually processed to final shape at the same time they polymerize. A non-polymerized mixture has its catalyst added just prior to filling a mold so that the polymerization occurs within the mold.

7.2.5 Composites

The materials known as composites include fiberglass, concrete, plywood, and gypsum board. In all these examples, different materials are brought together to form a new structure or material that is somehow better than any of the individual components. In a composite, the individual components remain visible, unlike in an alloy, where the various metallic and nonmetallic elements are mixed together to form a uniform solution.

One of the components in a composite will typically be a continuous phase called the matrix, i.e., it will be the mortar or glue that surrounds and holds the components together (Fig. 7.14). In fiberglass, the matrix is a resin polymer; in concrete, the matrix is Portland cement. The other component in a composite will be a discontinuous phase, i.e., present as separate pieces, and will also be considered the reinforcing phase, providing strength to the composite. In fiberglass, the reinforcing phase is the glass fibers, while in concrete, the reinforcing phase is gravel. The reinforcing phase may be in the form of particles, fibers, or woven cloth.

Composites are likely to have mechanical properties quite different than the individual phases. For example, fiberglass is used in many applications including the hulls of smaller boats, and it is the presence of the glass fibers that makes fiberglass strong enough for that purpose. Certainly no one would consider building a boat hull from a brittle material like glass or from a soft and weak material such as a polymer resin. And yet, the combination works very well. In designing composites, materials engineers purposely choose materials that have some desirable property, such as strength, and combine it with another material that can be easily processed or handled.

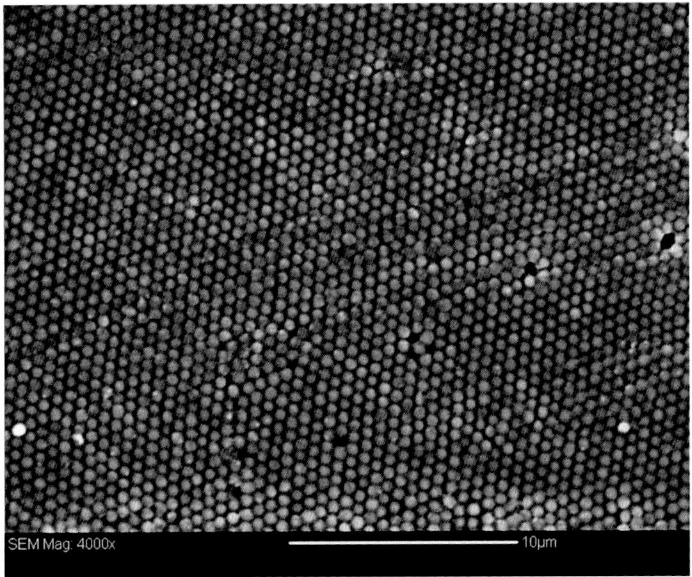

Fig. 7.14 A scanning electron microscope image of a particle reinforced composite. The *light spheres* are the reinforcing particles (made of glass), dispersed in a dark matrix phase (consisting of a polymer). Although in this case the particles have an ordered arrangement, in many composites the particles do not have an ordered arrangement

Today, composites are used in applications ranging from bicycle frames, golf club shafts, hockey sticks, airplane bodies (the Boeing Dreamliner 787), helicopter components, and body armor. In medical biotechnology, composites are used as dental restorative materials (the white filling material now used to repair fractured or decayed teeth), for orthopedic implants, and for rehabilitation equipment. The great advantage of composite materials as implants is that their modulus of elasticity may be closely matched to that of bone, so that the likelihood of stress shielding will be minimized.

7.3 Surface Properties

All implanted medical devices have surfaces which interact with physiologic fluids, particularly blood, as was discussed in Chap. 6. The surface of a piece of material is special; it has a free energy associated with it. Atoms in the interior of a piece of material are surrounded by other atoms of the same material, and as a result, they all coexist in a kind of equilibrium with a balance of attractive and repelling forces. The atoms on the surface, however, are missing neighbors on one side. This imbalance of forces results in an excess energy, and in order to reduce the surface free energy, a coating on the surface is energetically favored (to provide the missing neighbor atoms). Materials with high surface energies will be more easily coated than materials with a low surface energy (the reduction in energy being more dramatic for the high surface energy situation).

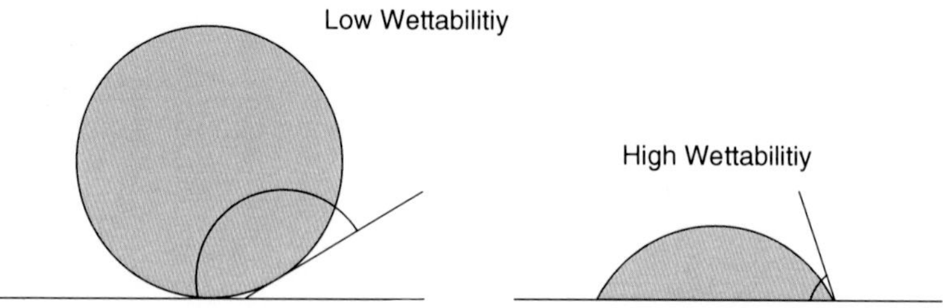

Fig. 7.15 The contact angle of a liquid with a solid is used as wettability index

The coating can occur either by adsorption (when the coating molecules adhere to only the surface) or by absorption (when the coating molecules are partially dissolved into the material and penetrate beyond the surface). In the body, implants are coated by adsorbed (not absorbed) proteins and other substances found in blood or cells. Proteins can be absorbed only if the material of the implant is porous or if the implant degrades and dissolves, permitting penetration of proteins into the interior.

The ease with which a surface can be coated is sometimes expressed as "wettability," although in this expression, the entire system (surface and coating agent) has to be considered. A way to think about wettability is to imagine placing a drop of the coating liquid onto a material surface and observing what happens (Fig. 7.15).

In Fig. 7.15, the system on the left exhibits a low wettability. The contact angle for that system is greater than 90°. In the system on the right, with high wettability, the contact angle is less than 90°, and you can imagine that adding more drops onto the surface will enable the entire surface to be easily covered. If we were to perform this experiment using water and obtained the same results, we would say that the surface in the system on the left is hydrophobic (water-fearing), while the surface in the system on the right is hydrophilic (water-loving).

Still another chemical characterization of a surface is its charge. We probably all recall school experiments with static electricity, when a balloon rubbed against a sweater accumulated a charge. Material surfaces can also carry an electrical charge, making them slightly positive (in which case they attract negatively charged molecules) or slightly negative (in which case they would attract positively charged molecules). Implant materials may also be given certain treatments, for example, by exposure to a gas plasma, which induces surface charges.

7.4 Mechanical Behavior of Materials

If we were to place an order to an implant manufacturer requesting that the implant had to be strong, what exactly would that mean? The word "strong" is as vague and unspecific to the materials scientist/engineer and to the manufacturing engineer as the word "blue" would be to a painter, or the word "fast" to an athlete, or the word "unfair" to an attorney. All professions have a vocabulary that is used to define precisely what is being discussed, and the field of biotechnology is no exception.

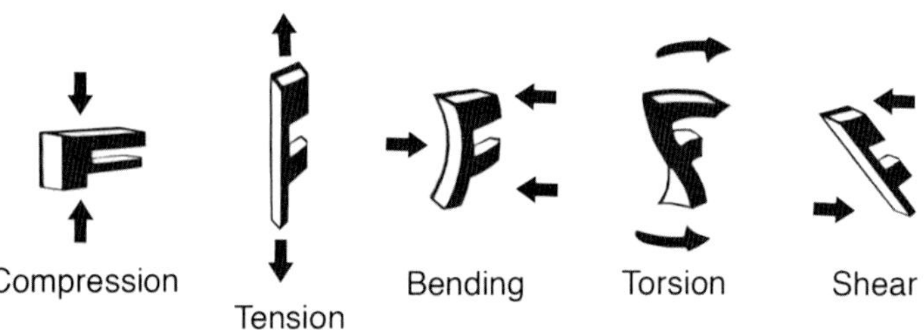

Fig. 7.16 Different modes of applying a load

7.4.1 Static (No Time Variable Involved) Mechanical Behavior

The mechanical behavior of materials is important in applications when an implant or device is subjected to forces in the body, and it is desirable that the implant or device remains stable in the face of these forces. Let's start by considering the ways in which forces can be applied (Fig. 7.16).

In "compression" loading, the atoms or molecules in a material are squeezed together. A consequence of compression is that the piece being compressed becomes shorter in the direction of compression and bulges out in a direction perpendicular to the compression direction. One can readily imagine that the long bones of the legs and the vertebrae of the spine undergo routine compression loading.

In "tensile" loading, the atoms or molecules in a material are pulled apart. A consequence of tension is that the material becomes longer (stretches) in the direction of loading and becomes smaller (thinner) perpendicular to the direction of tensile loading. However, in bending loading, one side of the beam (where a single arrow is providing the load) will get shorter, i.e., will be in compression, while the other side (where two arrows provide the load) will get longer, i.e., it will be in tension. There is a plane called the neutral axis in the middle of the beam that experiences neither tension nor compression. Our bones experience bending daily; anytime we lift with our arms while contracting the biceps muscle, the forearm bones (the radius and ulna) are loaded in bending mode.

Torsional loading applies a twist to the structure, while shear loading is similar to the action of shears (scissors). The vertebral column in the human spine experiences torsional loading regularly, while shear occurs when our teeth slide past each other during chewing.

Because many tissues in the body are loaded at one time or another by the weight of the body itself, perhaps the most obvious question an implant design engineer would ask is what is the required "strength" of the replacement material? To answer this question, it is necessary to first agree on a definition of strength, determine the strength of the tissue that is being replaced, and compare it with the strength of available biocompatible materials. These material properties serve as important factors used in computing the structural behavior of the specific implant design.

A relatively simple way to obtain information about the strength, stiffness, and deformation potential of a material is to conduct a tensile test. This procedure is

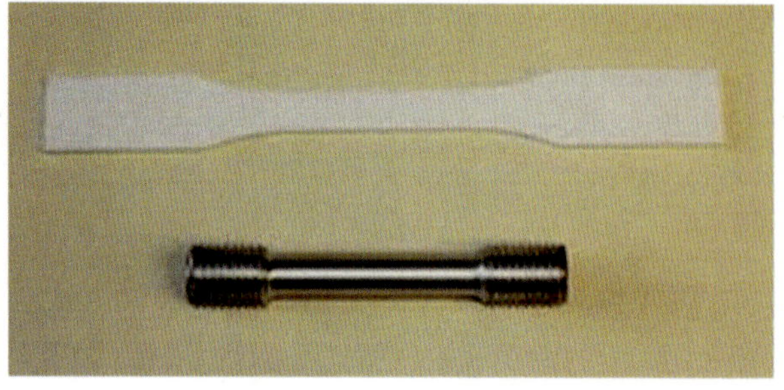

Fig. 7.17 Standard round metal and standard flat polymer tensile specimens

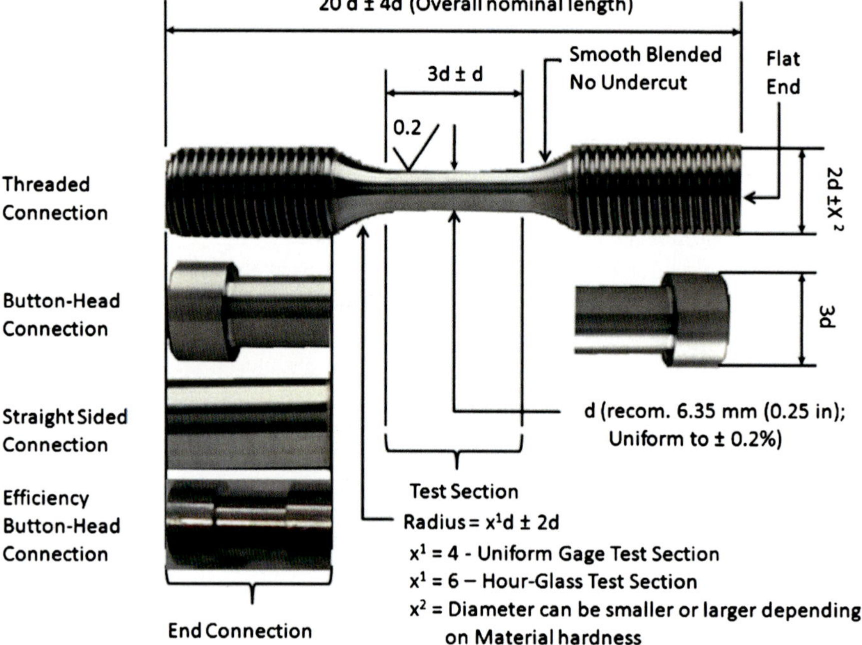

Fig. 7.18 Nomenclature for tensile test specimens. Photo courtesy of MTS Systems Corporation

most often used to characterize the mechanical properties of metals and polymers (plastics). It is a test that is used worldwide and therefore is part of a common vocabulary used by design and materials engineers everywhere. In this test, a specimen similar to that shown in Fig. 7.17 is prepared; although the specimen that is shown is round, flat specimens are also permitted.

All tensile test specimens are characterized using measured variables such as those shown in Fig. 7.18.

The ends of the specimen are designed to be gripped in a machine so that the specimen can be pulled apart in tension; a narrowed central zone is machined, and within it is a length of constant diameter or thickness; this is the gage length. A typical setup

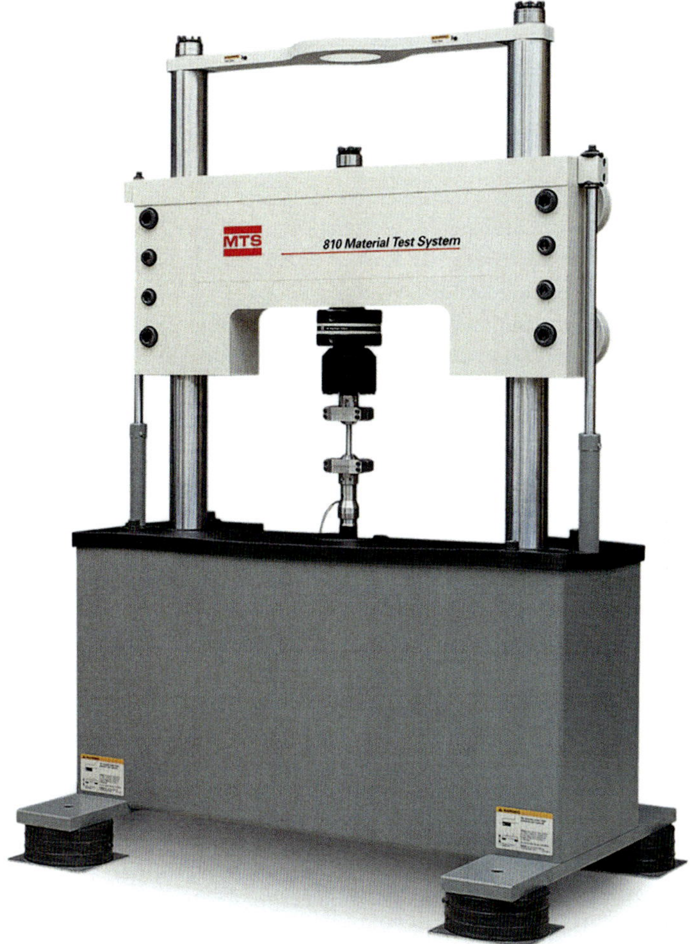

Fig. 7.19 Diagram showing the setup in a standard tensile test. Photo courtesy of MTS Systems Corporation

for tensile testing is shown in Fig. 7.19. As the crosshead moves upward and the lower holding grip remains stationary, a load is exerted on the tensile specimen.

Prior to testing, the specimen dimensions are carefully measured, and the cross-sectional area of the gage length portion of the specimen is calculated. This is the area where the load applied during testing will yield the highest stresses. As the specimen is pulled apart, the machine and the operator simultaneously monitor two variables: the length of the gage section (which is getting longer) and the load (which is steadily increasing). As the length of the gage section changes, a variable known as strain (ε) is computed using the following equation:

$\varepsilon = \Delta l / l_0$ where Δl is the change in gage length and l_0 is the original gage length or strain = change in length/original length

Strain is dimensionless, e.g., it has units of inches/inch, or centimeters/centimeter, and may be expressed as a percent. At the same time, as the load increases, it is possible to compute a variable called stress (σ) using the following equation:

$\sigma = F/A$, where F is load and A is the cross-sectional area of the gage portion of the test specimen, or

Stress = load/cross-sectional area

Stress is reported in units of force per unit area, e.g., pounds/square inch or kilograms/square meter. In the standard international scientific nomenclature system, stress is reported in units of Pascals (1 Pascal = 1 kilogram/square meter), so named after the French mathematician and physicist Blaise Pascal, who conducted many of the first experiments with an instrument called the barometer that measured atmospheric pressure.

The values of stress and strain that pair with each other may be plotted to yield a stress/strain curve as shown in Fig. 7.20.

While the exact shape of the stress–strain curve varies somewhat between different materials, Fig. 7.20 is representative of results obtained with many metals and polymers. Examination of this curve shows that there is an initial straight-line portion of the curve. In this area, the specimen is behaving elastically, like a spring. If the load were to suddenly be released and the stress fell back to zero, the specimen would shorten to its original length, to a strain of zero. If, however, the stress applied to the specimen exceeded the straight-line portion of the graph beyond the yield strength, a release of the load and stress would result in zero stress, but not in a zero strain. Instead, the residual strain would be found by drawing a straight line (parallel to the line of the elastic range) from the highest stress reached during the experiment to a value of zero stress.

The slope of the straight-line portion of the curve (shown in Fig. 7.20 next to the red line) is known as "Young's modulus" or "modulus of elasticity" and is an indication of the stiffness of the material. The higher the modulus, the stiffer (more difficult to deform) is the material. The yield strength is defined as the value of stress needed to reach 0.2 % strain (where the red line intersects the stress–strain curve); at this point, the material is said to have exceeded the elastic limit, and all additional stretching will result in a permanent deformation or plastic deformation.

What do you think? If you were making a spring, would you use a metal with a high modulus or a low modulus?

As the stress continues to rise during the test, a maximum point in the curve will be reached, and the stress at that point is considered to be the ultimate tensile strength. If one were to observe the shape of the tensile specimen, one would note that the specimen will begin to exhibit a change in shape; it will "neck." The tensile strength of a material is therefore the highest stress that may be applied before a material exhibits an instability that renders it less capable of sustaining higher stresses. Note that this is the first time that we have used the word "strength"; we now have a quantitative definition of strength instead of a vague description of that

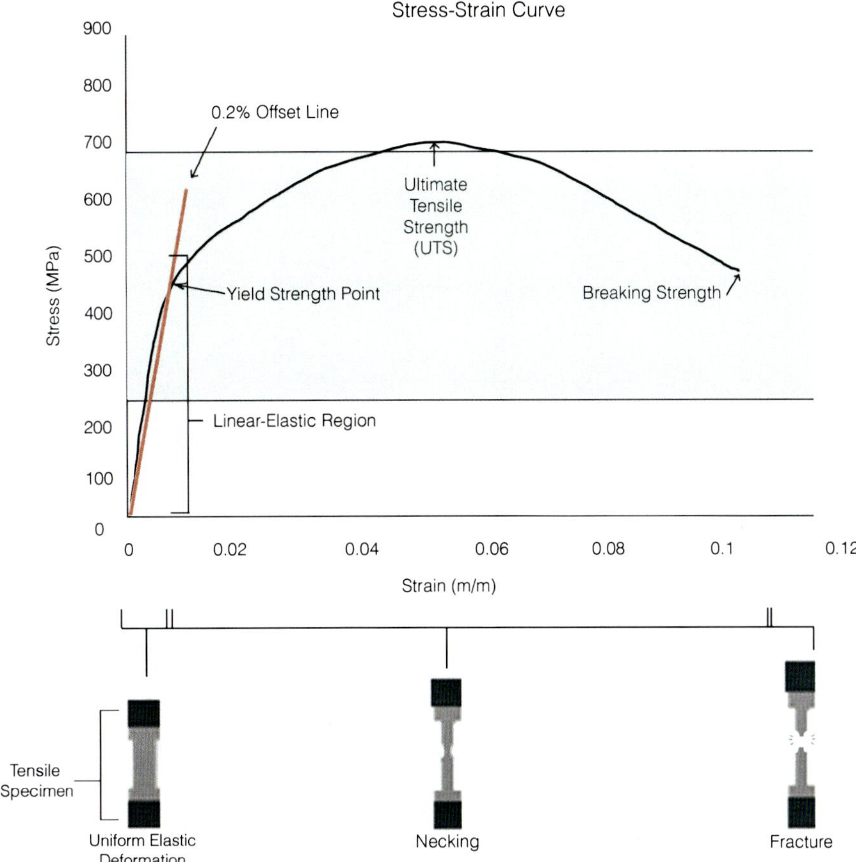

Fig. 7.20 A typical stress–strain curve with important properties labeled and the appearance of the tensile specimen at different times during testing

term. Continued stretching of the specimen will result in eventual failure at a stress called the breaking or fracture strength, but the total strain at failure is a measure of the material's ductility, expressed as a percent.

An interesting phenomenon that may not be noticeable at first is that the stress–strain curve shows that a material gets stronger as it deforms; that is the meaning and consequence of the rise in the curve until the ultimate tensile strength. This phenomenon is named "strain hardening" and may be observed by anyone while playing with a paper clip, bending the wire back and forth. With each successive bend, the wire requires more force to be bent. Eventually, the wire's strength reaches its failure strength, and the wire breaks.

As discussed in the following examples, understanding these material properties is critical for the proper design of implants when materials are chosen:

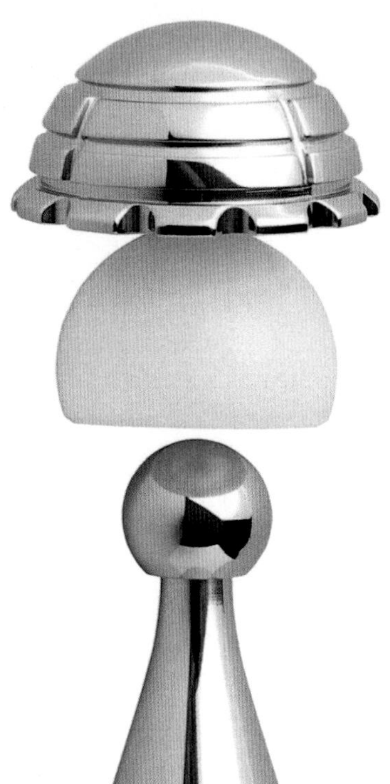

Fig. 7.21 An exploded view of a hip implant, showing a metallic femoral head (*bottom*), an ultrahigh molecular weight polyethylene liner, and a metallic acetabular cup. Copyright Springer Science+Business Media B.V.

- The elastic modulus or stiffness of a material, being a measure of how easily it deforms, must be considered important if the material is to be used as an implant that shares duties with another bone. In that situation, both the implant and the bone must deform equally in response to a load, i.e., their moduli of elasticity should be the same. In fact, a mismatch between the modulus of elasticity of bone and most implant materials is responsible for a phenomenon called "stress shielding." In this scenario, the metallic implants are typically stiffer than bone (see Table 7.3 at the end of this chapter). So, when an implant is placed in bone, the implant will be the component to carry any applied load; the bone will be "shielded" from stress. However, as we already know, bone requires mechanical stimulation in order to remain strong, and in the absence of a load, the bone will resorb. One consequence of bone resorption surrounding an implant is that the implant will become less anchored and more likely to eventually loosen, potentially leading to more bone destruction and requiring replacement of the implant.
- The yield strength of a metal used to replace the femoral head in a hip prosthesis (Fig. 7.21) must be high enough so that the head does not permanently deform and flatten, changing the fit of the implant.
- The ductility of a metal used for orthodontic wire must be high enough so that the wire may be drawn to its desired diameter without fracturing.

The hardness of a material is essentially a measure of how well the material responds to penetration by a sharp instrument called an indenter. In a test called the Brinell hardness test, a spherical indenter made of a hard material such as a carbide is forced into the surface of the test material using a standard load (F). After the load is released, the surface will show a circular indentation or permanent mark with a diameter "d"; the Brinell hardness is calculated using measured values of "d," the indenter diameter, and the indentation load. Other hardness tests utilize different shapes of indenters, including pyramids or diamond shapes, but the variables used to calculate hardness always include a shape parameter for the indenter, a measure of the size of the permanent indentation, and the force used. In an example of a biomedical need to specify hardness, a replacement for natural teeth should closely mimic the hardness of tooth enamel, otherwise it will likely be permanently indented through contact with the opposing tooth, and the restored tooth will no longer function, having lost its required anatomic shape.

Note that hardness is not the same as strength and that the two terms are defined differently and that the two properties are measured differently.

Ceramic materials (e.g., glass) do not easily lend themselves to tensile testing, as the process of gripping a tensile specimen made from glass or other ceramics typically causes the specimen to break before the test can even start. For brittle materials, it is customary to test specimens in bending mode, in either a three-point or a four-point configuration, as shown in Fig. 7.22.

In conducting a flexure test, stress and strain may also be calculated and a stress–strain curve plotted. However, it is more customary to calculate a property called "modulus of rupture" (MOR) that is an indicator of the material's strength. For the case of the four-point test setup shown here, the following formula is used to calculate MOR:

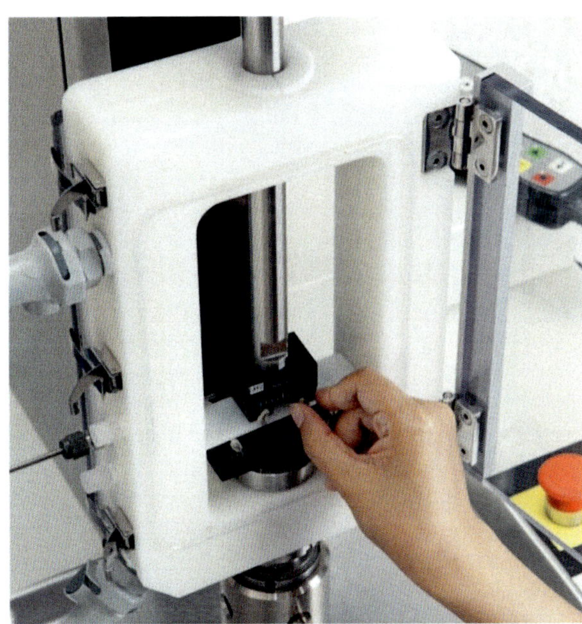

Fig. 7.22 Diagram of a four-point flexural strength test used for brittle or weak materials. The test specimen is the white flat piece inside the plastic housing and is loaded at two points on the top while being supported at two points on the bottom. Photo courtesy of MTS Systems Corporation

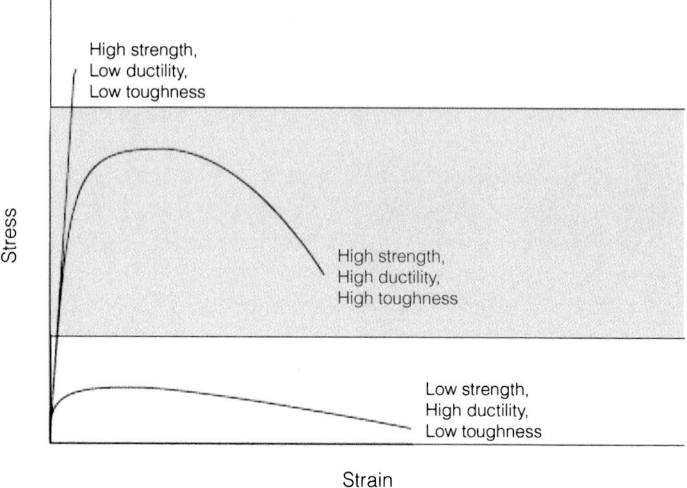

Fig. 7.23 Representative stress–strain curves for materials with different toughness

$$MOR = 3FL / 4bd^2$$

where F is the applied load at failure, L is the distance between the two lower supports, b is the width of the rectangular beam, and d is the height of the rectangular beam. (Think about the significance of the beam height, because its value is squared in this formula, having a greater influence on MOR than beam width.)

The toughness of a material is a measure of how difficult it is for a crack to travel through the material and can be derived from the area under a stress–strain curve.

In Fig. 7.23, consider the meaning of strength and toughness and how these two properties differ. The material with only a linear stress–strain curve has a high strength; it fractures at a high stress. The middle of the three curves breaks at a lower stress but has considerably greater ductility or ability to be plastically deformed. The lower curve has the greatest ductility but the lowest strength. Considering the areas underneath each of the curves, it becomes apparent that the high-strength material is least tough, the low strength material has an intermediate toughness, and the remaining material has the highest toughness. These curves are quite representative of a ceramic, a polymer, and a metal, respectively. We see, therefore, that the material with the highest breaking strength is not the toughest material; there is a clear distinction between toughness and strength, and the materials engineer and implant designer are routinely confounded by the inability to create materials that are simultaneously very strong and very tough; toughness demands an ability to deform.

An interesting fact about toughness is that its value can depend on temperature; many readers will have seen demonstrations of rubber balls shattering after being struck by a hammer if they have first been immersed in liquid nitrogen; the same rubber ball will simply bounce from the hammer blow if it has been kept at room temperature. Several metals also exhibit a so-called temperature-mediated "brittle–ductile" transition; below a certain temperature (which varies with the specific alloy in question), they shatter easily and cannot be plastically deformed, while above the transition temperature, they may be stretched and permanently deformed. Mild steel has a brittle–ductile transition temperature of approximately −50 °C, and the metal zinc has a brittle–ductile transition of approximately 40 °C.

To reiterate, modulus, ultimate tensile strength, hardness, toughness, and breaking strength are all measures of a material's resistance to stress, but they do not necessarily "scale" together (e.g., a strong material may not be tough; however, hard materials generally have high tensile strengths). And, though they may all be somewhat indicative of the "strength" of a material, they are not equivalent. All these properties include a contribution from the strength of the bond between the atoms that compose a material; the modulus of elasticity in particular is a material property that is dependent exclusively on the composition of the material. While strength, hardness, and toughness also are composition dependent, the exact values for any given material are also a function of the material's microstructure (e.g., grain size, etc.) which may be affected by processing techniques. For that reason, although the modulus of a material with a fixed composition cannot be manipulated, scientists and engineers are able to alter the strength, hardness, and toughness of materials.

7.4.2 Dynamic (Time Is a Variable) Mechanical Behavior of Materials

A. Mechanical "fatigue" is a process characterized by repeated loading and unloading of a structure. The maximum stresses experienced by the structure during fatigue are usually much lower than the ultimate tensile strength and usually lower than the yield strength too. Loading and unloading can occur periodically at a constant frequency or chaotically. Preexisting cracks that are oriented perpendicular to the direction of tensile stress will grow, getting longer. If no cracks are present, the application of stresses above some threshold stress will eventually initiate a crack in a local region where stress happens to be concentrated and continued load cycling will enable the usual crack growth which will ultimately lead to failure. Some materials have a lower stress limit called the endurance limit or fatigue limit and do not fail if cycled below that stress limit. However, it is often difficult to be certain that a fatigue limit exists, and so engineers design structures taking fatigue into account.

The particularly dangerous aspects of fatigue are that damage is cumulative (simply stopping cyclic application of stress will not heal any cracks that have already formed nor cause them to shrink), damage may remain undetected (cracks may form and grow in parts of the structure not easily visualized), failure occurs catastrophically without warning, and failure usually occurs at stresses well below the failure stress established in tensile test experiments. That's because in a tensile test, stresses increase continuously until failure with the crack responsible for failure getting longer in step with the stress; in fatigue, the crack grows a small amount

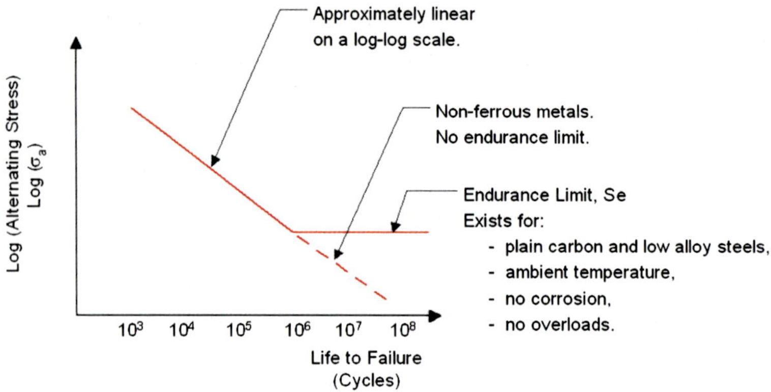

Fig. 7.24 A typical fatigue plot. Image courtesy of MTS Systems Corporation

during each stress cycle, and even though the stress is not high enough to cause the crack to grow to its critical length all at once, the cumulative effect of intermittent crack growth eventually causes the crack to reach the critical fracture length.

Even though fatigue conditions can be simulated in the laboratory, it is often impossible to exactly duplicate the environment where the structure will be placed and impractical to conduct testing for as long as the structure is planned to remain in service. If a hip implant is meant to last for 15–20 years in the body, should manufacturers perform 15-year-long fatigue tests? Were that to happen, new devices would hardly ever be introduced to the market, and manufacturers would go out of business waiting until tests were completed. These confounding needs: conducting realistic and meaningful fatigue tests and yet being able to introduce new materials and designs for patient care, are often difficult to reconcile. It is possible to shorten a test by increasing cycling frequency, but one cannot be certain that the higher frequency cycling over a shorter time period will enable the same failure mechanism as low frequency cycling over a longer period of time. For these reasons, the lifetime of implants (and other structures exposed to long-term cyclic stressing) cannot be known with 100 % certainty.

Laboratory fatigue tests are conducted using well-developed statistical protocols that eventually yield an estimate (not a certainty) of how long an implant or device will survive under simulated conditions of actual use, with stress or strain being the independent variable and lifetime in cycles being the dependent variable. The data collected are usually plotted as in Fig. 7.24. In this particular representation, note that an apparent endurance or fatigue limit exists, defined at the break in the red line. The endurance limit is a value of stress below which the material is deemed to have an infinite lifetime, i.e., will never break.

Recall, however, that the solid line is a "best-fit" line and that there will be scatter in the actual data. The scatter is one source of the uncertainty associated with any lifetime prediction made on the basis of these data. Note also that some metals have an endurance limit, and others do not. Polymers do not possess endurance limits, and ceramics are considered to not undergo fatigue because

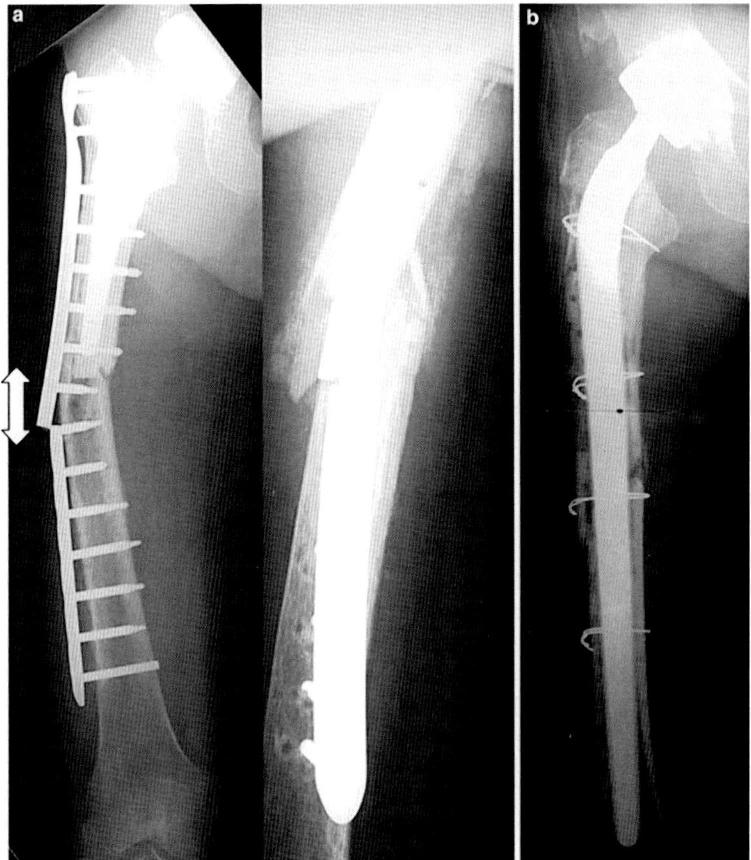

Fig. 7.25 Implant fractures in the hip resulting from fatigue stressing. The image on the *right* depicts the solution that was adopted, i.e., placing an implant with an internal femoral shaft. Copyright Springer-Verlag

they fail quite rapidly. Because it is important for the implant designer to incorporate a safety factor into biomedical devices, fatigue tests are carried out on many specimens, and a statistical basis is established that allows a specific degree of certainty for future lifetime predictions.

Implants that undergo cyclic stressing, such as those placed in the hip (Fig. 7.25) and stents placed in blood vessels (Fig. 7.26), are those most likely to undergo failure in service.

Because of the risk of catastrophic failure, these implants are often tested as completely fabricated devices, rather than as standard tensile specimens, and undergo laboratory testing under simulated conditions. In an example of such a test, shown in Fig. 7.27, the implant is secured in a holder and immersed in physiologic fluid kept at body temperature to simulate the in-service environment. The upper fixture applies cyclic loads, and testing may go on until the

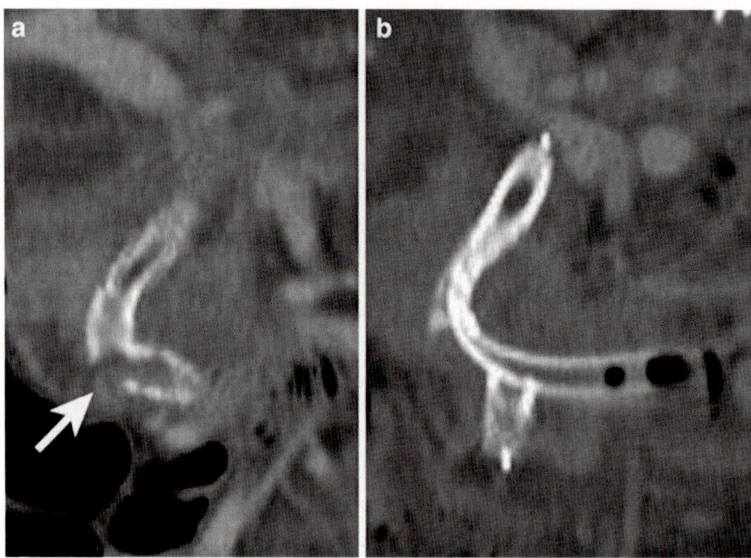

Fig. 7.26 Arterial stent fracture (*left*) due to fatigue (cyclic stressing at pulse rate). On the *right*, the stent has been replaced. Copyright Springer Science + Business Media New York

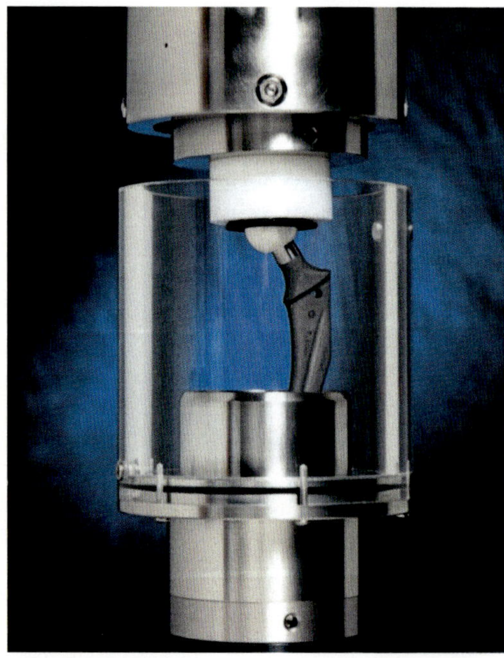

Fig. 7.27 Diagram of a fatigue test setup for a hip implant. The clear plastic chamber may be filled with saline or another liquid to simulate exposure in the physiologic environment. Photo courtesy of MTS Systems Corporation

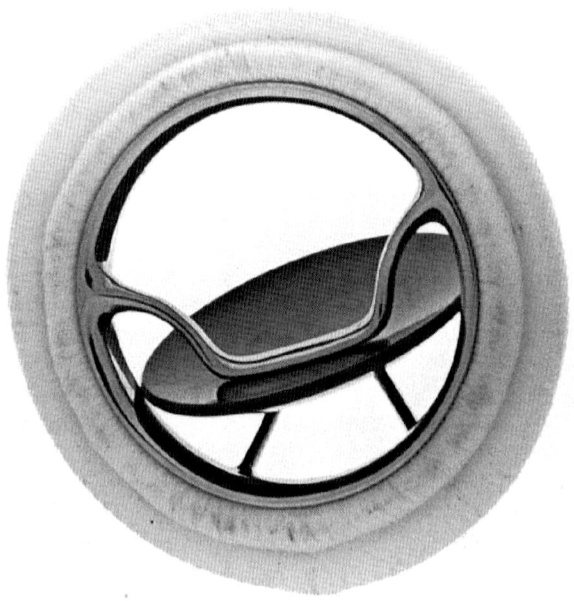

Fig. 7.28 The Bjork–Shiley convexo-concave heart valve which experienced failures in the outlet strut-support ring region because of mechanical fatigue. Copyright Current Medicine LLC

implant fails or for some predetermined amount of time believed to represent a reasonable service lifetime.

Heart valves are important devices subjected to high cycle fatigue. The heart reaches one million cycles of beats in less than 1 year, so the hope is that an artificial valve can survive a minimum of tens of millions of cycles during its lifetime. Just as an example, devices called the "Björk–Shiley convexo-concave" heart valve (Fig. 7.28) experienced a failure rate of only 0.75 % [2].

However, that degree of failure is somewhat misleading. It is not high in and of itself, but the facts are that the failures had a patient mortality rate of 70 %, the manufacturer was subjected to many lawsuits, and the valve was withdrawn from the market. Analysis of the failed components indicated that the outlet strut, which was welded to the support ring, could contain small flaws (cracks) in the weld region. As the occluder disc opened and closed during normal blood flow, it would hit the weld region with more force than the designers had anticipated. The higher-than-expected stresses caused eventual fatigue failure.

This example illustrates one of the ways in which fatigue life could be extended. Note that lifetime is a sum of the time needed to initiate a crack (if none are present), as well as the time needed for the crack to propagate to a critical size. If exceptional care had been taken to eliminate cracks or flaws during manufacturing, then lifetime would extended by the amount needed to initiate a crack. In the case of the valve, alternative strut-support ring attachment techniques may have been available that would have avoided the formation of welding flaws.

If cracks cannot be avoided, then it is possible to reduce their size so that more time is needed for them to achieve the critical, catastrophic propagation size.

For example, since many flaws are found on the surface of a device in the form of scratches, polishing will serve to reduce the average surface flaw size. And finally, because the driving force for crack propagation is an applied stress, a redesign of the piece (e.g., increase the cross-sectional area where loading occurs) could reduce the magnitude of the stress.

The time and expense associated with manufacturing processes to ensure that any inherent flaws are small and the requirement that all components have a similar flaw size distribution (and therefore fatigue lifetime) are two factors responsible for the high costs of critical components or devices used in medical technology, the space program, and some defense applications.

B. Temperature also is critical in determining several ways in which some materials behave mechanically; recall the blacksmith's ability to shape metals at high temperature. One can see from that example that materials are more inclined to deform at elevated temperature. Of course, the temperature range that enables visible deformation or flow is material dependent; iron and steel must be heated to over a 1,000 °F (Fahrenheit) before they may be easily deformed, but polymers such as Plexiglass™ require only 250–300 °F. The ability to flow at elevated temperatures is linked to a phenomenon known as "creep," which describes the permanent deformation of a material when subjected to a constant stress. Experiments may be easily carried out in which change in dimension is measured as a function of stress and temperature; the higher the applied stress and temperature, the higher the rate of creep. Fortunately for biomedical design engineers, creep becomes a significant factor for metals and ceramic only at temperatures greater than one-half their melting temperature, i.e., much higher than encountered in the human body, though perhaps within the temperature ranges used in some processing steps.

C. Viscoelasticity is another time-sensitive mechanical property of particular importance for glasses and amorphous (noncrystalline) polymers and for several natural tissues in the body. If we think of a spring as a perfectly elastic material (it instantly returns to its original shape when the load is removed) and of a substance such as heavy grease as a perfectly plastic material, then it is possible to imagine a viscoelastic material as being able to exhibit both types of behavior. Indeed, an elastic material may be modeled as a spring, a viscous material modeled as a dashpot (a damping device consisting of a piston inside a cylinder filled with a fluid such as air or oil), and a viscoelastic material as a spring and dashpot in series or in parallel (Fig. 7.29). If one imagines the application of a load, the spring would be expected to immediately stretch out, and the dashpot would slowly stretch out at a speed dependent on the viscosity of the fluid within the cylinder. The series model would be expected to show a rapid initial stretch followed by an additional slow stretch, and the parallel model would be expected to exhibit a slow stretch. If the load were to be removed, the spring would immediately return to its original length and the dashpot would remain at its elongated length, the series model would immediately recover some of its length but remain permanently deformed, and the parallel model would slowly recover to its original dimension. In this way, it is possible to model stress relaxation (all of the stress is recovered when the spring is allowed to contract) and creep (a slow

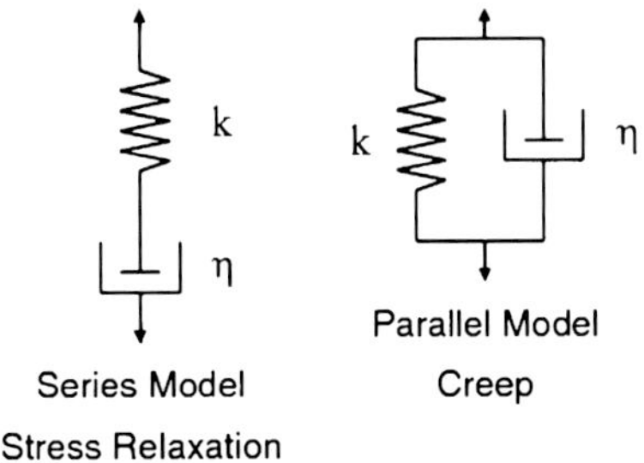

Fig. 7.29 Spring and dashpot models of viscoelastic behavior. The spring (zigzag line) is characterized by a spring constant (modulus of elasticity E), the dashpot (piston in open cylinder) by a viscosity ν. Copyright Springer Science and Business Media New York

change in dimension). The rate of creep increases with an increase in temperature and with an increase in applied load.

An excellent example of a viscoelastic material encountered by children and adults everywhere is "Silly Putty™." When this material is loaded quickly (as when rolled into a ball and thrown against a hard surface), it behaves elastically, because it bounces back; when a piece is grasped with two hands and stretched quickly, the putty breaks. However, when the putty is allowed to stand in place, it will flow and form a puddle, and if it is stretched slowly, it will yield and flow, forming a thin strand. In these cases, the constituent components of the material have not changed except that the speed of load application was varied.

It turns out that several biologic tissues such as skin, tendon, and bone are viscoelastic, as is the intervertebral disc found in the spine. Consider the consequences of this knowledge as it might apply to athletic activities; to ensure a quick start for a sprint, the elastic component of a viscoelastic tendon should be preserved. And yet, to avoid injury from an abrupt load, it is best to stretch to allow the dashpot component of a viscoelastic tendon to activate and elongate the tendon, guarding against a tendon rupture. The viscoelasticity of an intervertebral disc explains why a sudden impact, such as a fall taken without flexing the knees or a football tackle with the spine straightened, could cause disc herniation, while a slower application of force allows the disc to behave as a shock absorber. Blood vessels experience pulsatile loading, and the synthetic fabric grafts used to replace cholesterol-blocked arteries can also exhibit creep. Finally, because bones are viscoelastic, they can experience stress relaxation; screws inserted and tightened in bone will eventually loosen as the bone relaxes and the pressure holding the screws decreases [3].

It is important to remember that the mechanical properties of natural materials such as skin, muscle, tendon, ligament, and bone change with age. These materials degrade, and their elasticity decreases, as does their strength. These changes should be kept in mind when a patient considers the replacement of damaged tissue with donor tissue. For example, a young patient with a torn anterior cruciate ligament (ACL) can be offered a ligament from a deceased donor. The positive aspect of donor tissue is that it eliminates the need for the patient to undergo additional surgery when tendon is harvested from another site. On the other hand, the donors are typically older individuals, and the properties of those tendons are inferior to young tendon. The patient will likely live many more years, but the ACL repaired with donor tendon could be eventually compromised.

The viscoelastic behavior of amorphous materials is strongly dependent on temperature. The transition is gradual, because the structure of amorphous materials is nonuniform throughout their bulk, with some regions making the transition at a lower temperature than others (more on structure later in this chapter). Therefore, inorganic and organic glasses do not possess a true melting point. Instead, they gradually soften when heated, and the temperature associated with a certain degree of viscosity or a change in elastic modulus is called the "glass transition temperature" or T_g. Below T_g, inorganic glasses (e.g., window glass) are elastic and glassy; above T_g, they assume a more viscous nature, and eventually as temperature continues to rise, they reach their softening temperature when they are no longer able to support weight. For organic glassy polymers (e.g., Plexiglass), below T_g they are rigid; as temperature increases to approximately T_g, they transition to a leathery state; with further increases in temperature, they become rubbery state and eventually transition to a viscous state where they are able to flow.

7.5 Wear

Wear is not a true mechanical property of a material, because wear is dependent on the two materials in contact, the forces applied to these materials, their surface condition, and the environment (e.g., presence or absence of lubrication). However, wear is an important phenomenon associated with implants such as artificial hips and knees in which two surfaces are in contact and move relative to each other. Excessive wear and subsequent biologic reactions are the principal failure causes for hip and knee implants.

No matter how well machined and polished is a surface, on the microscopic level, it will be rough. Therefore, two surfaces in direct contact will actually only touch where their high points (asperities) meet (Fig. 7.30). As a load is applied to the surfaces, the asperities will deform (because the stresses are quite high in these small cross-sectional area features), and if the surface is sufficiently clean, they will weld together. If the surfaces attempt to move over each other, then the welded asperities provide a resistance to movement in the form of friction. The coefficient of friction, commonly labeled as μ, is defined as F/P, where F is the sliding force controlled by the yield strength of the asperity contacts and the asperity contact area and P is the pressure forcing the two materials together. The interesting point to this equation is that it implies that the coefficient of friction is independent of sliding speed, surface roughness, contact area, and load and is only dependent on the strength parameters of the material [3]; more specifically, on difficult it will be to tear off a piece of material from the surface.

It is interesting to note that the cartilage lining the surfaces of articulating hip and knee joints has extremely low coefficients of friction, but the synovial fluid which

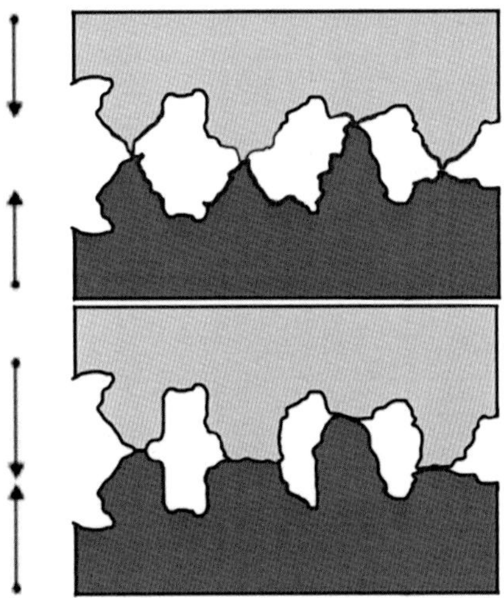

Fig. 7.30 Diagram of two surfaces in initial contact (*upper*) and after a load has been applied, showing how asperities can deform and pressure-weld

surrounds the joint also plays a valuable lubricating role. Lubricants not only cool the surfaces of materials in sliding contact, but a phenomenon called hydrodynamic lubrication occurs, which traps a thin layer of lubricant between the surfaces, making it less likely for the asperities on the materials' surfaces to come into contact and cold weld to each other. Of course, large asperities will be able to penetrate the lubricating film; that's why it is common practice to polish rubbing surfaces to the greatest degree possible, as the process reduces the average height of asperities.

Abrasive wear occurs when sharp particles or protrusions on one surface scratch the opposing surface. Sandpaper wears wood away by an abrasive wear mechanism. This mechanism could be important in some orthopedic implants, especially if the metal alloy contains hard particles that strengthen the alloy and which are markedly harder than the opposing surface. Fatigue wear is accompanied by repetitive loading, and an example usually given in engineering texts is that of a railcar wheel traveling over a rail, though fatigue wear occurs in the polymer linings of hip implants too. The starting point for fatigue wear is at or near the surface, because that is where the maximum tensile stresses occur, and then the crack propagates below the surface. Once below the surface, continued cyclic loading permits the crack to grow parallel to the surface, eventually turning upward so that it rejoins the surface. As the result of that process, a piece of material is freed, and falls off, producing a pit. Fatigue-induced wear yields relatively large pieces of wear debris and is minimized if tough materials are used.

Teeth that have been repaired with various materials can undergo wear when hard particles of food become trapped between chewing surfaces, and eventually some of the repair material is worn away. Similarly, in hip and knee implants, particles of material that have been produced by adhesion or abrasion wear can be trapped between the two contacting surfaces and cause additional wear to occur.

7.6 Material Degradation

7.6.1 Corrosion

Corrosion is an electrochemical process during which a material (usually a metal) reacts with its environment, new compounds are formed, and the material itself diminishes in size and weight. All metals placed in the human body run the risk of corroding, because the body is an aggressive environment. Metals are commonly used for hip and knee implants, bone plates and bone screws, artificial spinal discs, cardiovascular implants, shoulder implants, implants placed in blood vessels, and ear implants. In this section, we will discuss the chemical principles behind corrosion and ways in which corrosion can be prevented.

The most common form of corrosion, visible in everyday life, is rusting. In that instance, metal alloys containing iron react with moisture in the presence of oxygen in air to form a new compound, iron oxide, or red rust. Because the rust does not stay adherent to the metal but falls away, a fresh, noncorroded surface of metal is exposed and rusts in its turn. This sequence of events continues until the entire piece of metal has been converted to rust. But corrosion does not only occur in wet environments; the metal alloys used in boilers for the chimney exhaust stack also corrode through exposure to exhaust gases. And at home, everybody who owns sterling silver cutlery has to periodically clean off the silver sulfide tarnish. For our purposes, however, corrosion in the physiologic environment is of greatest concern.

Where does the "electro" part of the electrochemical process come in? If one studies the reactions that occur during corrosion, it becomes apparent that the reaction is an "oxidation/reduction" type. That is, some metal "M" (because that's the most typical scenario) is oxidized as shown here:

$$\mathrm{M} \rightarrow \mathrm{M}^{n+} + ne^{-}$$

This equation represents an oxidizing reaction in which a metal is oxidized to form a metal ion and that in the process some number "n" of electrons are freed. The superscripts + and – indicate the presence of a positive or negative charge, and their number indicates how many such charges are carried by each ion. In the case of iron, the reaction is:

$$Fe \rightarrow Fe^{2+} + 2\mathrm{e}^{-}$$

The iron atom changes to an iron ion, freeing two electrons, which now get involved in further reactions called reduction reactions. By agreement, the location where oxidation occurs is called the "anode," while the place where reduction occurs is called the "cathode."

Different metals differ by how easily they give up electrons and that property has been measured and listed in the "Standard Electromotive Force Series." In that table, an abbreviated form of which is shown here (Table 7.1), metals are ranked in comparison to each other (the more positive the volt value, the more resistant is the element to corrosion), and their electrode behavior is measured in a highly standardized manner which is not necessarily representative of the conditions in the human body.

Table 7.1 The electromotive force table

Metal	Standard volts
Magnesium	−2.37
Aluminum	−1.66
Titanium	−1.63
Zinc	−0.76
Iron	−0.44
Tin	−0.14
Lead	−0.13
Hydrogen	0.00
Copper	+0.4
Silver	+0.8
Platinum	+1.2
Gold	+1.6

Table 7.2 The galvanic series for selected metals

Platinum	Noble, cathodic end
Gold	
Graphite	
Titanium	
Silver	
Passivated stainless steel	
Passivated iron–chromium alloys	
Nickel	
Cupronickel alloys	
Bronzes	
Copper brasses	
Nickel	
Tin	
Lead	
Active stainless steel	
Cast iron	
Mild steel	
Aluminum alloys	
Zinc	
Magnesium alloys	Corroding, anodic end

Simply stated, the table shows that, for example, the metallic element magnesium (Mg) is very readily oxidized, while the metallic element gold (Au) is extremely resistant to oxidation. It would seem that neither aluminum, iron (steel), nor titanium would be particularly stable with respect to corrosion. And yet, we know that many metallic implants are made from stainless steel and many more from titanium; so, what information is missing?

The physiologic environment, i.e., body fluids, is known to contain salt. How can we estimate the corrosion behavior of metals in body fluids? It's possible to conduct experiments in the laboratory, but a more readily available answer may be found by consulting the galvanic series (Table 7.2) which is similar to the standard electromotive force series but is obtained with seawater as the electrolyte (the liquid in which the corrosion test is conducted).

The information about the behavior of aluminum in a salt-containing solution suggests that aluminum would not at all be a suitable candidate as a medical implant. Its corrosion resistance would be quite poor; in addition, aluminum has been linked to "osteomalacia," or softening of the bones. While corroding, aluminum will release aluminum ions into the body, possibly inducing or contributing to osteomalacia. On the other hand, stainless steel and titanium seem to be resistant to corrosion in a saline electrolyte, particularly if they have undergone "passivation."

Do all metals with a negative standard electrode potential dissolve in a corrosive environment? Not necessarily. The problem with iron rust is that it does not adhere to steel or iron; as the coating of rust gets thicker, it also tries to grow sideways. The stresses formed as the rust grows push it away from the metal surface so that it falls away exposing a fresh metallic surface. However, there are metals that form corrosion products such as oxides (compounds consisting of the metal and oxygen) that are adherent to the metal, and that do not fall away. These metals are said to be "passivated." Examples include aluminum, titanium, and stainless steel. In the case of titanium, there is a tightly adherent coating of titanium oxides on the surface. In the case of stainless steel, the metallic element chromium (Cr), which is a critically important component of stainless steel, forms a chromium oxide coating on the surface of the steel. The coating is so thin that it is invisible to the naked eye, but its presence is why stainless steel remains stainless, whereas ordinary steel (with less than approximately 18 % chromium) will rust readily. Aluminum also spontaneously forms a coating of aluminum oxide which protects it from further corrosion.

Although titanium and stainless steel spontaneously form an oxide layer, it is common practice to ensure that a minimum thickness of oxide has been formed. Metals and alloys may be purposely passivated. Aluminum is rinsed with dilute nitric acid and hydrogen peroxide in a process called "anodizing," which accelerates corrosion in a controlled manner and grows a thick passive film on the surface that is somewhat porous. That porosity is eventually filled with dyes, corrosion inhibitors, and sealers, and anodized aluminum articles often have colorful anodized surfaces. Stainless steel is passivated by dipping into a citric acid bath, thereby accelerating the growth of the protective chromium oxide film. Titanium can also be passivated in a citric acid bath, but it is often anodized just as aluminum is. During anodization, the titanium surface acquires a color which depends on the thickness of the oxide layer; it can range from clear to deep green and is formed as a result of interference of the light reflecting from the metal surface and passing through the oxide layer. Anodized titanium is sometimes used for jewelry, and in the medical device industry, it may also be used to color-code similar products so that different sizes may be easily distinguished, as, for example, the bone screws shown in Fig. 7.31.

When different metals are in contact, because they each have a different standard electrode potential, in the presence of a fluid that can conduct electrons (the electrolyte), a galvanic cell (battery) is completed. The metal that is less anodic (more inert) will be protected from corrosion by the presence of the more anodic metal, and an electric current will flow between the two metals. (A real-life confirmation of the electric current flow resulting from contacting dissimilar metals in the

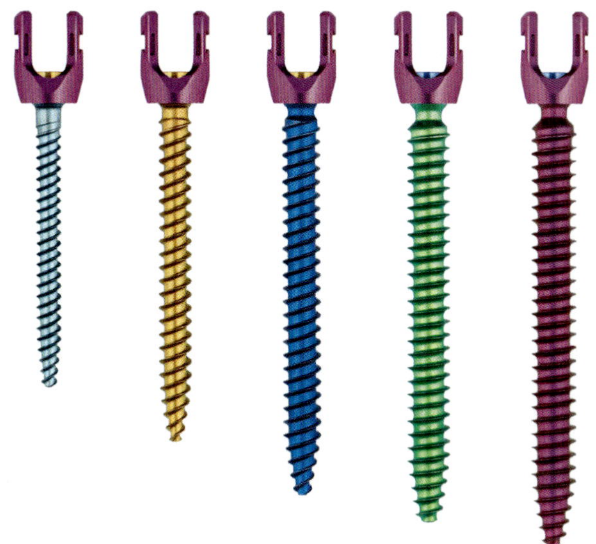

Fig. 7.31 Anodized titanium bone screws, color-coded for convenient size discrimination. Courtesy of Globus Medical

presence of an electrolyte can be provided to anyone who has silver fillings in their mouth; go ahead and chew on a piece of aluminum foil and see if you don't get energized.) The presence of an electrolyte is also important because electrolytes that contain ions will easily conduct the electric current that is a component of the corrosion process. A fluid containing salt (sodium chloride) which readily disassociates into sodium ions (Na^+) and chloride ions (Cl^-) will be more corrosion active than an electrolyte that contains only water. That's one reason why bodily fluids, such as saliva and blood, which contain dissolved ions, present a relatively harsh environment for implanted materials.

The complete dissolution of a metal is an extreme case of corrosion. Far more common but far less visible (and therefore dangerous) are the types of corrosion that confine themselves to only certain areas of a metallic implant.

The EMF series table has shown that the oxidation tendency depends on the composition of a metal alloy, and we have also learned that the environment influences corrosion. In metals, there are also small differences in composition on the surface, particularly in metals which have been cast rather than forged and where some alloy components segregated to grain boundaries during solidification. In the presence of an electrolyte, it is the grain boundaries that are most prone to be an active corrosion site.

Pitting corrosion and crevice corrosion are similar phenomena in that they both occur at the site of some defect on the surface of the metal. In pitting corrosion, the dissolution of the metal is confined to a small, approximately circular area (hence the name "pit"). The dangerous aspect of pitting corrosion is that the dissolution of the metal continues into the bulk rather than spreading across the surface; so, a small pinhole pit on the surface may actually hide a much wider and deeper hole under the surface. In crevice corrosion, the metal loss is confined to a scratch that keeps getting deeper. In the pit and in the crevice, it is likely that the electrolyte is markedly different in composition from its average composition outside the pit or crevice. That's because various impurities have a tendency to concentrate in these protected areas, and the fluid in the pit or crevice may become saturated with the impurities. Also, the fluid in the protected area is oxygen starved. The area within the crevice is anodic (dissolving), and the electrochemical activity there has to equal the electrochemical activity at the cathode, which is the relatively large and smooth surface area. The disparity in size further stimulates corrosion within the crevice and pit.

Fretting corrosion occurs where there is intimate mechanical contact between two pieces of metal in the presence of motion. For example, screws that are tightened against a flat metal surface form a crevice at the line of contact between the screw head and flat piece, possibly initiating crevice corrosion, but if there is simultaneous vibration causing movement of the screw relative to the flat piece, the corrosion will increase as any passive film or coating on either metal surface will be rubbed off. The motion does not have to be large, it can be less than a millimeter in range.

What can be done to avoid or prevent corrosion? Choosing noncorroding or corroding but passivating metals for medical device components is a good start. Controlling the environment usually helps, but that may not always be possible. If corrosion is a surface phenomenon, then protecting the surface is usually a good strategy. The surface may be coated with paint, or with a polymer coating such as medical grade silicone. The passivating process has already been referred to; aluminum is anodized, and stainless steel is passivated by dipping articles made of that metal into an acid bath, which quickly forms a protective chromium oxide layer on the metal. Sensitized stainless steel and other alloys with large differences in composition across the surface may be heated to permit the surface composition to come to a more homogeneous state. Metals with residual stresses may also be stress-relieved through heat treatment.

7.6.2 Polymer Degradation

The chemical process responsible for degrading metals in the body is corrosion, and as discussed earlier in this chapter, it results in release of metal ions and destruction of the structural integrity of a metallic implant. Ceramic materials, particularly bioglasses, also undergo corrosion, releasing calcium and phosphorus ions into the local environment. Polymers can degrade in the physiologic environment too, but because they have a different structure than metals and ceramics, they behave differently than metals and ceramics.

The principal mechanisms responsible for polymer degradation are swelling and chain scission (breaking of the polymer chain into shorter chain units). Swelling occurs if the polymer is in contact with physiologic fluid and is aided by the presence of hydrophilic regions or groups in the polymer chain. Water present in the physiologic fluid is a small molecule and can diffuse or penetrate into the polymer surface. As a result, an implant or device will swell, and the

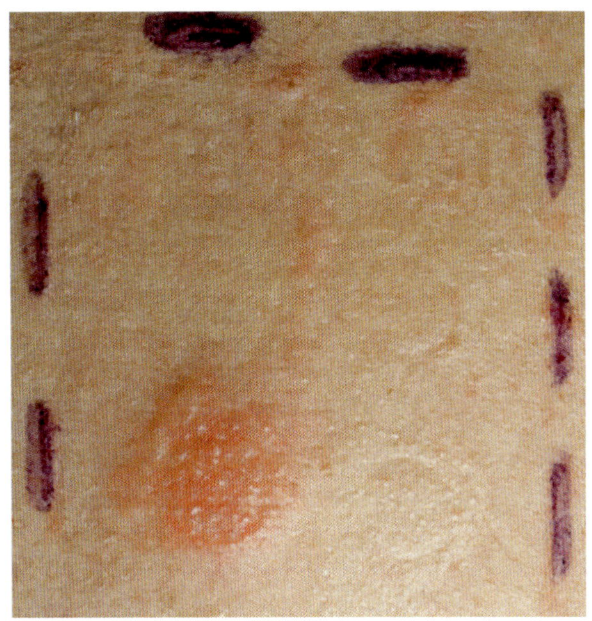

Fig. 7.32 Irritation caused by residual monomer during an allergy test; a similar irritation can occur when polymeric devices that have not been fully polymerized (cured) are placed in contact with skin. Unreacted monomer once caused irritation in fingers when certain compounds were used to make artificial finger nails

swelling can cause cracks to form because of the expansion of the material. Absorption of water also can make the polymer weaker and more deformable because the water interferes with the weak bonds between polymer chains, making it easier for the chains to slip past each other. At the same time that water enters the polymer's structure, small organic molecules can exit the polymer. During the polymerization process (discussed earlier), not all the monomer components are consumed or incorporated into a longer polymer chain; some monomer remains unreacted. These small molecules are readily able to enter the physiologic environment and interact with cells and tissues; it is these small molecules that are sometimes responsible for skin irritation near recently polymerized or reacted artificial nails (Fig. 7.32).

Other small molecules that may be released from polymers include additives such as coloring agents and plasticizers (compounds added to make the polymer softer, particularly with polyvinyl chloride, PVC, which is used for medical tubing).

Chain scission (cutting or breaking a polymer chain) can occur as a result of water sorption or oxidation reactions often through free radicals that are present because of inflammatory cells or because of nearby metallic corrosion. This latter process is responsible for the cracking of urethane insulation on pacemaker leads. Environmentally induced chain scission is also evident on polymers that have been exposed to ultraviolet rays such as are found in sunlight. As an example, plastic cups and glasses that have been left out in the sun show evidence of damage as yellowing and cracking.

7.7 Designing with Materials

Ever wonder why the long bones of humans are hollow? It's true that the hollow space contains bone marrow and other cells, so that design provides a convenient storage facility. However, there is another reason too, one that also explains why the bones of birds are hollow: hollow bones are lighter than if they were solid. It's easier for birds to fly and for humans to get around if they have less mass to carry. But what are the mechanical implications of hollow bones? If we consider the type of loads that the long bones in humans endure, we soon settle on compression and bending as the primary loading modes. In compression, a failure mode that should be avoided is buckling, which is a sudden collapse of the structure that can be brought about by an instability along the length of a compressed hollow structure. If you want to verify this for yourself, the next time you finish drinking from an aluminum can, try compressing it flat; it is quite difficult, even impossible for most of us. Now, introduce an instability; pinch the can, bending it somewhere in the middle. Try compressing the can again; it should easily flatten.

In 1757, a mathematician named Euler developed an equation that described the buckling resistance of a slender column (such as a long bone):

$$\mathrm{F} = \pi^2 EI / (KL)^2$$

where F is the maximum load on the column, E the modulus of elasticity, I the second moment of inertia, L the length of the column, and K a factor whose value depends on the conditions at the ends of the column. We need not be mathematicians to realize that the formula actually provides quite a bit of design information. First, it tells us that the critical (and only) material property we need to be concerned with is the modulus of elasticity, so when choosing a material for an implant that will replace a load-bearing long bone, we might look at materials with high elastic moduli if we wish to maximize resistance to buckling. If the modulus increases, the maximum permissible load also increases. Second, the maximum load is also dependent on the second moment of inertia; if the moment increases, the permissible load increases. The formula for the second moment of inertia for a tube (with two radii, one for inner wall and one for the outer wall) is $I = \pi(r_2^4 - r_1^4)/4$.

In order to increase the second moment of inertia (and thereby also the stability of the column), we need to distribute the material of the column as far from the principal axis (the center) as possible; the moment of inertia will increase by the fourth power of the radius! And if we want to keep the structure light, we want to make it hollow. If you were to do some calculations, you would find that a tubular section is much more efficient than a solid section of the same weight used as a column (or bone or implant for bone). Comparing a tube and rod with the same diameters will show the rod to be stiffer, but if the relative weights are taken into account, the tube is a more efficient shape at providing stiffness, yielding a higher "strength to weight" ratio. Incidentally, the second moment of inertia is also the reason why I-beams are designed the way they are (Fig. 7.33); note that much of the material is separated far away from the center!

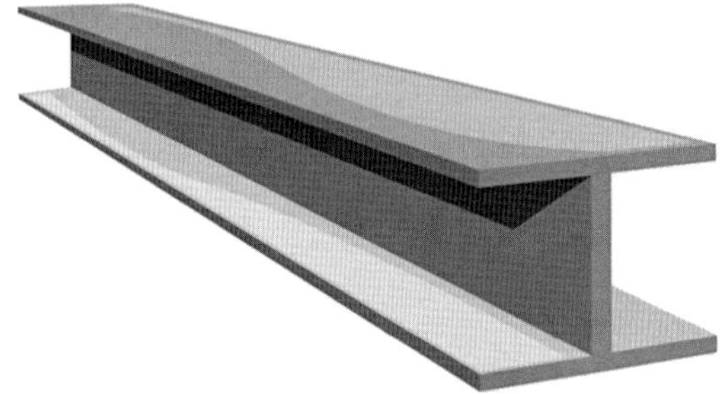

Fig. 7.33 I-beam. Note that much of the beam's mass is distributed away from the "middle" of the beam. The second moment of inertia is thus maximized, as is the resistance to bending

Table 7.3 lists several mechanical properties used by designers of medical devices when they decide which materials should be used to fabricate a device. This list is not exhaustive and will be supplemented when needed with additional property data. Nevertheless, it should provide the reader with a sense of the relative differences in mechanical behavior within and among groups of materials. It should also be pointed out that many of these properties are averages and there would be a statistical distribution associated with these values.

7.8 Summary

The three classes of materials used in medical devices and implants are metals, ceramics, and polymers; composites are combinations of two or more of these materials and are made in such a way that the individual components retain their identity while contributing to improved processing or mechanical properties. The type of interatomic bonding and the internal atomic and molecular structure in each of the three material classes is different and explains their very different chemical and mechanical characteristics.

Any discussion of which material is best suited for a medical device must first establish that the material will not degrade in the physiologic environment, and second, determine which mechanical properties are important in the given application; is strength, hardness, wear resistance, fatigue resistance, or toughness the most critical concern? Standard test methods have been developed to permit the device designer to specify the levels of performance that are needed.

7.9 Foundational Concepts

- The three general classes of materials are metals, ceramics, and polymers.
- Metals are composed of atoms distributed in a repeating order and are therefore crystalline materials. Defects in the order are called dislocations and generally are due to missing atoms. Dislocations make it possible for metals to undergo plastic

Table 7.3 Physical and mechanical properties of natural and synthetic materials used for biomedical applications

Material	T_g °C	Modulus of elasticity (GPa)	Tensile strength (MPa)	Ductility (%)	Toughness (MPa m$^{1/2}$)
Dental enamel		74	241		0.88
Dentin		21	138		1.97
Compact bone		12–18	120–150		≥5
Skin		0.07	7.6	78	
Tendon		1.2	53	9.4	
Cartilage		0.45–0.80	3	30	
Cardiac muscle		0.1E-3	0.11	64	
Collagen	120	1	50–100	10	
Pyrolytic carbon		28	493	1.58	4.8
Aluminum oxide		366	>500		4
Zirconium oxide		201	950		10.5
Hydroxyapatite		40–117	147		1.2
Bioglass		35	200		0.6
Calcium phosphate		40–117	147		0.52–1.24
Surgical stainless steel		200	1,000	9	100
Cobalt–chromium alloy		230	655–1,800	8	100
Titanium (pure)		110	799	15–24	66–140
Titanium–aluminum–vanadium alloy		116	1,103	10	80
Polyurethane	−73 to −23	1.5–2	28–40	600–720	0.2 (foam)
Poly(tetrafluoroethylene)	21	1–2	15–40	250–550	J_{IC}: 7.0 kJ/m^2
Poly(methyl methacrylate)	100–117	3–4.8	38–80	2.5–6	0.7–1.6
Poly(ethylene terephthalate)	67–207	3–4.9	42–80	50–500	1.01–1.7
Ultrahigh molecular weight polyethylene (UHMWPE)		0.5–1.3	30–42	130–500	J_{IC}: 27–238 kJ/m^2
Poly(lactic) acid	54–59	1.2–3	29–35	2–6	4.2
Poly(glycolic) acid	36	6.6	339–394	15–35	

(permanent) deformation. Alloys are made by dissolving one or more metallic elements into a host metal. Metals are strengthened as a result of alloying, because the atoms of the added elements do not exactly fit into the structure of the host metal.

- Ceramics are composed of metal and nonmetal ions distributed in a repeating order and are also crystalline. Because of ionic bonds and repulsive interactions between like-charged ions, ceramics do not readily undergo plastic deformation. If metal and nonmetal ions are arranged in a chaotic, disorderly structure, the material is considered to be noncrystalline or amorphous or a glass.
- Polymers are typically composed of atoms of light elements such as carbon, oxygen, hydrogen, and nitrogen. The atoms are covalently bonded and form groups of atoms called molecules. Monomers are the smallest representative grouping of atoms, and they are joined together in chemical reactions to form polymers.

Polymers can be thought of as long chains of assembled monomers and may be linear, branched, copolymerized, grafted, or cross-linked. All these changes in structure (but not composition) result in changes in mechanical properties.
- Composites consist of combinations of various materials in a way that preserves the identity of each component. The component that is continuous is called the matrix, and the components that are present in a separated form are usually provided to reinforce the matrix. Everyday composites include fiberglass and concrete.
- Materials are said to behave elastically if they return to their original shape after being subjected to a load that is removed, plastically if they show signs of permanent change in shape after removal of a load, and viscoelastically if they regain their shape over a period of time.
- Mechanical properties used in designing medical devices include the modulus of elasticity, the yield strength, ultimate tensile strength, ductility, hardness, and toughness. A standard tensile test can help to determine the modulus, ductility, yield strength, tensile strength, as well as an indication of toughness. Stress is defined as load divided by unit area, and strain is defined as the change in dimension (e.g., length) divided by the original value of that dimension.
- Materials undergo fatigue when they are loaded in a cyclic manner to stress levels below their yield strengths. In these circumstances, they will fracture after some number of loading cycles. Virtually all medical devices are subject to fatigue. Laboratory testing seeks to determine what the projected lifetime of a medical device will be in service by applying loads that simulate physiologic conditions. It is unfortunately not realistic to screen materials and devices for the length of time they are intended to be in service.
- During wear, two material surfaces slide past each other while they are forced together by some load. Resistance to sliding is caused by high spots on the surfaces interfering with each other, sometimes causing material to be torn out. Wear can be reduced by using lubricating fluids, but wear debris in the form of particles is released from artificial hip and knee joints.
- Metals degrade in a chemical process called corrosion, and their resistance to being dissolved may be predicted by consulting the galvanic series. Polymers degrade by a process of chain scission brought on by exposure to light and sorption of fluids from their environment.
- Hollow cylinders are stiffer than solid rods of the same weight.

References

1. Davis, J. (Ed.). (2003). *Overview of biomaterials and their use in medical devices* (Handbook of materials for medical devices). Materials Park, OH: ASM International.
2. Koppenhoefer, K., Cromption, J., & Dydo, J. (2007). Prediction of failure in existing heart valve designs. In M. Mitchell & K. Jerina (Eds.), *Fatigue and fracture of medical metallic materials and devices* (pp. 77–86). West Conshohocken, PA: ASTM.
3. Park, J., & Lakes, R. (2007). *Biomaterials. An introduction* (3rd ed.). New York, NY: Springer.

8 Biomaterials Applications in Medicine and Case Studies

I did not have implants. I just had a growth spurt.

Britney Spears

Discussion of anatomy and physiology and materials properties has set the stage for an exploration of the ways materials are used to construct biomedical devices.

8.1 Introduction

In the last two chapters, we have covered a considerable amount of foundational information and discussed how the human body protects itself from foreign bodies including bacteria and implants. Chapter 7 focused on understanding why different types of materials possess different properties, how these properties are measured, and we hope that you have come to understand why chemical and mechanical properties are important in biomedical technology applications. All implants and medical devices that interact with the body are made from materials, and the exact material used strongly influences implant and device performance.

In this chapter, we will discuss medical materials in greater depth, introduce you to specific types of implants, and present case studies that should help you understand the degree of design sophistication and analysis needed to apply a knowledge of materials and mechanical behavior to solve medical needs.

8.2 Examples of Implants

There is an astounding variety of implants manufactured today and approved for use. They include craniofacial implants used after trauma surgery (Fig. 8.1), made from a polymer called poly(etheretherketone), and fabricated using a laser melting

G.R. Baran et al., *Healthcare and Biomedical Technology in the 21st Century: An Introduction for Non-Science Majors*, DOI 10.1007/978-1-4614-8541-4_8,

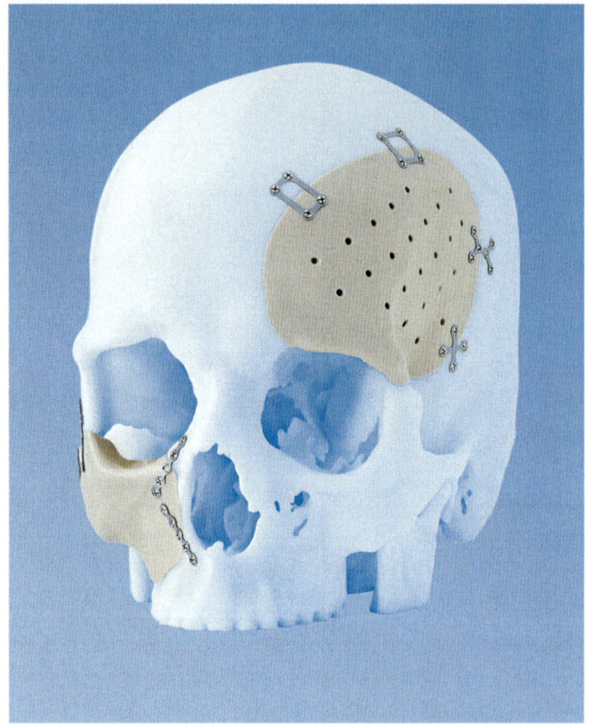

Fig. 8.1 Cranial implant made from poly(etheretherketone) polymer, customized by a laser fabrication process for the individual patient requiring posttraumatic reconstruction. Photo courtesy of DePuy Synthes Companies; used with permission

technique that permits surgeons to plan and obtain a customized implant for the individual patient.

Tooth implants that replace missing teeth (Fig. 8.2) have been available for several decades. They are made from titanium or a titanium alloy and can also be coated with hydroxyapatite, the mineral found in bones. They are inserted after the dentist drills a pilot hole in the jaw bone, and after the bone heals and secures the implant, its upper portion is restored with a crown to resemble a natural tooth. Titanium is capable of bonding directly to bone, and if the patient maintains good oral hygiene, the implant will remain in service for many years.

Perhaps the most widely known implants are artificial hip and knee replacements (Figs. 8.3 and 8.4). Both are multicomponent devices, and in both types of prostheses, the metals often chosen for the stem portions are either titanium or cobalt–chromium alloy, while the femoral head is most often made from cobalt–chromium.

During orthopedic surgery, the hip stem is inserted into the marrow cavity of the femur (the long bone in the thigh), and the femoral head is fitted into place over a metal peg at the top of the femoral component. The metal cup is fitted separately into the hip socket (acetabulum), secured with bone screws, and a plastic (polymer) liner made from ultrahigh molecular weight polyethylene is press-fitted into the metal cup. In service, the femoral head freely rotates within the lined cup. Critical design and medical issues associated with these implants include a choice of liner material (some designs use no liner and rely on metal-to-metal contact; other

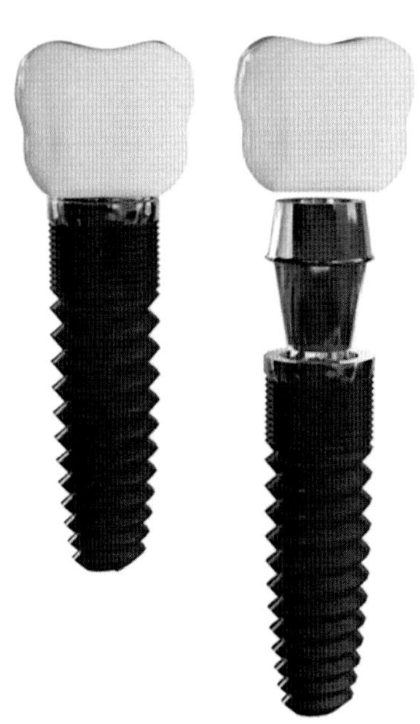

Fig. 8.2 Individual titanium dental implants

designs utilize a ceramic head and a ceramic liner), the size of the cup and femoral head, the length of the stem, and the choice of whether to use bone cement to secure the stem in the femur. Factors that influence the success and lifetime of the implant include surgical accuracy; the better the anatomic alignment of the stem and acetabular cup, the better the outcome.

The knee prosthesis is also a modular device. The surgery consists of preparing the tibia (the large long bone in the lower leg) by planing its head to yield a flat surface and inserting the short tibial stem into the tibial marrow cavity. The end of the femur is also surgically altered to receive the femoral component. This is usually done by first placing a template over the end of the femur to ensure that all the surgical cuts are made at the correct angle and that the depth of the cuts is appropriate. The femoral component may be cemented into place or held by pressure because when a patient walks, their weight prevents the implant from being displaced. The bearing surface is again made from ultrahigh molecular weight polyethylene. As with hip implant surgery, outcomes are strongly dependent on proper alignment and fit of the prosthesis, as well as matching the size of the implants to the patient's size and weight. A less appreciated design feature is the curvature of the femoral component. One can imagine that a sharply curved surface would cause the lower leg to swing at an unacceptably fast rate during walking; designers spend time ensuring that the kinematics of the joints movement will not be unnatural and coincide with the speed of the other foot.

Shoulder joint replacement implants are also available, as are artificial discs for the spine. The materials used for these devices are similar to those used in hip and knee replacements. Spinal disc prostheses such as shown in Fig. 8.5 are a relatively new development, and as of spring 2013 only two devices have been FDA approved for

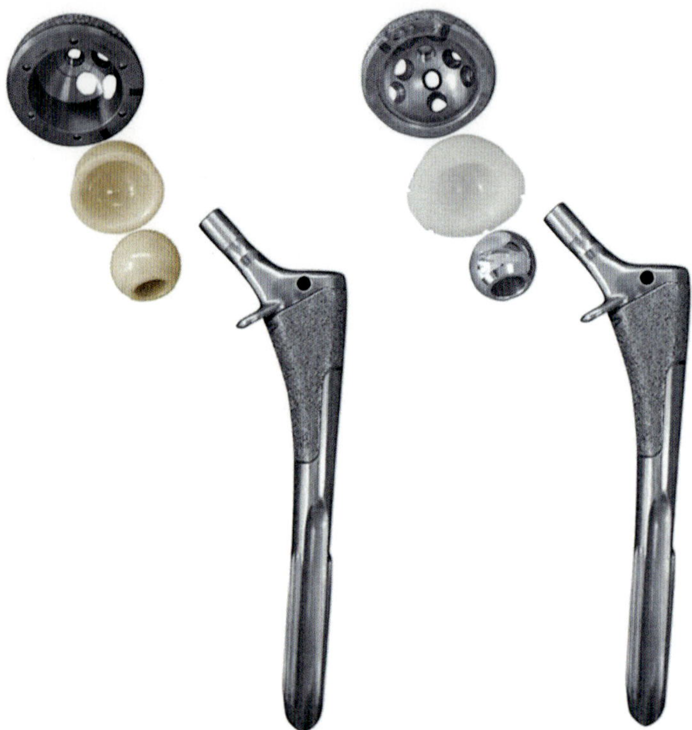

Fig. 8.3 Hip implants. On *left*, the femoral head and acetabular cup liner are made from the ceramic material aluminum oxide. On the *right*, the femoral head is made of metal; the acetabular cup liner is made from ultrahigh molecular weight polyethylene. Both of the femoral shafts have been partially coated with fibrous metal to enhance implant retention. Copyright Springer-Verlag

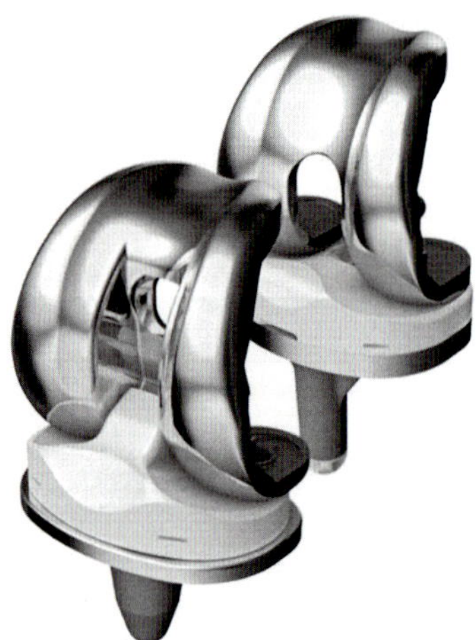

Fig. 8.4 Total knee replacement. Photo courtesy of DePuy Synthes Companies; used with permission

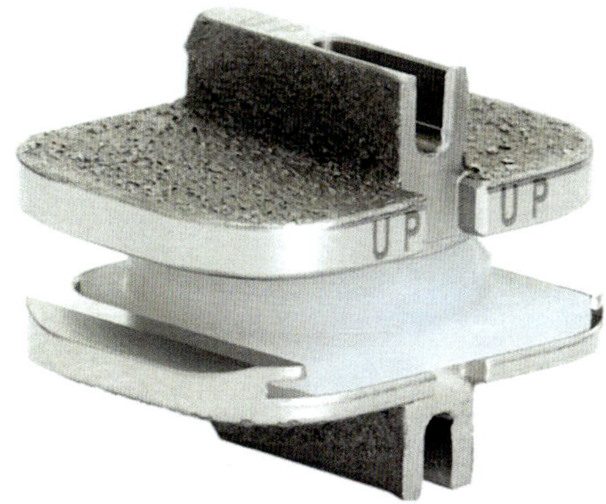

Fig. 8.5 An artificial disc for implantation into the spine to replace a badly deteriorated disc. Photo courtesy of DePuy Synthes Companies; used with permission

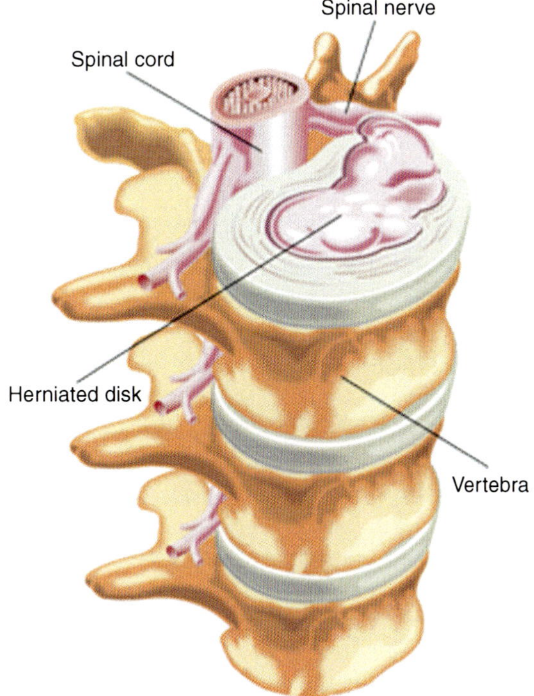

Fig. 8.6 Drawing of herniated disc showing compression of spinal cord

placement in the lower (lumbar) spine. They are used when the natural disc has herniated (sometimes also called a "slipped" disc), creating a bulge that irritates the spinal cord which is nearby (Fig. 8.6). The patient also loses some height as a result of this procedure. The interior of the disc consists of a nucleus that degenerates and loses volume as the patient ages, so that compression of the spinal cord almost always occurs eventually and surgery may be recommended as a last resort to control pain.

Fig. 8.7 Spine fusion utilizing screws, rods, and space-maintaining implant. Image courtesy of Globus Medical

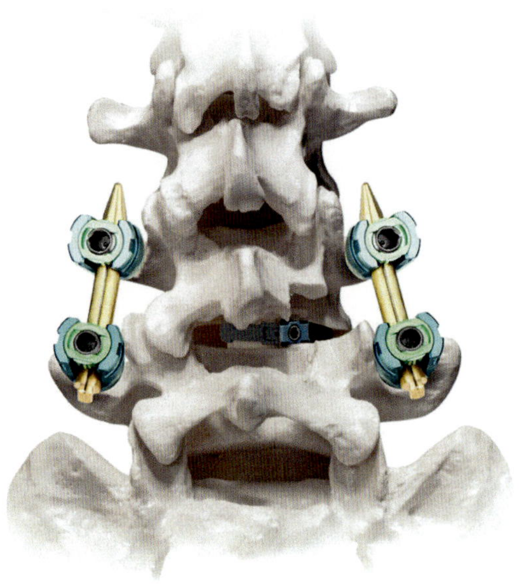

Another type of treatment for herniated discs, illustrated in Fig. 8.7, is for the surgeon to remove the herniated disc, replace it with a block of bone or a synthetic implant to maintain the appropriate intervertebral space, and then affix rods using pedicle screws to stabilize that portion of the spine. A potential advantage of the artificial disc is that it preserves motion of the spine, i.e., the patient may still bend and rotate at that level of the spine. Potential issues that may result with artificial discs include wear of the device and subsidence (the disc will sink into the vertebrae immediately above and below).

Subsidence has a greater probability of occurring in the lumbar spine (lower back) than in the cervical or thoracic spine (neck or chest), because the lumbar spine carries greater weight. Materials used for artificial discs include titanium and titanium alloys, as well as cobalt–chromium alloys; the bearing surface may be metal or ultrahigh molecular weight polyethylene.

Patients with severe rheumatoid arthritis and deformed finger joints may also require implants. Finger joint implants are made either from silicone (which has high flexibility enabling weakened ligaments to articulate the joint) or from pyrolytic carbon (which has excellent biocompatibility).

Stents (Fig. 8.8) are implanted to prop open clogged arteries, and breast implants (Fig. 8.9) are used for cosmetic reasons or postmastectomy (cancerous breast removal) reconstruction. Breast implants have a long and controversial history and originally were made of a silicone polymer envelope encasing a silicone gel. Today, however, breast implants may contain a saline solution to ease fears of the consequences of implant rupture.

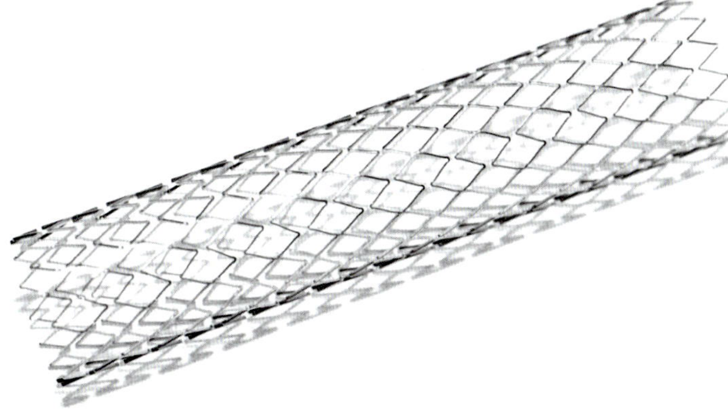

Fig. 8.8 An arterial stent that has been deployed (expanded)

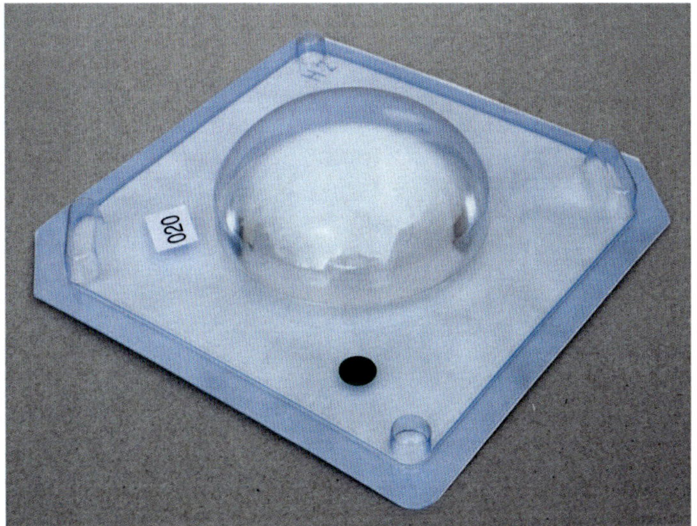

Fig. 8.9 A silicone breast implant in its package

Stents, which will be discussed again in Chap. 9, are origami-like devices usually made from nickel–titanium or stainless steel wire. Before they are inserted into an artery, their normal configuration is compressed. Once they have been guided into place, they are expanded using a mechanism attached to the catheter in a procedure called an angioplasty to restore normal blood flow by widening the diameter of a blood vessel that may have become clogged with plaque (Fig. 8.10). Sometimes, stents are coated with drugs that are slowly released in order to prevent restenosis (re-clogging or re-narrowing of the blood vessel).

Surgical mesh (Fig. 8.11), made from polypropylene, polytetrafluoroethylene, or polyester, is used to stabilize internal organs following surgical hernia repair

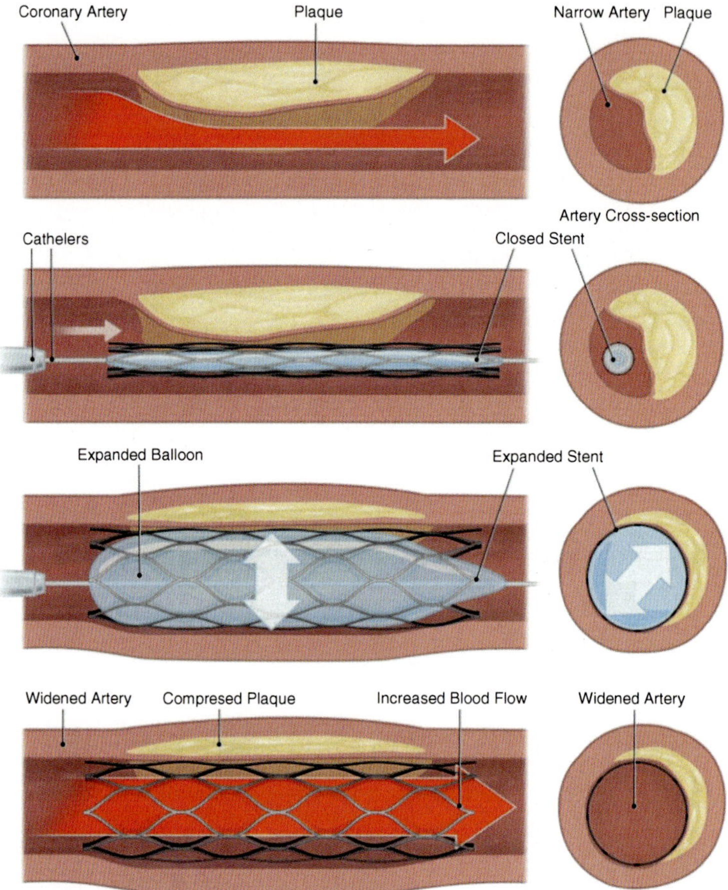

Fig. 8.10 Diagram of the function of a stent to widen a partially clogged blood vessel in a procedure called an angioplasty

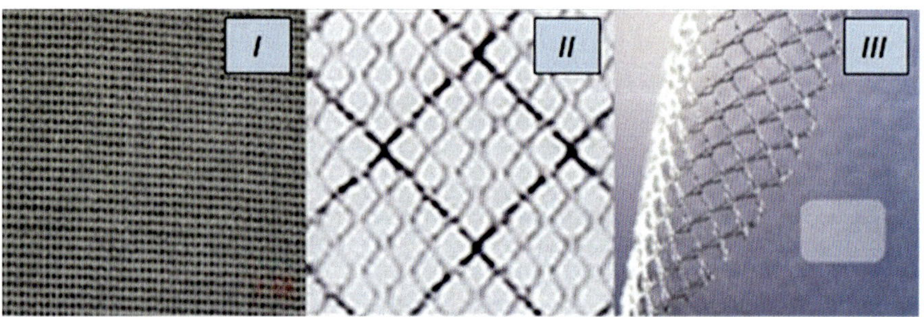

Fig. 8.11 Surgical meshes made from polypropylene (I), polypropylene and polyglactin (II), and polypropylene and titanium (III) used to repair hernia and pelvic organ prolapse. Copyright Springer-Verlag

(a hernia is a protrusion of an organ through a wall of tissue that is intended to contain the organ; commonly, hernias occur in the abdomen when a portion of the intestine penetrates through into the inguinal canal). The surgical mesh is placed underneath the skin to prevent recurrent penetration. Although most surgeries yield good results, potential complications can occur if portions of the intestine adhere to the mesh or to other portions of the intestine. An additional use for this type of mesh is treatment of pelvic organ prolapse, a condition in which the bladder, top of the vagina, uterus, rectum, or bowel descends from their normal position, probably because of a weakening of pelvic muscles due to childbirth and the aging process. During hysterectomy surgery, the mesh can be implanted by access through the abdomen or through the vagina.

8.3 Metals in Medicine

The requirement that an implant material be biocompatible and not corrode in the body restricts the range of metals that may be considered for implantation. Although gold and platinum possess excellent corrosion resistance and have adequate strength, the costs of these metals preclude them from being used except in the most demanding applications (e.g., electric contacts in a corrosive environment). The three most common alloys used as implants or medical devices are stainless steel, cobalt–chromium alloys, and titanium or titanium alloys.

There are many stainless steels used for cutlery, fermentation vessels, piping in pharmaceutical factories, etc., but the variety used in medicine is called 316L, surgical stainless steel. It is utilized for surgical tools, including scalpels and staples, and for implants. The composition of 316L is shown in Table 8.1.

An adequate content of the element Cr is essential, because it provides corrosion resistance, but carbon content must be kept low. Carbon is a remnant of the iron refining process, and it has a tendency to form compounds with Cr called carbides. The carbides are segregated to grain boundaries, and because carbides are very brittle materials, they can weaken the stainless steel alloy (carbides located within grains are not harmful). 316L is available as a cast only metal alloy, but its most frequent appearance is after processing into sheets or rods or wire.

Cobalt–chromium alloys were initially developed for aerospace applications as jet engine turbine components because of their ability to maintain strength at high temperature and their resistance to corrosion in engine exhaust gases. They are used

Table 8.1 Composition of 316L surgical stainless steel

Iron: 670–65 %
Chromium: 17–20 %
Nickel: 12–14 %
Molybdenum: 2–3 %
Carbon: 0.03 % maximum
Traces of manganese, copper, silicon, phosphorus, sulfur, nitrogen

Table 8.2 Composition of medical grade cobalt–chromium alloys

Cobalt: 58–69 %
Chromium: 26–30 %
Molybdenum: 5–10 %
Nickel: 0–11 %
Tungsten: 0–16 %
Carbon: 0.15–0.35 % maximum
Traces of manganese, phosphorus, sulfur, silicon, iron, nitrogen

Table 8.3 Common medical titanium alloy compositions

CpTi	Ti-6Al-4 V	Nitinol
99.96 % titanium	88–91 % titanium	50 % titanium
0.15–0.4 % oxygen	5.5–6.5 % aluminum, 3.5–4/5 % vanadium, traces of carbon, iron, nickel	50 % nickel

in hip and knee implants, dental partial denture frameworks, and for orthodontic wires. The composition of a typical cobalt–chromium alloy is provided in Table 8.2.

There are four families of Co–Cr alloys, grouped according to the presence or absence of W and Ni. The exact composition determines if the alloy is better suited to be used as a casting or to be processed by mechanical methods into sheet or bar stock. Co–Cr alloys are the strongest metals available for use in medical devices.

Titanium is available in the "cp" designation (commercially pure) and as alloys with aluminum (Al), vanadium (V), niobium (Nb), zirconium (Zr), and molybdenum (Mo). Because titanium is highly reactive with oxygen, every attempt is made to reduce the amount of that element in titanium or its alloys, because just as carbon does in steels and Co–Cr alloys, oxygen will make titanium brittle. Desirable characteristics of titanium and its alloys include its low modulus, which provides a better match with bone than cobalt–chromium alloys or stainless steel. This means that the stress shielding due to a titanium implant will not be as severe as it would be with a cobalt–chromium alloy implant. Titanium and its alloys also possess a high strength to weight ratio (titanium has a low density), good corrosion resistance, high fracture toughness, the ability to osseointegrate (bond with bone), and last but not the least, it is nonmagnetic. That means that implants or devices made from titanium will not interfere with MRI imaging.

Titanium or its alloys are used in hip implants, dental implants, orthodontic wires, medical devices such as pacemakers, artificial limbs, surgical instruments, and spinal implants and accessories. The composition of some common titanium alloys is given in Table 8.3.

Nitinol is an interesting titanium alloy, consisting of 50 % Ti and 50 % Ni. The alloy has "shape memory" made possible by a temperature-controlled transition (a martensitic transformation) between two different crystal structures. The transition temperature, which can range from approximately 70 °C to −50 °C, can itself be controlled by small changes in the amount of nickel in the alloy. Useful applications may be obtained by first shaping the alloy at a temperature above the transition temperature, then deforming the component while it is cooled below the transition temperature and placing it in service. If the transition temperature is exceeded in the new environment, the component spontaneously recovers its original shape. For example, a magician could bend a spoon in half while it is heated to above the transition temperature, then cool the spoon and straighten it while it is cool. By later placing the bent spoon in warm coffee or tea, the spoon will bend itself in half, allowing the magician to claim psychic powers. In a medical device application, nitinol may be formed into an expanded stent above the transition temperature then cooled and compressed into a narrow shape easily passed through a blood vessel until reaching the site where the vessel is partially clogged, where the elevated temperature of the human body will trigger the stent to return to its original expanded shape.

8.4 Ceramics and Glasses in Medicine

Various forms of ceramic and glass materials are used in biomedical technology. Some are inert and will become covered with a fibrous sheath (scar tissue) after implantation. Others, such as bioglasses and calcium phosphate ceramics, are designed to interact with the cells of the human body and can bond to bone and even soft tissue [1]. The composition of these materials is high in calcium and phosphorus, elements found in native bone, so they are capable of promoting bone growth by providing the necessary elements for bone hydroxyapatite. The precipitation of new bone mineral on bioactive ceramics is made possible either by the arrangement of the Ca^{2+} ions on surfaces of ceramics containing calcium (such as synthetic hydroxyapatite) or by the surface charge of the synthetic material, which must be negative and capable of attracting Ca^{2+} ions (as is the case with titanium implants, which are also capable of bonding to bone). However, precipitation of calcium and formation of crystalline hydroxyapatite from solution is itself not enough to form bone; for that, "osteoblasts" (bone building cells) need to be recruited to the implant surface site. Bone formation on an implant surface is a complex process, but it is thought that the proteins which absorb on bioactive surfaces somehow enable bone formation and that cells on bioactive surfaces that do not participate in bone formation die, leaving behind cells that do participate in bone formation [1].

Alumina (Al_2O_3) and zirconia (ZrO_2) are two inert (not degraded by the body and considered biocompatible) ceramics used as bearing materials in artificial hips (both femoral head and acetabular cup liner) and knee implants. (Note that alumina is a ceramic unlike aluminum which is a metal. The fact that aluminum corrodes has no bearing on the corrosion behavior of alumina because it is an altogether different kind of material.) These are the only ceramics used in load-bearing implants because they possess high strength and, more importantly, because they are resistant to crack propagation (they have a high fracture toughness). Alumina ceramic implants consist entirely of Al_2O_3 (>99.8 %), but zirconia materials contain small amounts of yttrium oxide (Y_2O_3). This compound is added because it stabilizes a particular crystalline form of zirconia which is exceptionally resistant to crack propagation. It may be easily understood that in artificial joint implants, cracking would lead immediately to total implant failure and the need for replacement. In order to achieve optimal performance, the contacting surfaces of alumina and zirconia total joint components are highly polished, not only to achieve the smoothest possible surface, but also to attain the desired shape. These additional manufacturing steps are performed to reduce the potential for stress concentrations that could lead to crack initiation. Alumina and zirconia have also been used as dental implant materials, but for that application, they may be made porous in the hope that bone will grow into the pores and anchor the implant.

The inorganic mineral phase naturally found in teeth and bones is hydroxyapatite, which has the chemical formula $Ca_{10}(PO_4)_6(OH)_2$. The two principal elements are calcium and phosphorus (suggesting why it is recommended that our diets include foods rich in calcium). Because the human body requires calcium for other physiologic processes such as impulse conduction in nerves and clotting of blood, a lack of adequate amount of calcium in the diet can lead to the loss of calcium from bones. The hydroxyl group (–OH) in this mineral can also be partly replaced with fluoride (–F) to form fluorapatite, which is particularly resistant to bacterial acid attack, so the incorporation of small amounts of fluorine from a water supply into growing teeth will provide them with resistance to tooth decay.

It is very useful to have materials available that can bond to bone; then, it is not necessary to stabilize implants by using screws, which can themselves eventually become potential failure sites. The different interactions of materials with bone include osteoinduction (inducing neighboring cells to become active bone-depositing cells even in locations where native bone is not found), osteoconduction (permitting bone to grow on the material surface), and osseointegration (or permitting bone to have direct contact to the implant).

Osteoinduction was demonstrated by implantation of demineralized bone matrix into the muscle of several animal species, and it was subsequently found that the principal substances responsible for the phenomenon of mineralization were a family of proteins called "bone morphogenetic proteins" or BMPs. These compounds have been synthesized, and two of them (BMP-2, BMP-7) are currently FDA approved for use in speeding the healing of bone fractures and in spinal fusion procedures.

However, osteoinduction has also been observed to occur in the presence of certain synthetic biomaterials, including polymers (polyhydroxyethylmethacrylate), metals (titanium), and ceramics (primarily calcium phosphates such as hydroxyapatite) [2]. Whereas it is somehow more intuitively acceptable for synthetic materials containing calcium and phosphorus to induce bone formation, scientists are less able to explain why the polymer and metal are able to do so; it is not presently known how to create new osteoinductive materials, only that the material's composition, structure, and surface structure all have a degree of influence.

Hydroxyapatite is usually synthesized using wet chemical methods into a powder form. It falls within the general category of calcium phosphate ceramics, a large and very diverse family of chemical compounds. The exact relative amounts of calcium and phosphorus, the amount of water, and the degree of crystallinity of the mineral all influence its reactivity and mechanical properties. The synthesized powder can be sintered into a dense form or used as a powder. Because hydroxyapatite is not a strong material, it is not used in applications where high stresses will be encountered, such as the bearing surfaces of artificial joints. In its dense form, it finds applications as an inner ear implant and as an alveolar ridge augmentation material (patients who lose teeth also lose the supporting bone structure; in order to eventually place a dental prosthesis that would enable normal function, it is necessary to replace the missing bone). Hydroxyapatite is also used as a coating over metal implants because it is "osteoinductive" (it induces bone growth). In this way, an implant coated with hydroxyapatite can become more firmly anchored in bone. Hydroxyapatite mineral may be deposited in several different ways, but a common method is to spray molten hydroxyapatite powder onto the metal surface; melting is accomplished with a plasma torch. The coating produced in this manner is adherent, and modifying the temperature and composition of the powder can change the degree of crystallinity of the coating, which in turn will affect its stability in physiologic fluid.

Hydroxyapatite is also used as a porous material for filling defects in bone. The porosity, which must be within a size range of approximately 100 μm, encourages native bone to grow into the hydroxyapatite. Suitable porous constructs may be made synthetically or obtained from certain species of coral which have pores of the desired size and connectivity. The coral, which initially consists of the compound calcium carbonate, is heated to transform into calcium hydroxyapatite.

Other uses for calcium and phosphorus ceramics are as bone cements. In this instance, di- or tricalcium phosphate powders are mixed with water to form a quickly setting (< 20 min) cement. The material is useful as a filler for bony defects in patients with arthritis, bone cancer, osteoporosis, or trauma. The cement is "osteoconductive"; it will eventually dissolve and be replaced with native bone. The speed with which the cement degrades depends on its exact composition, crystallinity, and grain size.

It should be apparent that in certain clinical applications, a material that is inert and non-biodegrading is required, while in others, a material that degrades and is replaced by native bone is desirable. In addition to resorbable calcium phosphates, certain glasses (e.g., Bioglass™) also are capable of resorbing and bonding to bone and even to soft tissue. These glasses consist of a mixture of SiO_2, CaO, Na_2O, and P_2O_5. Upon exposure to physiologic fluid, they begin to dissolve and a gel forms on their surface. The presence of the gel facilitates bonding to tissue, and the relative rates of the dissolution of the glass and the rate of new bone formation must match in order for the glassy construct to remain stable. Bioglasses are often used in a particle form, so that they can be dispensed and packed into bony defects in jaws, between molar teeth, or in the treatment of scoliosis (curvature of the spine). Powdered or granulated bioglass may be mixed with the patient's blood and packed into the defect site where it stimulates natural bone formation [3]. Another use for bioglass is as a porous material for tissue engineering applications where it may be hybridized with another material such as a polymer to counteract the brittle nature of the glass [3].

Although direct bonding of a load-bearing implant to bone is a desirable outcome, in practice this is not always possible to achieve. The techniques of applying hydroxyapatite coatings to metal substructures can sometimes be problematic;

the degree of crystallinity of the coating influences how quickly the synthetic hydroxyapatite is resorbed, and if the resorption process is much faster than the rate at which new bone forms, the implant can become unstable. Any motion of an implant in bone inevitably leads to ever-greater loosening, because bone resorbs under those conditions rather than growing onto the implant.

For this reason, mechanical means of implant fixation are often designed into load-bearing implants such as artificial hips, knees, and teeth. Although bone screws may be used to anchor components such as acetabular cups (hip portion of a total hip replacement) and spine instrumentation, other implants (replacing teeth and the femoral stem component of a hip implant) rely on bony ingrowth into a porous surface for stability. These porous coatings are achieved by deposition of a metal powder or small diameter wires onto the implant surface, then heating to achieve a weld of the powder to the implant body (Fig. 8.3).

The porous coating is designed with porosity large enough to permit healthy bone to grow into the spaces in the coating and thereby stabilize the implant in the long term. In the short term, as with all other implants, it is important to minimize micromotion at the implant–tissue interface because the tissue may form a fibrous sheath surrounding the implant rather than a bony layer.

8.5 Polymers in Medicine

8.5.1 Synthetic Polymers

A large variety of polymers is used in medical devices and as biomaterials. Poly(methyl methacrylate), abbreviated as PMMA and also known as Plexiglass™, is used for bone cements. It is dispensed as a powder and mixed with a catalyst just prior to being inserted in the cavity where an implant will be placed. It is also used as a replacement for diseased lenses in the surgical treatment of cataracts.

The discovery that PMMA could be used as a replacement for lenses was made by Sir Harold Ridley in the late 1930s. During World War II, British fighter pilots would return from sorties having sustained damage to the clear plastic canopy that covered the cockpit. Sir Ridley treated members of a Hurricane (Fig. 8.12) squadron for injuries.

Sir Ridley made the observation that pilots who had sustained eye injuries caused by debris from shattered canopies did not display a severe reaction to the polymer splinters, and decided to use this polymer (called Perspex in the UK) as an implant material for cataract surgeries. PMMA eventually became widely used as a lens replacement, but softer polymers are now preferred.

Soft contact lenses are made from a polymer somewhat similar to PMMA, but the replacement of one of the chemical groups makes the polymer more hydrophilic and able to absorb moisture. When dry, the material is fabricated into a lens, but soaking in saline causes the absorbed liquid to soften the lens. Polyethylene is used for medical tubing and in its ultrahigh molecular weight form as a bearing surface in artificial hip and knee implants. Polytetrafluoroethylene (PTFE, trade name

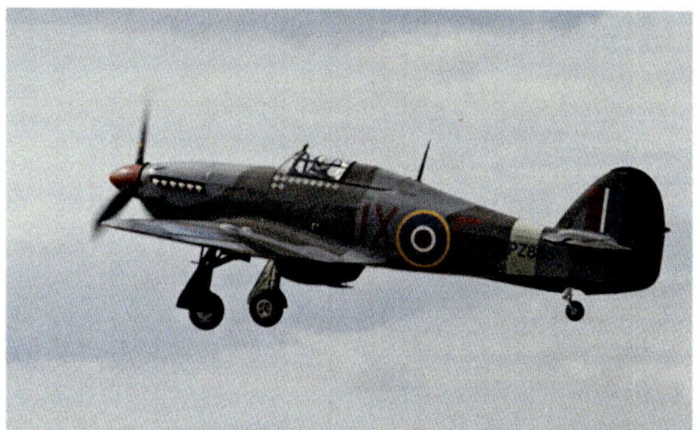

Fig. 8.12 A World War II era British fighter airplane, the "Hurricane"

Teflon™) is used in the manufacture of vascular grafts (replacements for blood vessels) and also in surgeries as a barrier to prevent excessive overgrowth of tissue.

Polydimethylsiloxane, or PDMS, is unique in that it has no carbon atoms in the backbone of the chain. Instead, silicon atoms alternate with oxygen atoms, and different chemical groups can be attached to the two remaining available silicon bonds. This transparent polymer can be modified to have a high refractive index (ability to bend light), and therefore this formulation is useful for manufacture of thin contact lenses. The structure of PDMS allows the material to absorb liquids and gases, and so it has also found use as a drug reservoir for drug delivery applications. The polymer's flexibility and biocompatibility also makes it ideal for finger joint prostheses and for cartilage replacement in the ear and nose. PDMS also has the ability to accurately reproduce surface features and has found use as a mold material for stamping out components of lab-on-a-chip devices.

Polyethylene terephthalate (PET) is used to fabricate vascular grafts and is easily woven into fabrics (Dacron™) useful for hernia repair and ligament reconstruction. Polyethylene glycol (PEG), also known as polyethylene oxide (PEO), is an extremely hydrophilic polymer and is highly effective as a coating material; its high water absorption enables its antifouling (it prevents bacterial adhesion) ability. PEO is also lubricious when it adsorbs water; the strip on low friction or easy-glide razor blade inserts is made from PEO. These polymers are soluble in water; after some period of time, the comfort strip on these razor blades disappears.

Hydrogels constitute a particular category of water-sorbing polymers used for tissue engineering and drug delivery applications [4]. These materials are generally biocompatible, easily synthesized, and may possess a wide range of physical characteristics [5]. Their structure is based on a cross-linked network of hydrophilic polymer chains, and they may be amorphous or crystalline. When dry, hydrogels occupy a small volume; when allowed to come into contact with water, they swell and can have an equilibrium water content of up to 90 %. By changing the composition of the organic groups attached to the main polymer chain, hydrogels can be made to be responsive to temperature, acidity, electric or magnetic stimuli, and the composition of the swelling fluid [6].

Release of drugs from hydrogels can be controlled; the rate with which the drug becomes available, and the stimulus prompting drug release can be tailored for specific applications [5]. Hydrogels can also be positioned in locations where delivery of the drug is needed, for example, on the inner surface of blood vessels. In the simplest method of incorporating a drug into a hydrogel, a dry hydrogel is first immersed into a solution containing a dissolved drug. The hydrogel swells, taking up the solution, and then is dried, losing water but retaining the drug. It may then be implanted at a site where physiologic fluid or saliva re-swells the hydrogel, and the drug slowly diffuses outward to perform its therapy.

Hydrogels also are useful as carriers for cell transplantation. Because the gel is permeable to oxygen and nutrients, the cells can be maintained in a healthy state but be isolated from the body's immune system components so that they are not targeted and destroyed.

Polymers which form hydrogels include PEG, poly(vinyl alcohol) or PVA, and polyhydroxyethylmethacrylate (PHEMA). The latter is used frequently as a soft contact lens material. Hyaluronic acid hydrogels are components of cosmetics and are said to hydrate dry skin, while somewhat more cross-linked varieties are used as dermal fillers to plump up skin wrinkles (e.g., Restylane™, Juvederm™).

Not all materials are designed to remain in the human body unchanged; on some occasions, it is desirable that they degrade and permit the natural tissues of the body to take over that space. Biodegrading implants also eliminate concerns about the long-term compatibility of the implant material. Perhaps the best-known examples of biodegradable or bio-dissolving polymers are those used in suture materials (stitches for closing a wound). Poly(lactic acid) or PLA and poly(glycolic acid) or PGA are the two most frequently used materials in this application. They are not degraded by the body per se; in other words, the enzymes and cells of the body do not participate in their dissolution. Rather, the presence of water eventually destroys the backbone of these polymers. Because of the long history of successful use and approval by regulatory agencies such as the Food and Drug Administration, PLA and PGA and mixtures of these two materials have been also exploited as scaffold materials in tissue engineering. In this application, porous constructs of the polymer are used as carriers for cells and implanted in the body where it is hoped the cells survive and regenerate tissue. Eventually, the construct disappears and is replaced by natural tissue. The trick is of course to adjust the composition in order to ensure that the construct does not degrade too quickly nor too slowly. PLA and PGA are not ideal materials for scaffolds, as their degradation produces lactic acid and glycolic acid, respectively, which tend to cause inflammation; as new scaffold materials also gain FDA approval, it is likely that PLA and PGA will no longer be chosen for scaffolds.

8.5.2 Natural Polymers

Naturally occurring polymers are also useful in medical biotechnology; after all, our bodies and those of other animal organisms are essentially composed of polymers called proteins. Natural polymers can function biologically at the molecular, microscopic, and macroscopic levels. They can potentially be metabolized by the

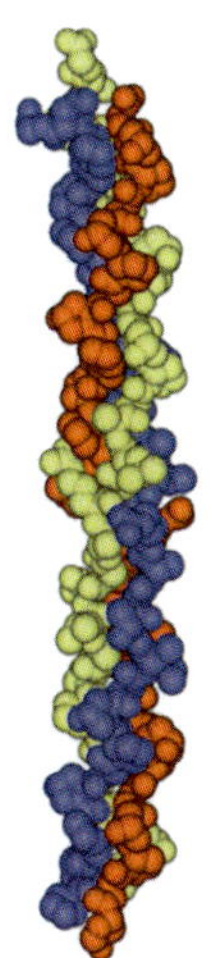

Fig. 8.13 The triple helix structure of the collagen molecule

body so that they will eventually disappear to be replaced by our own tissues. Several proteins may be obtained from animals (e.g., collagen, keratin, silk, elastin); recall that animal sinews and cat gut were once the only materials used for sutures. Other natural polymers used in biomedical applications include polysaccharides (sugars) such as cellulose, dextran, chitin, and glycosaminoglycans. The difficulties associated with natural polymers (i.e., they trigger the body's immune response and there are few processing techniques that can be used with these essentially delicate materials) have limited wider adoption of natural polymers.

Collagen is an essential component of the extracellular matrix (ECM) in our bodies and accounts for 25–35 % of all the proteins within us. It is produced by cells called fibroblasts (cells that make the collagen found in skin and muscle) and chondrocytes (cells that make the collagen found in cartilage). There are at least 29 different types of collagen found in different tissues and organs. Collagen occurs as a fibrous protein and may be thought of as a reinforcement for the polysaccharides and proteoglycan constituents of ECM, just as fibers of glass are used as reinforcements in the material known as fiberglass. The collagen molecule is a triple helix formed by coiling three individual chains of polypeptides (polymers made from short chains of three different amino acids, Fig. 8.13). Interestingly, the synthesis of one of these amino acids (hydroxyproline) cannot be accomplished in the absence of vitamin C.

The complex structure of collagen contributes to the difficulty in its processing. The individual triple helix collagen molecules link together with other collagen molecules to form fibrils, and many fibrils organized together form a collagen fiber. This organization is somewhat similar to the way a rope is constructed. When collagen degrades through the action of chemicals called proteases or because of sun damage, the organization of the collagen molecule is changed; as a result, it shrinks…causing skin wrinkles to occur.

Examples of tissue-based collagen used as implants in humans are heart valves obtained from pigs; these are treated with cross-linking agents such as glutaraldehyde to strengthen the collagen and to remove compounds that could produce an immune response by the implant recipient and can last for 10 years or more in the body. Interestingly, although these valves are not thrombogenic (they do not induce blood clotting), valves from pigs or from cattle are susceptible to calcification and failure just as human heart valves are. The exact reason for this phenomenon is not clear, but it may involve aspects of the tissue preparation/cross-linking process.

Collagen derived from minced tissue that has been treated with enzymes may also be purified and chemically modified and processed into a variety of shapes including sheets, tubes, foams, powders, and injectable solutions. This purified collagen "format" also has low immunogenicity and has the added advantage of being readily processed. If added strength is desirable, it can be cross-linked. It was this characteristic that was exploited during World War II to meet the demand for wound and burn dressings. Collagen was used in a variety of applications, including hemostatic agents (sponges or powder to stop bleeding), as blood vessels (either human or animal origin), heart valves (from pigs or cattle), tendons and ligaments, nerve grafts, dialysis membranes, retinal reattachment, plastic surgery, and drug delivery applications [7, 8].

A uniquely processed collagen-based implant is the Omniflow™ vascular prosthesis. This device consists of a silicone mandrel or tube which is covered in polyester fiber, then inserted into a live sheep, which covers the "implant" with a fibrous collagen sheath as part of its foreign body response [8].

8.6 Surface Modification

We have emphasized the importance of the body's interaction with the surfaces of implants several times in Chap. 6. Because of the importance of this interaction and its influence on the subsequent response of the body, it should come as no surprise that engineers have developed ways in which to modify surfaces to obtain a desired behavior. Why is this necessary? Well, cobalt–chromium alloys are extremely strong and could be useful for a load-bearing implant. However, they do not bond to bone, and so they have to be secured to bone using bone screws. If the cobalt–chrome surface could be modified, perhaps with a coating of hydroxyapatite, then bone could bond and anchor the implant in place.

Several surface modification methods involve the use of a gas plasma. A sample of material is placed into a container flooded with nitrogen, oxygen, or a reactive hydrocarbon gas at low pressure and at room temperature. A voltage is applied, and the gas disassociates into ions and free electrons (a plasma). The gas ions are useful in cleaning the sample or can also be deposited onto the sample surface to prepare it for additional chemical treatments. A related treatment, the plasma spray process, operates at high temperatures at normal pressure; a hot plasma gas is initiated by a high voltage discharge in a nozzle, and as the plasma exits the nozzle, powdered coating material is dispensed to be included within the plasma. The high temperature of the plasma melts the coating material (e.g., ceramics such as hydroxyapatite or titanium oxide) and carries it onto the surface of the sample. The molten powder cools and solidifies as it is deposited on the metal sample surface (Fig. 8.14).

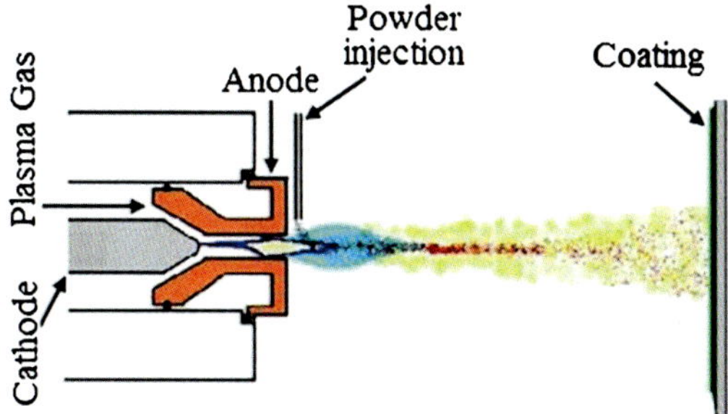

Fig. 8.14 The plasma flame spray process for depositing a bioceramic coating onto an implant. Copyright Springer Verlag

Other gas phase coating technologies include Chemical Vapor Deposition (CVD); in the medical device field, this method is used to deposit pyrolytic carbon, a material that resists clot formation and is therefore useful in artificial heart valves, and diamond, a material with high hardness and good wear resistance, making it useful in orthopedic implants that undergo sliding when the patient walks. In these instances, a metal is the substrate onto which carbon is deposited.

"Grafting" is a method useful for modifying polymers or plastics [9]. In this technique, the surface of a polymer is first made reactive by irradiation with electrons, gamma rays or ultraviolet light. A second polymer is then brought into contact with the energized surface and chemically bonds to it. In this way it is possible to bond together polymers that may not otherwise be compatible. Medical devices may undergo grafting coating methods to render their surfaces non-fouling (i.e., proteins will not adsorb onto such surfaces).

Ion beam implantation is still another coating method, used to render orthopedic implants more wear resistant. In this method, a gas such as nitrogen is ionized and used to bombard a metal sample. The nitrogen ions have sufficient energy to penetrate into the surface of the implant to the depth of one micron.

A technique that requires little in the way of high-energy equipment relies on the formation of self-assembled monolayers (SAMs). This method utilizes a substrate such as a thin layer of gold, or silicon dioxide, onto which a long, three-part molecule is adsorbed. The head of the molecule is designed to attach to the sample surface; the body of the molecule is a chain of linked atoms whose length is varied by the material designer and the functional end of the molecule is the portion designed to interact with cells, bacteria, or bodily fluids (Fig. 8.15). The solid substrate is immersed into a container with the molecule dissolved in an alcohol, and over a period of time ranging from minutes to days, the molecules adsorb onto the sample surface. Because only the head of the molecule has affinity for the substrate surface, all the molecules line up in the same way, with heads on the surface and functional ends extending away from the surface. SAMs are particularly useful in devices called biosensors, where they can be used to bind a substance that is being monitored, for example, glucose in a diabetic patient, or in defense-related applications such as bioweapons.

Attaching specific molecules called polypeptides (compounds similar to proteins but smaller) or sugars to implantable surfaces which bind directly to cell receptors represents a higher degree of sophistication in controlling bioactivity [10].

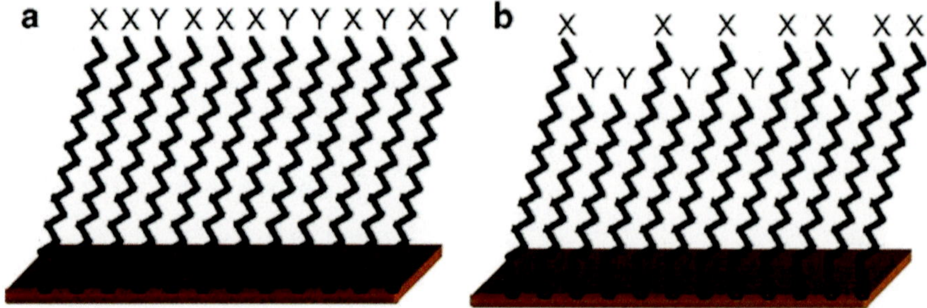

Fig. 8.15 A self-assembled monolayer showing a three-part adsorbed molecule. Note that the spacer lengths can be varied to vary the accessibility of the functional ends. Copyright Springer-Verlag Berlin Heidelberg

This strategy avoids the indirect way of communicating with a cell, i.e., through the conformation of an adsorbed protein, and is used for antimicrobial coatings.

8.7 Antimicrobial Coatings

An important use of surface modification technology is the development of antimicrobial surfaces. The World Health Organization, as well as other institutions and individual scientists, has warned about the development of antimicrobial resistance in certain bacteria [11]. In hospital settings, where implants are surgically placed, the risk of infection by so-called super bugs such as MRSA is particularly high. Under appropriate conditions, bacteria can attach to a surface, adhere, aggregate forming a slimy biofilm, and disperse as portions of the biofilm detach and relocate [12]. Once the biofilm has formed, it is difficult for drugs to gain access to bacteria; for that reason too, it is best to avoid exposure to and colonization by bacteria in the first place. An implant that has been colonized by bacteria and covered by biofilm is best removed from the patient, because it is often not possible to disinfect the implant while it is in place.

In general, bacteria are more adherent to hydrophobic surfaces than to hydrophilic surfaces. Rough surfaces also provide a favorable environment, because bacteria are trapped in the grooves and pits of a rough surface, making them difficult to dislodge. Ways of increasing the hydrophilicity of titanium (thereby rendering it less hospitable to bacterial adhesion) include irradiation with ultraviolet light or deposition of polymer coatings such as poly(ethylene) glycol (a material that always is “wet” and too slippery for bacteria to adhere). Surfaces with directly attached antibiotics such as vancomycin have been shown to maintain antimicrobial behavior, but this strategy is limited by the spectrum of bacteria susceptible to the antibiotic and the potential development of drug tolerance in a short period of time [13]. An alternative solution that is gaining ground is to directly attach antimicrobial peptides to implant surfaces; these peptides are able to prevent biofilm formation by effectively killing bacteria shortly after contact [13].

Other active antibacterial substances can also be incorporated into coatings on implant surfaces. For example, the chemical chlorhexidine, which is also used in mouthwash and in contact lens solutions, can be bound within ceramic and polymer (plastic) coatings. The metallic elements copper and silver also possess antimicrobial activity. The process by which copper hinders bacterial growth and adhesion is still under study, but this metal has a long history as a potent inhibitor of biomass growth; the wooden hulls of sailing ships were once lined with copper sheet, and copper-containing paint is still sold for use on the hulls of smaller wooden boats, as the growth of marine algae on the submerged hull is prevented in the presence of copper. There have been reports that brass or bronze (both alloys contain copper) water jars can effectively eliminate bacteria in water contaminated with *E. coli*. Today, surfaces in hospitals that are often touched (and therefore likely contaminated), such as bed rails, may be made using copper components in an effort to reduce the presence of bacterial. The US Environmental Protection Agency (EPA) has funded studies that confirm copper's effectiveness as an antimicrobial.

The use of silver in health and medicine technology also has a long history. Silver apparently interferes with bacterial enzymes; with the replication of DNA, it inhibits bacterial growth and affects the properties of the cell membrane [14]. Ancient cultures such as the Phoenicians used silver linings in their water jars to keep water safe to drink. Perhaps the idea that silver bullets could kill supernatural creatures such as werewolves and vampires was based on the medicinal properties of silver? In any case, today silver is used for its bactericidal properties in a large number of products. Samsung™ washing machines inject silver ions into a wash; home humidifiers contain silver in the water tank to prevent bacteria from being dispersed in the mist spray; Kohler™ has incorporated silver into toilet seats; a company called Nanohorizons™ incorporates silver into clothing fabrics, rendering them active in the fight against body odor; and both Curad™ and Elastoplast™ brand bandages contain silver to reduce wound infections. Silver is also found in catheters and burn wound ointments. In an interesting Philadelphia connection, Dr. Alfred Barnes, the man who assembled a world-class collection of Impressionist art now housed in a museum in downtown Philadelphia, made his fortune by selling an ointment called Argyrol™, which was used to treat gonorrhea in adults and was also applied to the eyes of infants born to women infected with gonorrhea or chlamydia to prevent blindness.

Still another strategy for fabricating antimicrobial surfaces is to make them "superhydrophobic." These types of surfaces are not wetted by the fluids in which some bacteria are dispersed, and therefore bacteria do not contact the surface and cannot adhere. Surfaces may be made superhydrophobic either by altering the surface composition, for example, by adding a fluorocarbon coating such as polytetrafluoroethylene (Teflon™) or by changing the physical structure of the surface. This latter strategy is borrowed from nature, where it has been observed that lotus leaves, springtails (small insects), and termite wings exhibit self-cleaning, bacterial resistance. Shark skin also resists adhesion of marine organisms, in contrast to whale skin, which often exhibits colonization by barnacles and other microorganisms. The structural characteristic shared by all these surfaces is roughness. This roughness effect which prevents adhesion of larger organisms and water is in some contrast to

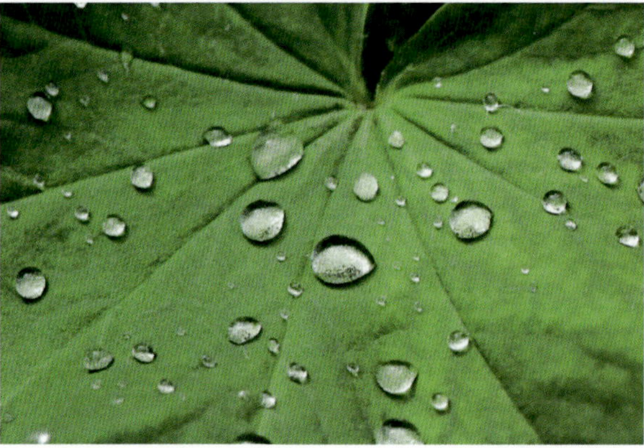

Fig. 8.16 Droplets of water on a leaf; note that the droplets do not spread. The surface of the leaf is hydrophobic because of microscopic roughness

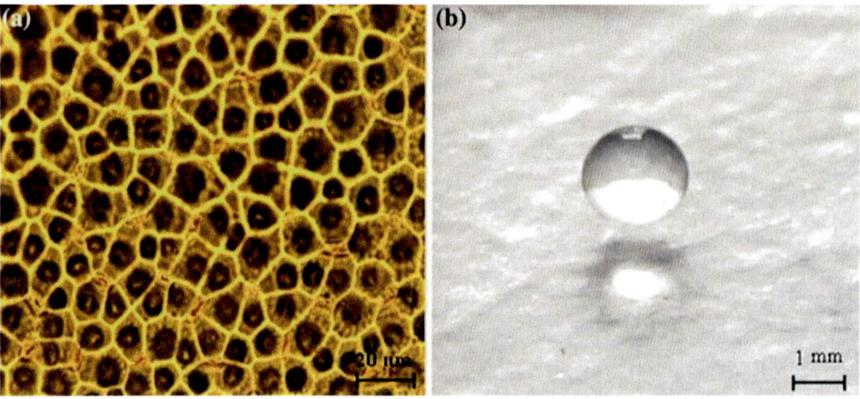

Fig. 8.17 On (**a**) an artificial rubbery superhydrophobic lotus leaf surface. On the (**b**) a water droplet does not wet the surface

bacterial adhesion, where it is found that if the surface roughness is of the size of a bacterium, bacterial adhesion increases because the bacteria are able to "shelter" among the roughness features. Note in Fig. 8.16 that the small protrusions on the leaf hold the water droplet suspended so that it does not wet the leaf.

A significant advantage of physically altered superhydrophobic surfaces is that the bacteria cannot adapt to overcome the superhydrophobic effect, whereas they can develop a resistance to chemicals used to make antibacterial surfaces. And, it is possible to manufacture such structurally altered surfaces in the laboratory using a variety of methods (Fig. 8.17). Recently, a simple technique for altering surfaces was revived that relies on temperature-induced buckling of metal-coated shrink wrap (like Saran™ wrap) [15]. When the film of wrap is heated, it shrinks, and in doing so it forms small raised features on the surface. Because the film has been metal-coated, these features are relatively stable and can be used as a pattern for making a mold. To do this, a rubbery plastic solution is poured on top of the wrinkled surface, allowed to harden, and removed. That mold may then be used to make copies of the rough, superhydrophobic surface on a variety of polymers used in medical technologies. These surfaces have been shown to resist bacterial colonization [15].

8.8 Designing Medical Devices

Medical device manufacturers produce many different devices. How do they go about deciding what type of device is needed and what should be its size and shape? How do they select a specific material, when there are so many biocompatible materials to choose from? Manufacturers study anatomy and consult with surgeons in order to learn what sizes and shapes are needed. For example, pedicle screws (screws for anchoring spine implants to vertebrae) need to be available in several lengths; a spine surgeon might express the need for screws ranging from 2.5 to 4.5 cm in length, and the manufacturer will comply, providing a kit containing several sizes (Fig. 8.18). Similar kits are provided for other types of implants too.

However, there is still a need to design (specify the material and the dimensions) of more complex implants. Fortunately, engineers have a tool called "finite element analysis," originally used to design aeronautical and automotive components with strict strength and low weight specifications (the new Boeing Dreamliner jet, the 787, was designed using this method). The finite element method utilizes a 2- or 3-dimensional model of the component or device, such as shown in Fig. 8.19 (the example here is an intramedullary nail implant, used to hold a broken tibia (lower leg bone) in place), and segments the model into small volumes called "elements." Each element is provided with a set of mechanical properties; then, when the model is "told" that a force is being applied from a specific direction and focused on a

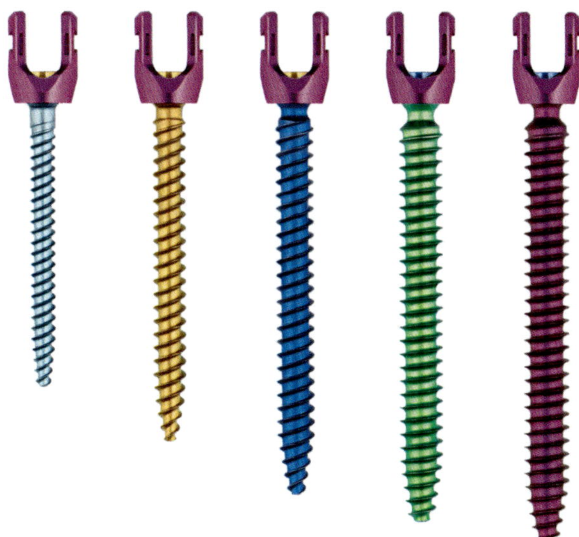

Fig. 8.18 Pedicle screws used in spine surgeries. Photo courtesy of Globus Medical

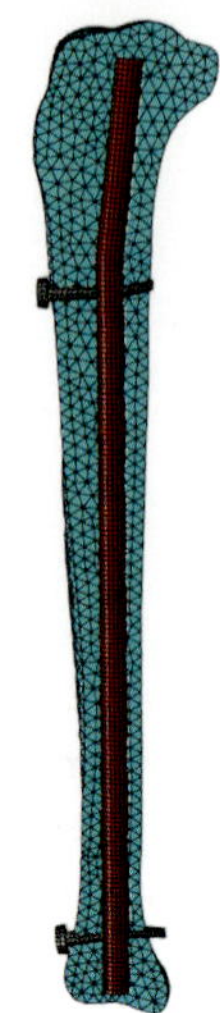

Fig. 8.19 Finite element model of an intramedullary nail in a tibia

particular portion of the model, the finite element analysis software performs a number of calculations yielding the stress distribution throughout the model. So, for example, if the manufacturer wishes to know the stresses in the intramedullary nail and in the bone when stainless steel is used, the mechanical properties of stainless steel are input to the finite elements. If the manufacturer wishes to then estimate the stresses in the intramedullary nail if it were to be made from titanium instead, then the mechanical properties of titanium are input to the elements, and the calculations performed again. It should be apparent that the finite element method allows great freedom in design; not only is it possible to predict the component's mechanical behavior characteristics if different materials are used, but the method also makes it is possible to change the shape and size of the component in order to reduce areas of stress concentration. In fact, the finite element method is now routinely used in medical device research to design implant or device components such as spinal implants, blood pumps, artificial heart valves, artificial joints, and pacemaker leads.

A more recent application of finite element analysis is to estimate the effects of different surgical techniques on patient outcomes. For example, a spine surgeon is interested in attaching a long stabilizing rod to a patient with scoliosis (curvature of the spine). How many screws should be used to fasten the rod to ensure that it does not become loose, and yet not jeopardize the strength of individual vertebrae? This question can be easily answered using finite element analysis as long as the mechanical properties of the vertebrae and the pullout strength of the screws are known. The finite element method can also be used for dynamic fluid flow analysis; so, for example, it would be possible to model different ways of performing a bypass surgery (where the arteries supplying the heart muscle are clogged and blood flow needs to be rerouted).

Might there be other specific design, mechanical property, or performance requirements for intramedullary nails? The role of the FDA has been discussed in an earlier chapter, and the standard ways in which materials and design engineers communicate using specific names for different mechanical properties were discussed in

Chap. 6, but it is sometimes not appreciated that the *way* properties are measured has an influence on testing outcomes. The FDA does not always specify which tests are to be used, but ASTM International, an organization previously called the American Society for Testing and Materials, concerns itself with developing standards and test procedures for thousands of materials applications.

ASTM standards are prepared by various committees, with each committee focusing on certain materials or on certain applications. For example, there will be a committee on surgical cobalt–chromium alloys. That committee will concern itself with specifying the elements such alloys should contain, the mechanical properties that should be measured for these alloys, how the properties should be determined, etc. Membership on the committee is purely voluntary, and open to all interested parties. Typically, every manufacturer making a product that is the subject of a standard will have a representative on the committee. There may also be a few academic members who do research on the material or device that is the subject of the standard, as well as representatives of consulting organizations that might be involved in lawsuits pertaining to failures of the material components. Finally, representatives of consumers, or of organizations that purchase significant quantities of the components (e.g. hospitals) might also be members of such committees.

If a new alloy or polymer is developed and becomes widely used in a given application (e.g., a carbon fiber–epoxy composite used as an intramedullary nail), the committee on surgical fracture fixation devices might choose to develop a new standard for composite nails. The committee's work would begin by calling on its members to submit proposals for the new standard. The suggestions would be distributed to all members, and the committee would meet to discuss individual experiences with testing and data collection, and the proposed new standard would begin to take shape. Committee members would then try the new proposed tests in their own laboratories and then gather again to discuss the strengths and weaknesses of the test procedures. Eventually, a consensus will be developed and a Draft standard published, which can be referred to by composite nail manufacturers used while other interested parties comment. The draft may change again in response to the comments, but eventually a final version will emerge, be voted on, and adopted by the full membership of the committee.

The process for developing and adopting a standard usually requires several years.

Other standards organization exist worldwide, but in 2009 a new common source for over 1,300 medical device standards was created called the Medical Device Standards Portal. The critical documents from AAMI (Association for Advancement of Medical Instrumentation), ASTM, DIN (German Institute for Standards), the US Food and Drug Administration (FDA), the International Electrotechnical Commission (IEC), and the International Organization for Standardization (ISO) can be found easily using this portal. This action was taken in recognition of the global reach of the medical devices industry and the need for common standards whenever possible.

Getting back to the intramedullary nail, consulting the 2012 ASTM list of standards reveals that approximately eight standards have been adopted and applied to intramedullary nails, covering topics such as how to conduct relevant fatigue tests, how to measure critical dimensions, and how to evaluate the nail strength in bending. Manufacturers of intramedullary nails will use these standards to design and evaluate their particular products and advertise the fact that their products adhere to ASTM guidelines and meet ASTM standards. Of course, standards exist for most other implants and medical devices.

It is important to recognize, however, that the standards do not prescribe which material or design is to be used in a specific clinical application. For example, one simulated biomechanical study found that titanium nails were more stable than stainless steel in torsion and axial compression and would provide superior results [16], another that stainless steel nails were less expensive and resulted in a lower incidence of bony nonunion than titanium [17], and still others have made the point that removal of titanium nails takes more time than removal of stainless steel nails because the titanium has a tendency to bond to the bone. These types of reports, with apparently contradictory findings, are often the reasons why getting a second, third, and even fourth opinion from surgeons leaves the patient confused; the surgeon will recommend an option that is most reasonable to him in his/her experience. Because the experiences of other surgeons may be quite different, they will provide other recommendations.

8.9 Implant Case Studies

8.9.1 Case 1: Femoral Bone Fracture Treated Using Intramedullary Nail

A 27-year-old male amateur soccer player with no history of smoking, alcohol, or drug abuse was admitted to a local emergency center with severe swelling and deformity of the right leg. He was playing a recreational match for a local soccer team. While being tackled by an opposing team player, he fell to the ground with severe pain in the leg. The patient was unable to stand and was transported to an emergency center. Bone mineral density measured using DEXA was normal at the femoral neck. Radiographic (X-ray) images of his right leg showed a simple fracture without much comminution (crushed bone) in the right tibia with fibula intact. To keep the bone fracture fragments together and promote healing, a locked intramedullary nailing was performed. Intramedullary nailing is a technique where a metal rod is forced into the medullary (marrow) cavity of the long bones to keep the broken bones close to each other, promoting healing (Fig. 8.20). Callus formation was observed 4 weeks postoperatively, suggesting a normal pattern of bone fracture healing. Tibial bone fusion was complete 6 months postoperatively. The patient was seen 4 years after the surgery during a regular physical examination and he reported returning to recreational soccer.

The process that provided the physician in this case with a way of treating the patient began many years earlier. In 1939 during World War II, an orthopedic surgeon seized on the idea that using an intramedullary nail (actually, it looks more like a rod) could provide a better healing environment than simple casting; the two ends of the broken bone could be held together in such a way that they would not move relative to each other, and importantly, the patient would be somewhat mobile during the approximately 6 week recovery period. It's conceivable that the first attempts to use such a device were tried on a cadaver, with a rod borrowed from a machine shop, in order to practice the surgical method. Then, once the surgeon had gained

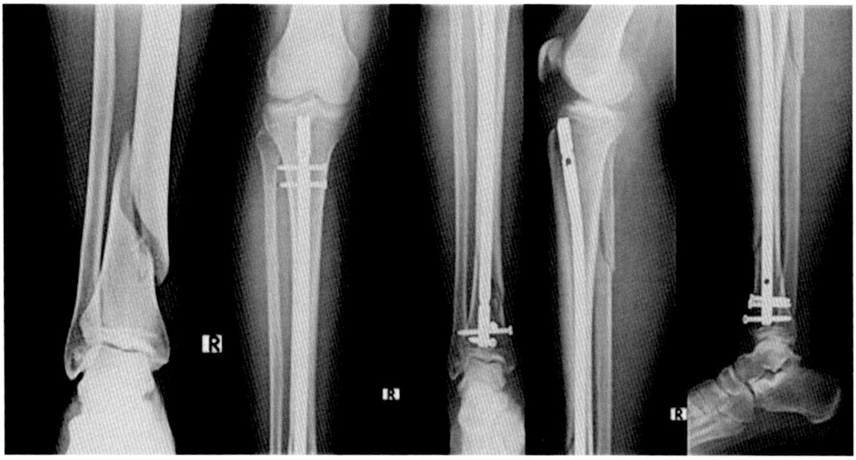

Fig. 8.20 Radiographs of treatment and outcome of intramedullary rod fixation of tibial fracture. Copyrighted by Springer-Verlag

confidence in the technique, he may have approached a surgical supply company or manufacturer of surgical and implant devices for help with designing a nail.

It was known already, from analyses covered in Chap. 7, that the optimum design for a high stiffness to weight ratio is a hollow tube, so the only decision a manufacturer would have to make is which biocompatible metal to use: titanium, stainless steel, or cobalt–chromium alloy. There are many implant manufacturers, and it is likely that they would have carried out the implant design and material specification process using finite element analysis. The approximate dimensions are known, because the nails have to fit into the medullary canal of the tibia, where the average diameters are approximately 8–10 mm and the length of the cavity is approximately 30 cm. However, there is considerable variation in the diameter of the cavity; some have a diameter of 6 mm. Also, examination of the shape of the tibia marrow cavity shows that there is a slight angle to the bone, so any nail designed to fit into the cavity will either have to be no longer than the straight portion of the cavity or be angled to correspond to the anatomic angle. Implant manufacturers are therefore able to offer slightly different versions of these nails, using different biocompatible materials. The choice of a particular brand of nail might be made by the surgeon based on personal preference or by a hospital purchasing agent.

8.9.2 Case 2: Total Knee Replacement

A 56-year-old obese Caucasian woman presented to an arthritis center with an 8-year history of increasing knee pain and stiffness of both knees. She also had a known history of peripheral vascular disease. After radiographic images and blood work, she was diagnosed with osteoarthritis. At that time, the rheumatologist decided to treat the patient with intra-articular corticosteroid injections to relieve pain and inflammation. Not satisfied with the outcome of the injections, the patient

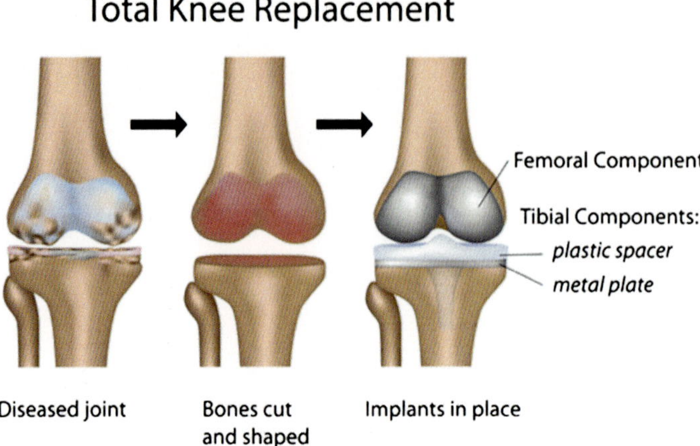

Fig. 8.21 The origin and progression of arthritis was discussed in Chap. 6, and to summarize, osteoarthritis is a disease that is responsible for the destruction of joint cartilage. The loss of cartilage can be provoked or accelerated by several factors, but patients that are overweight place a high load requirement on this tissue, causing the cartilage to crack and to wear away. Because cartilage cannot heal itself, the current standard treatment (once pain-reducing measures are exhausted) is replacement of the entire joint

decided to see an orthopedic surgeon 4 months after the initial corticosteroid injection. The orthopedic surgeon recommended total knee arthroplasty to replace both knee joints. During the surgery, the patient's diseased knee joints were removed and replaced with a total artificial knee (Figs. 8.4 and 8.21). The patient was also treated with an anticoagulation drug to prevent any blood clots (e.g., deep vein thrombosis) after surgery. The surgery and the postoperation recovery were uneventful. The patient was able to flex her knees without pain after 8 weeks. A 3-year follow-up showed no bone resorption.

In examining the design of an artificial knee after implantation, the tibial plate component is held in place by a shaft, whose length can vary depending on the patient's needs, that intrudes into the marrow cavity in the tibia. The plate may be held in place with bone screws, or a bone cement may be inserted into the tibial marrow cavity and eventually harden around the shaft of the tibial plate. The surface of the shaft is usually treated to increase its roughness so that the bone cement will achieve better mechanical adhesion. The femoral component is placed after the femur has been prepared by the surgeon who has cut away unnecessary bone and cartilage. There is a short stub on the femoral component that helps to keep it in place, and either frictional force or bone cement is used to keep the component in place during service. An interesting design aspect of knee prostheses is that the shape and angulation of the femoral component surface have a significant effect on the patient's comfort while walking. Great care is taken by manufacturers to ensure that the surface permits a normal rate of bending at the knee.

Table 8.4 Friction coefficients of selected medical materials combinations

Combination	Coefficient
Cobalt–chromium alloy/UHMWPE	0.1–0.24
Titanium/UHMWPE	0.2
Nitrogen implanted titanium/UHMWPE	0.06
Cobalt–chromium alloys/itself	0.3
Aluminum oxide/itself	0.007
Teflon/itself	0.04

Examining the relevant ASTM specifications for total knee implants reveals that manufacturers are concerned with implant wear, fatigue, and stability of the components are the critical topics of concern. Many of these tests require specialized equipment and fixtures that would be found in the laboratories of a manufacturer or a consulting testing service.

The list of alloys available for knee implants includes titanium, stainless steel, and cobalt–chromium alloys. Because wear resistance has to be a critical requirement of this implant (and of any other implants where sliding movement occurs in the presence of a load or force, e.g., hip, shoulder, teeth), it is reasonable to examine the factors involved in providing a material combination with good wear resistance. Friction coefficients, even though they are only one of the factors affecting wear, can serve as an initial screening tool and are determined experimentally using a "tribometer." The coefficients for some relevant material couples are shown in Table 8.4, which indicates that a combination of a nitrided titanium (titanium that has been bombarded with nitrogen ions to form a wear-resistant coating of titanium nitride) femoral plate on ultrahigh molecular weight polyethylene (UHMWPE) is a promising combination. UHMWPE was also chosen as a bearing surface because of its toughness (it is the material used for the bottom of skis and snowboards). Because it is softer than the metal that it contacts, however, most of the wear particles produced in service consist of UHMWPE. A new treatment that involves radiation cross-linking (and additional toughening) of this polymer has yielded improved wear characteristics.

Perhaps because the tribometer only determines coefficients of friction, the medical device industry has pioneered the design and use of simulators for hip (Fig. 8.22) and knee implants. In these devices, both halves of the implant are immersed in a chamber filled with serum (serum is blood plasma with fibrinogen, a component of the clotting process, removed) to simulate body fluids, because it has been found that wear test results are influenced by the kind of lubricating fluid that is used; saline yields different results than serum. The implant is loaded by a computer-controlled arm which simulates the movements made by the implant in service.

After testing, the serum is drained and examined for the presence of polymer or metal wear particles, and both halves of the implant are examined for evidence of wear-induced scarring. These measurements determine how wear resistant the particular combination of materials is when subjected to a more clinically relevant exposure than in a tribometer.

In the continuing quest to reduce wear, ceramic-bearing components have been introduced consisting of a ceramic femoral head and acetabular cup liner. This material combination exhibits very low wear and acceptable strength characteristics.

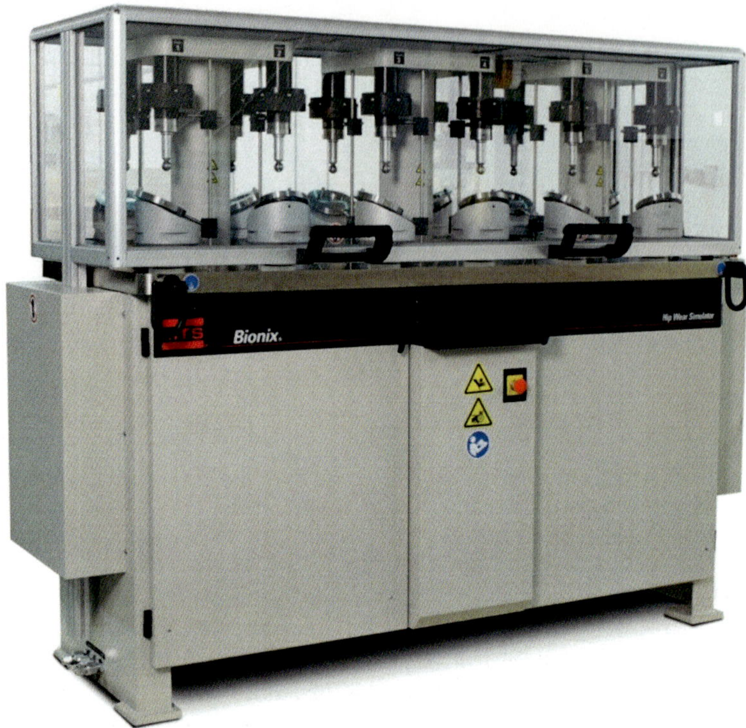

Fig. 8.22 A view of an opened hip simulator station exposing the femoral heads (*top*) and the acetabular cups (at *bottom*) of the implants. During testing, the implants are submerged in a lubricating fluid containing serum. Testing many implants at the same time speeds up the testing process. Photo courtesy of MTS Systems Corporation

Unfortunately, the sliding of two ceramic components produces squeaking noises in 3–7 % of patients, and while there are several theories proposed as to the reason, at this time there is no obvious remedy available [18].

There are also nonmaterial factors that significantly influence implant performance. For example, femoral heads and acetabular cups and liners are available in a variety of different sizes (femoral head range in diameter from 22 to 36 mm and acetabular cups ranging from 46 to 63 mm in diameter). The surgeon is in control of choosing implant size, and while the cup size is dictated by the patient's hip size, there is some flexibility in choosing the matching femoral head. The patient's gait also influences implant performance, as the extent to which the leg is bent while walking determines the range of movement of the femoral head within the liner. Finally, the skill of the surgeon also plays a role in eventual success, not only because he chooses the implant size, but because proper alignment of implant components is critical. A misaligned or improperly placed implant can lead to leg length discrepancies. Misalignment occurs because during surgery, the patient is on a surgical bed, positions of the bones shift and the patient's muscles relax, so the 3-D leg–hip relationship is different than when the patient standing or walking. There are computer image-guided systems (discussed in Chap. 5) now available that assist the surgeon in achieving optimal alignment, and an additional benefit is that surgical incisions may be smaller because the surgeon has a more precise idea where to cut.

8.9.3 Case 3: Chronic Low Back Pain Treated Using Posterior Lumbar Interbody Fusion (PLIF) Surgery

A 56-year-old male, who works as a software engineer and is a recreational golf player, presented with a 5-year history of chronic low back pain. The pain was refractory (not responding) to conservative treatments such as medication with NSAIDS (nonsteroidal anti-inflammatory drugs, e.g., Motrin™), injections of steroids, or physical therapy. The patient was sent for lumbar magnetic resonance imaging (MRI) and was diagnosed with degenerative lumbar disease. Degeneration of the lumbar disc is fairly common in humans and is due to degeneration of the disc nucleus and weakening of the annulus, a band of tough tissue that wraps around the viscoelastic nucleus. The annulus can rupture and allow the internal material, the nucleus, to flow out, leading to pain and to a loss of height between the vertebrae above and below the ruptured disc. An orthopedic surgeon who specializes in spine surgery recommended that the patient undergo an "elective" spinal fusion surgery to alleviate his condition. During this Posterior Lumbar Interbody Fusion (PLIF) Surgery, the patient's intervertebral disc was removed and replaced with a cage implant containing a growth factor called recombinant human bone morphogenic protein (BMP) soaked in a collagen sponge. The cage is used to restore the height lost by the removal of the intervertebral disc. The growth factor allows the bones to fuse more rapidly by stimulating new bone growth. The operation and the recovery went without incident. Successful fusion of the lumbar L4–L5 vertebra was observed at 1-year follow-up, and the patient reported complete pain relief.

In the case described here, the patient's intervertebral disc between the fourth and fifth lumbar vertebrae had collapsed. This is commonly known as a herniated disc; the disc material extrudes out into the space occupied by the spinal cord, and it is this pressure on the nerves which produces pain. In this patient, herniation occurred in the lumbar portion of the spine, between the vertebrae in the lower back (Fig. 8.23).

This patient filled out the Oswestry questionnaire and scored 50 %. The Oswestry index is a standardized form that has been in use for approximately 25 years and is used by surgeons to quantify and understand the degree of impairment of a patient's life, i.e., to learn how intense are the pain and discomfort [19]. A score of 50 % signifies severe disability. It's important for patients in this position to be quite certain that the procedure will be worthwhile, because spine surgery is not without complications.

The nonsurgical options for managing back pain have apparently not been effective in this case, so the surgeon and patient can select from two alternatives that vary in the range of motion the patient will have after surgery. The first is a fusion procedure, which permanently joins vertebrae together, preventing their further independent motion. In one type of fusion surgery, an implant is inserted between the

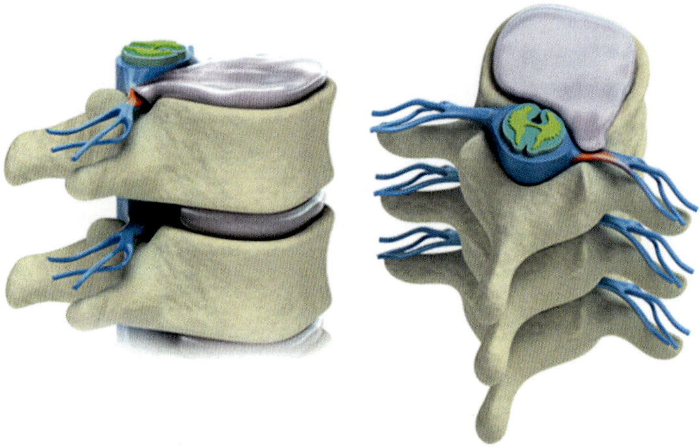

Fig. 8.23 Diagram of a herniated disc process with the disc pressing on nerves and causing pain

transverse processes (two bony projections from a vertebra) and the spine stabilized in that region with screws set into the vertebrae holding a rod (Fig. 8.24).

In another type of spinal fusion, the surgeon will use instruments to separate the two vertebrae and, while they are separated, remove any remains of the intervertebral disc. Access to the damaged area may be gained from the anterior (through the abdomen, in a procedure called an anterior lumbar interbody fusion or ALIF) or from the posterior (the back, in a procedure called a posterior lumbar interbody fusion or PLIF). The anterior approach requires that the surgeon navigates past the stomach and various muscles, while the posterior approach is more direct. Once that space is gained, the surgeon will insert an implant that will be positioned between the endplates of the two vertebrae and remain permanently in place while maintaining the appropriate spacing (height) between the two vertebrae. There are various and many designs for these implants, commonly called cages; the one shown in Fig. 8.25 has a feature that allows its height to be set and optimized during surgery.

Common features of these implants include a toothlike surface designed to prevent migration of the cage, and an empty space throughout the cage. Because these implants are designed to remain permanently in place, the surgeon will attempt to accelerate bone formation throughout the implant in order to reinforce its load-carrying capacity and to help hold it in place. Often, the surgeon will pack blood and bone chips into the spaces within the implant to provide a starter material for bone growth. The implanted bone material can be autogenous (obtained from the patient), taken from another location such as the iliac crest (the outer edge of the pelvis or hip bone), or it may be allogeneic (obtained from a donor, usually a cadaver).

To further accelerate bone growth (and the spine stabilization process), the surgeon may implant a source of bone morphogenetic protein, BMP. These substances were discovered in 1965 to be found in demineralized bone and proved to be potent stimulators of bone and cartilage growth. Research has identified approximately 20 different types of BMP's, and BMP-2 has been approved for use by the FDA in

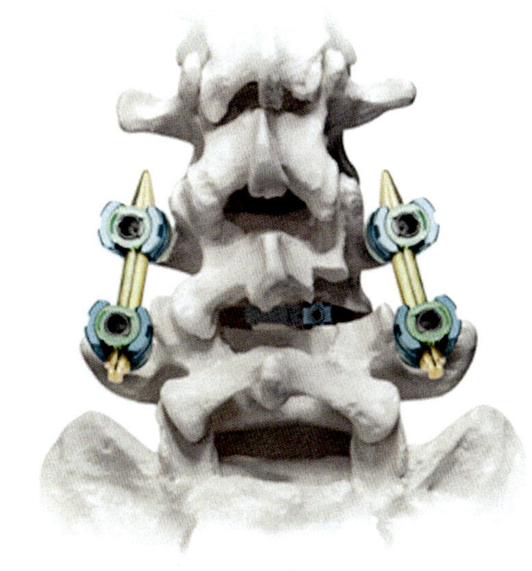

Fig. 8.24 Drawing of a two unit spinal fusion. The height-restoring implant is visible between vertebrae in *blue*. Image courtesy of Globus Medical

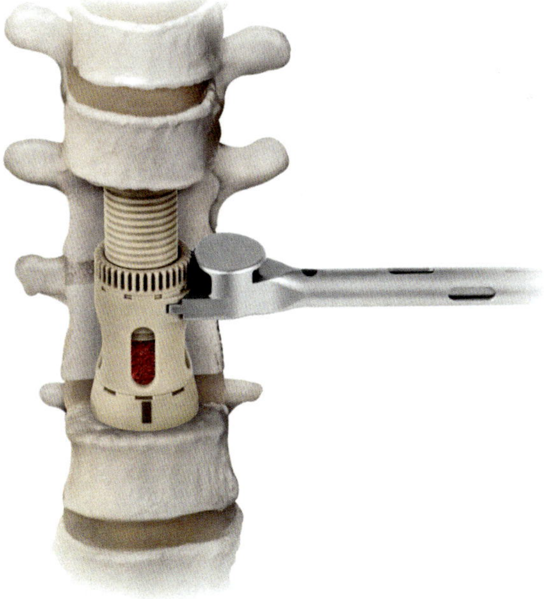

Fig. 8.25 A spacer used in fusion surgery of the spine. The height of the device may be adjusted when it is placed. Image courtesy of Globus Medical

ALIF procedures; that means that in the case just described, where a PLIF was performed, the BMP was used off-label. In order to provide BMP at the site where bone growth is desired, the substance is typically delivered in a resorbable carrier such as a collagen sponge. The use of this technology in spine surgery has recently been questioned, because although it adds significant costs to the surgery, clinical studies have not shown there to be significant benefits to the majority of spine fusion patients, and side effects can occur. It is likely that routine use of BMP in these applications will no longer continue, and it will be reserved for patients who demonstrate delayed bone growth.

Although the outcomes of spinal fusion have been proven effective in reducing back pain and permitting patients to resume at least some of their normal activities, there are some less attractive consequences. First, the degree of mobility of the spine is somewhat reduced; the patient simply cannot bend or rotate as before. Second, the spine segments immediately above and below the fusion will experience abnormally high biomechanical loads, and it is possible that they will begin to suffer degenerative changes also, possibly leading to an eventual need for additional fusion surgeries.

For these reasons, an alternative, motion-preserving type of implant has been developed, the artificial intervertebral disc. The (FDA) has currently approved two artificial discs for lumbar disc replacement and five artificial discs for cervical disc replacement. All these devices are intended for single-level surgeries only. In other words, the disc is inserted to replace one intervertebral. Only fusion accompanied with rod instrumentation is approved for multilevel spine stabilization.

An example of an artificial disc as it is placed in the cervical spine (neck) is shown in Fig. 8.26. A close-up view of the disc is shown in Fig. 8.27

After consulting the relevant ASTM standards and specifications for spinal cages, it becomes apparent that manufacturers are concerned with the stability of these devices in compression and with their resistance to fatigue loading. Additionally, manufacturers (and patients!) are concerned with the likelihood that the teeth intended to keep the cage in place (see Figure again) can cause the endplate of the vertebra to rupture.

The relevant ASTM standards and specifications for artificial discs reveal concerns with the fatigue resistance of these devices, as well as the potential for generating wear debris. The lumbar spine is a particularly dangerous for artificial disc replacements when it is considered that all the weight of the upper body is carried through L5 before it is redistributed in the pelvis.

8.10 Summary

Implants have been designed to replace soft or hard tissues and to perform in static or dynamic environments. The FDA and ASTM have developed and continue to update rules and specifications for adopting new materials and devices. Scientists and engineers have discovered ways of modifying material surfaces to elicit favorable or minimal responses from the implant host, and ways of avoiding bacterial

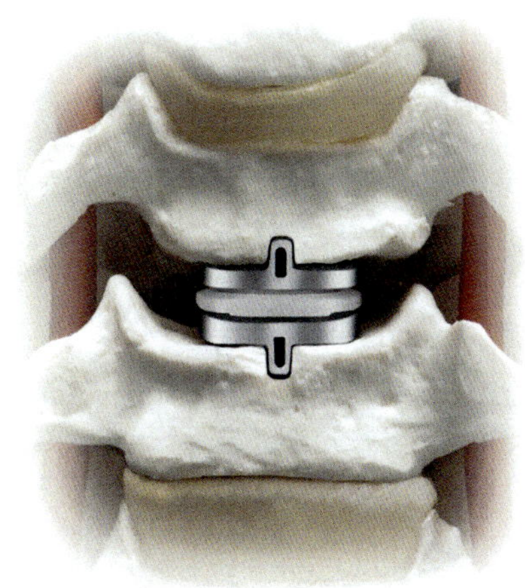

Fig. 8.26 An artificial disc in the cervical spine. Image courtesy of Globus Medical

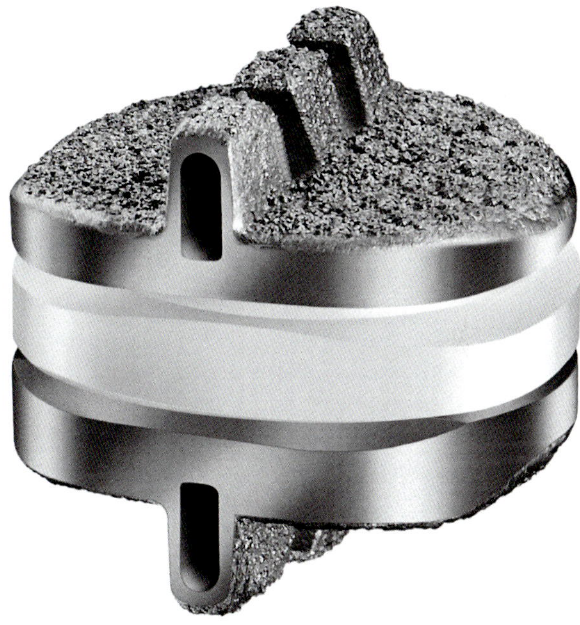

Fig. 8.27 A close-up view of an artificial disc designed for use in the cervical spine (the neck). Note the surface roughening that aids retention of the disc after it has been placed. Image courtesy of Globus Medical

contamination have become reasonably well understood. Laboratory test methods have become more sophisticated at simulating physiologic conditions. Today, physicians are able to draw on the expertise of scientists working in academic institutions, medical device manufacturing, regulatory bodies, and surgical experience when choosing between the many varieties of implants available today.

8.11 Foundational Concepts

- The metals most commonly used in biomedical applications are stainless steel, titanium, and cobalt–chromium alloy. All are biocompatible, but titanium has the ability to osseointegrate (bond with bone). They are all primarily used in applications requiring adequate strength.
- Ceramic materials used in implants are aluminum oxide and zirconium oxide. These two compounds are extremely stiff and hard and have high toughness (for ceramics). Calcium phosphate compounds are used in short-term cases, because they dissolve in the body; they also can serve as fillers for defects in bone. Hydroxyapatite, the mineral component of bone, can be synthesized as deposited as a coating on metallic implants to provide additional biocompatibility.
- A great variety of synthetic and natural polymers are used for biomedical purposes. Applications include vascular grafts, contact lenses, drug reservoirs, catheters, sutures, dermal fillers, and allogeneic heart valves.
- Material surfaces can be chemically modified to enhance their biocompatibility, resistance to wear, antibacterial potential, and the ability to capture analytes in biosensor applications.
- Finite element modeling is an engineering method that enables design of complex devices because it provides estimates of structural stability and permits virtual modifications of size and shape. Various materials may be simulated in this technique, saving device development time.
- Artificial hip and knee joints are implanted when the patient has severe arthritis limiting mobility. The bearing surfaces of these implants typically consist of a cobalt–chromium alloy piece articulating with a surface of ultrahigh molecular weight polyethylene. During service, wear is highly likely to occur and generate particles of wear debris which can cause bone resorption in the area of the implant. The long-term performance of these implants often depends on the surgical skills and experience of the surgeon, because choosing the right size of implant and ensuring that it is accurately aligned with respect to the bone are critical determinants of success.
- Herniated discs in the spine may be repaired by fusing the vertebrae above and below the herniation together; an implant is placed in the space formerly occupied by the disc, and a rigid fixation device consisting of rods held in place with pedicle screws is implanted. Because the patient loses range of motion following this surgery, artificial disc devices have recently been introduced to the market.

References

1. Cerruti, M., & Sahai, N. (2006). Silicate biomaterials for orthopedic and dental implants. *Reviews in Minerology and Geochemistry, 64*, 283–313.
2. Barradas, A.M., Yuan, H., van Blitterswijk, C.A. & Habibovic, P. et al. (2011). Osteoinductive biomaterials: Current knowledge of properties, experimental models, and biological mechanisms. *European Cells and Materials, 21*, 407–429.

3. Jones, J. (2013). Review of bioactive glass: From hench to hybrids. *Acta Biomaterialia, 9*, 4457–4486.
4. Ratner, B., & Bryant, S. (2004). Biomaterials: Where we have been and where we are going. *Annual Reviews in Biomedical Engineering, 6*, 41–75.
5. Slaughter, B.V., Khurshid, S.S., Fisher, O.Z., Khademhosseini, A. & Peppas N.A. et al. (2009). Hydrogels in regenerative medicine. *Advanced Materials, 21*, 3307–3329.
6. Peppas, N. (1987). *Hydrogels in medicine and pharmacy*. Boca Raton, FL: CRC Press.
7. Yannas, I. (2004). Natural materials. In B. Ratner et al. (Eds.), *Biomaterials science*. San Diego, CA: Elsevier.
8. Ramshaw, J., Werkmeister, J., & Glattauer, V. (1995). Collagen-based biomaterials. *Biotechnology and Genetic Engineering Reviews, 13*, 335–382.
9. Bhattacharya, A., & Misra, B. (2004). Grafting: A versatile means to modify polymers. Techniques, factors, and applications. *Progress in Polymer Science, 29*, 767–814.
10. Hubbell, J. (1999). Bioactive biomaterials. *Current Opinion in Biotechnology, 10*, 123–129.
11. World Health Organization. (2013). *Antimicrobial resistance*. Fact Sheet No. 194. http://www.who.int/mediacentre/factsheets/fs194/en/.
12. Temenoff, J., & Mikos, A. (2008). *Biomaterials the intersection of biology and materials science*. Upper Saddle River, NJ: Pearson Prentice Hall.
13. Costa, F., Carvalho, I.F., Montelaro, R.C., Gomes, P. & Martins, M.C. et al. (2011). Covalent immobilization of antimicrobial peptides (AMPs) onto biomaterial surfaces. *Acta Biomaterialia, 7*, 1431–1440.
14. Jung, W.K., Koo, H.C., Kim, K.W., Shin, S., Kim, S.H. & Park, Y.H. et al. (2008). Antibacterial activity and mechanism of action of the silver ion in Staphylococcus aureus and Escherichia coli. *Applied and Environmental Microbiology, 74*, 2171–2178.
15. Freschauf, L.R., McLane, J., Sharma, H. & Khine, M. et al. (2012). Shrink-induced superhydrophobic and antibacterial surfaces in consumer plastics. *PLoS ONE, 7*. doi:10.1371/journal.pone.0040987
16. Mahar, A.T., Lee, S.S., Lalonde, F.D., Impelluso, T. & Newton, P.Q. et al. (2004). Biomechanical comparison of stainless steel and titanium nails for fixation of simulated femoral fractures. *Journal of Pediatric Orthopedics, 24*, 638–641.
17. Wall, E., Jain, V., Vora, V., Mehlman, C.T. & Crawford, A.H. et al. (2008). Complications of titanium and stainless steel elastic nail fixation of pediatric femoral fractures. *Journal of Bone and Joint Surgery (American edition), 90*, 1305–1313.
18. Currier, J., Anderson, D., & Van Citters, D. (2010). A proposed mechanism for squeaking of ceramic-on-ceramic hips. *Wear, 269*, 782–789.
19. Fiarbank, J., Couper, J., & Davies, J. (1980). The oswestry low back pain questionnaire. *Physiotherapy, 66*, 271–273.

Cardiovascular Devices: Getting to the Heart of the Matter

9

"Hearts will never be made practical until they are made unbreakable."

The Tinman in "The Wizard of Oz"

Most of us have family members who have had at least a brush with heart disease. In this chapter, we will discuss the anatomy of the heart and how this remarkable organ works. Many technological advances have been made in the treatment of heart disease, though the ultimate goal remains development of a fully implantable artificial or tissue engineered heart. We will make sense of the current standard of care and learn how engineering techniques have been used to repair and maintain the body's pump.

9.1 Introduction

The term cardiovascular disease (CVD) is used to describe a variety of different illnesses affecting the heart and the vascular system. CVD is the leading cause of death in the USA and throughout the world for both men and women. According to the American Heart Association, an estimated 80,000,000 adult Americans (one in three) have one or more types of cardiovascular disease. CVD contributes to approximately 40 % of all deaths in the USA. Risk factors for cardiovascular disease include advancing age, gender, heredity (including race), smoking tobacco, high blood cholesterol, elevated blood pressure, physical inactivity, obesity and being overweight, and diabetes mellitus; all of us are likely to have at least one of these risk factors eventually. In general, older people are at a significantly higher risk of dying from CVD, and men have a greater risk of being inflicted with heart disease than women. Individuals with a family history of heart disease and/or high blood pressure are more likely to develop heart disease, and certain communities, e.g., African-Americans, are more likely to develop heart

G.R. Baran et al., *Healthcare and Biomedical Technology in the 21st Century: An Introduction for Non-Science Majors*, DOI 10.1007/978-1-4614-8541-4_9,

disease than others. Research has also shown that while moderate alcohol consumption may reduce the risk of heart disease and stroke, heavy or binge drinking may be risk factors for heart disease and can cause other pathologies (e.g., cirrhosis of the liver). The combined risk of coronary heart disease increases dramatically in an individual having several risk factors.

The danger of heart disease can be reduced by changes in lifestyle, including increased physical activity, weight loss, and adopting a healthier diet. Nevertheless, as the general population ages, the incidence of heart disease is rising rapidly, and clinical treatment has become an important component of modern healthcare. These treatments often start with pharmacological management of the disease but often require more invasive interventions ranging from implantation of pacemakers to cardiac bypass surgery. In this chapter, after briefly reviewing the basic anatomy and function of the heart, we will present several examples of cardiac devices that have revolutionized the treatment of heart disease.

9.2 Heart Anatomy and Function

Figure 9.1 shows a cross-sectional view of the inside of a heart. There are four chambers: the two upper chambers are the atria and the two lower chambers are the ventricles. The atria receive blood, and the ventricles are the main pumps that propel blood either to the lungs (pulmonary circulation) or to the rest of the body (peripheral circulation). The right atrium and right ventricle circulate blood to the lungs, and the left atrium and left ventricle circulate blood to the body. Normally, blood continually flows through veins into the atria. About 80 % of the blood flows directly through the atria into the ventricles without atrial contraction; an additional 20 % of the blood is pumped into the ventricles by atrial contraction. Thus, the atria act as primer pumps for the ventricles, and the ventricles serve as the major pumps moving blood out to the circulatory system. The deoxygenated blood returns to the heart through the vena cava into the right atrium. The blood then enters the right ventricle, which pumps the blood to the lungs. After exchanging carbon dioxide with oxygen in the lungs, the reoxygenated blood flows into the left atrium and then into the left ventricle. The left ventricle then pumps the blood out to the body.

The heart rate of a normal healthy adult usually is about 60–100 times/min. One heartbeat consists of a period of cardiac muscle relaxation (diastole) and followed by a period of cardiac muscle contraction (systole). During ventricular systole, large amounts of blood accumulate in the right and left atria. As soon as systole is over, blood rapidly flows into the ventricles. At the end of the ventricular diastole (when blood fills the ventricles), the amount of the blood in each ventricle is the end-diastolic volume. Then, the ventricles contract to pump blood out. The amount of blood pumped out of the ventricle is the stroke volume output. The remaining volume in each ventricle is called the end-systolic volume. The amount of the end-diastolic volume that is ejected is called the ejection fraction. These parameters are clinically used to assess the health of the heart; so, for

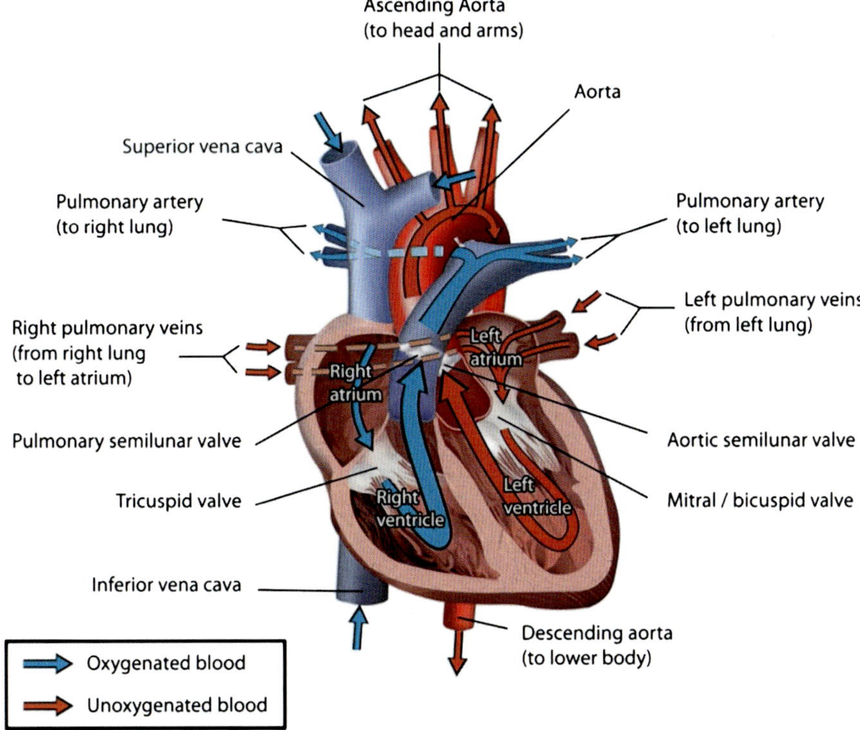

Fig. 9.1 Cross section of the heart

example, an adult with an ejection fraction that is significantly less than 50 % may be diagnosed with heart failure.

The pumping force of the heart is generated by the contraction of cardiac muscle. Cardiac muscle is one of the three major types of muscle in our body; the other two are skeletal and smooth muscle. About 40 % of the body is skeletal muscle, and perhaps another 10 % is smooth and cardiac muscle. Skeletal muscle is connected to the bone by tendons and is responsible for the coordinated movement of the limbs, trunk, jaws, eyes, etc. Smooth muscle is located in the walls of hollow internal structures such as blood vessels, stomach, intestines, and urinary bladder. The slow movements of the stomach and intestines are controlled by the contraction and relaxation of the smooth muscle in their walls. The smooth muscle in the walls of arteries regulates blood flow and pressure by changing the diameter of the vessels.

Although all three types of muscle contract, they do not contract in the same way. Voluntary muscle contractions are initiated consciously in the brain. A command signal is generated in the brain, conducted through the nervous system to a motor neuron, with the result that muscle fibers contract or relax. A movement such as walking is the product of voluntary contractions in skeletal muscles. Involuntary muscle contractions are initiated in the spinal cord or by a local stimulus and cannot be consciously controlled. Smooth muscles in the gut and vascular system are usually involuntary muscles. Skeletal muscle tissue can be made to contract or relax by voluntary conscious or involuntary, nonconscious control (e.g., the patellar reflex is a good example of involuntary contraction). When the patellar tendon is hit by a hammer (as when a physician tests your reflexes), an impulse is triggered in a sensory neuron leading to the spinal cord. There, the sensory neuron connects directly to a motor neuron which conducts an impulse to contract the quadriceps muscle. At the same time, the sensory neuron conducts an impulse through another motor neuron to relax the hamstring muscle, with the result that the leg kicks forward. The entire process happens without conscious control.

Cardiac muscle is an involuntary muscle and shares some common properties with smooth and skeletal muscle. However, several unique features of contraction in cardiac muscle distinguish it from the other two muscle types. Like them, cardiac muscle contraction can be stimulated by nerves or adrenalin with the result that, cardiac muscle will work harder to increase the heart rate. At the same time, smooth muscle surrounding blood vessels contracts, raising blood pressure, and skeletal muscle contracts in the "fight or flight" response.

Unlike other muscle types, cardiac muscle also has the property of automaticity in that it is self-excitable for contraction and relaxation and it contracts as a unit. Skeletal muscle and smooth muscle contraction is initiated by either the brain or by local stimuli, whereas cardiac muscle contraction is regulated by the unique electrical system of the heart, shown in Fig. 9.2. Cardiac muscle contraction is initiated by the spontaneous generation of an action potential, approximately 75 times/min, by a special group of cells in the heart called the sinus node (also called the sinoatrial or S-A node). The node, the heart's natural pacemaker, is located in the superior (upper) lateral wall of the right atrium near the opening of the superior vena cava. Electrical signals generated by the S-A node travel through the intermodal pathways in the atrium to the atrioventricular (A-V) node, where the impulse from the atrium is delayed before passing into the ventricle. Electrical signals exit the A-V node and travel through the A-V bundle to the His–Purkinje system. The A-V bundle is a group of special cells between the heart's upper and lower chambers and serves as an electrical bridge between the atrium and the ventricle.

The heart's electrical system: the S-A node, the A-V node, and the His–Purkinje system, triggers and carries electrical signals through the heart, making cardiac muscle contract and relax. The special arrangement of the conducting system from the atria into the ventricles causes a delay of more than 0.1 s during passage of the cardiac impulse from the atria into the ventricles. This delay of the impulse conduction allows the atria to contract ahead of the ventricular contraction, and therefore, the atria can pump blood into the ventricles before the ventricles contract and pump blood into the pulmonary or systemic circulation. Another unique feature of this system is that all portions of the atria contract at the same time and all portions of the ventricles contract at the same time. This is essential for the most effective pressure generation in the chambers.

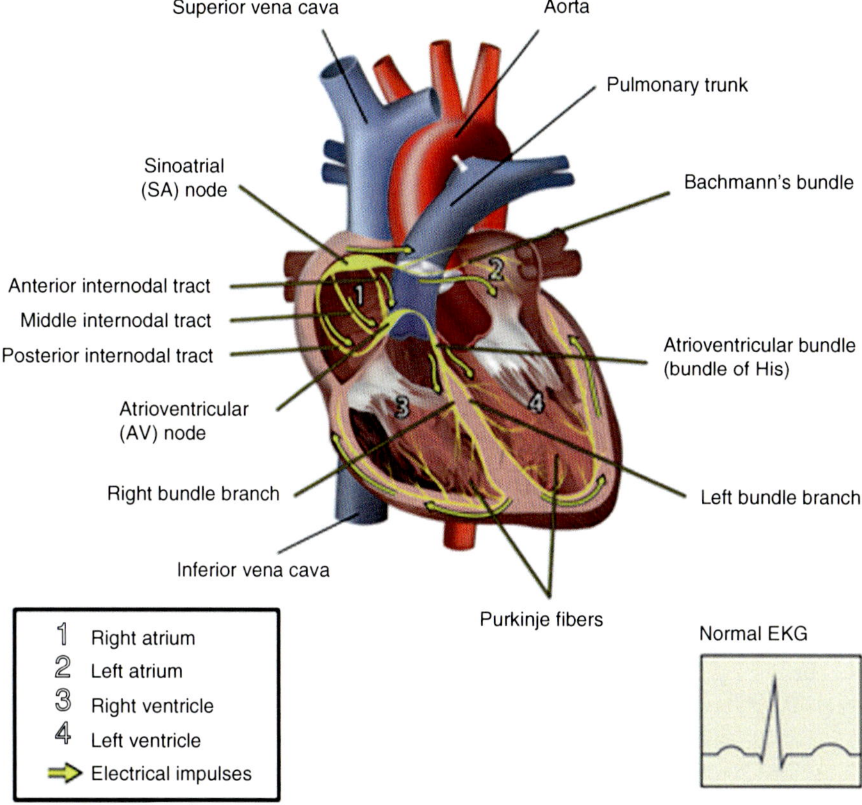

Fig. 9.2 The electrical system of the heart

9.3 Malfunctions of the Cardiac Electric System and Remedies

9.3.1 Arrhythmia

The unique electrical system in the heart can generate electrical impulses and conduct these impulses rapidly through heart muscle to cause the heart's rhythmic beat (rhythmicity). Heart diseases such as a myocardial infarction, which causes heart tissue damage by ischemia (a restriction of blood supply, oxygen, and glucose to heart muscle) and is commonly referred to as a "heart attack," may impair the rhythmical and conductive system of the heart, resulting in abnormal heart rhythm and abnormal contraction action of the heart chambers. Abnormalities in heart rhythm including arrhythmia, bradycardia, and fibrillation can significantly reduce the pumping efficiency of the heart and even lead to death.

An abnormal heart rhythm is called an arrhythmia. Cardiac arrhythmias result from abnormalities in the rhythmicity–conduction system of the heart. An abnormal pacemaker in a patient with diseased heart tissue may generate impulses which are intermittent, irregular, or at an inappropriate rate for the patient's metabolic demand or may not generate an impulse at all. An abnormality can occur at any point within the S-A node, A-V node, His bundle, or distal conduction system.

During bradycardia, the heart beats too slowly because either the heart's native pacemaker cannot generate an impulse at the proper time or the heart's electrical conduction system is blocked. Electrical cardiac pacing for the management of bradycardia through a small medical device such as an artificial pacemaker was first described in 1952. In the 1960s, permanent transvenous pacing devices were introduced. A pacemaker system typically includes two components, a pulse generator and a pacing electrode. Multiple electrodes may be needed to stimulate different positions within the heart to improve synchronization of heart muscle contraction. In operation, the pacemaker monitors the heart's native electrical rhythm. When the pacemaker senses that the heartbeat is below the normal heart rate range, it generates a short low-voltage pulse to stimulate the cardiac muscle and initiate the contraction in the atria and/or ventricles of the heart. This sensing and stimulating activity continues on a beat-by-beat basis. By measuring physiologic parameters such as oxygen and carbon dioxide in blood, body temperature, or ATP levels, newer pacemakers can even adjust the pacing level, and hence the heartbeat, to meet the changing metabolic demands of a person who, for example, is jogging. Currently, over 400,000 pacemakers are installed annually in the USA, and the great majority is placed in patients 65 years of age and older.

A pacemaker implantation uses local anesthesia. The procedure is performed by incision of a suitable vein near the collarbone, and then one or more pacing electrodes are inserted and gently steered inside the vein, through the valve of the heart, and positioned in the chamber, as shown in Fig. 9.3. The procedure is monitored by fluoroscopy, which enables the physician to view passage of the electrode lead. The leads should be fixed in a stable manner with no risk of being dislodged after implantation. Some leads are "actively fixated" with small hooks that act like mini-harpoons to stabilize the electrode. Others are made of porous metal, or shaped like the letter "J" in a passive fixation approach, and placed in the right atrial appendage. Once the electrode is lodged successfully, the opposite end of the pacing electrode is connected to the pulse generator and is tested to make sure the system works together to deliver the impulse. Generally, the pulse generator is placed below the skin, above the muscles and bones of the chest. The outer casing of pacemakers is usually made of biocompatible materials such as titanium and may be covered with a biocompatible polyurethane, to cause only minimal rejection by the body's immune system. Even though pacemakers consume very little power, their batteries don't last forever; every 7–10 years, patients will undergo another surgery to replace the battery. Research is in progress along several lines, seeking to eliminate the need for batteries. One approach tries to harness blood glucose to fuel the pacemaker; another harnesses the energy of lung motion as they expand and contract while the patient is breathing.

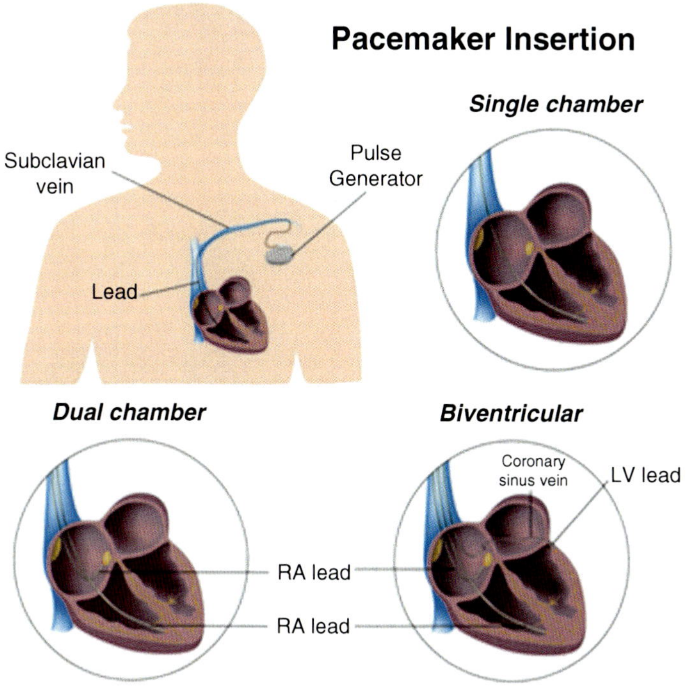

Fig. 9.3 Insertion of a pacemaker

Infection is always a concern after surgery and implantation of a device. The infection can originate in the pocket where the pacemaker was placed and travel along the leads to the heart. If the leads themselves become a site for bacterial colonization, they need to be removed, but given that they have been firmly encased in fibrous tissue, removal may require additional surgery. The failure mode often encountered with pacemakers involves the leads. The lead wires are encased in a biocompatible and flexible polyurethane coating, which has the potential to degrade in the body, and allow the wire to break and puncture the coating. Broken wires cannot conduct a pacing signal and can also cause other injuries to the heart and blood vessels. Class-action lawsuits have been initiated against pacemaker manufacturers as a result of lead or insulation failures [1]. Other issues associated with the leads involve formation of fibrotic tissue at the lead tip, where both the sensing and pacing signals are delivered. During the electrode lead maturation process that follows fixation, the body often reacts to the presence of this foreign material by surrounding the electrode with immune cells which cause swelling (edema) and eventual development of a fibrotic capsule around the location where the electrode has been implanted. The development of this capsule, which is not excitable, reduces the current at the electrode-cardiac tissue interface, requiring more energy to pace or defibrillate the heart.

Pacemakers often incorporate a diagnostic protocol or test method that permits a physician to check for proper operation during a patient visit to the office or to a special pacemaker clinic. In addition, pacemaker function may be evaluated telephonically. The patient is given a transmitter which converts cardiac signals into signals that are transmitted over telephone lines or to a monitoring facility which can print out an ECG tracing that may be reviewed for a sign of heart problems [2]. An advantage of remote sensing of this sort is that the patient is not required to travel and may be prompted to report problems more readily than if calling for an appointment was necessary. Remote monitoring should occur every 2–12 weeks depending on how long the pacemaker has been implanted.

Inevitably, patients are concerned with the possibility that pacemaker function can be affected by other, nearby electrical devices. Older pacemakers were interfered with by electric tooth brushes, microwave ovens, or electric razors. Newer pacemaker models have better electromagnetic shielding, and it has been found that home appliances such as radios, televisions and remote controls, electric blankets, electric shavers, metal detectors, and normally functioning microwave ovens do not interfere with pacemakers. Cell phones should not be carried while "on" in the breast pocket of a shirt. Although airport security gates do not interfere with pacemakers, the handheld metal detectors contain magnets and can affect pacemaker function. Anti-shoplifting gates in some stores can interfere with pacemakers. Questions about safe pacemaker function are addressed at www.hrsonline.org.

9.3.2 Fibrillation

Fibrillation is defined as an abnormally fast and chaotic heartbeat. When fibrillation occurs in ventricles, it is called ventricular fibrillation. Ventricular fibrillation often begins with a rapid rhythm (ventricular tachycardia). Sometimes, ventricular tachycardia stops on its own after a few seconds, while at other times, the fast rhythm continues and progresses to an even more rapid and more dangerous rhythm called ventricular fibrillation. Fibrillation is often caused by problems in the heart's electrical system due to ischemia of the heart muscle. During ventricular fibrillation the ventricular muscle is not able to contract as a unit. Instead, some portions of the ventricular muscle contract, while other portions relax. Therefore, the ventricles are quivering rather than pumping, resulting in no clear cardiac cycle with diastole or systole periods. The heart under this condition barely pumps any blood out. Within 4–5 s after the onset of fibrillation, the patient becomes unconscious due to the lack of blood flow to the brain, and irreversible tissue damage begins to occur throughout the body within a few minutes.

If the fibrillation occurs in atria, it is called atrial fibrillation, the most common form of cardiac arrhythmia. Atrial fibrillation can occur without ventricular fibrillation, and vice-versa, because atria are separated from ventricles by fibrous tissue. The only connection in the electrical conduction system between atria and ventricles is the A-V bundle. The mechanism of atrial fibrillation is the same as that of ventricular fibrillation. Even though atrial fibrillation is usually not life threatening, it may result in complications such as chest pain or heart failure.

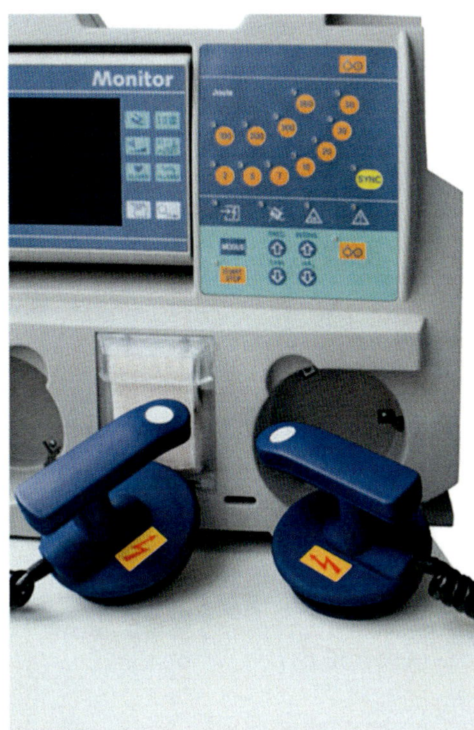

Fig. 9.4 A heart defibrillator

Ventricular fibrillation is the most serious of all cardiac arrhythmias. If not stopped within 3 min, it can result in serious injury or death. Ventricular fibrillation often leads to sudden cardiac arrest and sudden cardiac death. Cardiac arrest results from an abrupt stop of the heartbeat due to the cessation of all electrical signals in the heart. With defibrillation treatment, the heart can return to a normal rhythm.

A defibrillator (Fig. 9.4) is a battery-powered electrical impulse generator that is designed to treat fibrillation and cardiac arrest. It delivers a therapeutic dose of electrical energy for a short period of time to stop fibrillation and to restart the heart. This strong electrical current stops the heartbeat. Several seconds after defibrillation, the heart starts to beat again. Defibrillators can be external, transvenous, or implanted. Some patients who have conditions that cause permanent fibrillation or cardiac arrest can be treated by rhythmical electrical impulses from an implantable defibrillator. Implantable defibrillators are surgically placed in patients in a way similar to pacemakers and can accurately sense the heart's electrical activity to determine if fibrillation has occurred. When it does, a defibrillating pulse is generated to restart the heart. Although implantable defibrillators keep patients alive, many complain of the pain and discomfort when the defibrillator provides an electric shock. External defibrillators are often used in hospitals to revive patients experiencing cardiac fibrillation [3]. These are the devices often shown on television and in the movies when a doctor takes two paddles to the chest of a patient whose heart has stopped, shouts "clear !,"and delivers a shock to the patient. Usually, the first attempt fails to revive the patient, and the energy is increased for the second attempt. The discharge voltage to the patient is often close to several thousand volts! Recently, and thanks in part to the recommendations of public health officials and the American Heart Association, external defibrillators have been installed in many public areas, including government buildings and airports that can be used by untrained personnel to help in the resuscitation of people who may be experiencing fibrillation.

9.4 Malfunction of the Vascular Network and Remedies

9.4.1 Stents and Cardiac Bypass Surgery

Just as all other muscles in the body, the heart muscle requires oxygen and nutrients to remain viable and to function properly. Coronary arteries deliver oxygenated blood to the myocardium, and coronary veins remove deoxygenated blood from the heart muscle. There are two main coronary arteries: the right coronary artery and the left coronary artery. Both originate from the root of the aorta, immediately above the aortic valve. When the blood supply to a part of the heart is interrupted, the downstream cardiac muscle cells may die from a lack of oxygen through myocardial infarction, commonly known as a heart attack. The most common cause of the interruption of blood flow to the heart is the blockage of a coronary artery by ruptured plaque. Plaque is a substance consisting of fats (lipids) and white blood cells in the wall of an artery. If a plaque ruptures, a blood clot can form blocking blood flow and resulting in cardiac muscle tissue death. The damaged heart muscle can lead to other heart conditions.

A normal artery wall consists of three layers (Fig. 9.5). The inner layer, the tunica intima, consists of a single layer of endothelial cells that line the lumen (the inside space) of the vessel. This layer is in direct contact with the blood. The middle layer, the tunica media, is composed of smooth muscle cells and elastic fibers. This layer is responsible for the regulation of blood flow through smooth muscle contractions or relaxations based on oxygen demand. The outer layer consists of collagen fibers that hold the vessel together. During the development of atherosclerosis (thickening of the artery), fatty materials such as cholesterol build up on an artery wall. The body's immune system responds to this by attracting white blood cells to the diseased site, often forming a fibrous cap over the affected area. This "plaque" often causes wall thickening, narrows the artery, and reduces blood flow (Fig. 9.6).

By the way, do you know what cholesterol is? This organic compound, found in all animals and even in some plants, is a kind of a steroid that is essential to the formation and function of cell membranes and is continually being synthesized by our bodies. It is therefore neither possible nor desirable to have no cholesterol whatsoever in the human body. It turns out too that most foods, except for eggs and shellfish, are not high in cholesterol. The problem has to do with our fat intake. Animal fats, such as those found in cheese and meat, are converted into cholesterol in our bodies. Cholesterol is carried by substances called "lipoproteins" between the liver via blood circulation and the cells of the body. Low-density lipoprotein (LDL) carries cholesterol from the liver, and high-density lipoprotein (HDL) carries cholesterol

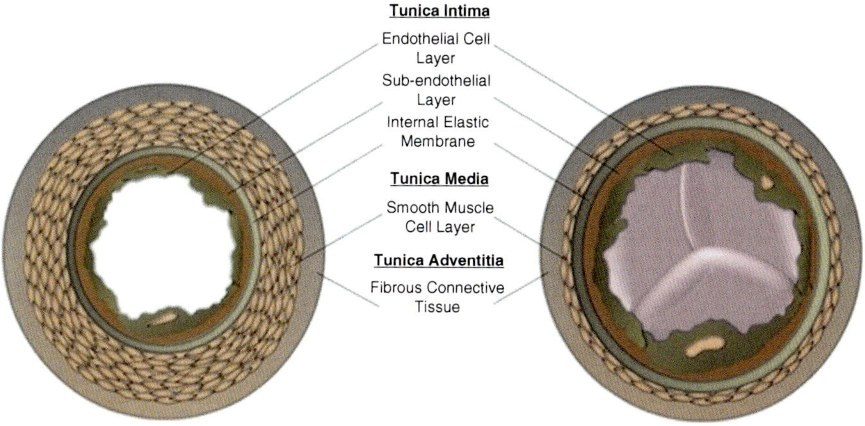

Fig. 9.5 Diagram of the components of an artery (*left*) and vein (*right*). Copyrighted by Springer Science + Business Media LLC

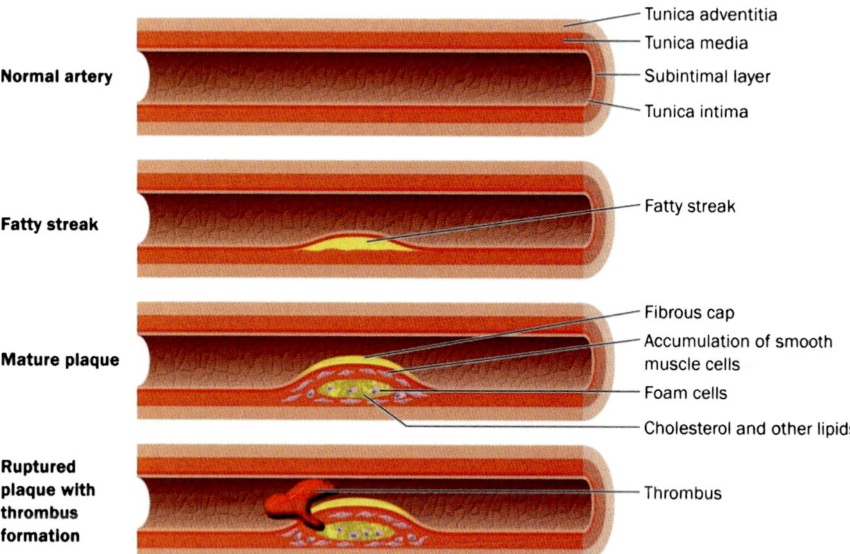

Fig. 9.6 Atherosclerotic artery

from the cells to the liver where it is broken down and eventually excreted. If the demand for cholesterol by cells is exceeded by the supply of cholesterol, the LDL which transports cholesterol will eventually form deposits on the walls of blood vessels and contribute to heart disease. A blood test will typically determine the overall cholesterol level, the amount of LDL, and the amount of HDL. It is preferred to have a low amount of LDL and a high amount of HDL. It also appears that there is a link between high triglyceride levels and low HDL levels. Triglycerides are compounds in the blood that are the product of refined carbohydrate metabolism.

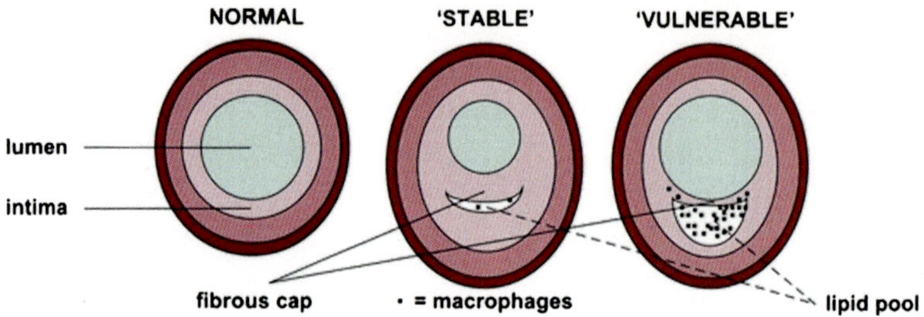

Fig. 9.7 Diagram of vulnerable and stable plaques. The vulnerable plaque has a thin fibrous coating over a fatty deposit. Copyrighted by Springer Science + Business Media LLC

> Although high cholesterol may be easily treated by drugs called "statins" (e.g., Lipitor™, Crestor™), a diet low in saturated animal fats and refined carbohydrates will normally result in low LDL and high HDL blood levels without the need for medication. And even though there are some skeptics out there who do not believe in a direct link between mortality and high cholesterol levels, the consensus is that high cholesterol contributes to heart disease.

There are two types of plaques: vulnerable plaque and stable plaque (Fig. 9.7). A vulnerable plaque is lipid rich and has a thin fibrous cap. The thin fibrous cap can rupture easily, and when ruptured, blood platelets rapidly accumulate at the site to form a clot (thrombus), which can rapidly slow or stop blood flow. If left untreated for approximately 5 min, the downstream cardiac tissue dies, resulting in a myocardial infarction. Such a blockage of vessels in the brain may result in a stroke. If a blood clot detaches from the plaque before it has fully blocked the artery, the blood clot will move through the vessel until it reaches and blocks a smaller diameter vessel in the heart or other tissue. This blood clot can completely block small vessels and reduce or stop blood flow in that region. Usually, only a small amount of tissue is affected, and the patient may not exhibit any symptoms (a clinically silent infarction). On the other hand, stable plaque is a lipid-poor plaque, with a thick fibrous cap which does not rupture easily. A stable plaque slowly narrows the artery and reduces blood flow to the tissue downstream. Clinically, most myocardial infarctions are caused by low-grade stenosis (blockage of the blood vessel) caused by stable plaques.

Even small reductions in vessel diameter resulting from stenosis can result in large changes in blood flow through the vessel. This process can be modeled using Poiseuille's law, which states that flow in a vessel decreases in proportion to the fourth power of the diameter (i.e., even small changes in the diameter of a vessel cause tremendous changes in the rate of blood flow in the vessel). Jean Louis Marie Poiseuille was a French physician and physiologist who was interested in blood flow in the aorta and who published his law in 1840. The following is a simplified equation derived from Poiseuille's law:

$$F = C \times D^4$$

where F is the rate of blood flow, D is the diameter of the vessel, and C is vessel conductance which in turn depends on the pressure difference between the ends of the vessel, length of the vessel, and viscosity of blood.

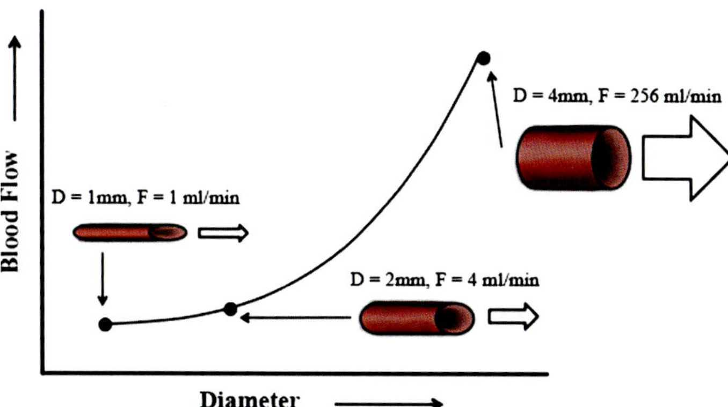

Fig. 9.8 The effect of vessel diameter on blood flow

To further illustrate this point, take as an example a portion of a blood vessel blocked by a plaque and assume that the pressure difference between the ends of the vessel remains constant. Furthermore, since the vessel does not change its length and the blood in the vessel does not change its viscosity, the parameter C will be constant. In this case, if the vessel diameter decreases to half of the original diameter due to the presence of plaque, the flow rate will decrease to 1/16 of the original flow rate. Figure 9.8 shows the relationship between vessel diameter and blood flow. Note that the rate of blood flow is directly proportional to the fourth power of the diameter of the vessel, which demonstrates that the diameter plays the most important role of all factors in determining the rate of blood flow through a vessel.

Currently, interventional treatments for coronary heart disease include balloon angioplasty and bypass surgery. Angioplasty is a minimally invasive technique that mechanically reopens the narrowed or blocked blood vessel. The patient is given either local anesthesia or light general anesthesia depending on the location of the narrowed vessel. An incision is made at either the femoral artery in the groin or the brachial artery in the arm. A catheter and guide wire is passed through the incision in the chosen vessel and into the narrowed artery. A type of video X-ray imaging called fluoroscopy is utilized to visualize the wire movement in the vessel in real time enabling the physician to move the wire to the precise location of the blockage. Once the wire is in place, a tightly folded deflated balloon is passed over the guide wire into the narrowed location. The balloon is inflated using water pressure, pushing the plaque against the vessel wall, and flattening the vessel wall. Once the vessel wall is flattened, the balloon is deflated and withdrawn from the vessel. An angiogram is performed to determine if any more ballooning is needed. Since there is no supportive material to keep the vessel wall from opening, the artery may eventually begin to close again (restenosis), which is a common problem after a balloon angioplasty.

A device called a stent can be used to reduce the possibility of restenosis. The stent is made of metal processed into a mesh-like form and which is delivered over the guide wire to the diseased location. Stents are often made of biocompatible, inert metals such as stainless steel or titanium or, more recently, from biocompatible

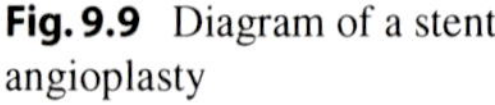

Fig. 9.9 Diagram of a stent angioplasty

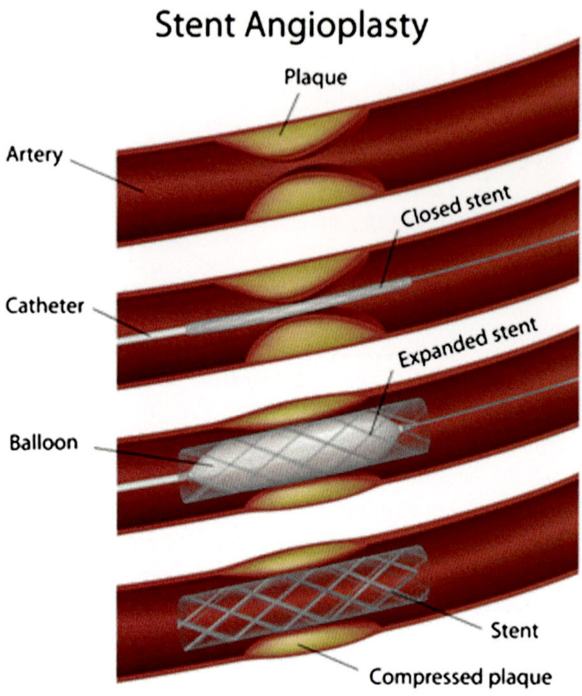

polymers. Once in place, the balloon is inflated, pushing open both the vessel and the stent (Fig. 9.9). The balloon and the guide wire are then retreated, leaving the opened stent in the location to permanently keep the vessel from closing. Drugs may be applied to the surfaces of the stents, creating "drug-eluting stents" that reduce the risk of restenosis and thrombosis. Angioplasty surgery usually lasts about 20 min after anesthesia and the patient usually recovers quickly and does not need to stay in the hospital for long. However, some patients may still have chest pain and may need another angioplasty or bypass surgery in the future.

Stents were initially designed to be placed in arteries, but now are also placed in veins. They are considered to be permanent devices, and so the materials used to make them must not only be biocompatible, but also resistant to fatigue. As the blood pulses within the blood vessel, the stent is stressed in a cyclic manner, and failure of the thin metal segments can occur. Other concerns associated with stents include the risk of blood clot formation and occlusion (closure) of the blood vessel. The surfaces of the wires in the stent are highly polished to reduce this risk, and some stents are coated with polymers with an anticlotting chemical attached to further minimize the possibility of blood clot formation. Also, the wall of the blood vessel undergoes a healing response after stent placement. The more metal there is in contact with the wall, the greater the intensity of the healing response. As part of this response, the stent becomes covered with tissue, and if the tissue is too thick, it too can block the flow of blood. Regular follow-up visits are recommended to image and evaluate the stent placement site for evidence that the stent remains mechanically sound and that restenosis of the blood vessel has not occurred.

Atherectomy is another minimally invasive technique used to remove the plaque in the artery. A laser or a rotating razor is inserted over a guide wire into the narrowed artery. The plaque is cut off by the rotor razor or vaporized by a laser. A stent may be placed following an atherectomy.

9.4.2 Intravascular Filters

During long periods of inactivity, e.g., bed rest in a hospital or long airplane flights, older patients and travelers are often told to wear tight socks or stockings, or to move about the airplane cabin, in order to reduce the possibility of developing deep-vein thrombosis. This condition is responsible for the formation of blood clots in the lower legs. The danger arises from the possibility that the clot will break free and travel to the heart, lungs, or brain, where it can cause serious medical problems. During periods of inactivity, the blood in the extremities is not as well oxygenated and has a tendency to pool, and these factors contribute to clot formation. Walking or performing leg exercises while sitting produces an increase in circulation and reduces the risk of clot formation, while wearing compression socks also forces the blood out of the legs and toward the heart.

Patients at risk of developing blood clots because of age, recent surgery, or other medical risk factors may also have a blood filter (Fig. 9.10) implanted in the inferior vena cava (the large vein that travels from the legs to the right atrium). These filters are made of stainless steel or titanium alloy wires with small hooks that are used to fix the device into the wall of the vein. Filters may be permanent or removable. Approximately 25,000 filters are placed each year in the USA, and the procedure may be performed by a heart surgeon or by an interventional radiologist. After placement, the filters may be imaged from time to time to determine if they themselves have been infiltrated with large clots; approximately 8 % of patients have a filter that is at least partially blocked by clots.

9.4.3 Heart Bypass Surgery and Vascular Grafts

As discussed earlier, atherosclerosis (thickening of the artery wall due to the accumulation of cholesterol and triglyceride deposits) is often characterized by coronary vessel blockage, which may result in angina (chest pain) and loss of cardiac function. In cases of significant vessel blockage where stenting is not possible, bypass surgery may be recommended. A more serious form of this surgery is sometimes referred to as a "quadruple bypass," which means that four coronary arteries were bypassed in the operation; anywhere from one to five arteries may be treated in this way. The cardiac surgeon usually harvests a vein or artery from the leg or chest of the patient and sutures it so that it provides a bypass route for blood around the occluded portion of the artery; the new blood vessel is called a vascular graft.

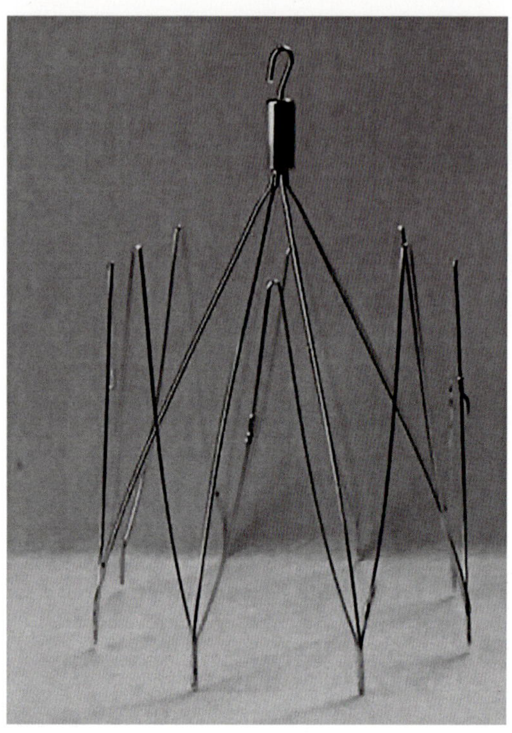

Fig. 9.10 A Guenther Tulip inferior vena cava filter. Copyright by Springer Science+Media Inc.

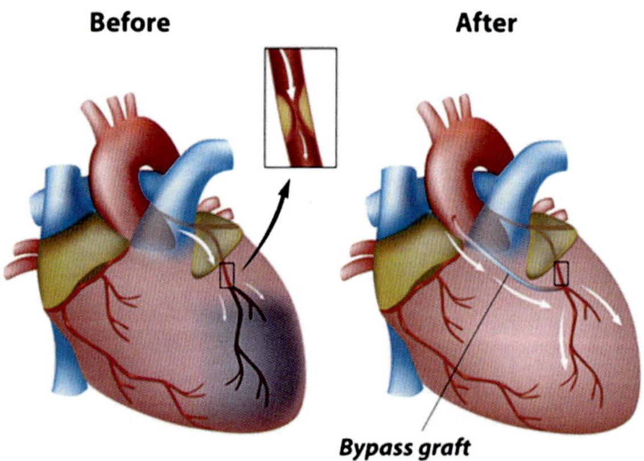

Fig. 9.11 Diagram of a bypass surgery. Note the new blood vessel that has been inserted

The patient's own vessels are used for the bypass in order to minimize the immune system responses. Since there are few suitable vessels in the patient's body, artificial vessels (e.g., synthetic tubing made of biocompatible polymers) can also be used in bypass surgery (Fig. 9.11).

Materials used to fabricate artificial vessels include knitted or woven Dacron polyester, expanded poly(tetrafluoroethylene), and human umbilical veins. Tightly woven Dacron grafts have high strength and low porosity, but as a result are stiff and the ends fray after cutting to fit the surgical site; also, the low porosity can lead to poor healing at the site where the synthetic graft encounters the natural blood vessel. Knitted Dacron grafts have higher porosity, and the risk of blood leakage through the graft is reduced by impregnating the graft with natural polymers such as collagen or gelatin. Poly(tetrafluoroethylene) grafts are inert, and their porosity can be controlled during the manufacturing process. Bleeding through the suture holes is a product of the inert character of this material. Human umbilical veins (the vein that carries blood from the placenta to a fetus, normally discarded after birth) are harvested, placed on a tool called a mandrel so that they keep their shape, and treated with the chemical glutaraldehyde to strengthen them and to eliminate their potential to cause an immune response in the recipient patient.

Bypass surgery is an open chest procedure performed under general anesthesia. The patient is first given a dose of an anticoagulant (heparin). Then, the chest is opened (resulting in the collapse of the lungs), and blood traveling to the right atrium of the heart is diverted into a reservoir in a heart–lung machine. Heart–lung machines are possibly the most dramatic pieces of equipment in an operating room (Fig. 9.12). Because the patient's heart has been stopped to allow the cardiac

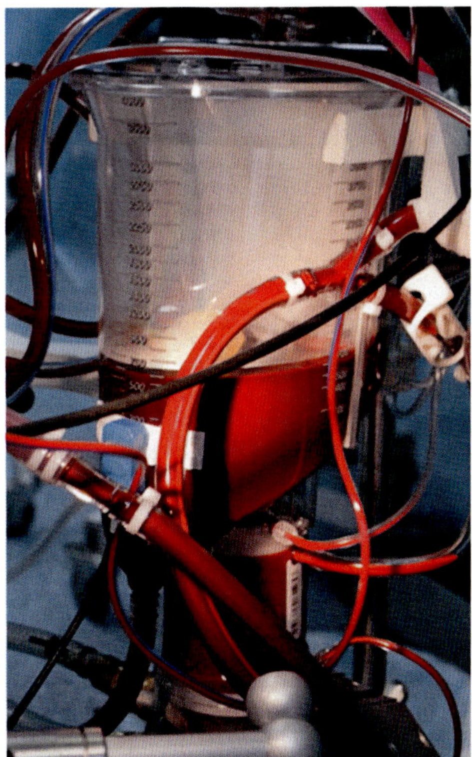

Fig. 9.12 The blood reservoir in a heart–lung machine. The tubing conducts blood through filters where it is cleaned and oxygenated

surgeon to do the operation, the machine takes over the job of the heart and lungs, pumping and oxygenating the blood. It consists of several pumps (called peristaltic pumps) that "massage" surgical silicone tubing to force blood to keep moving, an oxygenator which delivers oxygen to the blood and removes carbon dioxide from blood taken from veins, and multiple tubes (cannulae) that are inserted into various parts of the patient's body depending on the specific surgery or disease condition. Heart–lung machines also include various sensors that monitor blood temperature, blood chemistry, and filters. Interestingly, heart–lung machines can be used not only during heart surgery but also in cases where the patient has been exposed to extreme cold.

The blood taken from the patient is then pumped into an oxygenator, where oxygen is diffused through a synthetic membrane made of polypropylene or silicone into the blood and carbon dioxide (the product of cell metabolism) diffuses through the membrane out of the blood [4]. In other words, the two gases are exchanged through the membrane which is permeable to gases but not to liquids. The newly oxygenated blood passes through a heat exchanger and then directed into the patient's aorta. The blood is cooled to help lower the core temperature of the body and decrease its metabolic needs. The heart is stopped to perform the bypass surgery during which the harvested vessel is sewn into place as a new conduit for blood to flow around the blocked area. Upon completion of the procedure, blood flow is returned to the heart from the heart–lung machine and is now warmed to normal body temperature, and a defibrillating shock is given to revive the normal heartbeat. The surgery usually lasts 2–3 h, and compared to balloon angioplasty, patients with bypass surgery usually need a longer recovery time and require 4–5 days of monitoring in the hospital. After recovery, patients are less likely to have chest pain, to need medication, and to need another bypass procedure.

Extracorporeal membrane oxygenation (ECMO) machines are similar to heart–lung machines, but are designed for longer-term (a few months) use in patients, both adults and children, whose hearts and lungs can no longer function. Very young children, e.g., newborns under four and half pounds in weight, cannot take advantage of ECMO because their blood vessels are too narrow. As with a heart–lung machine, the patient has tubes inserted into the large blood vessels, and the machine pumps blood through a "membrane oxygenator" that performs the oxygen–carbon dioxide exchange. Anticlotting drugs are added to maintain blood flow. These machines are used in an ICU after heart surgery in a transition to the use of a ventilator and for patients who have not responded to treatment with a traditional ventilator. However, ECMOs are not a long-term solution, and there are risks to the patient from infection and clotting.

Potential problems associated with bypass surgery include infection and, in the case of knitted Dacron grafts, gradual enlargement. More severe failures of synthetic grafts, such as fiber breakdown, have been found to occur in fewer than 3 % of patients. Older models of heart–lung machines also caused damage to red blood cells (hemolysis) and to blood platelets, sometimes resulting in bleeding problems. New pump designs and use of membrane oxygenators rather than bubble oxygenators have reduced the degree of damage.

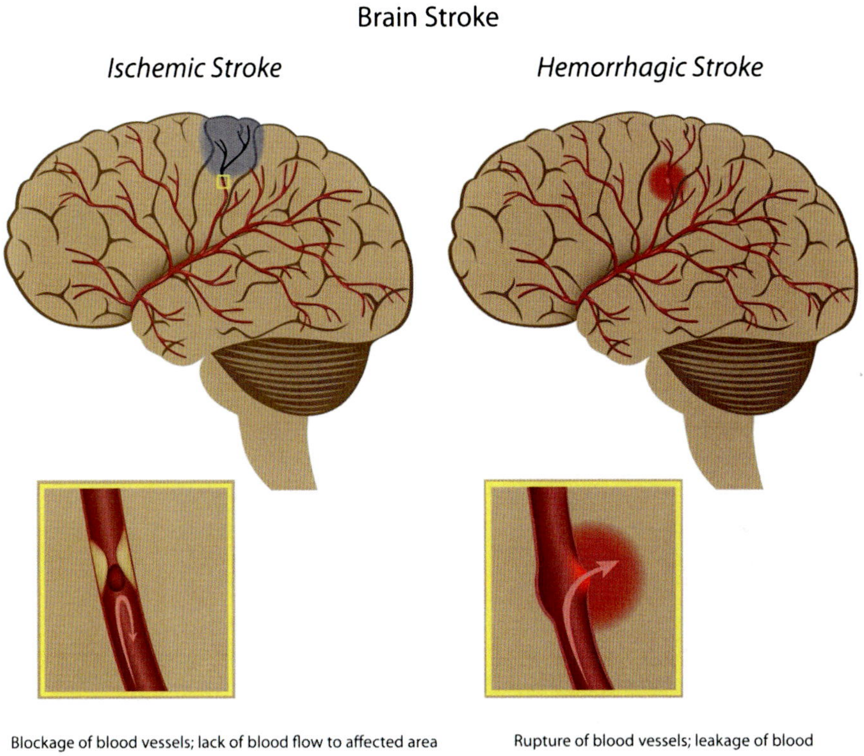

Brain Stroke

Ischemic Stroke

Hemorrhagic Stroke

Blockage of blood vessels; lack of blood flow to affected area

Rupture of blood vessels; leakage of blood

Fig. 9.13 Diagram of two causes of stroke

Stroke is the third leading cause of death after cancer and heart disease, and approximately 20–30 % of stroke is caused by stenosis of the carotid artery followed by a piece of the plaque breaking off and traveling to the brain [5]. Complete or significant blockage (50–90 %) can cause a stroke, but even partial blockage, which restricts the flow of oxygenated blood to the brain, can be responsible for a gradual loss of brain function. The loss of small pieces of plaque that cause blockage of narrow brain arteries can cause transient ischemic attacks (TIA or mini-strokes), which do not cause death, but may subsequently impair various bodily functions such as speech, swallowing, and mobility. Strokes are also caused by hemorrhage, when the wall of a blood vessel ruptures, spilling blood into the brain (Fig. 9.13)

The surgical treatment for restoring unimpeded blood flow through the carotid artery is a "carotid endarterectomy." In this procedure, the surgeon clamps two ends of the artery on both sides of the blockage and places a shunt (an alternative path for blood to continue flowing to the brain). The carotid artery is opened, and the plaque is removed. If the artery is found to be damaged, a graft is placed consisting of either the patient's own vein or one of the synthetic alternatives described earlier.

Still another use of stents and vascular grafts is described in the following case study.

9.4.4 Case 1: Traumatic Aortic Rupture Treated Using Endovascular Stent Grafting

A 69-year-old woman with a history of hypertension was walking back from a grocery store and suddenly lost balance and fell. She denied previous dizziness, difficulty walking, leg weakness, and numbness of her feet. She was rushed to the emergency room and upon examination (using contrast-enhanced computed tomography (CT)) was found to have sustained a traumatic aortic rupture. Thoracic aortic injury remains a leading cause of death after blunt trauma such as a fall and automobile accident. After obtaining informed consent from her husband, the patient underwent a minimally invasive procedure to repair the ruptured aorta. The minimally invasive procedure involved the use of an endograft (endovascular stent grafting, meaning that the graft remained on the inside of the blood vessel). The surgery was performed under general anesthesia in an angiographic operating room with fixed fluoroscopic equipment. The endograft was introduced through the left common femoral artery into the proximal descending thoracic aorta into the region of rupture and deployed. The 1-month follow-up using contrast-enhanced computed tomography (CT) showed a well-placed graft and no blood leakage. The long-term outcome of this graft is unknown.

Traumatic aortic rupture occurs when the largest artery in the body, the aorta, is torn as the result of a blow to the chest. It is believed that the sudden deceleration of the body leads to differential rates of deceleration of the heart and aorta and the sudden stresses cause rupture. It would seem that death should be instantaneous or rapid, and in cases where the tear is large, some 75–80 % of patients die, but in others when there is only a partial tear or when the aortic wall is not completely torn through the patients can continue living for hours. The condition often is diagnosed only after an angiogram or CT imaging is performed when the patient starts to complain about pain or shortness of breath after an accident or fall.

After the condition is diagnosed, the primary action is to manage the patient's blood pressure to reduce the likelihood of additional damage occurring to the fragile artery, to be followed by surgical repair. Surgery may not always be possible because some patients may also be suffering from severe injuries to the abdomen and to the head. The aorta may be repaired by directly suturing the tear closed or by using a graft. Complications may arise during and after surgery because of ischemia (restriction of blood supply), occurring after the aorta is clamped while the repair is occurring. Severe damage to the brain and spinal cord tissues can result in paraplegia, and lack of blood supply to the kidneys results in renal failure.

The difficulties that may follow clamping of the aorta are the reasons why in this case a minimally invasive repair was made. In this procedure, the physician makes an incision in the groin area and uses an endoscope (Fig. 9.14) to guide a stented graft to the site of the injured artery. There, the stent is deployed (opened; Fig. 9.15) and remains in place. A stented graft is used because the natural blood vessel, the aorta, has been damaged and a replacement blood vessel is needed. Recovery time

Fig. 9.14 A cardiac catheter used to introduce a stent

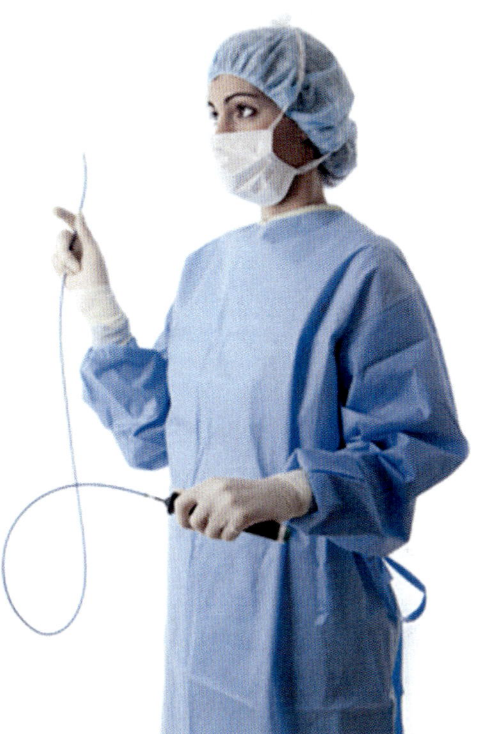

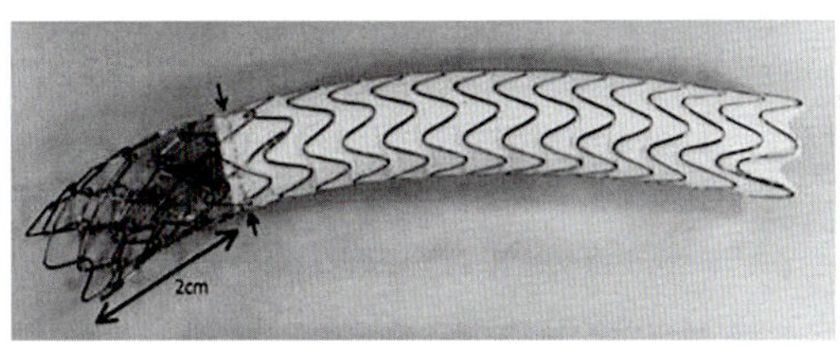

Fig. 9.15 A grafted stent; the device consists of a vascular graft (the white fabric material) with a stent providing structural support. Sometimes, the stent is located inside the graft. Copyright Springer-Verlag

postsurgery is 1–2 days as compared with a week for open repair of the aorta, although operating time is somewhat longer for laparoscopic surgery [6].

A key issue is the choice of material through which the blood will be flowing, i.e., for the vascular graft. For bypass surgeries, which also can include the aorta, a variety of materials are used: natural vein taken from the long vein of the leg and thigh or one of the synthetic materials described earlier. Small blood vessels with diameters narrower than 6 mm can be replaced with decellularized umbilical vein, but the aorta is too large (approximately 3 cm). At one time, grafts made of PTFE were preferred, as these were highly resistant to formation of blood clots. Dacron fabric grafts needed to be pre-clotted prior to insertion, but remained somewhat popular because of the ease of suturing with Dacron. As surface modification techniques advanced, it was possible to coat or impregnate Dacron fabric with collagen, albumin or gelatin, and a platelet inhibitory drug (heparin). This advance made it more convenient to use Dacron rather than PTFE and allowed the surgeon to preserve the patient's natural veins for potential future use [7]. The frequency of reports of failures of Dacron grafts because of fatigue-induced fabric degeneration and creation of false aneurisms (bulging out of the graft wall) has been reduced with greater care observed during preoperative handling of the grafts and better quality control during manufacturing [8]. At the present time, Dacron grafts are preferred for replacement of larger blood vessels, and PTFE grafts are preferred for replacing smaller diameter blood vessels. Narrower grafts appear to have lower patency rates (how long they remain open or non-clogged).

Dacron grafts are one-piece knitted fabrics in the shape of a tube and are available in various diameters. The configuration of the tube is often ribbed, to permit easier bending of the graft while avoiding crimping or buckling of the graft. The porosity of the fabric is controlled by the type of weave, with the goal being the intimate adaptation of the graft to natural tissue, and the hope that endothelial cells will readily colonize the velour-like surface of the artificial graft, although cells appear to colonize only a short distance into the graft, 10–15 mm. Antibiotics can be deposited onto the surface of the graft to reduce postsurgical infection risks. Future versions of vascular grafts may be engineered not only to include medications, but the surfaces of the grafts could be seeded with endothelial cells to provide a highly natural synthetic graft.

Grafts are typically used for bypass or repair procedures. In order to use a graft endovascularly (inside the blood vessel), the graft must incorporate a framework. Stents have been used without grafts to strengthen weakened blood vessels, and because the technology is well understood, it was reasonable to combine stents with grafts. The stent portion may be made of stainless steel or Nitinol wire and is normally collapsed; after expansion, the stent has a larger diameter, enabling it to press against the inside wall of a partially blocked blood vessel (Fig. 9.9).

A stent is attached to a graft and deployed either as a self-expanding unit or over a balloon, which inflates when the stent graft is delivered to the appropriate location and activates the stent (Fig. 9.16). The graft may be located inside or outside the stent.

Concerns about the longevity of stent grafts involve both biological and materials design factors. Mechanical fatigue is the major culprit that can cause failure of the struts of the stent or separation of the fabric. The ASTM lists a test method for in vitro pulsatile durability testing of vascular stents, which is concerned with the effect of fatigue loading caused by pulsing blood flow on the durability of the fabric, particularly its resistance to perforation.

In addition, the FDA provides guidance for industry as to the recommended nonclinical engineering tests that should be conducted by a manufacturer seeking FDA approval for intravascular stents. The list in the updated document dated April 18, 2010,

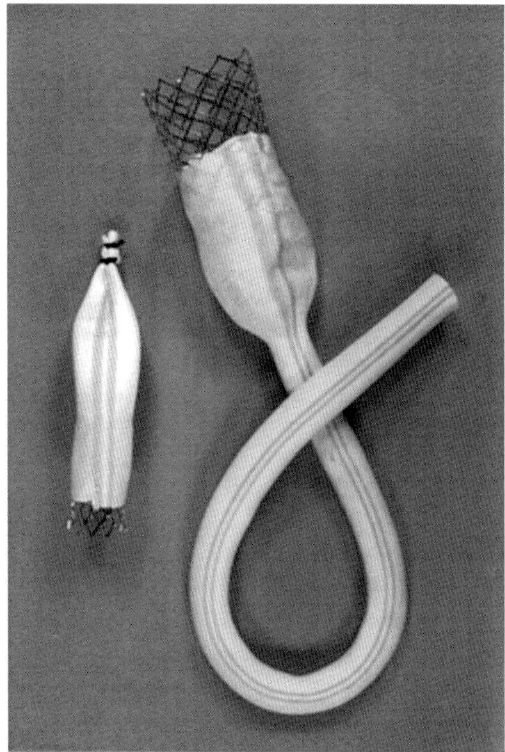

Fig. 9.16 Two stented grafts, on the *right* is also shown a length of synthetic vascular graft extending beyond the stented portion. Copyrighted by Springer Science + Business Media New York

includes material characterization (composition and corrosion resistance) and functional attributes (radial stiffness and strength, mechanical properties, stress–strain analysis, fatigue analysis, accelerated durability testing, MRI safety and compatibility, radiopacity, crush resistance, and kink resistance).

9.4.5 Peripheral Vascular Disease

Peripheral vascular disease (PVD), also known as peripheral arterial disease or "hardening of the arteries," is a disease caused by formation of plaques on the interior wall of arteries. However, the arteries involved are in the lower legs. Because of the reduced circulation, patients will begin to experience pain in their calves after walking (also called "intermittent claudication"). As the disease progresses, pain at night becomes a problem too, because when lying down, the gravity-assisted blood flow to the legs disappears. Unless the progress of the disease is halted or reversed, the arteries may become fully blocked, and the tissue of the legs and feet will begin to die; skin ulcers form and will not heal. If left untreated, amputation becomes a treatment option. Before that occurs, however, it is often possible to treat the disease by surgically removing the plaque, bypass surgery, or sympathectomy (removing the nerves that cause arteries to contract).

Risk factors for peripheral vascular disease include smoking, lack of physical activity, obesity, and excess alcohol consumption. Hypertension, diabetes, and high cholesterol also contribute to this disease. Males are more likely to develop PVD than females, and people from India, Pakistan, and Bangladesh appear to be more prone to suffer from PVD.

9.4.6 Vascular Access Devices

There are a number of medical conditions that require treatment by directly infusing medication into the blood supply using a central venous catheter. Examples include providing intravenous fluids, blood, intravenous medication such as during chemotherapy, and repeated blood sampling; these are short-term needs. Long-term applications include intravenous fluids, blood, medications, total parenteral nutrition (intravenous feeding), hemodialysis, plasmapheresis (removal, treatment, and return of blood components), and bone marrow transplantation [9]. Catheters are usually made from polyurethane or silastic (a type of silicone polymer).

Venous access ports are devices made from polymeric or metal chambers implanted subcutaneously and connected to an internally located catheter. The medication is delivered by needle during an injection through the skin directly into the access port. A similar approach is taken by implantable infusion pumps, which are devices implanted subcutaneously and designed to continuously deliver chemotherapy to the liver, opioids to the spine in cases of chronic pain, insulin for diabetics, and heparin to patients who continue to develop blood clots [9]. The pumps are accessed in the same way as venous access ports, by a needle through the skin.

9.5 Malfunction of Heart Valves and Remedies

9.5.1 Heart Valves

The heart valves' primary function is to ensure that blood flows mostly in one direction. The valves behave similarly to one-way doors in order to prevent backflow. Without this one-way feature, the heart would have to work much harder to push blood into adjacent chambers or major arteries. Your doctor can often learn much about the functioning of your heart by putting a stethoscope to the left side of your chest and listening to the thumping sound of the heart valves opening and closing.

The heart has four valves: tricuspid, mitral, pulmonary, and aortic see Fig. 9.1. The tricuspid valve is the valve between the right ventricle and right atrium. The mitral valve is between the left ventricle and left atrium. These two valves prevent backflow of blood from the ventricles to the atria during systole. The aortic valve is positioned between the left ventricle and the aorta, and the pulmonary artery valve is between the right ventricle and the pulmonary artery. These two valves prevent blood backflow from the aorta and pulmonary arteries into the ventricles during diastole. The opening and closing of these valves are not driven by muscle contraction or relaxation, but rather passively by the pressure gradient of blood. When a backward pressure gradient pushes blood backward, the valves close, and when a forward pressure gradient pushes blood in the forward direction, the valves open.

There are several heart valve diseases that prevent the proper flow of blood. Many of these valvular pathologies often result in turbulent blood flow and heart murmur, which is the change in the thumping sound of your heartbeat. These diseases can be grouped into two general types according to the functional changes that they cause. In the first type, the diseased valve is unable to open completely due to stiffening of the valve tissue through deposition of calcium. In this type of heart valve disease, which primarily affects the elderly, the heart must work harder to pump blood through the ailing valve. In the second type of heart valve disease, the valve is unable to close completely, which causes backflow ("regurgitation") of blood in the heart. In this latter type of disease, the heart has to work harder to compensate for the inefficiency of the valves. Some heart valve diseases are caused by genetic deficiency and are present from birth; others are often caused by damage from infections or illnesses suffered in childhood, like rheumatic fever.

Although in most cases medication is the best treatment for heart valve disease, sometimes the defective valves have to be replaced with prosthetic valves to restore normal valve function and prevent other complications induced by the defective valves such as heart failure. The idea of replacing the diseased valve by a prosthetic valve became widely accepted in the 1960s. However, at that time, mortality and complication rates associated with replacing heart valves were unacceptably high. Since then, engineers and scientists have been developing and designing better prosthetic valves resulting in the saving of many thousands of lives [10].

Before describing some of the prosthetic heart valves currently in use, let us discuss the characteristics that are desirable for a heart valve. Given that the primary function of the heart valve is preventing the backward flow of blood, the most important characteristic of an ideal prosthetic heart valve is to create a non-backflow system over the full range of physiologic heart function. Natural heart valves have a low transvalvular pressure gradient. They present little obstruction to the flow through the valves. Therefore, the prosthetic valve must be able to open and close easily by only a minimal pressure gradient, so that the valve itself does not induce much resistance. As the outer layer of natural heart valves consists of endothelial cells and is continuous with the endothelium lining of the heart chambers and hence not normally thrombogenic, the desirable prosthetic valve must be designed so that it also has no or minimal thrombogenic potential. Any blood clot (thrombus) can lead to serious complications; the detached fragments of the thrombus may travel with the blood flow and lodge in arteries blocking the downstream vasculature. This blockage may in turn lead to a myocardial infarction if the coronary arteries are blocked or a stroke if the cerebral arteries in the brain are blocked. The prosthetic valve must also be durable, as a damaged or broken valve may rapidly endanger the patient's life.

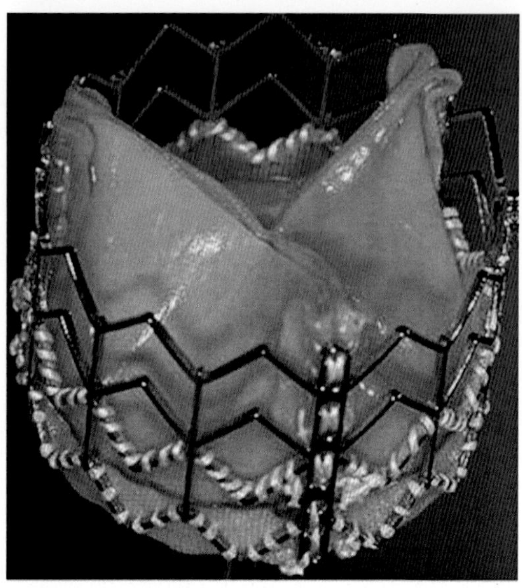

Fig. 9.17 A bioprosthetic heart valve made from bovine (cow) pericardial tissue mounted in a stainless steel frame, with polyethylene terephthalate (PET) fabric. This valve is designed to be introduced with a catheter and expanded once it is in place. Copyrighted by Springer Science + Business Media LLC

9.5.2 Prosthetic Valves

The two types of prosthetic valves currently in clinical use are tissue valves and mechanical valves. Tissue valves, of the type shown in Fig. 9.17, are obtained entirely from animals or made of tissue from animals. These valves are treated to remove the biological markers (mainly proteins) that might cause a response from the host's immune system. Sometimes, medication is used to retard this immune response. Given that the porcine heart is most similar to the human heart in anatomy, porcine valves are one of the most commonly used types of tissue valves for valve replacement. In another approach, pericardial animal tissue is utilized to make leaflets that are sewn into a metal frame. This tissue is typically harvested from either cows or horses.

The tissue heart valve is an extremely effective means of valve replacement and has many advantages over mechanical valves. Tissue valves are flexible and have better hemodynamics (blood flow characteristics), so they do not damage red cells while blood flows through them and hence cause less clot formation. Patients implanted with tissue heart valves are usually not required to take anticoagulant drugs. Tissue valves have almost no regurgitation volume. The most common cause of tissue valve failure is stiffening of the tissue due to the buildup of calcium. Calcification may cause narrowing of the opening through the valve, thus restricting blood flow. Calcification may also cause a collapse in the valve leaflets. Since younger patients have a greater calcium metabolism, tissue valves tend to last longer in older patients. These valves last approximately 15 years once transplanted to the human heart. Compared to mechanical valves, their limited lifespan is their main weakness.

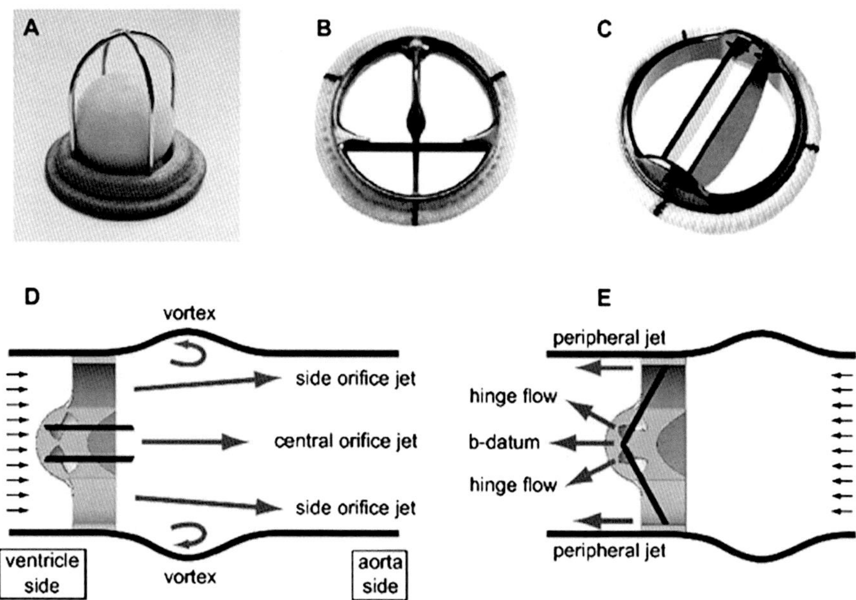

Fig. 9.18 Three mechanical heart valves. **a** is the ball in cage design, **b** is the tilting-disc design, and **c** is the bileaflet design. When open, the bileaflet design permits unimpeded blood flow (**d**), and when closed, some regurgitation is present (**e**). Copyrighted by Springer Science+Business Media LLC

Mechanical heart valves (MHV) are made of substances such as titanium, Teflon™, chromium–cobalt alloy, and pyrolytic carbon and are designed to replicate the function of the natural valves of the human heart. They are much more durable than tissue valves. However, because of the rigidity of the material they are made from, red blood cells may hit the leaflets as they traverse through the valves and rupture. The ruptured red blood cells then release their contents, which may induce blood clot formation. Therefore, patients with a mechanical heart valve replacement are required to take anticoagulant drugs throughout their lifetime to stop blood from clotting. Monthly blood tests to monitor coagulation are also required. Obviously, a potential complication of taking anticoagulant drugs is that the patient may not be able to easily stop bleeding in case of external or internal injury.

The caged-ball design is one of the early mechanical heart valves and consists of a ring attached to a cage composed of curved struts made of a cobalt–chromium alloy containing a free-floating ball made of silicone polymer (Fig. 9.18a). During systole, the pressure gradient opens the valve by pushing the ball up and allows blood flow through the valve. At the end of systole, the ball falls back in the ring and closes the valve to prevent the backflow of blood. Natural heart valves allow blood to flow straight through the center of the valve. However, the caged-ball valves completely block central flow, requiring more energy for blood to flow around the central ball/disc, which in turn requires a higher valvular pressure gradient. In addition, because of the change in direction of the blood flow, a large number of red blood cells are damaged due to collisions. A patient implanted with a caged-ball or caged-disc valve needs to take a large dose of anticoagulants throughout his or her life. There is only one version of this design still available.

To overcome the problems of the caged-ball/caged-disc design, a new class of prosthetic valves (the tilting-disc valve) was developed (Fig. 9.18b). These valves consist of a metal ring and a single circular disc held in place by two metal struts. The metal ring is covered by a Dacron fabric, and the suture threads are stitched through the fabric and into heart tissue to hold the valve in place. The disc is usually made of an extremely hard material (pyrolytic carbon) to reduce wear and prolong the life cycle of the valve. The disc swings between open and closed positions and is held in place by the two struts. When the blood flows forward, the pressure gradient pushes the tilting disc open at an angle of 60°. As the blood begins to travel backward, the tilting disc closes completely, preventing backflow. This tilting-disc design provides a large opening angle, improves central flow, and reduces the mechanical damage to blood cells and clotting and infection. Nevertheless, a low level of anticoagulant is still needed for the patient. A major problem with this design is the tendency for the outlet struts to fracture as a result of fatigue from the repeated ramming of the struts by the disc. There are three models of such valves still available; a fourth, the Björk–Shiley valve, was withdrawn from the market.

In 1979, a new mechanical heart valve design known as a bileaflet valve was introduced (Fig. 9.18c). These valves consist of two semicircular leaflets attached to a circular sewing ring. The leaflets swing open and closed to regulate blood flow. When open, the two leaflets are almost parallel to the direction of the blood flow, providing a large opening angle for unimpeded flow (Fig. 9.18d). This design provides the closest approximation to central flow achieved in a natural heart valve and has minimal turbulence and lower thrombogenicity compared with other types of mechanical valves. Therefore, patients implanted with a bileaflet valve only need to take a very low dose of anticoagulants to prevent clotting of the blood. However, this design is not considered ideal because it is vulnerable to backflow when the leaflets do not close completely, even though some regurgitation is desirable because it reduces the chance of clot formation in the valve. Nevertheless, this design is the most widely used type now. More than one million of these valves were implanted by the year 2000 [10]. They have excellent survival, approximately 94 % at 10-year post-insertion.

The main advantage of modern mechanical valves is that they are very reliable and can often last for the lifetime of the patient. However, the main disadvantage of these valves is their thrombogenicity, which can lead to very serious consequences such as heart attack or stroke. Therefore, patients implanted with mechanical heart valves must take anticoagulant drugs for the rest of their lives, which may lead to other complications, including uncontrolled bleeding. Another disadvantage of mechanical valves is regurgitation. The caged-ball/caged-disc design has a low level of leakage, but the tilting-disc and bileaflet valves have a larger regurgitation volume. The reported incidence of freedom from thromboembolism is 72 % for the bileaflet valve [10]. Mechanical valves are usually chosen for young patients and patients who already are on anticoagulation medication, while the bioprosthetic valves are indicated for patients who do not comply with anticoagulation therapy or the elderly with limited life expectancy. However, some surgeons believe that even young patients should be presented with bioprosthetic valves, because long-term anticoagulation is not viewed as desirable. Along with the general aging of the population in developed countries, the trend seems to be toward an increased use of bioprosthetic valves, more porcine than bovine.

Wear and fracture of the silicone ball in caged-ball artificial valves has been the subject of several lawsuits. This type of valve has not been sold after 2007 even though the wear and fracture problem has been resolved by heat curing of the silicone used in the manufacture of the valve. By far, the most well-known lawsuits were directed against the manufacturer of the Björk–Shiley tilting-disc valve (Pfizer). Although this valve was developed after the FDA had adopted a PMA process for evaluating devices, the FDA had not yet formulated the extensive procedures needed today for approval, and so the valve was not as thoroughly tested as it would be if it were to be introduced today. In any case, the valve failed for structural reasons. It turns out that engineers had not foreseen the possibility of the disc over-rotating and placing excessive stress on the struts holding it in place. When the struts failed, the disc was free to escape, and the result was uncontrolled blood flow through the heart followed by death. In the lawsuit, the manufacturer was accused of shoddy manufacturing practices, a faulty inspection process, and an unwillingness to spend money to improve its control over fabrication of the valve. The manufacturer appears to have also attempted to hide the extent of the problem [1]. Eventually, Pfizer lost the case and a few hundred million dollars as well.

What do you think: if a manufacturer loses a lawsuit where it is proven that a device was poorly designed, should patients in whom the device was implanted (but who have suffered no damage because their device continues to perform well) receive any payments?

After implantation of a heart valve, visits to the physician include examination by auscultation; recall that this is the procedure when a physician listens through a stethoscope. It is particularly applicable to mechanical heart valve recipients because the valves make noise and the type of noise can suggest a problem in their functioning. Complications associated with heart valves include structural failure, valve thrombosis, bleeding, endocarditis (infection), and nonstructural dysfunctions such as hemolysis (abnormal breakdown of red blood cells), paravalvular leaks (blood leakage through the valve), or pannus formation (ingrowth of fibrous tissue that interferes with valve function).

9.6 Life-Sustaining Cardiac Devices

9.6.1 Heart Failure

Heart failure is a condition in which the heart is unable to pump sufficient blood to meet the body's needs. As a diseased heart becomes incapable of providing enough blood to the body and tries to pump harder, the heart muscle fibers often increase in size resulting in a condition referred to as myocardial hypertrophy. That is the reason why a heart failure heart is larger than a normal heart. Despite its misleading name, heart failure does not mean that the heart has stopped working, is about to stop working, or that the patient has necessarily had a heart attack. Instead, heart failure develops slowly over time as the heart muscle gradually weakens. In fact, millions of people are living with heart failure.

Heart failure affects nearly five million Americans. It is the only major cardiovascular disorder on the rise as more people are surviving heart attacks and other cardiac pathologies, but are left with weakened hearts. There are approximately a half-million new cases of heart failure diagnosed each year, and heart failure is the most frequent cause of hospitalization in people age 65 and older. An estimated 700,000 Americans annually die of heart failure every year. While there is no cure for heart failure, heart transplantation can be used to treat this disease. However, there are only about 2,500 hearts available for transplant every year. Therefore, various drugs, artificial hearts, and left ventricular assist devices have become attractive alternative treatments for heart failure.

Heart failure can be caused by any disease that weakens the ability of the heart muscle to pump blood. Muscle damage and scarring caused by a heart attack is the greatest risk factor for heart failure. Cardiac arrhythmia (irregular heartbeat) also increases heart failure risk. Uncontrolled high blood pressure may increase the risk of heart failure by 200 %, and the degree of heart failure risk is directly related to the severity of high blood pressure. People with diabetes also have a two- to eight-fold greater risk of heart failure, and women with diabetes have a greater risk than men with diabetes. A single risk factor is enough to cause heart failure, but multiple risk factors greatly increase the overall risk. Advanced age also adds to the potential impact of any heart failure risk. The diagram in Fig. 9.19 portrays both risk factors and the aging process as contributing to heart failure and eventual death.

A large variety of symptoms is typical of heart failure, including fatigue, the ability to perform only limited activities, chest congestion, edema or ankle swelling, and shortness of breath. Many people are not aware they have heart failure because the most common symptoms are often confused with normal signs of aging.

Heart failure can be diagnosed by several tests. One of the most important diagnostic tools for detecting heart failure is an echocardiogram or "echo" for short. It is a painless and noninvasive procedure that allows the doctor to use an ultrasound signal to image the heart and detect how vigorously the heart is pumping. During the echo, a parameter called ejection fraction (EF) is often obtained, which measures how well a heart is pumping. Ejection fraction represents the percentage of blood squeezed out of the left ventricle with every beat. The healthy heart does not pump 100 % of the blood out of the left ventricle, and normally people have an ejection fraction of about 55–65 %. People with heart failure often have an ejection fraction of 40 % or lower. Another painless and noninvasive diagnostic test for detecting heart failure is an electrocardiogram or EKG. During an EKG, electrical wires are attached to the patient's chest, arms, and legs to measure the electrical activity of the heart, the pattern of which is

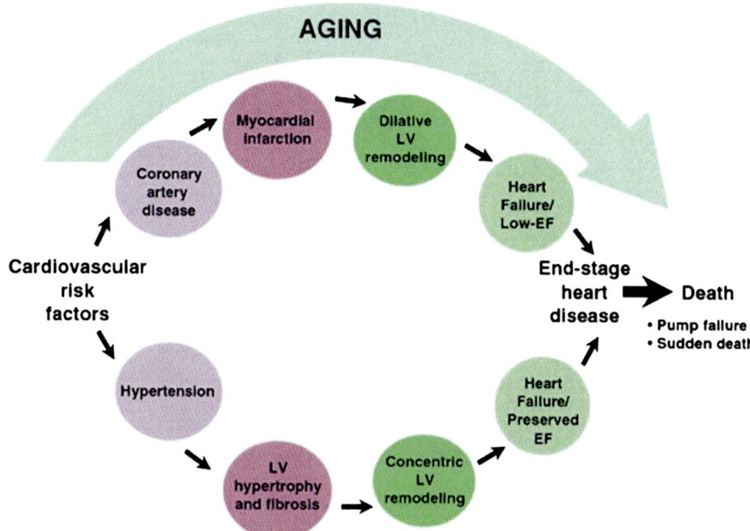

Fig. 9.19 Heart failure, aging, and cardiovascular disease. Risk factors such as hypertension, obesity, type 2 diabetes, and high cholesterol levels contribute to hypertrophy of the left ventricle and concentric remodeling of the left ventricle (thickening of the wall of the left ventricle). The ejection fraction is unaffected. In the aging process, heart attack leads to dilative left ventricle remodeling (enlargement of the left ventricle), and the ejection fraction is lowered. Copyrighted by Springer Science + Business Media LLC

often altered if there has been any damage to the heart muscle. The doctor may also take a chest X-ray to measure the size of the heart to determine if the heart muscle has been enlarged. A chest X-ray may also show fluid accumulation in the lungs, another sign and symptom of heart failure.

9.6.2 Left Ventricular Assist Devices (LVADs) and Artificial Hearts

Approximately 23.0 million patients suffer from heart failure worldwide with 2.0 million new cases diagnosed each year. In the USA, there are approximately 5 million patients with 550,000 new cases each year. Each year, only 2,000–2,500 patients in the USA receive a heart transplant, while more than 25,000 die waiting for a donor heart. The National Institutes of Health estimates 100,000 US patients per year would benefit from left ventricular assist device (LVAD) technology, but this population is extremely underserved with LVADs being implanted in only about 3,000 of these patients annually.

The left ventricle is the chamber of the heart that pumps blood out to the body. A patient can live with a right ventricular failure, but left ventricular failure can often lead to early death. A left ventricular assist device can help maintain the pumping ability of a heart that cannot effectively work on its own. Left ventricular assist

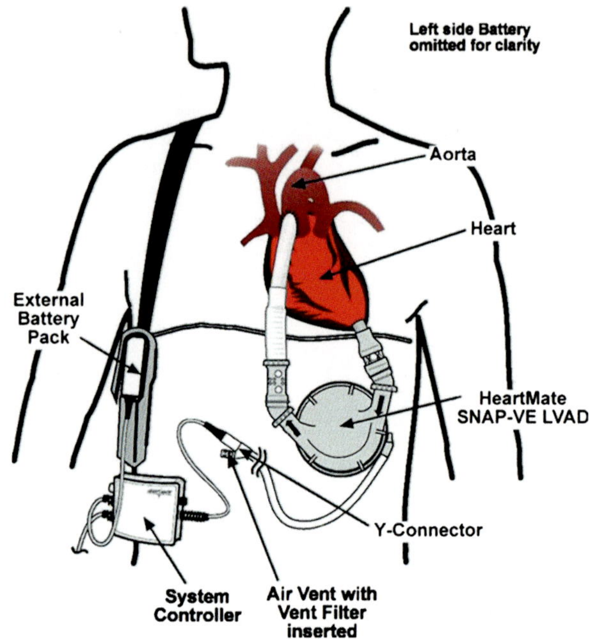

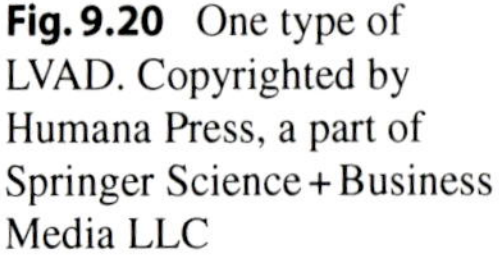
Fig. 9.20 One type of LVAD. Copyrighted by Humana Press, a part of Springer Science + Business Media LLC

devices (LVADs), originally developed in the early 1960s, are generally battery-powered, mechanical pumps that are implanted in the chest cavity of the patient. An LVAD does not replace the diseased heart but provides assistance to the diseased heart. Currently, LVADs are used either in cases of potentially reversible heart failure ("bridge to recovery") or for end-stage heart failure as a "bridge to transplant" for short-term applications in patients awaiting a suitable heart for transplantation. However, in some cases heart failure patients implanted with an LVAD have shown significant improvements in the heart muscle to a level where the diseased heart can pump sufficient blood on its own and does not require mechanical augmentation. In other cases, such as for patients with metastatic cancer who are not eligible for transplant, the LVAD becomes "destination therapy."

A typical LVAD (Fig. 9.20) has a mechanical pump that at the input end is connected to and receives blood from the bottom of the left ventricle. The output end of this pump is attached to the aorta, so that the pump moves blood from the left ventricle to the aorta. The pump, which may be pulsatile or continuous, is placed in the upper part of the abdomen, and a wire connected to the pump passes through the abdominal wall to the outside of the body and is attached to the pump's battery and control system. The pumps have mechanical valves to ensure that the blood flow is unidirectional and can be driven by air pumped from the outside or electrically. The inside of the tubes and the outside surface of the device are designed to minimize thrombogenesis and rejection by the immune system. A modern LVAD is small enough, and generally contains a rechargeable internal battery and controller, to allow the patient to move freely without being connected to an external power source

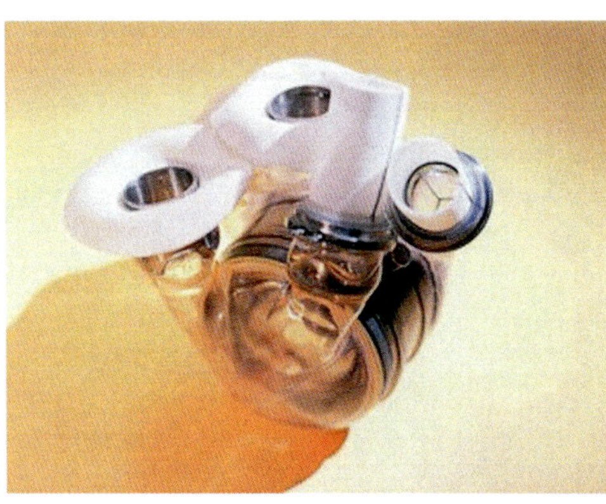
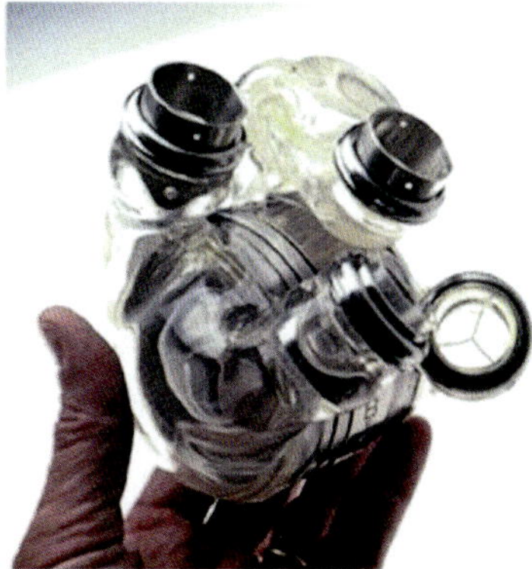

Fig. 9.21 Two models of artificial hearts. On the *left*, the CardioWest, FDA approved in 2004 as a bridge-to-transplant device; it is not self-contained, as tubing exits the patient's chest. On the *right*, the AbioCor device, FDA approved in 2006; it is self-contained, with no external connections. Copyrighted by Humana Press, a part of Springer Science+Business Media LLC

and controller at all times. The goal is to eliminate all through-the-skin connections, and the pumps can be charged with transmitted radio frequency energy which passes through the skin. Patients with LVADs can be discharged from the hospital and have an acceptable quality of life while waiting for a donor heart to become available.

An artificial heart is a mechanical device that is designed to replace the biological heart in a patient with heart failure (Fig. 9.21). AbioCor produced the first completely self-contained total artificial heart, with a hydraulic pump transporting fluid from side to side. This device is approximately the size of a grapefruit and weighs 1 kg. Blood is received from the body and pumped to the lungs from the right chamber and pumped to the rest of the body from the left chamber. A valve opens and closes to control fluid motion between left and right. The device has internal and external components. The internal component includes the artificial heart, a rechargeable battery, and a controller unit. The external component consists of a battery pack worn on a waist belt. A wireless transcutaneous energy transfer coil is used to power the pump and to charge the internal rechargeable battery. The external battery pack can pump the artificial heart for 4 h, whereas the internal battery can maintain the heart function for only 30 min. The ability of this system to function in an "untethered" manner for 30 min significantly increases the quality of the patient's life by, for example, allowing them to shower without being attached to a large external power source.

As stated above, LVADs may pump blood in pulses (like the heart itself) or continuously. Interestingly, the use of continuous pumps to replace a heart could result in individuals who no longer have a pulse! For example, in several recent experimental cases, the patient's severely diseased heart was completely replaced with two modified HeartMate II continuous pumps (manufactured by Thoratec Corp), with the patients surviving with no heartbeat and no pulse. [http://www.dailymail.co.uk/health/article-2211679/Former-fighter-man-live-pulse-SIX-MONTHS-thanks-revolutionary-artificial-heart.html#ixzz2RiSZ8Cea].

Both LVADs and artificial hearts have many potential complications. These devices have limitations that are similar to artificial valves, including infections, thrombogenesis, hemorrhage (uncontrolled bleeding; recall that these patients are all on blood thinner medications), and hemocompatibility. In addition, other characteristics such as the constant pumping noise of the device may cause psychological problems for the patient. Furthermore, these devices are very expensive, with the current cost of a LVAD exceeding $250,000. However, the fact that up to 35 % of these devices may fail within 2 years of implantation is a serious concern with these devices. A failed device can cause sudden death if the patient cannot receive treatment within minutes.

9.7 Summary

Heart disease is a major cause of mortality in the developed world, and its incidence is rising in the developing world too. Many of the specific types of heart disease can be avoided by making lifestyle changes that are constantly repeated by doctors to their patients: do not smoke, reduce the intake of saturated animal fats, maintain a normal body weight, and exercise regularly. Many cardiac diseases originate in the electrical or pacing system of the heart, the vascular or arterial–venous system, and the heart valves or focus on a generalized weakening of the heart muscle called heart failure. Surgical and medical device options to treat many of these diseases are available, but they are often expensive. Heart failure, on the other hand, is best treated by transplantation of another human heart (though there are shortages of these organs) or by powered devices such as LVADs or artificial hearts. These latter two treatment modalities are also extremely expensive, not available to patients who do not have comprehensive medical insurance, and currently are not intended to replace or augment cardiac function on a long-term basis.

9.8 Foundational Concepts

- The human heart has four chambers: left and right atria (these receive blood) and left and right ventricles (these pump blood; the left ventricle pumps blood to the body, the right ventricle pumps blood to the lungs). Valves between the chambers and out to the principal arteries ensure that blood flows in one direction. The heart is really a large hollow muscle, which has the attribute of automaticity (it contracts on its own, without the need for control by conscious thought).
- The heart rate of a normal adult is 60–100 beats/min. The heartbeat is composed of a period of relaxation (diastole) and a period of contraction (systole). Blood pressure is measured as both the systolic and diastolic pressure. The timing of contraction is governed by electrical signals originating in the sinoatrial node and traveling through the atrioventricular node to the His–Purkinje system for distribution to all parts of the ventricles.
- Patients with arrhythmia may be treated by implantation of a pacemaker or, if their heartbeat is chaotic and too rapid, by implantation of a defibrillator.

- Patients suffering from valve disease may have valve replacement surgery. The new valves are either bioprosthetic, made from porcine or bovine tissue, or all synthetic, made from corrosion-resistant metal, Dacron fabric, and pyrolytic carbon.
- Deposits of fatty compounds on the inside of blood vessels are called plaque. They cause narrowing of blood vessels and thereby restrict the blood flow. Occasionally, in unstable plaques, pieces may break off and block a smaller blood vessel downstream, leading to death of the tissue served by the blocked artery. When the tissue without a blood supply is cardiac muscle, the patient may suffer a heart attack. When the tissue that dies is brain tissue, the patient can have a stroke. Blood vessels that are partially occluded by deposits may be reopened with balloon angioplasty and stenting. Blood vessels that are blocked by deposits may be replaced with synthetic Dacron vascular grafts or by segments of the patient's own veins taken from another location in the body. Drugs called statins also reduce the amount of lipoprotein circulating in the blood which would be available for plaque formation.
- Heart failure is a degenerative disease caused by the gradual weakening of the heart. There is currently no cure for heart disease other than transplant of a healthy human heart or the use for a limited time of a left ventricular assist device or an artificial heart.

References

1. Mayesh, J., & Scranton, M. (2004). Legal aspects of biomaterials. In B. Ratner et al. (Eds.), *Biomaterials science*. San Diego, CA: Elsevier Academic Press.
2. Bjerregaard, P., & El-Shafei, A. (2006). Cardiac pacemakers. In F. Johnson & K. Virgo (Eds.), *The bionic human* (pp. 633–644). Totowa, NJ: Humana Press.
3. Street, L. (2012). *Introduction to biomedical engineering technology*. Boca Raton, FL: CRC Press.
4. Padera, R., & Schoen, F. (2004). Cardiovascular medical devices. In B. Ratner et al. (Eds.), *Biomaterials science*. San Diego, CA: Elsevier Academic Press.
5. Kasirajan, K., Matteson, B., Marke, J. & Langsfeld, M. et al. (2006). Vascular prostheses. In F. Johnson & K. Virgo (Eds.), *The bionic human*. Totowa, NJ: Humana Press.
6. Rouers, A., Meurisse, N., Lavigne, J.P., Francart, D., Quaniers, J., Desiron & Limet, R. et al. (2005). Potential benefits of laparoscopic aorto-bifemoral bypass surgery. *Acta Chirurgica Belgica, 105*, 610–615.
7. Devine, C., & McCollum, C. (2004). Heparin-bonded Dacron or polytetrafluoroethylene for femoropopliteal bypass: Five-year results of a prospective randomized multicenter clinical trial. *Journal of Vascular Surgery, 40*, 924–931.
8. Van Damme, H., Deprez, M., Creemers, E. & Limet, R. et al. (2005). Intrinsic structural failure of polyester (Dacron) vascular grafts. A general review. *Acta Chirurgica Belgica, 105*, 249–255.
9. Compton, C., & Raaf, J. (2006). Vascular access devices. In F. Johnson & K. Virgo (Eds.), *The bionic human* (pp. 561–587). Totowa, NJ: The Humana Press.
10. David Arya, M., & Labovitz, A. (2006). Cardiac valves. In F. Johnson & K. Virgo (Eds.), *The bionic human*. Totowa, NJ: Humana Press.

10 Clever Strategies for Controlled Drug Release and Targeted Drug Delivery

"Drugs are not always necessary, but belief in recovery always is."

Norman Cousins

The large gains in knowledge of molecular biology have made it possible for pharmaceutical companies and researchers to make "designer" drugs and to target the drugs at specific disease points in the body rather than subjecting the entire organism to the effects of the drug. In this way, drugs may act much more efficiently.

In this chapter, we will discuss how drugs are packaged and aimed at specific tissues and designed to be released in a controlled manner so that they are able to do the most good.

10.1 Introduction

While most diseases are localized in a specific area of the body (e.g., brain tumors), very few drugs are administered locally to the diseased tissue. Instead, most drugs are administered systemically (they are dispersed throughout the entire body), and so they are often given at high concentrations to ensure that a sufficient dose of the drug will reach the target even in a diluted condition. Administration of drugs in elevated concentrations can induce significant side effects, which sometimes result in lower efficacy, reduced patient compliance with treatment, and lower quality of life. For example, hair loss, which is a readily recognizable side effect of chemotherapy for treating cancer, results from the systemic administration of chemotherapeutic agents which not only kill tumor cells (the desirable effect), but also damage other tissues including hair follicles. These and other side effects limit the amount of drug that can be safely administered; it would be better to increase the drug amount in order to increase its effectiveness.

G.R. Baran et al., *Healthcare and Biomedical Technology in the 21st Century: An Introduction for Non-Science Majors*, DOI 10.1007/978-1-4614-8541-4_10,

It is frustrating to know that delivery of a drug to a diseased tissue could improve a patient's health if only a number of inconvenient and potentially dangerous side effects and biological strategies used by our bodies for self-protection could be avoided [1]. Drug designers and drug-delivery specialists try to outsmart the body and develop drugs that:

- Target and bind preferentially to diseased tissue
- Avoid being destroyed by or eliminated from the body before they can perform their therapeutic function
- Be able to travel to the targeted tissue site without being trapped in other locations
- Are dispensed at a constant rate, avoiding an initial surge in local or systemic concentration followed by a rapid decrease in concentration

Treatment of disease through drug therapy has improved dramatically over the past 50 years, thanks in most part to the hard work of many scientists. However, while a large number of new drugs have been discovered and successfully implemented in the clinic, the development of targeted drug-delivery systems has lagged far behind [2]. Many advantages of targeted delivery and controlled release of drugs in the body can only be achieved if the target tissue is easily accessible and biologically responsive. The desired target tissue is generally removed from the site of administration; e.g., medication to relieve headaches is normally taken orally but has to be absorbed into the bloodstream in the intestine after passage through the oral cavity and stomach. Therefore, having the drug reach the desired target tissue, while avoiding nontargeted normal tissue within the sought-after time course, has been a main obstacle for developing more effective targeted treatments. Nevertheless, a number of controlled-release formulations and several targeted drug-delivery systems have already been approved for patient use as over-the-counter formulations or in a clinical setting. The names of such commercially available formulations may carry extensions such as "CR" for controlled release (e.g., Ambien CR®), "ER" for extended release (e.g., Depakote ER®), or "XR" for, again, extended release (e.g., Effexor XR®).

10.2 The Goals of Controlled-Release Systems

A controlled-release system may have a number of components, including the drug to be delivered, the carrier system (e.g., nanoparticles), and recognition molecules that target various tissues (e.g., antibodies). For example, a sleep-aid medication may be encapsulated in a large number of nanoparticles which are dissolved at different rates in the stomach; taking such a formulation orally will result in the slow release of the drug into the stomach over an extended period of time, helping to keep the person asleep for a longer period as compared to taking the drug in a single dose (e.g., a conventional pill).

The overall goal of the controlled-release system is to allow control of drug concentrations throughout the body, either maintaining a certain drug concentration or limiting the rate of drug release in particular parts of the body or organs. Ideally, a controlled/targeted delivery system should have the following properties:

1. Sustained drug action: a sufficient and constant drug level in the body should be maintained so that the drug can effectively perform its therapeutic function with minimal undesirable side effects.
2. Localized drug action: the drug should be preferentially released near or inside the diseased tissue or organ.
3. Targeted drug action: certain carriers or chemical derivatives are used to preferentially deliver drugs to a desired location where the drugs can perform their therapeutic action with minimal undesirable side effects.
4. Protected drug action: drugs should be protected from being degraded and/or eliminated in the hostile environment of the body before reaching the disease tissue.

A key and desirable characteristic is that the controlled/targeted release system must be able to maintain a therapeutically effective drug level in target tissue over an extended period of time and ideally leave the rest of the body drug free, or at least with a significantly lower drug concentration. In addition, the drug-delivery method should readily pass the drug through biological barriers in the body, such as the digestive system for drugs taken orally or the blood–brain barrier if the drug targets the brain via systemic administration. It is also desirable that the drugs or the vehicle that carries the drug can preferentially target the diseased tissue to eliminate or minimize undesirable side effects to other tissues.

Obviously, it is very difficult to create a controlled-release system that meets all these requirements. In this chapter, we will review the basic concepts and principles of controlled release and targeted drug delivery and describe the factors that influence the design of such systems.

10.3 The Basic Mechanism of Drug Dispersion: Fick's Law

Most conventional drugs are water-soluble. They disperse in tissue by a mechanism called diffusion, modeled by Fick's law of diffusion. Imagine that the drug is like a drop of dye placed in a container of still water (mimicking tissue). With time, the color dye molecules gradually diffuse (travel) throughout the water slowly, with a high color intensity where the drop of dye was first placed and a gradual lowering color intensity moving away from the spot where the drop of dye was placed. Eventually, of course, given enough time, the color will be uniform throughout the water but at a much lower intensity than the site of the original drop.

The drop of dye contains many molecules of dye, and each one can, in principle, move randomly in any direction with equal probability. However, as you have observed in many situations, the molecules preferentially move away from the center of the drop of dye in the water, not toward the center. That is because in the center of the drop, the dye molecules are concentrated and they bump into each other. The bumping causes them to move apart from each other in a process called the "random walk," and as they keep moving apart from each other, they naturally migrate from an area of high concentration to an area of low concentration. Eventually, the dye molecules are evenly distributed throughout the water.

Adolf Fick was a physiologist who reported his laws of diffusion (there are two laws) in 1865. His work focused on diffusion in fluids, even though we know today that diffusion occurs in solids too, and Fick's laws apply to liquids, solids, and gases.

Fick's first law of diffusion mathematically describes this molecular diffusion process by the following equation:

$$J = -D \times \Delta C / \Delta X$$

where "J" is the mass flux in units of mol/m^2/s (the amount of substance that diffuses through a unit area per unit time), "D" is the diffusion coefficient or diffusivity in units of m^2/s, ΔC is the change in concentration (mol/m^3) with distance, and ΔX is the distance from the source of the material.

The diffusion coefficient (D) depends on the material properties of the fluid (including temperature and viscosity) and the size of the molecules or diffusing particles. The rate of diffusion (J) depends on the diffusion coefficient (D), the concentration of the diffusing substance, and the distance from the point of release (X). The driving force for diffusion is the concentration gradient ($\Delta C/\Delta X$), so the greater the concentration gradient (the difference between concentrations at two locations), the more rapidly the substance will diffuse. After reaching equilibrium, the concentration gradient drops to zero, and so does net diffusion.

The amount of a drug reaching a tissue generally depends on its diffusion from blood plasma but is also affected by drug elimination from blood plasma. The plasma half-life of a drug is defined as the time it takes for half of the original quantity of drug to be removed from the plasma by the body and is the result of both the drug diffusion rate into tissue and the elimination rate of the drug from plasma. In general, if the plasma concentration of a given drug is below a certain level, the drug will not have any therapeutic efficacy. Taking a large dose of a drug to maintain the plasma drug concentration above the minimal effective concentration level may result in a toxic plasma drug concentration which may be harmful (Fig. 10.1).

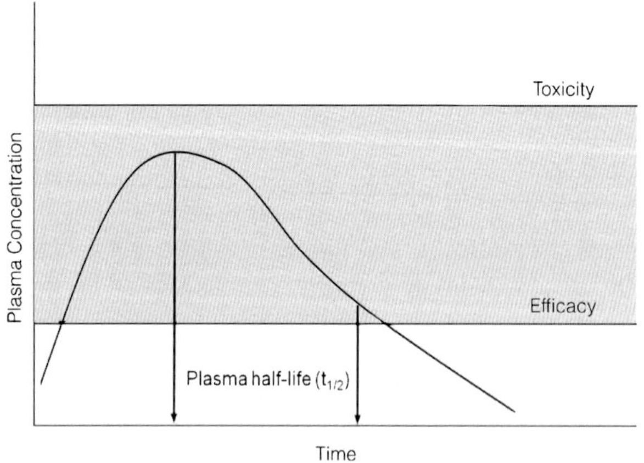

Fig. 10.1 Drug concentration in plasma versus time. If the plasma concentration of a given drug is below a certain level (efficacy level), the drug will not have therapeutic efficacy; a very high concentration of the drug (toxicity level) may be toxic for the body

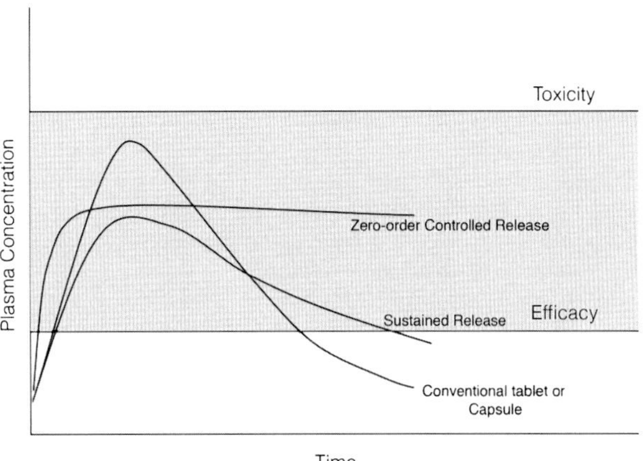

Fig. 10.2 Plasma drug concentration profiles for a conventional tablet or capsule, a sustained-release form, and an ideal "zero-order" controlled-release form

In most cases, the plasma concentration of a drug should remain between the toxicity level and the minimal effective level for as long as possible so that the drug can treat the diseased tissue over a long period of time without tissue damage. As a matter of fact, one of the main purposes of controlled-release systems is to extend the time that the drug is at the therapeutically effective concentration without raising the concentration above the toxicity level. Figure 10.2 shows plasma drug concentration profiles for a conventional tablet or capsule, a sustained-release formulation, and an ideal "zero-order" controlled-release form. In a conventional tablet or capsule, the plasma concentration of the drug reaches its peak and then quickly decreases below the efficacy level, so that it only has a short window of time during which it can act on the target tissue. A sustained drug formulation can maintain a relatively sufficient and constant drug level in the body over a longer period of time without necessarily increasing the total drug concentration in plasma. A zero-order controlled-release (prolonged-release) formulation slowly releases the drug at a rate equal to the elimination rate, so that the concentration of the drug is held constant in plasma. Unfortunately, a true "zero-order" controlled-release system cannot be achieved in practice because all drugs are eventually removed from the body resulting in a drop in their plasma concentration.

10.4 Advantages and Disadvantages of Targeted Drug-Delivery and Controlled-Release Systems

As mentioned before, controlled/targeted release systems have a number of advantages but also disadvantages compared to conventional drug formulations. These are described in Table 10.1.

Table 10.1 Advantages and disadvantages of controlled or targeted drug-delivery systems

Advantages	Disadvantages
Reduced undesirable systemic side effects; can control drug release rate and/ or release location	Targeted delivery and controlled-release systems are complex and difficult and costly to produce
Reduction in the total drug dose; can selectively deliver high concentration of drugs to the diseased site while keeping the systemic drug concentration low	The complexity of these systems makes them very difficult to characterize in the laboratory and in animal or human studies
Reduced dosing frequency; drug release rate may be controlled	Dose dumping: controlled-release systems usually contain large amounts of drugs. If changes in environmental factors (e.g., patient diet) cause an early and sudden release of the drug, the large sudden dose can pose a serious threat to health
Reduced drug plasma level fluctuation; drug release rate may be controlled so the drug concentration in the plasma is maintained at a relatively constant level	Dose adjustment in a controlled-release system is often determined during its production, so it's hard to change release rate after the medication is taken
Improved treatment efficiency; drug can be delivered to the diseased site in a high concentration	Increased potential for first-pass metabolism; much of the drug is excreted in the liver, so it does not reach the circulatory system
Improved patient compliance; minimized undesirable side effects	The drug in a controlled-release system may be released at a much slower rate than originally designed, which could result in a plasma concentration that is too low
Improved bioavailability for some drugs; the controlled-release system can protect the drug from degradation in the body	

10.5 Fine-Tuning Drug-Delivery Systems

In designing controlled/targeted drug release systems, drug properties, the molecular structure of the drug, and the carrier are often modified to improve drug pharmacodynamics (physiologic effects of the drug on the body) and pharmacokinetics (the time course of drug absorption, bioavailability, distribution, metabolism, and excretion). In this approach, a number of variables must be considered:

1. Drug properties: properties such as plasma half-life, drug stability, solubility, charge, and protein binding play an important role in the design and performance of controlled/targeted release systems.
2. Side effects/safety: biodistribution and safety of the drug carrier usually play important roles in determining the toxicity level of the system.
3. Routes of delivery: an orally administered formulation, for example, the drug has to survive the acidic environment of the stomach in comparison to an intravenous formulation.
4. Target site: the drug should accumulate at the disease site while keeping the systemic drug concentration low to reduce undesirable side effects.
5. Acute (occasional) and chronic (long-term and continuing) therapy: the length of drug therapy often depends on the type of disease being treated. For example,

antibiotic drugs are often administered for a short time, whereas antihypertension (high blood pressure) drugs are usually taken chronically.

6. The disease: changes in the body during the course of a disease can affect the effectiveness of the drug being delivered. For example, diabetic patients may often have associated heart disease, which should be taken into consideration when designing drug-delivery systems for treating diabetes.
7. The patient: the patient's age, gender, physical condition, etc. can significantly influence the design of a controlled-release system. For example, older patients usually have slow stomach movements, which result in longer transit time of drugs through their gastrointestinal systems. So, a controlled-release system for older patients with colon cancer has to be designed in a way that the drug is protected for a longer time in the stomach before it reaches the intestine where it is absorbed.

10.6 Routes of Drug Administration

Drugs can be administered through various routes, including oral, sublingual, mucosal, nasal, pulmonary, ocular, transdermal, vaginal, rectal, intrauterine, and parenteral (subcutaneous, intramuscular, intraperitoneal, intrathecal, or intraventricular injections).

The rate-limiting step is defined as the slowest step in a process. The rate-limiting step for drug delivery is different for traditional drugs versus controlled-release formulations. In conventional drug-delivery systems, the barrier that limits the drug from reaching the targeted tissue is usually a biological membrane, and crossing this membrane is the rate-limiting step. For example, for orally administered drugs, the intestinal membrane often controls the overall rate of drug absorption into the bloodstream. In a controlled-release system, however, drug availability is controlled by the release properties of the drug carrier. For instance, a nanoparticle-based drug-delivery system can be designed so that it would release its drug content in a predetermined manner only after rapidly crossing the intestinal wall.

The route of administration plays an important role in determining the therapeutic efficacy of a drug-delivery system. For example, because stomach acid degrades proteins such as insulin, these compounds cannot be taken orally. Furthermore, an increasing number of recently developed drugs can be toxic if they are not administered through proper routes. Let's consider examples of some of the more common routes of drug administration.

10.6.1 Oral Controlled-Release Formulations

The oral route is by far the oldest and most commonly used route of drug delivery. It is convenient, flexible, and well characterized compared with other routes, and therefore, oral formulations may receive FDA regulatory approval much more easily than if the drug is to be delivered via another route. The oral and gastrointestinal tract provides opportunities for many mechanisms for controlled-release and multiple pathways for adsorption of the drug.

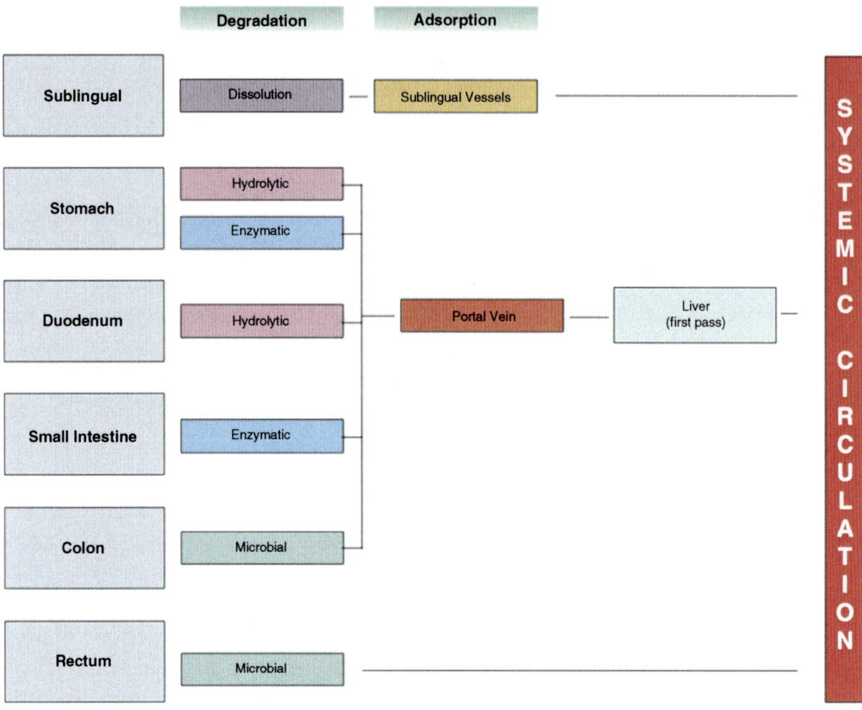

Fig. 10.3 A drug taken by the oral route passes through a series of different microenvironments, including sublingual, stomach, duodenum, small intestine, colon, and rectum, in which the degradation and adsorption of the drug can occur through various mechanisms

A drug taken by the oral route passes through a series of different microenvironments, including sublingual (under the tongue), the stomach, duodenum, intestine, colon, and rectum, in which the degradation and adsorption of the drug can occur through various mechanisms (Fig. 10.3). Please note that except for the sublingual and rectal routes, drugs taken orally must pass through the liver ("first pass") before reaching the systemic circulation. This presents a challenge if the liver has an affinity for the drug being administered, as much of the drug may be metabolized by the liver and therefore, never reach the target tissue.

The residence time of a drug in the gastrointestinal tract for healthy individuals is approximately 24 h and depends largely on the rate of gastric emptying and intestinal motility. Therefore, to increase absorption of the drug, the residence time of the drug in the gastrointestinal tract can be maximized by slowing gastric emptying. Alternatively, the degradation rate of the drug may be reduced by encapsulating a drug with a biocompatible material that is not easily degraded by the stomach fluid. Most commercially available extended-release capsules are examples of sustained-release formulations, which use slowly dissolving capsules to enclose a drug so that the drug is released slowly over time (Fig. 10.4).

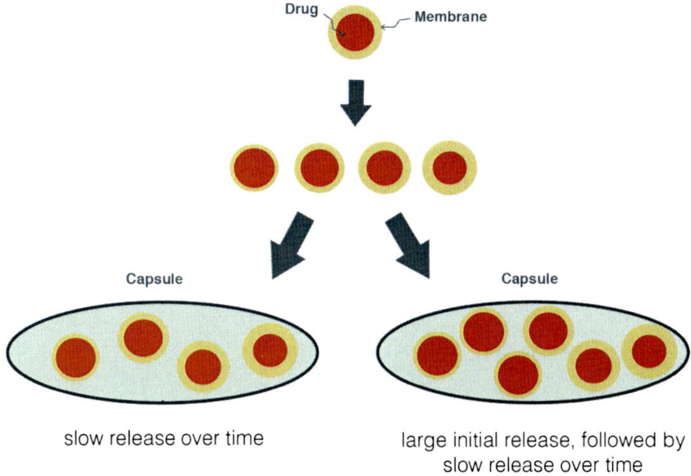

Fig. 10.4 An example of an extended-release formulation (*top panel*) which uses different biocompatible polymeric membrane thicknesses (*middle panel*) to program a different release rate of the encapsulated drug. This formulation can be used to ensure that the drug is released slowly over time (*bottom left panel*) or that there is a large initial release of the drug, followed by slow release over time (*bottom right panel*)

Because of the special features of the GI tract, orally administrated drugs encounter several pH (basic or acidic) environments before being absorbed or excreted. The drug is first exposed to a neutral pH of 7 in the mouth, then to an acidic pH of 1–4 in the stomach, followed by a basic pH of 5–7 in the small intestine. In the gastrointestinal tract, drugs can be released via a pH-dependent mechanism by, for example, utilizing microporous membranes to manage drug release. This type of formulation is prepared by coating a core tablet of the drug with a mixture of polymers, including some that dissolve in the acidic gastric fluid and others that dissolve in the intestinal fluid. A special group of these formulations, the so-called "enteric-coated" drugs, is coated with a polymer that stays intact in the stomach and will only release the encapsulated drug after it arrives in the intestinal tract (Fig. 10.5). Enteric-coated drugs have several functions, including protecting drugs from gastric liquids, preventing stomach discomfort for drugs such as aspirin, and ensuring that the drug is released at the proper site.

Figure 10.6 depicts two examples of orally administered controlled-release formulations. In a diffusion-controlled release drug-delivery system, the drug is coated with a polymeric membrane that allows gastrointestinal fluids to freely cross the membrane, and the drug is dissolved in place. The dissolved drug then diffuses down a concentration gradient across the membrane into the surrounding gastrointestinal environment. In this delivery system, the rate-limiting step is determined by the diffusion coefficient of the drug through the polymeric membrane. In an erosion-controlled release system, the drug is uniformly mixed with a slowly dissolving polymeric or other material. The drug release rate for this system then relies on the dissolution rate of the encapsulating material. Both of above systems control the

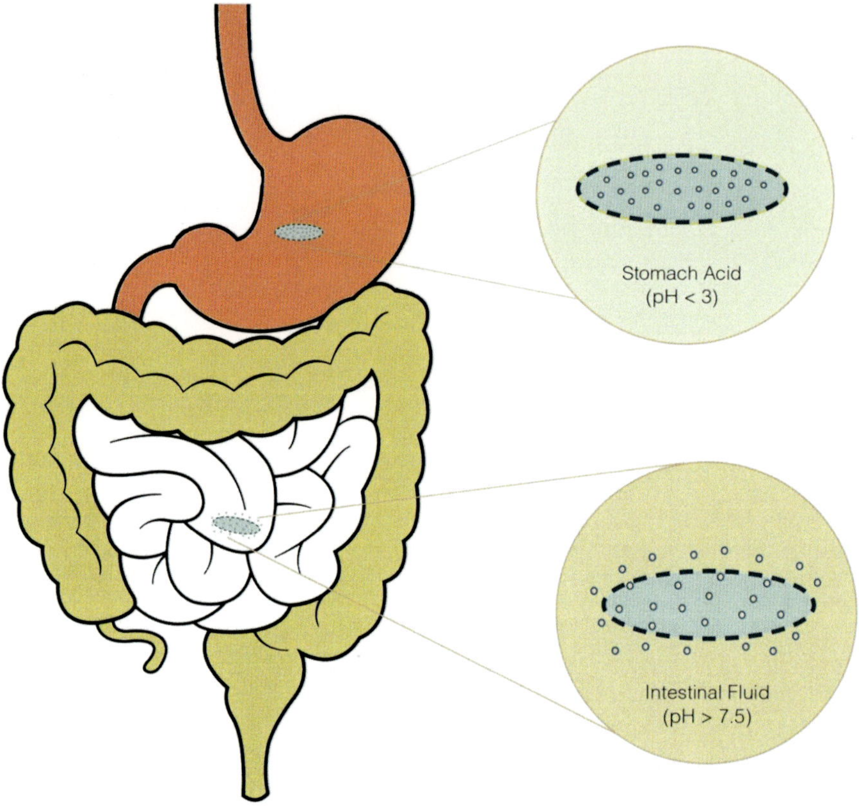

Fig. 10.5 Enteric-coated formulations are often used to prevent side effects of drugs such as aspirin that could be damaging to the stomach. This formulation utilizes a microporous membrane that does not dissolve in gastric fluid. As a result, this gastrointestinal delivery system stays intact in the stomach and will only release the encapsulated drug after it arrives in the intestine

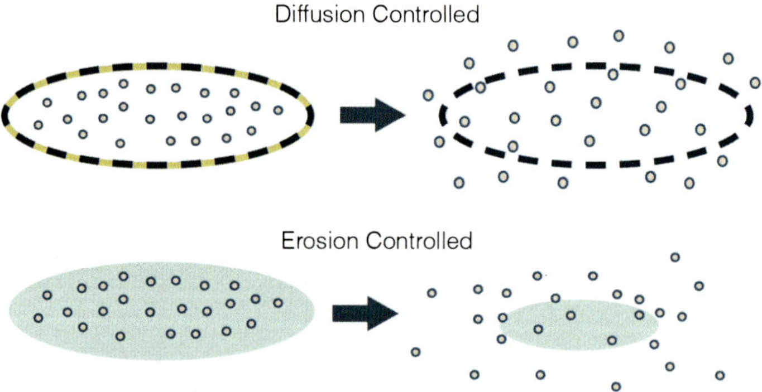

Fig. 10.6 Examples of two different mechanisms for controlled release in oral formulations. In the diffusion-controlled formulation (*upper panel*), rate of drug release depends on the porosity of the membrane, while in the erosion-controlled formulation (*lower panel*) rate of drug release depends on the breakdown of filler material

Table 10.2 Advantages and disadvantages of transdermal-controlled drug release systems

Advantages	Disadvantages
The system avoids the first-pass problem in which the drug is metabolized by the liver before reaching its target	The patches may fall off the skin if the adhesive is too weak
The skin is the most extensive and readily accessible organ of the body through which an adequate amount of drug can be absorbed into the circulatory system	The system may cause skin irritation
Administration of the drug is simple and easy resulting in increased patient compliance	The system may not be able to deliver an adequate drug concentration into the bloodstream
The drug can be delivered to the patient continually, even overnight	
The delivery of the drug can be stopped immediately if need be, simply by removing the delivery system from the skin surface	

drug release rate by the dissolution rate of the polymeric materials. A number of other mechanisms for the oral administration route, including combined diffusion- and erosion-controlled release, osmotically controlled-release, and chemically controlled-release formulations, can also be used to affect drug release rate, increase drug stability, and lengthen transit time through the gastrointestinal tract.

10.6.2 Transdermal Controlled-Release Systems

Transdermal controlled-release systems, such as nicotine patches, are specifically designed to deliver a drug through intact skin layers into systemic circulation. As with all drug-delivery methods, there are both advantages and disadvantages to transdermal controlled-release systems (Table 10.2).

When designing a transdermal controlled-release system, variables such as the bioactivity of the drug, skin characteristics, drug formulation, adhesion, and system design must be taken into consideration. The skin of an adult in most locations on the body is only a few millimeters thick, has a total surface area of approximately 2 m^2, and receives one-third of all circulating blood in the body (Fig. 10.7). It serves as a shield to protect the body from physical, chemical, and microbial attacks. The skin has three layers: the epidermis, the dermis, and subcutaneous fat tissue. The epidermal layer is the outmost layer of the skin which is in direct contact with the outside environment and is composed of stratified squamous epithelial cells. The stratum corneum is the outermost component in this layer and consists of many layers of compacted, flattened, dehydrated, keratinized cells in stratified sections. The epidermis, which serves as a barrier to percutaneous absorption, is considered to provide the rate-limiting step in the drug adsorption process. The thickness of the epidermal layer varies according to the extent of skin surface abrasion and the load applied to the skin. The dermis is composed of a network of robust collagen fibers

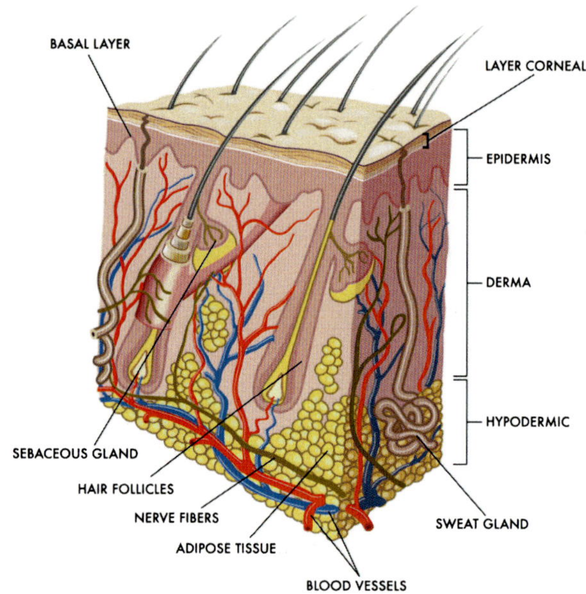

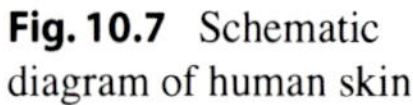
Fig. 10.7 Schematic diagram of human skin

and has a uniform thickness and contains blood vessels, lymphatics, and nerve endings. Beneath the dermis, there is a sheet of fat-containing tissue, which attaches the dermis to the underlying structures.

In general, only small, lipophilic, low-dose drugs can diffuse across intact skin. Transdermal transport of drugs is thought to be through two pathways: first, across the stratum corneum intracellularly and intercellularly and second, via the hair follicles and sweat glands. After passing through the epidermis, the drug is absorbed into the capillaries in the dermis, from which it enters systemic circulation, and is transported to the target tissue. One example of a transdermal drug-delivery system is the birth control patch for females, which usually delivers a combination of estradiol and progesterone into the systemic circulation. If taken orally, these drugs (especially estradiol) are converted to the less-active metabolite estrone by the first-pass mechanism when intestinal blood traverses the liver before entering the systemic circulation. Transdermal administration of these drugs protects estradiol from being degraded.

Several technologies have been developed to control the release rate of a drug by transdermal drug-delivery systems. The simplest design is a two-part system which includes a drug-impermeable backing laminate and a drug-containing adhesive. The drug-containing adhesive attaches directly to the skin, and the drug molecules permeated through the skin. The penetration rate of the drug through the stratum corneum is the rate-limiting step in this delivery system. In the so-called matrix dispersion drug-delivery system, the drug is mixed with a polymeric material that controls the release rate of the drug. In a polymer membrane permeation-controlled system, the drug reservoir is sandwiched between a drug-impermeable backing and a rate-controlling membrane, so that the drug release rate depends on the rate of the drug passing through the membrane. A transdermal microreservoir drug-delivery system is a combination of the reservoir and matrix dispersion drug-delivery systems. In this system, the drug reservoir is formed by homogeneously dispersing the drug suspension in a lipophilic (fat-loving) polymer to form thousands of unleachable microscopic spheres, which serve as drug reservoirs. An adhesive rim is then used to surround the medicated disc, and a drug-impermeable backing is attached to the outside of the disc. This approach stabilizes the unstable dispersion by cross-linking it with the polymer.

Second-generation transdermal drug-delivery systems utilize various chemical enhancers (e.g., ethanol) to increase skin permeability. In general, chemical enhancers effectively disrupt the highly ordered bilayer structures of the stratum corneum by creating nanometer-scale defects in the skin. This process then increases skin permeability, which provides an added driving force for drug transport across the skin by increasing the concentration gradient driving diffusion. A disadvantage of chemical enhancers is that they often increase skin irritation.

All the transdermal delivery systems mentioned above are based on passive diffusion of the drug through the stratum corneum layer. An alternate strategy, iontophoresis, uses an electric current to facilitate movement of charged drugs through the skin. In this method, two electrodes are connected to the delivery system, and the ionized drug penetrates through the skin along the voltage gradient, then diffusing through the capillary system to enter the systemic circulation. Iontophoresis can also be used to transport weakly charged and uncharged compounds across the skin by enhancing electroosmotic flow of water in the stratum corneum, but their transport is often inefficient. Compared to the passive transdermal controlled-release systems discussed above, iontophoresis allows for transport of higher molecular weight compounds across the skin with better controlled input kinetics (e.g., microprocess controlled) and minimum intersubject variability.

10.6.3 Implantable Controlled-Release Systems

Implantable therapeutic systems for long-term, continuous drug administration are controlled drug-delivery systems which can have much higher drug release rates when compared to transdermal controlled-release systems because the drug does not need to penetrate the skin [3]. In these systems, the drug-delivery device is implanted in the subcutaneous tissue, directly underneath the skin layers, so that the drug is directly released from the device into the subcutaneous tissue, entering its capillaries and the systemic circulation without encountering the high resistance to transport in the top layer of the skin. For example, in a membrane permeation-controlled drug-delivery system, the drug reservoir is encapsulated within a compartment, with a small opening covered by a rate-controlling polymeric membrane. The release rate of the drug is then dependent on the diffusion rate of the drug through the membrane. In an osmotic pressure-activated drug-delivery system, the liquid drug formulation is housed within an absorbent/

swellable hydrophilic layer laminate, which is contained in a shape-retaining housing. The drug-delivery orifice is opened to the outside, and as the laminate absorbs water from the body and swells, the drug solution is released at a controlled, constant rate under an osmotic pressure gradient.

10.6.4 Pulmonary Controlled-Release Systems

Pulmonary controlled release is another approach by which the hepato(liver)–gastrointestinal first-pass elimination associated with oral administration can be avoided. In this approach, the drug is delivered into the lungs by inhalation and then is absorbed through mucosal membranes into the systemic circulation. The large surface area of the mucosal membrane in the lungs allows for adequate drug to be delivered into the circulatory system. Adapting a drug for administration by a pulmonary controlled-release system provides a noninvasive route of administration for many drugs including many asthma and anti-allergy agents. These systems can also reduce dosing frequency, which improves patient compliance and convenience. Use of pulmonary delivery systems has been even extended to inhalable insulin, which was introduced in 2007 by Pfizer. However, this system was quickly removed from the market due to serious potential complications, including the increased incidence of lung cancer in patients using this therapy compared with the control population.

10.6.5 Parenteral Controlled-Release Systems

Parenteral administration of drugs involves piercing the skin or mucous membrane and includes intravenous (into a blood vessel such as a vein), subcutaneous (just under the skin surface), intramuscular (into a muscle), intraperitoneal (into the body cavity), and intrathecal (into the spinal canal) injections. Compared to transdermal and pulmonary routes, parenteral drug delivery has the advantage that the systemic bioavailability of a drug is not limited by its permeability across a barrier (e.g., the mucosal membrane or stratum corneum). Compared to the oral route, parenteral routes can avoid first-pass metabolism in the liver. Parenteral drug delivery via intramuscular or subcutaneous administration results in the formation of a drug depot at the injection site, which can serve as a drug reservoir that over time releases the drug into the systemic circulation through the surrounding capillary network. The delivery system can provide a prolonged release of the drug from the vehicle, which is dependent on the characteristics of the formulation. The rate of drug absorption is determined by the physicochemical characteristics of the drug and the interaction of the drug with vehicle and the tissue microenvironment. The advantages of this delivery system are that it reduces the needed drug dose, improves patient compliance, decreases side effects, and enhances drug utilization.

Hypodermic needles have been used for a long time to bypass the skin and deliver drugs such as insulin to muscular tissue, which serves as a depot for slow release of the drug. Alternatively, various types of needles can be used to directly access arteries or veins for injecting drugs, removing blood, and other procedures. In the intravenous injection route, a drug can easily and rapidly access the systemic circulation and reach the targeted site. Continuous intravenous infusion can deliver a drug with a constant and sustained therapeutic concentration for as long as required for effective treatment.

An obvious disadvantage of traditional hypodermic needles is the inherent discomfort they cause when piercing the patient's skin and the small amount of bleeding that may result from the injection. This problem, however, can be overcome with a new generation of polymeric biodegradable microneedles that are coated or impregnated with drugs. In one example of such a system, patches coated on one side with microscopic solid biodegradable needles painlessly punch a series of microscopic holes in the outer layer of skin, separate from the patch, and remain in the skin to release their payload while degrading, thereby facilitating transdermal delivery of a drug that normally cannot pass through the skin. Hollow microneedles can also be used for injection of drugs from a patch to the subcutaneous tissue. If these microneedles are less than 50 μm in length, in most cases they will not reach the nerve endings in the skin and will not cause pain.

10.7 Nanoparticles in Targeted Drug Delivery

Nanotechnology has been used for targeted drug delivery to improve the therapeutic efficacy and decrease the systemic toxicity of many conventional drugs. Carriers such as fluorescent or magnetic nanoparticles are also used to selectively deliver contrast agents for diagnostic imaging. A large number of intravascular drug carriers can be synthetized from naturally occurring (e.g., albumin) or synthetic compounds (dendrimers). However, these drug carriers should generally be small enough to be able to traverse the smallest capillaries in the body, which are a few micrometers in diameter. Therefore, the size of the intravascular drug carriers is usually in the nanometer to micrometer range (biodegradable natural polymers (<50 nm), micelles (50–100 nm), liposomes (50–1,000 nm), dendrimers (approximately 500 nm), and biodegradable synthetic polymers (tens of nanometers to few micrometers)). Even though intravascular drug carriers do not generally pass through barriers such as mucosal membranes or the stratum corneum, there are several mechanisms that may affect the half-life of intravascular drug carriers after they are injected into the bloodstream. For example, the reticuloendothelial system, which removes foreign substances from the body, tends to eliminate drug carriers from the body. Drug carriers may also be removed from the circulation by the liver, spleen, and lungs, in a size and surface chemistry-dependent manner. Inappropriate surface charges and/or surface hydrophobicity may also cause faster elimination of the drug carriers by interaction with other substances in the bloodstream. However, the surface chemistry of the drug carriers can be modified so that their elimination rate from the body can be significantly reduced.

A number of strategies are employed to target intravascular drug carriers to sites of disease and to control release of drug from the drug carrier to the diseased tissue.

In intravascular controlled-release drug-delivery systems, the systemic drug level can be controlled by the release rate of the drug from its carrier. Furthermore, adding environmental sensors (e.g., pH) allows the drug to be released only when the formulation reaches the target tissue where the environment is different than in normal tissue. For example, pH-sensitive formulations can be preferentially released in tumor tissue, where pH is often significantly lower than in normal tissue.

The surface and cytoplasmic proteins (ligands) of diseased cells are often different from those of normal cells. An antibody that can specifically bind to the surface ligands of the diseased cells in a lock-and-key fashion can be used as a site-targeting warhead. The site-targeting antibody is chemically linked to the surface of the delivery vehicle, which could then result in the accumulation of the drug carrier at the disease site by interaction of the antibody with its targeting ligands. If successful, this approach will result in preferential delivery of the drug to target tissue while keeping drug concentration in normal tissue at a very low level. Targeted drug delivery can reduce total drug dosage, improve patient compliance, decrease side effects, and enhance drug efficacy. These targeted drug-delivery systems range from preferential delivery of chemotherapeutic agents to tumors to direct delivery of drugs or genes to our DNA. In this section we will review several examples of nanocarriers that are currently used for targeted drug delivery.

10.7.1 Polymers

Both natural and chemically synthesized polymers are extensively used for developing nanoparticles for targeted drug delivery. Different polymer formulations have been designed to activate in a number of different ways. Polymers can simply degrade in physiologic fluid, they may respond to temperature changes (the difference between room temperature and the temperature of the body), and they may be designed to adhere to mucous membranes such as the eye or the gastrointestinal tract. Recently, a nanoparticle formulation of paclitaxel has been successfully applied clinically for the treatment of metastatic breast cancer. The carrier of this formulation is nontoxic, nonhemolytic, and non-immunogenic (does not cause a foreign body response in the body). If designed appropriately, polymeric nanoparticles may serve as a drug carrier which may specifically deliver the drug to tumor tissue or cells. Targeting molecules such as antibodies may be attached onto the surface of nanoparticles to improve the specificity to the targeted site. Polymeric nanoparticles can also be designed to control the release profile of the drug by adding properties such as positive charge or pH sensitivity.

10.7.2 Liposomes

Liposomes, discovered in the 1960s, are one of the most popular and well-investigated drug carriers [4]. Liposomes are spherical nanoparticles made of lipid (fatty molecule) bilayer membranes with an aqueous interior (Fig. 10.8). Liposomal

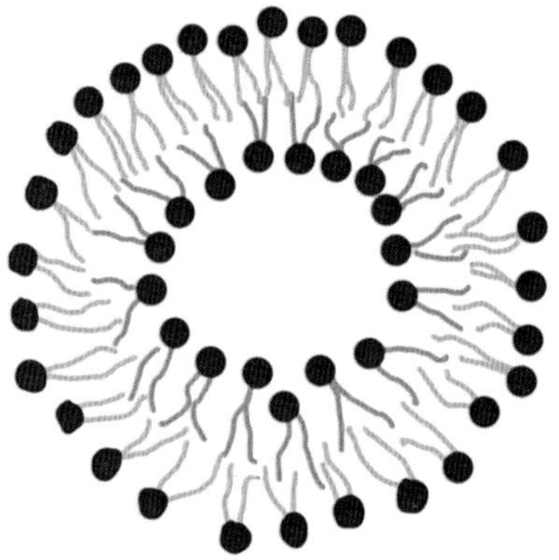

Fig. 10.8 Liposomes are spherical nanoparticles made of lipid bilayer membranes with an aqueous interior. In this illustration, the membrane is composed of two layers (a bilayer) of molecules called phospholipids. The molecules have a "head" that is hydrophilic and a "tail" that is hydrophobic. The tail ends spontaneously attract each other in the presence of water, and the result is a particle that has an empty volume interior suitable for carrying a drug

drug-delivery vehicles have been studied intensively in the past several decades because the biodistribution of therapeutic agents can be tailored for the needs of the targeted tissue. Drug carriers such as DOXIL, which is an FDA-approved liposomal formulation of doxorubicin (an anticancer drug), can effectively control the pharmacokinetics and biodistribution of the drug, in order to avoid or target specific tissues, thus achieving therapeutic enhancement via both toxicity reduction and/or efficacy enhancement. Drugs can be loaded either into the internal, trapped aqueous space (hydrophilic drugs) or between the lipid bilayer membranes (hydrophobic drugs). The grafting of molecules such as PEG (polyethylene glycol) on the liposome surface results in "stealth" liposomes which helps them evade the reticuloendothelial system (a part of the immune system that consists of cells that engulf foreign particulate matter) and have been shown to prolong circulation half-life. Antibodies or ligands can be conjugated to these long circulating liposomes to improve the specificity to the targeted tissue. Liposomes are not ideal drug carriers; just like any other drug-delivery technique, they have some drawbacks. Liposomes are not stable, and some encapsulated drugs may leak out of liposomes before the liposomes reach the diseased area.

10.7.3 Nanotubes

Nanotubes, usually made of carbon, have large internal volumes and external surfaces which allow more drugs or biomolecules to be loaded onto the nanotubes. Nanotubes can be either single-walled or multi-walled. The multi-walled nanotubes are useful as drug carriers since they have greater strength and stability. Drugs and biomolecules can be loaded either inside the nanotube, attached to the side of the nanotube wall, or trail behind the nanotube. Since nanotubes have the ability to carry DNA across a cell membrane, they are a very useful tool in gene therapy. Nanotubes have a very high optical absorbance in the near infrared (NIR) region, and this property allows them to be imaged using infrared fluorescence microscopy. Moreover, with continuous NIR irradiation, these nanotubes may be heated up, which could result in thermal destruction of cells if the nanotubes have been preferentially delivered into the diseased cells. The surface of the nanotube may be chemically modified to be hydrophilic and functionalized and linked to a wide variety of molecules such as antibodies, peptides, imaging agents, or therapeutic agents to facilitate the targeted delivery of anticancer agents to the cancer cells and enhance the endocytosis (incorporation into the cell) process. However, nanotubes are non-biodegradable, have a strong tendency to clump together, and may be toxic to humans.

10.7.4 Quantum Dots

Nanoparticle size quantum dots (QDs) have recently been established as a model for molecular, cellular, and in vivo imaging. QDs are nanocrystals of semiconductor material measuring approximately 1–10 nm, which can be made to fluoresce when stimulated by light. They are made of an aqueous organic coating over an inorganic shell, and beneath that is an inorganic core. QDs with a protective hydrophobic bilayer can be dispersed in aqueous solution and remain stable over long periods of time. They can be delivered into cells passively via endocytosis (the cell engulfs the QD) or actively by receptor-induced internalization. Targeting moieties (a part or a functioning group of a molecule), such as antibodies, oligonucleotides, or small-molecule ligands, can be linked to water-soluble QDs. QDs have also been studied as a delivery vehicle for cancer imaging and therapy by conjugating (linking) a QD with an anticancer drug such as doxorubicin. However, because of their chemical composition, which includes toxic heavy metals (e.g., Cd, Hg, Ph, As), using QDs in humans raises a number of safety issues. Compared to other drug vehicles, QDs have the advantage of fluorescence (they may be easily seen) and do not have to be modified to serve as imaging agents. However, QDs are solid particles, which means that drugs cannot be loaded inside them, but must be attached to the outside.

10.8 Commercially Available Drug-Delivery Systems

Devices that contain a reservoir of drug sealed in by a permeable membrane have been in use since the late 1970s and include the Ocusert™, which is inserted between the eye and the lower eyelid and releases a drug for controlling glaucoma, and a birth control device, the Norplant™ which releases levonorgestrel. A number of transdermal patch systems are available, including some that release testosterone (Testoderm™, Androderm™), estradiol (a female hormone used in hormone-replacement therapy and present in FemPatch™ and Vivelle™), nicotine (Nicoderm™), nitroglycerin (Deponit™ and Mitodisc™; used to treat the heart-related disease angina), and fentanyl (Duragesic™; used for relief of pain) [5]. Stents, which are implanted in partially occluded blood vessels, may be coated with drugs that prevent growth of smooth muscle cells that can cause a new blockage to form (Cypher™).

In osmotically controlled devices, the rate of drug release is controlled by how quickly water enters the device and then forces the drug out by osmotic pressure. An example of such a device is Oros™, which consists of a tablet covered with a water-permeable coating and small holes drilled into the tablet. Water entering the tablet eventually forces the medication out through the holes. A variety of different drugs may be used in this type of formulation.

Drugs that are dispersed with bioeroding or biodegrading polymers include synthetic suture materials such as poly(lactic acid) and poly(lactic-co-glycolic acid that are used in microsphere systems (Enantone LP™ and Lupron™; both for treating prostate cancer) and in systems where the drug is dispersed in a polymer strand (Zoladex™, used to dispense drugs treating breast or prostate cancer).

Clinically available liposomal delivery systems include vaccine formulations for Newcastle virus (a bird disease transmittable to humans), avian flu, hepatitis A, influenza, as well as the antileukemia chemotherapeutic medication daunorubicin (DaunoXome™) and severe fungal infections such as leishmaniasis and meningitis (amphotericin B) [6].

10.9 Summary

The development of new drugs usually follows new biological discoveries, because knowing how and why a disease progresses provides an insight into possible methods to cure it. For example, if it is known that a particular cancer metastasizes when a specific protein is synthesized, then interfering with that protein's synthesis using a drug will, in principle, prevent metastasis. Because of the increasing rate at which new biological discoveries are being made, it is likely that new drug development will also accelerate. New drugs are often powerful because they target difficult diseases (the "easy" diseases have been cured). It is simply a good strategy to ensure that the drugs will be delivered to the diseased tissue and that their release rate is calibrated to remain above the minimally effective level but below the toxicity level.

10.10 Foundation Concepts

- Most drugs are administered systemically (they travel through the entire human system), and it is therefore necessary to deliver high doses that often cause unwanted side effects. Targeting diseased tissues with "smart" delivery systems will ensure a higher dose at the diseased site and avoid most side effects.
- The goals of targeted drug delivery are to maintain a constant and effective level of the drug, deliver the drug locally at the correct location, and protect the drug from premature degradation or elimination by the body.

- Drugs disperse through tissue by diffusion, a process that is modeled by Fick's first law of diffusion, and the speed with which a drug diffuses is proportional to the concentration gradient.
- There are advantages and disadvantages to targeted drug-delivery systems, listed in Table 10.1; the advantages and disadvantages of transdermal delivery systems are listed in Table 10.2. Pharmacodynamics refers to the physiologic effects of a drug, while pharmacokinetics refers to the time course for drug absorption, metabolism, and excretion.
- Drugs can be administered through various routes, including oral, sublingual, mucosal, nasal, pulmonary, ocular, transdermal, vaginal, rectal, intrauterine, and parenteral (subcutaneous, intramuscular, intraperitoneal, intrathecal, or intraventricular injections).
- Orally administered drugs must be protected from changes in pH as the drug moves through the gastrointestinal system and from premature clearance by the liver.
- Only small lipophilic (fat molecule-friendly) low-dose drugs can diffuse through the skin, and chemical enhancers such as ethanol to increase skin permeability are sometimes used in transdermal delivery systems.
- Nanoparticles can be modified to become fluorescent or magnetic and are made from polymers, liposomes, and nanotubes. Their small size makes it possible for them to travel in the smallest capillaries and reach all vascularized tissues. Nanoparticles and some other drug carriers may be functionalized with antibodies that can target specific tissue types, thereby delivering the drug to the diseased site.

References

1. Langer, R. (2003). Where a pill won't reach. *Scientific American, 288*, 50–57.
2. Langer, R. (1998). Drug delivery and targeting. *Nature, 392*(Suppl), 5–10.
3. Langer, R. (1990). New methods of drug delivery. *Science, 249*, 1527–1533.
4. Torchilin, V. (2005). Recent advances with liposomes as pharmaceutical carriers. *Nature Reviews in Drug Discovery, 4*, 145–160.
5. Ratner, B.D., Hoffman, A.S., Schoen, F.J. & Lemons, J.E. et al. (Eds.). (2004). Drug delivery systems. In *Biomaterials science: An introduction to materials in medicine*. Elsevier: San Diego.
6. Gregoriadis, G. (Ed.). (2007). Liposome Technology 3rd edition, volumes I-III. Informa Healthcare: New York.

Tissue Engineering: Growing Replacement Human Tissue in the Lab

11

"Human bones grown from fat in laboratory."

Headline in Daily Telegraph (UK), June 10, 2011

In the last few chapters, we have discussed the state-of-the-art treatments for replacing missing or diseased tissues and organs. For the most part, synthetic or processed natural materials are used to design implants, etc. None of the treatments resemble or approach the sophistication of the body's own original tissue. Over the past two decades or so, scientists and engineers have begun to create tissues and organs in the laboratory, with the aim of eventually using those constructs for treatment of disease. Although simple tissues like skin substitutes are already available, more complex tissues and organs are still under development. Nevertheless, this field of tissue engineering or regenerative medicine holds the promise of someday being capable of producing body parts which will be fully integrated into the patient's body and alleviate the shortage of transplantable organs.

11.1 Introduction

How about that for an attention-grabbing headline? It serves both as an example of the tendency of the popular press to sensationalize scientific discoveries and the genuine excitement surrounding the field of tissue engineering. In its May 22, 2000, issue, Time magazine listed "tissue engineer" as the number 1 hottest job option in the twenty-first century; even the name sounds as if it could be an occupation found in science-fiction movie scripts.

Where did all that buzz come from? The term "tissue engineering" is reported to have first been introduced in 1987 by members of a scientific review panel convened by the US National Science Foundation (NSF). Y.C. Fung, a research scientist, suggested the name to identify research proposals that sought to grow tissue in the

G.R. Baran et al., *Healthcare and Biomedical Technology in the 21st Century: An Introduction for Non-Science Majors*, DOI 10.1007/978-1-4614-8541-4_11,

laboratory rather than on or in a live host. Subsequently, it was suggested that the name "tissue engineering should be applied to a new inter-disciplinary initiative which has the goal of growing tissues or organs directly from a single cell taken from an individual." Although it was recognized even then that it would be more practical to use many cells (not a single cell) and that the "individual" could be an animal or human, the definition did convey the potential power of the new technology. It was also important that from the very outset, tissue engineering was perceived to be an interdisciplinary effort, needing the coordinated efforts of physicians, chemical engineers, materials engineers, and biologists to make progress. In fact, most research programs that focus on tissue-engineered technology include large teams of scientists and engineers, because the specialized knowledge of many individuals with different backgrounds is needed. One of the first publications in this area that piqued the interest of many scientists in tissue engineering was coauthored by a chemical engineer and a surgeon [1].

Expanding a bit on the original definition, we can say that tissue engineering is the process of exploiting living cells to regenerate diseased or lost tissues inside a patient's body or to grow tissue structures outside the body in special laboratory facilities on a large scale. The tissue structures that are grown outside the body can eventually be used for a variety of purposes including replacing diseased tissues, diagnostics, or drug discovery. In 1998, a new term was coined when a paper was published reporting the ability to successfully grow embryonic stem cells in the laboratory. This new term, "regenerative medicine," refers to reestablish the structure and function of tissue and organs, in contrast to repair of damaged tissue.

The significance of being able to grow useful tissues (and eventually organs) should be obvious now that we have discussed a variety of synthetic implants and the complex devices that are needed to maintain a patient with a failing heart or with kidney failure. In the USA it was estimated that approximately 27,000 people died in 2009 from liver disease,120,000 died in 2010 from kidney failure, and 597,000 died in 2010 from heart disease [2, 3]. It is not known how many of these patients could have been saved if it had been possible to replace their failing organs, but certainly the majority of these individuals would have had their lives prolonged.

During the past two decades, significant advances have been made in the field of synthetic materials; however, many of these materials deteriorate in the body, do not self-heal, and cannot remodel (adjust their size or function in response to demand as natural tissues can). And while it is true that future therapeutic approaches such as genetic engineering hold great promise for improved therapies, there are still serious social and ethical issues that have yet to be overcome to make these technologies widely available. Now, just imagine if it were possible to grow heart tissue in the lab that would replace damaged heart tissue by implantation or if a new kidney could be grown in the lab and replace a failing one! Admittedly, the field of tissue engineering is not yet advanced enough to accomplish these goals, and in the present economic conditions, it is not clear if governments and the private sector have the will and the means to provide the large research budgets needed to move the field forward. The demand is certainly there: in the USA alone at the turn of the century, there were 58 million heart patients, 16 million diabetics, 10 million with osteoporosis, 5.5 million diagnosed with Parkinson's disease, 300,000 severe burn victims, and 250,000 spinal cord injury patients that could be helped if tissue engineering technology achieves its full potential [4].

11.2 The History of Tissue Engineering

Humans have been fascinated with the idea of tissue regeneration for a long time. In classical Greek mythology, Prometheus, after stealing the secret of fire and introducing it to humans, was chained to a mountain peak and punished by Zeus who sent an eagle to feast daily on his liver. Prometheus' liver regenerated overnight, and his torture resumed the next morning. Numerous observations about the regenerative potential of limbs, claws, liver, and antlers have also been recorded in the ancient literature. For example, Aristotle (384–322 BC) observed that salamanders could regrow amputated parts. In 1740 Abraham Trembley created a nine-headed hydra (a small, few millimeter-long animal that lives in freshwater ponds and streams). Rudolf Virchow (1821–1902), a pathologist who studied the cell, confirmed that tissue regeneration is dependent on cell proliferation.

Progress in biology and tissue engineering is only possible because of the important advances in knowledge that occurred in the past. Until the mid-seventeenth century, scientists were unaware that cells even existed. Only after the microscope was invented in the 1600s was Robert Hooke able to actually see cells. In 1838, the German botanist Matthias Jakob Schleiden and the German zoologist Theodor Schwann proposed the cell theory which eventually gave rise to modern biology.

The Cell Theory:

- All living organisms are composed of one or more cells.
- The cell is the basic unit of structure, function, and organization in all organisms.
- All cells come from preexisting, living cells.

The ability to grow mammalian animal cells in test tubes, developed in the early nineteenth century, was another major step that has made tissue engineering possible. Other significant advances included the discovery of antibiotics (to inhibit bacterial growth) and learning how to maintain a sterile environment. In the 1930s, Carrel and Lindberg invented a system that could maintain adult tissues (including the heart) alive for several weeks. Growth factors, chemicals that made possible the continuing survival of adult cells in laboratory glassware, were discovered in the 1960s. And inventions in fields outside medicine have also played a key role in the advancement of tissue engineering. For example, growing cells in test tubes or plastic containers requires a constant temperature of 37 °C, which would not have been possible to achieve on a large scale without advances in the fields of electrical and mechanical engineering.

11.3 Basic Concepts of Tissue Engineering

11.3.1 Cells and Cell Culture

The essential components of tissue engineering include a population of cells, a scaffold, growth factors that signal cells to proliferate and differentiate, and in some instances, a bioreactor (Fig. 11.1).

To understand the tissue engineering approach to therapy, we need to appreciate how living organisms are assembled and how they function. Cells are the basic building blocks of life. They produce, build, maintain, and repair substances such as the extracellular matrix (ECM) that make up the bulk of tissues and organs. Examples of different types of cells are listed in Table 11.1 and their shapes are illustrated in Fig. 11.2. Tissue (e.g., muscle, skin) is a collection of specialized cells; organs are made of several different types of tissue and have a specific function within the body. For example, the heart (an organ) is made up of muscle, ligaments, nerves, and blood vessels (all different tissues).

Diseases often begin with cell malfunction. Examples include arthritis or diabetes, which can be triggered by the body's immune system mistakenly attacking its own cells. Cancer results from the unchecked growth of cells that have genetically mutated and become immortal. Tissue or organ damage can also occur when cells

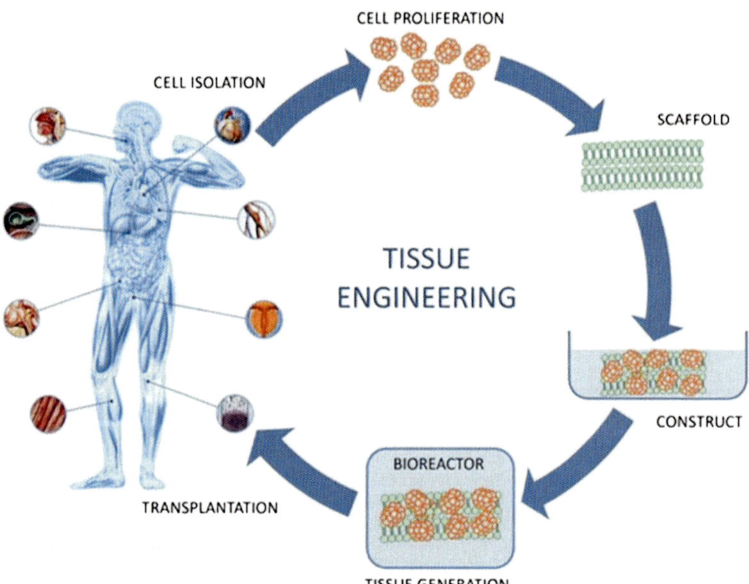

Fig. 11.1 A diagram of the tissue engineering process. It begins with identifying and isolating a group of cells that is separated and grown in the laboratory under conditions that enable the cells to replicate and expand their population. The cells are eventually placed or seeded onto a scaffold and placed in a reactor where they continue to proliferate. Eventually, the scaffold is transplanted back into a patient's body. Copyright Springer Verlag

Table 11.1 Tissue is composed of specialized cell types

Native cell type	Tissue
Chondrocytes	Cartilage
Red blood cells	Blood
Osteoblasts	Bone
Osteoclasts	Bone
Keratinocytes	Epidermis (skin)
Endothelial cells	These line the entire circulatory system, from the heart to the smallest capillary
Hepatocytes	Liver
Beta cells	Pancreatic cells called islets of Langerhans that produce insulin
Mesenchymal stem cells	Present in almost every tissue

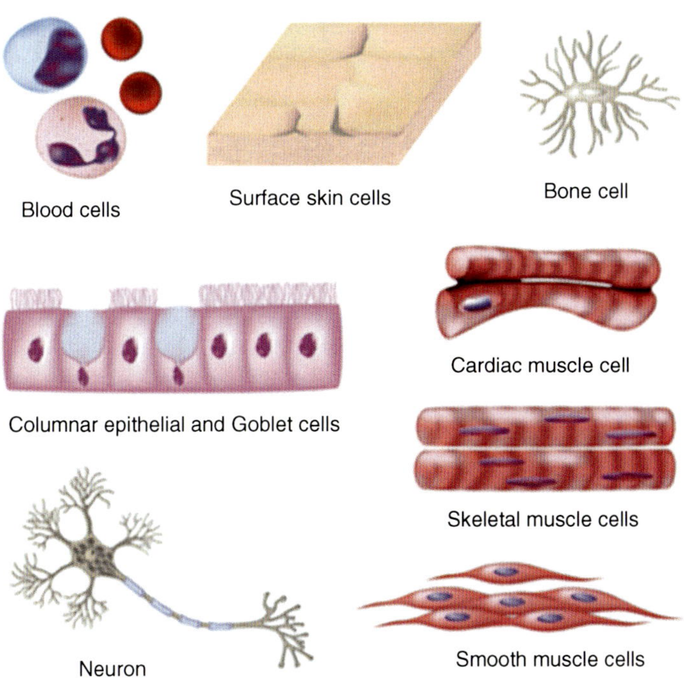

Fig. 11.2 Illustration of different types of human cells

in a particular tissue or organ begin to die; for example, Alzheimer's disease is due in part to the death of brain cells. Other reasons for major tissue or organ damage include physical trauma or burns.

In many cases, the dead or diseased cells or tissues can theoretically be replaced by healthy cells taken from the patient or from other human donors. These transplanted cells can be integrated in the patient's body and resume producing the proteins required for the proper functioning of the diseased tissue. In some situations, it is difficult to

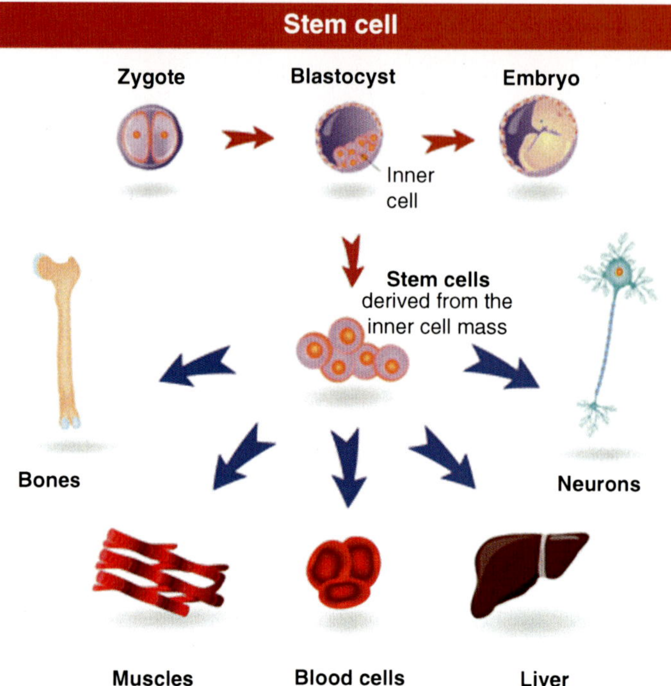

Fig. 11.3 The source of embryonic stem cells and the potential of such cells to differentiate into various types of tissue

obtain and grow differentiated (specialized) cells such as nerve or beta (pancreatic) cells in a test tube. However, it may be feasible to grow stem cells and then coax them into becoming nerve or beta cells. Stem cells, which are undifferentiated or nonspecialized, have the ability to develop into many different types of mature cells (Fig. 11.3).

Stem cells can also be isolated from many adult tissues, including the brain and the fat left over from liposuction procedures, umbilical cord blood, or the pulp under baby teeth. However, the most common source of adult stem cells is the bone marrow. The other source of stem cells is the embryo. Embryonic stem cells are generally more potent than adult stem cells and can transform into any kind of tissue. Currently, embryonic stem cells are usually obtained from stored embryos created as part of in vitro fertilization (IVF) procedures for infertile couples.

At the present time, there are several ways in which tissue engineering is foreseen to provide therapeutic benefits. The first is to grow human tissue outside the body, in vitro (in glassware, as shown in Fig. 11.4), and in a well-controlled environment in a process called "cell culture" and eventually implant that tissue to replace diseased or missing tissue in the body. The cells taken from the primary source (an animal or a human) are carefully isolated from other components, such as fat, blood, and skin cells, placed in sterile containers, and encouraged to grow and replicate (proliferate). They are monitored from time to time to see if they are healthy.

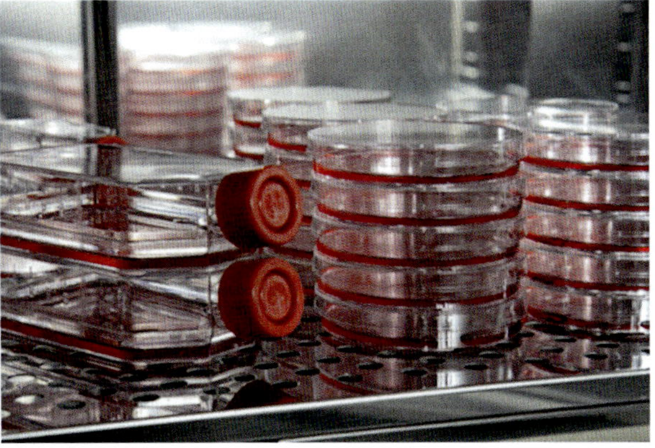

Fig. 11.4 Millions of cells are dispersed in the pink-colored tissue culture fluid, which also contains nutrients for the cells. The flasks containing the cells are stored in incubators such as the one depicted above

The laboratory or facility where this is done houses incubators (devices that maintain a desired temperature, usually 37 °C, and a humid atmosphere rich in carbon dioxide). You would think that the atmosphere should be oxygen rich; after all, don't humans need oxygen to survive? However, although the oxygen content in the earth's atmosphere is 21 %, the oxygen content in the body is between 1 and 12 %. It turns out that human tissue cells do better (live longer, grow faster, and show less stress) when they are cultured in an environment that is more like that of the body, i.e., lower in oxygen than the atmosphere. The laboratory or facility will also contain liquid nitrogen freezers that maintain a temperature of −196 °C and store cells in a state of "cryopreservation." Cells stored this way do not die; all their biological processes stop, and they can be brought back to normal function when they are thawed. Why don't the frozen cells die? It's because the freezing process is carefully controlled and is done slowly enough, so the cell is dehydrated before ice crystals can form inside the cell and cause damage to organelles or rupture the cell membrane.

Additional equipment found in a tissue culture facility includes liquid nitrogen storage rooms, microscopes (to observe the cells for signs they are growing normally), and storage for chemicals and for the containers where the cells "live." Cells also need "media" or a source of nutrients. You may have grown bacteria in a Petri dish where the bacteria were grown on an agar gel substrate. Tissue cells are grown in a liquid media, because they require not only nutrients, but also other substances such as hormones and growth factors (chemicals that encourage growth). Tissue cells grown in liquid media usually adhere to the bottom of the container in which they are grown, and the media is replaced when the nutrients are exhausted. Cells are normally cultured in sterilized plastic containers in special hoods that maintain a "laminar flow" (the air mixture inside the hood flows in such a way that prevents outside air from entering the space where the cells are being cultured). Of course, transfer equipment and supplies such as pipettes are needed to move the cells from one container to another (Fig. 11.5).

After the cells have occupied all available space on the bottom of the container (reached "confluence"), this primary cell culture is subdivided, and a portion of

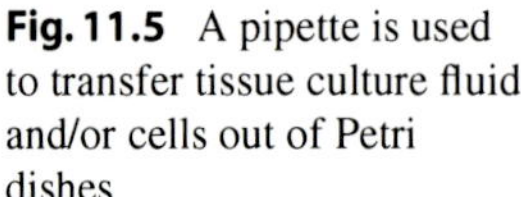

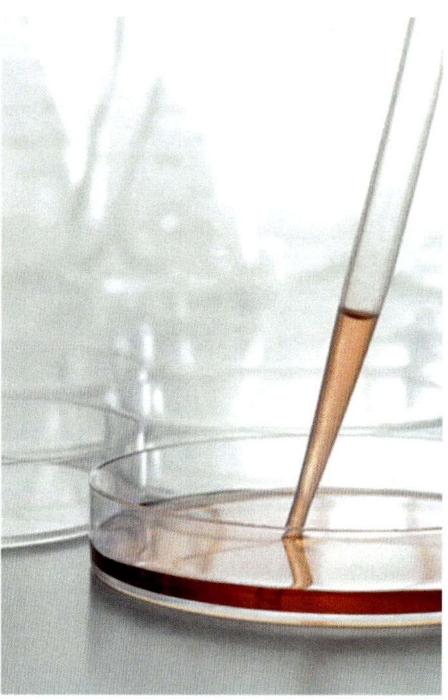

Fig. 11.5 A pipette is used to transfer tissue culture fluid and/or cells out of Petri dishes

the cells is transferred to other containers ("passaged") where the process of proliferation continues and further passages eventually become necessary. The advantage of this method is that only the "strongest" individual cells survive each passage, so those that are left become members of what is called a "cell line" and are eventually either used or placed in cryogenic storage. This cell culture process is one way in which cells for a tissue can be grown and maintained. Eventually, some may be taken for use in seeding a "scaffold" and making a tissue replacement such as human skin, but more on that later.

It should be noted that this list constitutes the bare necessities for a tissue culture facility; in reality, most laboratories will have cell sorters, pumps, pH meters, and centrifuges. Also, certain cells may require additional special handling to ensure the safety of those who work in the tissue culture lab.

A second way in which tissue engineering can provide a therapeutic benefit is to culture cells on a structure (called a "scaffold") having a shape and size suited for the damaged or missing tissue it is intended to replace, and when an adequate amount of tissue has formed, implant construct into the patient's body. After implantation, the entire construct enables the cells it contains to continue proliferating inside the body and keeps them together. A variation of this approach is to make devices that remain outside the body and contain cells that perform some specific function, for example, an artificial liver.

The third way that tissue engineering can provide a benefit is to begin by implanting a "place holder" kind of construct, which does not contain any cells, but instead

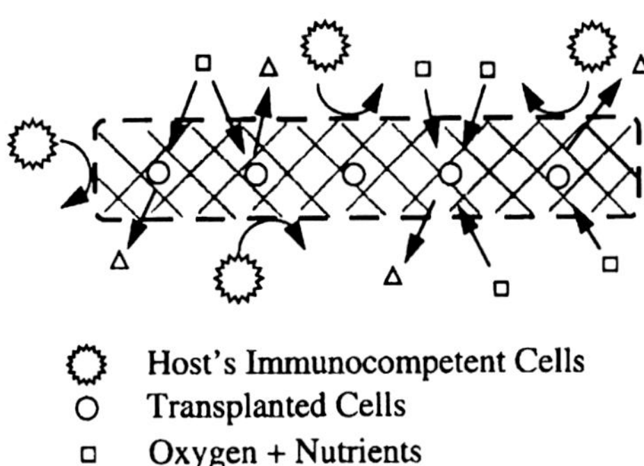

Fig. 11.6 Diagram of the strategy behind immunoisolation. The transplanted cells receive oxygen and nutrients through the polymer membrane but are kept from communicating with the cells of the host's immune system. Copyright Humana Press

maintains space and provides some mechanical support to neighboring tissue. The cells of the tissue where the device has been implanted are induced to proliferate and expand. The scaffold often has growth factors (signaling molecules such as drugs or proteins that stimulate the recruitment and growth of natural cells to the site) attached to its surface. Biodegradable materials such as polylactic acid are often used to make scaffolds.

We discussed transplants briefly in Chap. 5 and learned that they may be autogeneic or autologous (the patient's own tissue), allogeneic (tissue from a human other than the patient), and xenogeneic (tissue from a species other than human). For purposes of tissue engineering, autologous cells are preferred, because the patient will not need immunosuppressive therapy when implanted with a device containing living cells. On the other hand, it may be difficult to obtain sufficient numbers of these cells; for example, a patient who has had a heart attack is not likely to be in a condition to donate heart cells. It is also possible to use allogeneic cells called mesenchymal stem cells (adult stem cells found in bone marrow, cord blood, peripheral blood, fallopian tubes, and fetal liver and lung) in applications such as tissue-engineered skin; because this product is used to treat severe burn victims, there is often not enough natural skin remaining and inadequate time to proliferate the patient's own cells. If the cells are to be used for delivery of cell-synthesized molecules, rather than for production of tissue, it is possible to utilize allogeneic cells if they are immunoisolated (Fig. 11.6) [5].

This approach has been pursued while designing an "artificial pancreas" in the treatment of diabetic patients. If the host immune system reacts to interactions with the foreign cells, then an obvious strategy to prevent a foreign body response is to physically prevent that interaction. Accordingly, allogeneic islet cells are encapsulated in a semipermeable polymer membrane, which prevents them from encountering the host cells but still allows cell products (e.g., insulin) to diffuse out of the encapsulated cells and through the membrane. A number of different polymers including cellulose acetate, polytetrafluoroethylene, and alginate may be used as encapsulating films. This technology has shown promise, and a company called "TheraCyte" is seeking to exploit this approach.

Cells used for tissue engineering can also differ in their degree of differentiation (specialization). While skin cells, hepatocytes (liver cells), muscle, and bone cells are fully differentiated, embryonic and adult stem cells have the potential to differentiate and become various types of tissues. Embryonic stem cells are more "powerful" than the adult stem cells, but if they are sourced from a fertilized embryo, they will be allogeneic when used in a patient in a tissue engineering approach. Adult hematopoietic stem cells (HSCs) are found in the bone marrow and can differentiate into various blood cell types (red and white blood cells), osteoclasts (cells that break down bone), and specialized immune system cells, while adult mesenchymal stem cells (MSCs) can differentiate into tissue cells such as osteocytes (bone precursors), chondrocytes (cartilage cells), adipocytes (fat cells), and myocytes (muscle cells). Recently, the development of induced pluripotent stem cells (iSCs) has been reported, which are adult cells that are forced to become like embryonic stem cells, and this discovery could add to the repertoire of cells available for tissue engineering purposes. MSCs are exciting to bioengineers because they can be potentially useful in regenerating most of the tissues that most often require repair or replacement, such as bone, muscle, and skin (not fat!). If stem cells are to be used, then the tissue-engineered construct (device) must include appropriate growth factors and other substances called "cytokines" that stimulate differentiation into specific types of tissue. A practical difficulty with using MSCs is that it is practically impossible to harvest an adequate number of such cells from a patient; instead, the cells that are harvested must have their population expanded in tissue culture. Not only does this require additional time, but some cells differentiate, then undifferentiate in culture, and there is some concern that because the media used to culture these cells contain fetal calf serum, eventual immune system activation could occur.

11.3.2 Tissue Engineering Scaffolds

If tissue engineering is being utilized to replace missing tissue, a structural framework or scaffold is eventually needed to support proliferating and differentiating cells. The scaffold is often designed and constructed to resemble the tissue or organ it will replace (Fig. 11.7). Once it is implanted, the scaffold needs to possess sufficient structural stability to resist forces that might dislodge it.

The requirements for a scaffold material begin with biocompatibility. Not only must the scaffold not cause a toxic reaction or provoke an immune response from the host, but the cells that adhere to the scaffold must function normally, be capable of producing the tissue that is needed, and continue to proliferate. The products of degradation cannot be toxic themselves and must be readily disposed of by the normal excretory mechanisms. Scaffolds have mechanical property requirements that differ depending on the location where they are implanted. For example, a scaffold intended for tissue engineering of bone will need to withstand the normal forces that bone experiences, that is not to say that scaffolds are placed in areas experiencing high stresses. However, tissue-engineered constructs for cartilage are intentionally subjected to stress, because the cartilage cells (chondrocytes) require mechanical

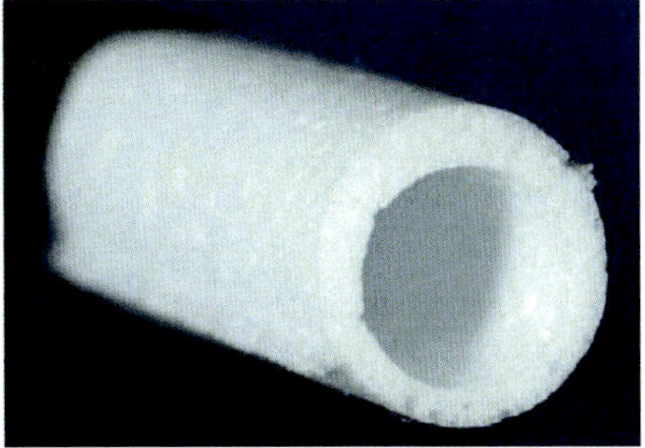

Fig. 11.7 A biodegradable scaffold intended for tissue engineering of blood vessels. Copyright Springer Science + Business Media, LLC

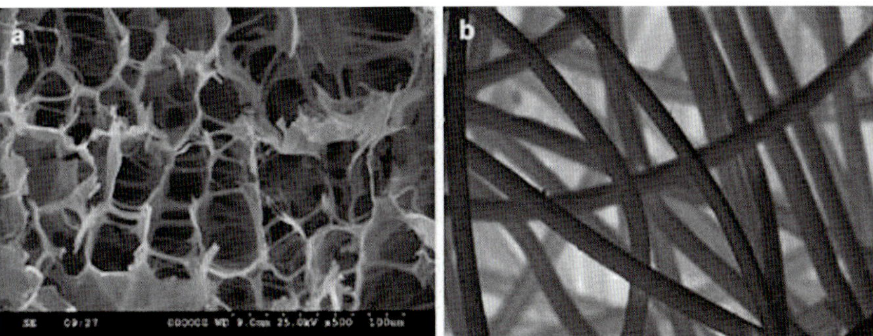

Fig. 11.8 Images of two tissue engineering scaffolds. On the *left* is a porous collagen scaffold; on the *right* is a fibrous hyaluronic acid scaffold. Copyright Springer Medizin Verlag

stimulation to retain phenotype (their characteristics as cartilage). All scaffolds must be robust enough to withstand handling by the surgeon as well as any alterations to their size and shape which may be needed at the surgical site.

There is a wide variety of materials and microstructures used in the design of scaffolds (Fig. 11.8). Because they are intended to be eventually replaced by natural tissues, bioresorbable scaffold materials are often preferred. We have discussed bioresorbable polymers in Chap. 5, but to briefly review these again, the synthetic polymers include polylactide (PLA), polyglycolide (PGA), polylactide-co-glycolide (PLGA), and poly-3-hydroxybutyrate, lactide-ε-caprolactone, among others. The degradation or dissolution of these materials is dependent on the pH of the environment, and the degradation products are lactic and glycolic acid. Both are normal products of muscle metabolism and pose no special challenges to the human body.

The degradation rates of scaffolds must be closely matched to the growth rate of the invading natural tissue. Glycolide and lactide–glycolide polymers degrade quickly, losing half of their tensile strength within 2 weeks; lactide polymers, on the other hand, degrade slowly, taking 3–6 years for the resorption process to be completed [6].

Naturally occurring polymers can also be used as scaffold materials, and these include collagen (obtained from cows), polyhyaluronic acid (derived from rooster

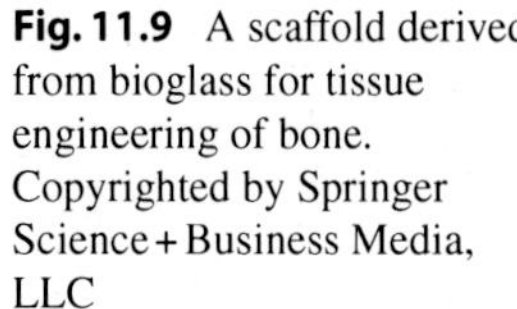

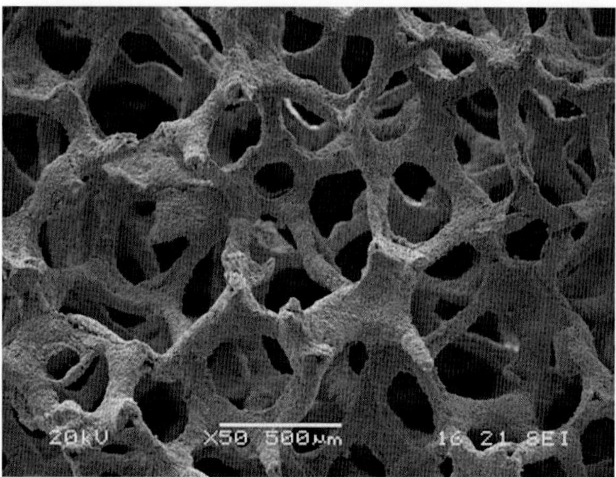

Fig. 11.9 A scaffold derived from bioglass for tissue engineering of bone. Copyrighted by Springer Science+Business Media, LLC

combs), chitin (derived from shellfish), gelatin, and alginate (derived from the cell walls of brown algae). With the exception of chitin, these materials have low mechanical strengths, and even chitin needs reinforcement with inorganic additives.

Inorganic scaffold materials based on calcium and phosphorus containing compounds such as human or bovine bone (with all organic content removed), calcium phosphates, and hydroxyapatites are sometimes used as tissue engineering scaffolds for bone applications (Fig. 11.9). The calcium phosphates are brittle, as are all ceramic materials, and may be reinforced with polymers for added toughness.

All scaffolds must be fabricated with a high degree of porosity, usually greater than 95 %. After all, when cells are being seeded onto the scaffold, they must be able to penetrate throughout the entire construct. The porosity must also be interconnected, not isolated. The differences in the two types of porosity are illustrated by soap and sponges; soap forms bubbles which enclose isolated pores; in contrast, the pores in sponges are interconnected. Interconnected pores are needed in scaffolds because nutrient-containing media must be allowed to circulate freely in a tissue-engineered construct. The pores must also be large enough to permit ingrowth of blood vessels; the cells will eventually rely on blood-borne delivery of oxygen and nutrients and extraction of metabolic wastes to survive. Oxygen supply is a critical factor, because cells in the body should be close enough to a blood vessel to obtain oxygen by diffusion. Most cells will tolerate a distance of slightly less than 200 μm from a blood vessel, but cells with higher metabolic rates such as islet cells require shorter distances on the order of 100 μm, while cartilage cells can maintain viability at a distance of 1 mm [7].

A balance must be struck between the degree of porosity and pore size in a scaffold. The greater the amount of porosity, the lower the mechanical strength of the scaffold, but the greater the availability of space for blood vessels and surface area for cells to adhere. The larger the pore size, the greater the availability of space for blood vessels, but the lower the pore surface area for cell adhesion.

Because there are many scaffold materials available, all with different processing needs, there are also many scaffold processing techniques that produce

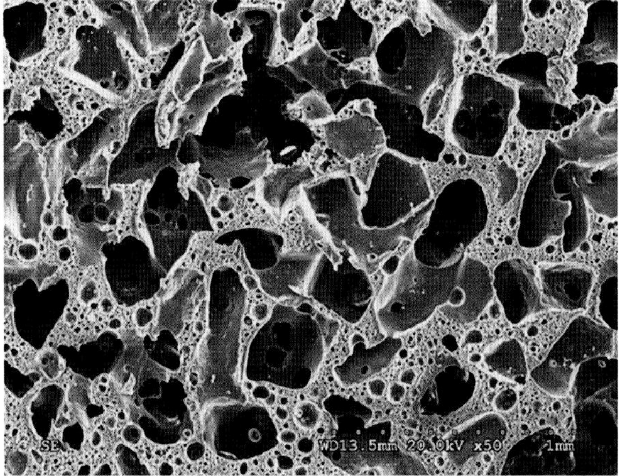

Fig. 11.10 A porous scaffold for tissue engineering made using a modified salt-leaching technique. Copyright Springer Science + Business Media, LLC

interconnected porosity. Fibers of synthetic biodegradable polymers such as PGA can be loosely assembled together and fused at contact points. Another method consists of dissolving PLA in an organic solvent such as methylene chloride and pouring the solution over a loose mesh of PGA fibers. The solvent does not attack the PGA; after the solvent has evaporated, the "composite" is heated slightly above the melting temperature of PGA, at which time the PGA fibers fuse together wherever they touch each other. After cooling, the composite is once again immersed in methylene chloride, which dissolves the PLA, leaving behind a mesh of PGA [8]. This technique unfortunately does not permit tight control of pore size and degree of porosity.

Another means of preparing porous structures is called the solvent casting and particulate leaching method. The protocol consists of first isolating sodium chloride (table salt) crystals of 300–500 μm in size; these particles will serve as a "porogen," or the substance that induces porosity. Then, the salt is dispersed in a PLA–chloroform solution, and the chloroform is allowed to evaporate, with any residual solvent being eliminated by using a vacuum. The dried construct is subsequently immersed in water, and the salt crystals dissolve, leaving behind pores (Fig. 11.10). The ratio of salt to solution determines the degree of porosity in the scaffold, and the size of the initial salt crystals determines the pore size. This casting/leaching technique cannot be used to produce thick constructs, and it is also necessary to ensure complete removal of the organic solvents, because these can have toxic effects on cells.

Both methods using PLA and PGA yield hydrophobic scaffolds, and cells dispersed in an aqueous medium sometimes will not distribute themselves evenly when they attempt to infiltrate the scaffold. To avoid this problem, the interior pores may be coated with polyvinyl alcohol or presoaked in ethanol then water.

A gas-foaming method wherein carbon dioxide is forced into a disc of polymer over a period of several days has also been employed to create porosity. When the polymer disc is withdrawn from the high-pressure chamber, the gas inside the polymer expands, forming bubbles (pores). Another technique often used for scaffold fabrication when a specific shape is desired involves dispersing a dissolved polymer

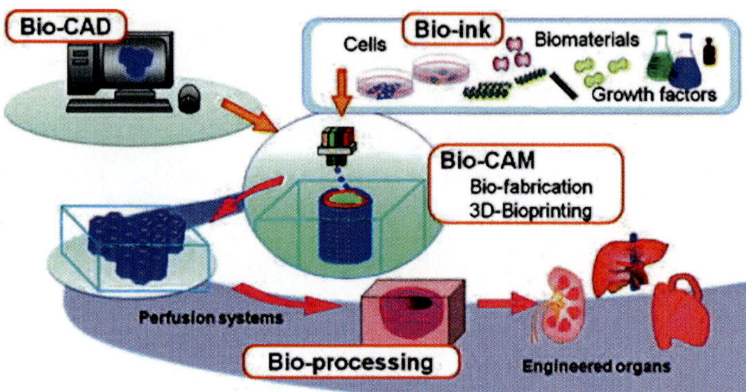

Fig. 11.11 Schematic of rapid prototyping equipment. A computer and software are used to control the "printing" of the "bio-ink" (the cells and growth factors and sometimes the biomaterials used for scaffolds) into a bioreactor where the cells replicate themselves and eventually occupy the scaffold. Subsequent processing may result in a tissue-engineered organ. Copyright Springer Science + Business Media, LLC

in water and stirring rapidly to form an emulsion which is poured into a mold and frozen using liquid nitrogen. When a vacuum is applied, the water and solvent vaporize, leaving behind a porous polymer in the shape of the mold.

Many of the methods described here result in constructs that are not large, because their size is limited by the distance a solvent has to diffuse in order to leach out the porogen. Also, control of pore size and pore distribution is not easily achieved. An alternative method called "rapid prototyping" can produce three-dimensional objects of virtually any size and dimension, with good control of pore size and pore distribution.

Rapid prototyping is achieved using a laser to sinter polymer or metal particles. The particles are placed on a platform, and the laser is scanned across the surface, being activated in response to a signal from a computer and sintering the particles only when it is activated. After one scan across the surface of the powder, the platform is slightly lowered and additional powder added onto the surface that has already been scanned, and the loose particle surface is smoothed. The laser then again scans across the surface and again sinters particles when it is activated. This sequence of events is repeated many (hundreds) times, and eventually a solid object is produced.

Ink-jet printing can also be used to fabricate scaffolds and simultaneously deposit cells and growth factors, the other necessary components of a tissue-engineered construct (Fig. 11.11). The printing is done on a substrate, but instead of using ink, the ink-jet head deposits liquid monomer in a pattern specified by the controlling computer. After the monomer is rapidly polymerized, the ink-jet printer head then goes over the same area again, and the construct continues to be built up. This process is repeated many times and eventually results in a three-dimensional scaffold. Ink-jet printers with multiple nozzles can deposit cells and growth factors at the same time and ensure an even distribution of these materials.

The description of scaffold fabrication techniques provided above is highly condensed, and many issues have not been discussed. For example, it is known from

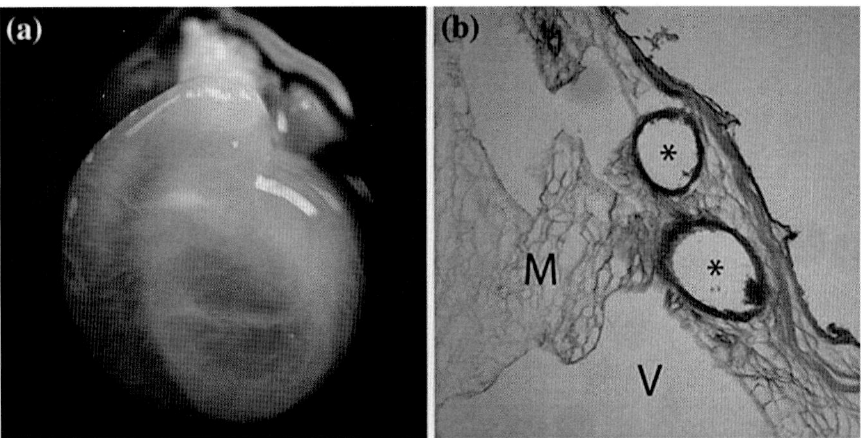

Fig. 11.12 Image of a decellularized rat heart (**a**). The microscopic view of the tissue (**b**) shows no cells present, only extracellular matrix (primarily collagen), and the *asterisks* indicate pores where blood vessels were found. Copyright Springer-Verlag Berlin Heidelberg

studying the interactions between tissues and implants that the morphology and roughness of the implant surface can affect tissue (cell) response. So, it is reasonable to hypothesize that the roughness of the scaffold will also influence how adherent cells behave. In fact, there is a growing realization that just as the natural tissues of the body have a hierarchical structure (meaning that the structure consists of multiple levels), so too should tissue engineering scaffolds. In other words, there ought to be a particular structure at the nanoscale (where molecules on the cell surface can interact with nano-sized features on the scaffold), at the microscale (where larger scaffold surface features such as roughness can interact with micron-size cells), and at the macroscale (where the size and shape of pores and their distribution can dictate cell organization into a specific tissue).

Research has also shown that cells cultured in proximity to other cells, and in a spatial distribution that mimics the natural tissue or organ, readily maintain their phenotype (maintain their distinctive character) while proliferating. Because it is difficult to construct a scaffold in the shape of an organ or complex tissue, there is a great deal of interest in using a natural scaffold (Fig. 11.12). If an organ such as a heart, liver, or lungs can be decellularized (all the muscle, liver, and lung cells removed), then what remains is a scaffold made of extracellular matrix (ECM) proteins and growth factors that is a perfect three-dimensional framework ready to be seeded with new cells. After all, the acellular matrix was originally constructed by the cells that populated it (i.e., the ECM matrix for a liver was tailored by liver cells (hepatocytes), and therefore it will possess the shape, anatomy, and mechanical properties that are optimized for hepatocyte culture). These matrices provide a virtually ideal microenvironment for new cells and provide cells with subtle cues that will help them to function. We currently cannot do better using synthetic materials or fabrication techniques!

An important requirement when decellularizing tissue is to maintain the composition and structure of the native natural ECM to the greatest degree possible.

Several processing steps are involved, including the use of chemicals that must effectively remove any traces of the original cells (and their antigens) in order to avoid or minimize the foreign body response. To begin, it is helpful to rupture the membranes of the original cells to enable the intracellular contents to be released, and this can be accomplished with freeze/thaw cycles and mechanical or ultrasonic agitation. Enzymes are used to digest remaining cellular material, and finally, detergents wash away cellular fragments. The organ is typically perfused (washed internally) with the liquid cleansing solutions. The exact protocols for the specific organs of interest (currently, the heart, liver, and lungs) vary by organ type.

The cells used to seed these natural scaffolds come from a variety of sources and include embryonic and adult stem cells from bone marrow and umbilical cord blood cells. One would think that the ideal cell type for seeding would be a cell obtained from the organ or tissue that is being replaced, i.e., use liver cells to seed a scaffold meant for a liver, but it turns out that the cells from organs don't have the ability to proliferate in adequate numbers to provide a supply for seeding an entire scaffold [3].

How many cells are needed to seed a scaffold? It depends on what is being replicated. If an organ is required to perform a mechanical function (e.g., heart), then the scaffold needs to be almost completely fully grown or recellularized at the time it is implanted into a new host. The heart contains approximately 100 million cells per cubic centimeter, so in order to grow a heart, a large number of starter cells are needed, together with a long period of time in vitro while the cells are proliferating. In contrast, organs such as the liver that do not perform mechanical functions can be effective with a fraction of their eventual cell numbers.

11.3.3 Growth Factors

If natural ECM scaffolds and synthetic scaffolds are usually seeded with stem cells, how can these stem cells be programmed to differentiate into the desired phenotype, and how can they be prompted to proliferate? Those functions are fulfilled by the action of signaling substances called "growth factors," which induce cells to migrate, to proliferate, and to differentiate. Examples of specific growth factors include bone morphogenetic protein (BMP, sometimes used in bone or spine surgeries to stimulate formation of reparative bone or cartilage), fibroblast growth factor (FGF, used to stimulate skin, nerve, and muscle growth), vascular endothelial growth factor (VEGF stimulates growth of blood vessels), and transforming growth factor-β (TGF-β, involved in proliferation of bone and cartilage cells). In addition, we have previously touched on the growth factors EPO (which stimulates formation of red blood cells) and HGF (human growth factor) in our discussion of drugs taken systemically to enhance athletic performance. Although these molecules provide powerful stimuli, as with any signaling process, the signals have to be delivered in the proper place and in the proper manner. Growth factors that are simply washed over the cell locations (a so-called bolus injection) are ineffective, because they quickly diffuse away. Also, growth factors may need to be available at different times in the maturation of the cell-seeded scaffold, and the presentation of one growth factor may be followed some time later by the presentation of another, different growth factor.

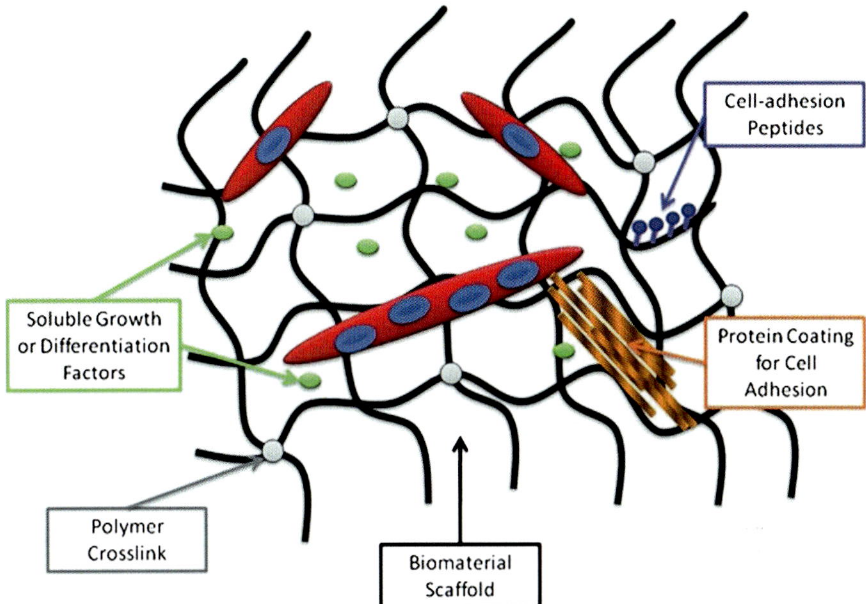

Fig. 11.13 A cartoon of a tissue engineering scaffold with adherent cells (*red*); other compounds have been deposited onto the scaffold to enhance cell adhesion and differentiation. Copyright Springer-Verlag Berlin Heidelberg

The two strategies that have been found effective in delivering growth factors are first to immobilize the growth factor into or onto the scaffold (Fig. 11.13) and second to encapsulate the growth factor in a delivery system [9]. In the first strategy, the growth factors may either be physically adsorbed through electrostatic interactions (the growth factor and scaffold have opposite charges) or held on the scaffold by the action of an intermediary molecule such as a protein. Scaffolds made of hydrogels can directly incorporate a growth factor, or in another variation of the first strategy, growth factors may be chemically bonded to scaffold materials. In this latter instance, there are potential advantages to the growth factor being released over a longer period of time (weeks to months) than if it had been physically adsorbed.

In order to take advantage of the second strategy, the growth factors are used in combination with techniques similar to those used in targeted drug delivery. That is, they are incorporated into synthetic or natural polymers and are slowly released via diffusion or erosion mechanisms. And, in other ways similar to targeted drug delivery, they may be released on demand when appropriate triggering mechanisms are designed into the carrier materials.

Much of the research on growth factor technology has been performed using animal models, and it is currently unclear how easily or effectively it will someday translate into human applications [9].

11.3.4 Bioreactors

Once cells are successfully dispersed into or onto a natural or synthetic scaffold, the scaffold may either be kept in vitro (outside the host body) or implanted directly into the host. If it is desired that the cell population be expanded and the scaffold conditioned, the scaffold is maintained in a "bioreactor" (Fig. 11.14). This is a device that maintains a physiologically conducive environment (temperature, atmosphere, and nutrient media) for optimal proliferation and differentiation of the cells seeded onto the scaffold. In certain instances, dynamic mechanical cues may be provided, as, for example, to chondrocytes (cartilage cells) in culture to help maintain their phenotype or to vascular endothelial graft constructs (where pulsatile loading that simulates the pumping action of the heart assists endothelial cells to maintain phenotype). The reliance on bioreactors to grow a virtually complete tissue and only then implant it into a host has been termed "functional tissue engineering" [10].

The importance of mechanical signals for the proper development of engineered tissue is supported by research showing that vascular cell morphology, proliferation, and orientation are affected by fluid-induced shear stress; that long-term cyclic stressing can lead to improved mechanical properties of muscle tissue; that cyclic compression of cartilage constructs at frequencies similar to walking speed enhances synthesis of cartilage (Fig. 11.15); and that tensile stresses are important in the tissue engineering of tendons and ligaments [10]. In addition to providing the proper chemical and biomechanical environment, bioreactors must be designed so that they permit periodic monitoring and examination of the growing tissue.

Bioreactors also require pumping systems to circulate the nutrient and oxygen-carrying media through the scaffold so that cells can survive. Depending on the cell type, pumping may be carried out continuously or be pulsatile as for heart muscle and endothelial cell constructs. For heart constructs, an electrical pacing stimulus may be needed for the cells to begin contracting in a way similar to normal heart muscle cells do. For lung tissue constructs, which are typically based on natural decellularized scaffolds, a ventilation system is also required so that the cells can achieve the ability to exchange oxygen, a minimum requirement for a "successful" engineered organ.

11.4 Examples of Engineered Tissue Currently Available for Patient Treatment

11.4.1 Tissue Engineering Skin

There are no commercially available skin graft constructs that emulate the dermal and epidermal layers together [6]. As listed in Table 11.2, fewer than ten products that are currently sold and reimbursed by health insurers are dermal replacements onto which an epidermis must be grafted. Essentially, they are based either on a combination of fibroblasts (connective tissue cells that synthesize collagen, found in

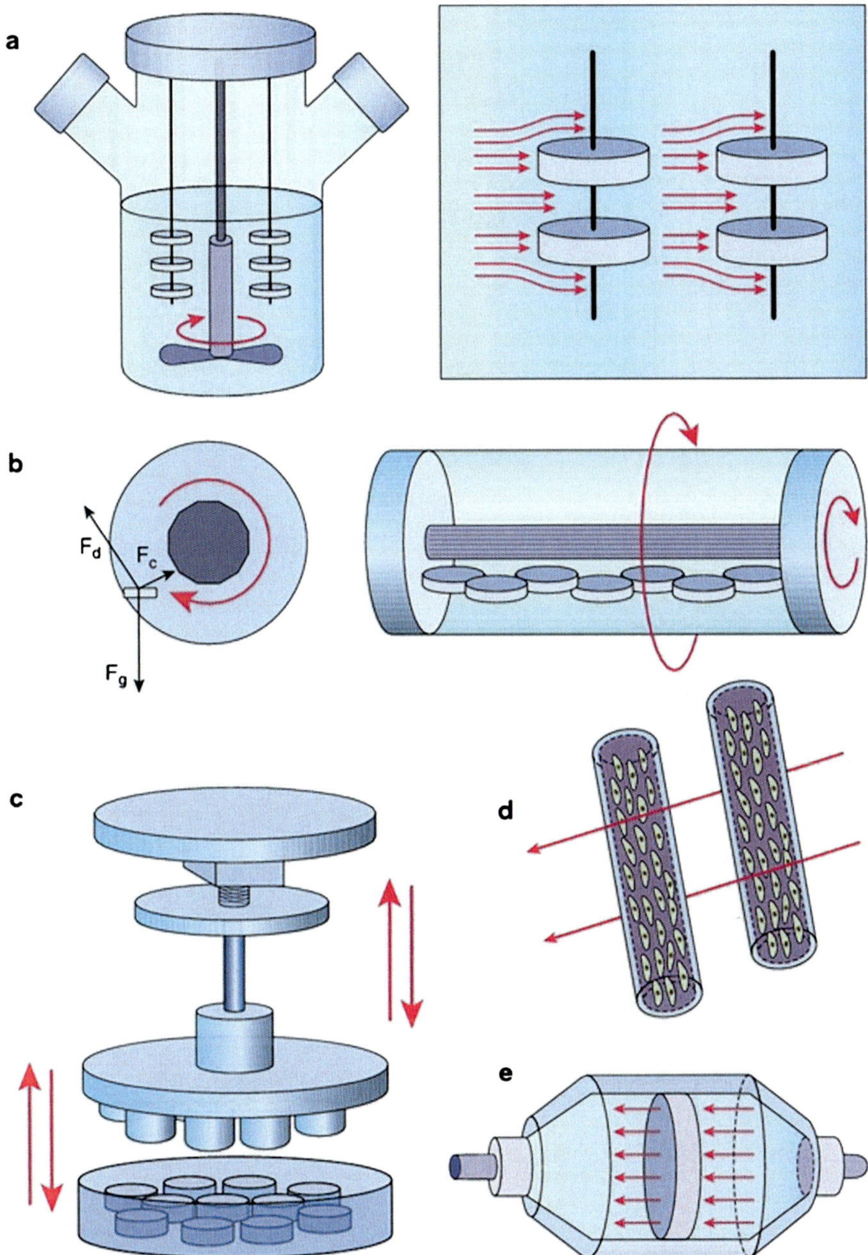

Fig. 11.14 Diagrams of various types of bioreactor: (**a**) Stirrers incorporated into the bioreactor (cells cultured in the flat dishes); (**b**) rotating vessel bioreactor (the rotation permits stirring of the nutrient fluid without causing damage to the cells); (**c**) hollow fiber bioreactors (media is flushed through the inside of the fibers while cells adhere to the outside of the fibers); (**d**) perfusion bioreactors (cells obtain nutrients and cell products are collected continuously); (**e**) dynamic force-applying bioreactors (appropriate for chondrocyte and vascular epithelial cell culture). Copyright Springer-Verlag Berlin Heidelberg

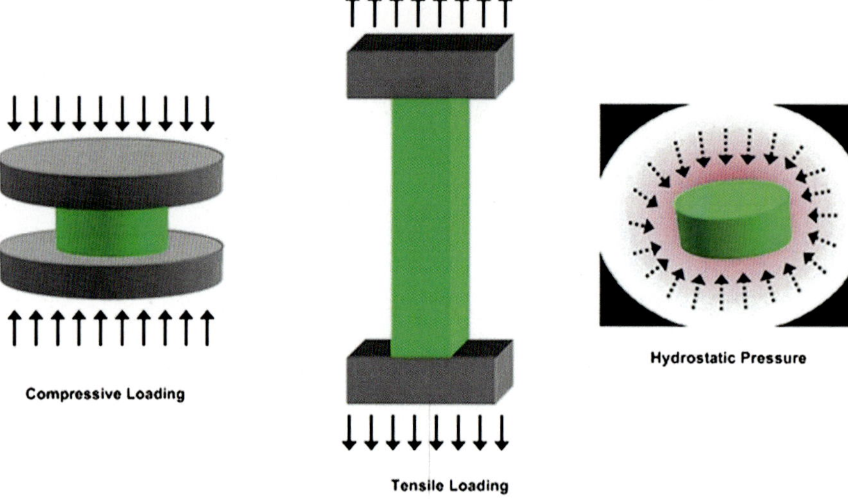

Fig. 11.15 Types of loading schemes applied to tissue-engineered cartilage constructs in a bioreactor. Copyright Springer Berlin Heidelberg

Table 11.2 Examples of commercially available skin replacement products

Name	Description	Indications for use
Dermagraft	Contains human fibroblasts and resorbable polymer mesh	Chronic diabetic foot ulcers
Apligraf	Contains fibroblasts and keratinocytes in a collagen matrix	Venous leg ulcers and diabetic foot ulcers
TransCyte	Contains human fibroblasts on a nylon mesh, with a synthetic epidermal layer	Temporary covering for burns
OrCel	Contains human dermal fibroblasts in a bovine collagen matrix	Burns
OASIS	Contains a porcine collagen matrix	Leg ulcers, wounds, pressure ulcers
Integra dermal regenerative template	Contains bovine collagen and glycosaminoglycans (a sugar) with a silicone protective layer	Burns
Graftjacket regenerative tissue matrix	Acellular matrix derived from human donor tissue	Diabetic foot ulcers
AlloDerm	Acellular matrix derived from human donor tissue	Hernia and abdominal wall repair and postmastectomy breast reconstruction

the dermis and elsewhere in the body) and keratinocytes (the cells that comprise the epidermis, the outermost layer of the skin) with a carrier (a polymer or collagen) or matrix alone without a cell component.

If the dermis layer is involved in the wound, healing is accompanied by scar formation and shrinkage of the skin, which can interfere with tissue regeneration.

11.4.2 Tissue Engineering Cartilage, Bone, Teeth, Tendons, and Muscle

Musculoskeletal regenerative products are designed to either replace damaged cartilage or missing bone. Cartilage tissue does not self-heal, and the tissue lost as the result of trauma caused by accidents or sports activities, or because of arthritis, does not regenerate. A common treatment for athletes who have suffered torn, dislodged, and missing cartilage is the "microfracture" procedure. In this surgery, small holes 2–3 mm deep are punched in the bone plate with an awl (a sharp, pointed instrument). Blood and bone marrow that contains stem cells slowly ooze out through the holes, eventually forming a clot. During the rehabilitation procedure, which requires approximately 6 months, mechanical stresses placed on the clot are believed to induce the stem cells to differentiate into cartilage. However, it should be noted that there are different types of cartilage: elastic, hyaline, and fibrous cartilage. Elastic cartilage is found in the outer ear and has no weight-bearing functions. Hyaline cartilage is the type found in joints; articular cartilage is hyaline cartilage that is on articulating surfaces (surfaces that are moving over each other). Fibrous cartilage contains fibrous tissue with cartilage and is found in some portions of the spine. Although all forms of cartilage have some mechanical integrity, it is only the hyaline cartilage that is able to withstand the forces that accompany joint movement and function. So, what kind of cartilage forms after microfracture surgery? Not hyaline cartilage, unfortunately, but rather the fibrous form. The extent and duration of beneficial effects of microfracture depend on patient age (the younger the better the result) and on the location where the replacement cartilage is formed. The rehabilitation process is long and complex and suited for professional athletes who have powerful financial incentives to return to sport or to individuals who can devote much of their day to rehabilitation.

Some of the currently available musculoskeletal repair products are listed in Table 11.3.

This listing is not intended to be inclusive, but it is representative of the types of products that are available. Note that there is only one FDA-approved product for treating cartilage loss, and it is not indicated for patients with osteoarthritis (the costs of the procedure are not reimbursed by insurers); and yet, those are the patients who most often require cartilage replacement. The reason for this exclusion is presumably that the product will not last for long in osteoarthritic patients who are often overweight and are candidates for total hip or knee replacement. There are approximately eight tissue-engineered cartilage replacement products in various stages of clinical testing. The control group used for comparison in these clinical trials often consists of microfracture patients.

The scaffolds used in cartilage tissue engineering for products in various stages of development include natural materials such as collagen, gelatin, and fibrin, and synthetic materials such as polylactic acid and polycaprolactone (Fig. 11.16). Because of the complexity of natural cartilage extracellular matrix (ECM), which includes several types of collagen and proteoglycans in addition to growth factors and other signaling molecules, some scientists believe that decellularized natural ECM will

Table 11.3 Commercially available bone and cartilage cell-based or regenerative treatment products

Name	Description	Indications for use
Corticel	Autogeneic chondrocytes reimplanted after expansion in culture	In regions of cartilage loss due to trauma, not osteoarthritis
DeNovo NT graft	Minced cartilage obtained from juvenile donors, mixed with fibrin glue, reimplanted	Repair of articular cartilage lesions
Grafton	Demineralized bone matrix and glycerol. Putty formulation includes alginate for mixing with water. Bone chips may be added	Osseous defects, regenerating bone for improved tooth implant retention, bone cysts in children, spinal fusion
Infuse	Collagen sponge "infused" with BMP-2 bone morphogenesis growth factor	Sinus lift (associated with dental implant placement), accelerated healing of tibial fracture (but with intramedullary nail)
Vitoss	Porous tricalcium phosphate, another formulation includes bioglass; may be combined with blood, bone marrow, or saline	Voids or gaps in skeletal system
Augment (sold in Canada, Australia, and New Zealand, awaiting approval in USA)	Tricalcium phosphate with human platelet-derived growth factor	Used internationally for foot and ankle fusion
Pro Osteon 200R	Coral-derived, thin hydroxyapatite coating over a calcium carbonate core	Bone void filler

yield better results than synthetic and simple natural material scaffolds [11]. They point to the successful use of natural ECM in tissue engineering heart valves, muscle, tendon, and gastrointestinal tissues such as the trachea and abdominal walls. Because natural ECM already contains many growth factors, it should provide an environment more suitable for growth and differentiation of chondrocytes.

The matrix for cartilage tissue engineering may be derived, as it is for other tissues, from allogeneic or xenogeneic sources, though the decellularization protocol for cartilage from those sources is somewhat vigorous and may affect the signaling molecules naturally occurring in cartilage ECM. An alternative is to use patient's own cells in culture to produce a matrix. In order to ensure that a cartilage construct possesses adequate mechanical strength, it may be reasonable to design hybrid matrices that include both natural ECM and a high-strength synthetic material [11].

Bone graft products typically include a source of calcium and phosphorous (either bone chips, hydroxyapatite, or tricalcium phosphate), a vehicle (glycerol, saline), and a growth factor (BMP-2 or human platelet-derived growth factor) to accelerate bone growth and repair. It should be noted that the bone graft products are not indicated for use in any "structural" (load-bearing) sites. Additional information about other FDA-approved bone graft materials can be found at http://www.aaos.org/research/committee/biologic/BI_SE_2003-1.pdf.

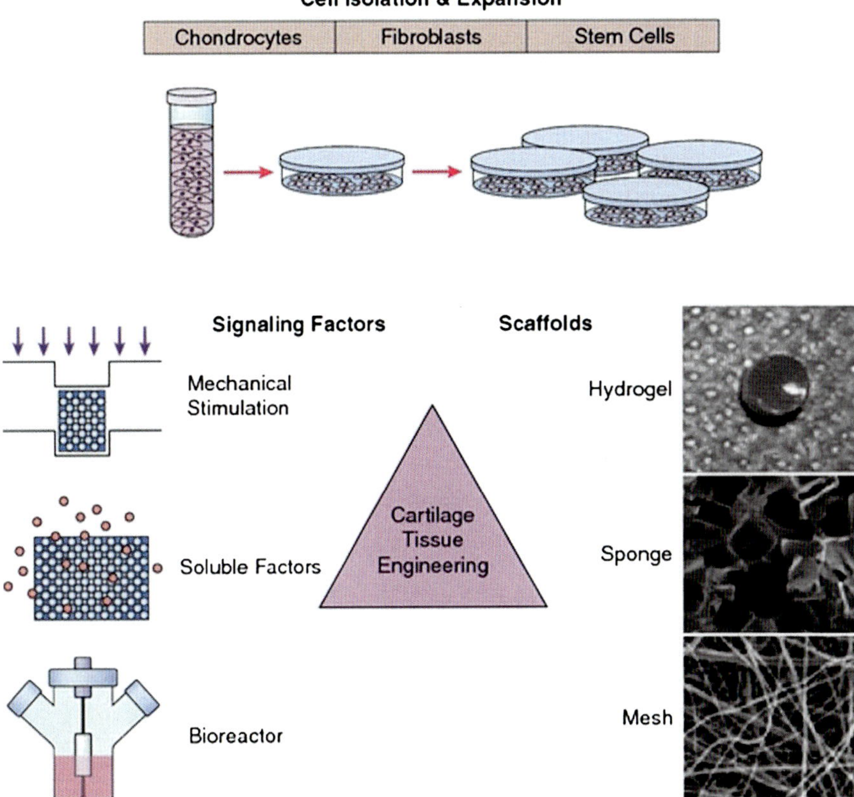

Fig. 11.16 A summary diagram of the process for tissue engineering of cartilage. The cells needed (chondrocytes, fibroblasts, or stem cells) are deposited onto one of a variety of scaffolds (hydrogel, sponge, or mesh format) and signaled to proliferate by mechanical and chemical stimuli in a bioreactor. Copyright Springer Berlin Heidelberg

Another hard tissue that has been the focus of regenerative medicine efforts is the tooth (Fig. 11.17). Researchers have been able to reconstitute a tooth germ (also known as the tooth bud), and when implanted into the jawbone of a mouse, the germ eventually grew into a fully functioning tooth [12]. The tooth had all the anatomic and structural features of other natural mouse teeth and responded to stimuli in the same manner as did the existing teeth, meaning that nerve growth into the new tooth had also occurred. These findings have given rise to the expectation that someday, it will be possible to create "teeth in a test tube."

Tendons are tissues transmitting forces from muscle to bone, and thereby they make movement possible. Their function is primarily biomechanical; their own mechanical properties are intermediate between bone and muscle, and so they can buffer the sudden stresses that can arise during sudden or strenuous movement, protecting the softer muscle tissue from tearing and injury.

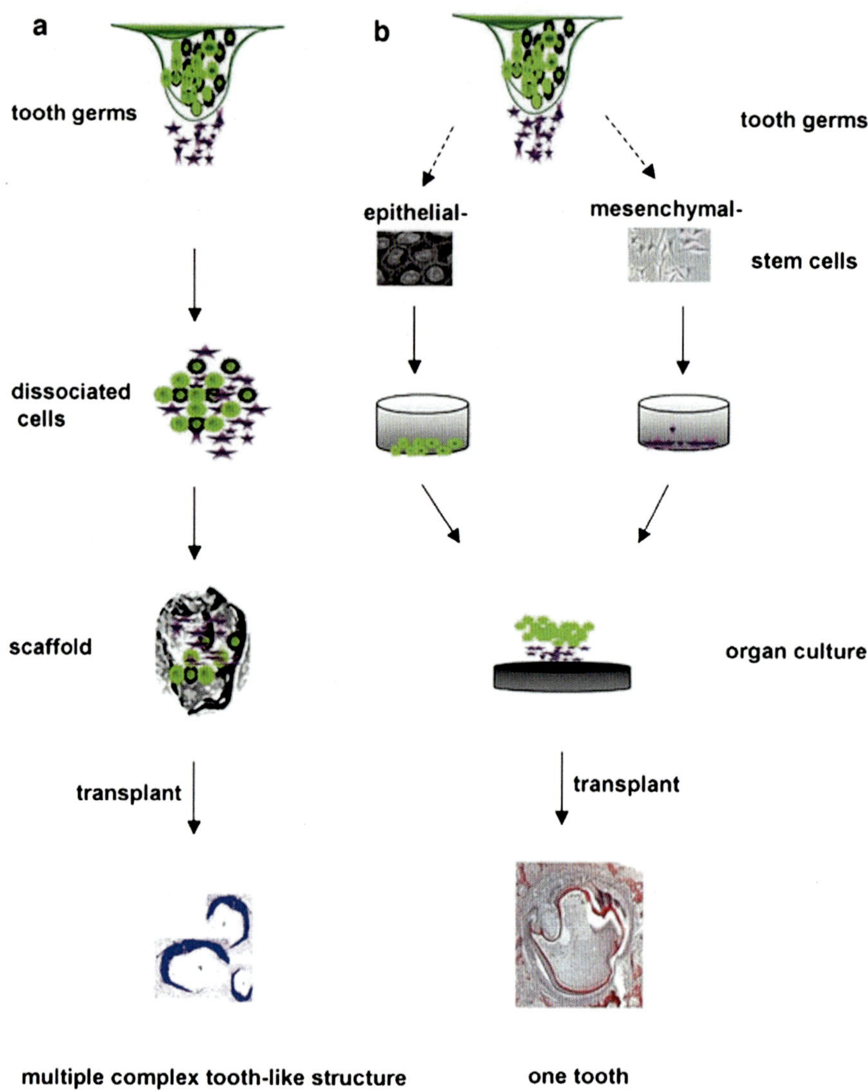

Fig. 11.17 Tissue engineering of teeth. The two approaches illustrated describe a process wherein tooth germs (primitive cells that eventually develop into a tooth) are (**a**) dissociated, seeded onto a toothlike scaffold, and form several toothlike structures or (**b**) stem cells are co-cultured and the interactions between the cells result in a tooth that can be implanted into the patient. Copyright Springer-Verlag

Tendons are viscoelastic materials, and they dissipate energy by responding in a viscous manner; they can stretch and yield, becoming "longer" in the process. The warm-up exercises done prior to athletic activity involve stretching, and tendons are said to "loosen up" as a consequence of lengthening. Because tendons are viscoelastic, stretching is to be done slowly, not with a rapid application of stress. As with all

Table 11.4 Commercially available tendon repair augmentation products

Name	Description	Indications for use
Graftjacket	Allogeneic, acellular tissue matrix provided in sheets for application to site	Diabetic foot ulcers, Achilles tendon and rotator cuff repair, hand tendon repair
TissueMend	Acellular non-cross-linked collagen from fetal bovine dermis	Reinforcement of the rotator cuff, patella, Achilles, biceps, quadriceps, or other tendons
Collagen repair patch	Acellular cross-linked collagen and elastin scaffold from porcine dermis	Rotator cuff repair
Restore orthobiologic soft tissue implant	Collagen from porcine small intestine submucosa	Rotator cuff repair
CuffPatch	Acellular allogeneic patch from human amniotic membrane (the sac holding the fetus) containing collagen I, III, IV, V, and VII and various growth factors	Rotator cuff repair

viscoelastic materials, a rapid stress or strain rate results in a purely elastic (springy) response by tendon rather than the desired viscous behavior. However, sports and other vigorous activities do sometimes include sudden movement, and the accumulation of damage to tendons caused by aging and extreme load application leads to tendon damage (accompanied by pain and inflammation) and potentially tearing. It is estimated that 10 % of the public and 50 % of runners could be diagnosed with Achilles tendinopathy (pain, etc.) [13].

After tendon injury, which typically involves at least some local tearing of the tissue, healing proceeds in three stages. In the first few days after an injury occurs, the site is inflamed, injured cells are cleared away by macrophages, and tendon cells called "tenocytes" begin to congregate. Approximately 2–3 days after the injury, cells begin to repair the tendon and to produce collagen III, which forms a temporary matrix for the tenocytes. In the final stage of healing, which begins 1–2 months after injury, the tenocytes become more aligned and collagen III is replaced by collagen I. This stage can last more than a year; the repaired tissue is scar like, and the tendon will never regain the properties it possessed prior to the injury. Repair of the tendon does not always occur, in part because there is often impatience on the part of patients who do not comply with instructions, remove the splint, lift heavy objects, etc.

In addition to surgical tendon repair strategies, which include (1) suturing torn tendon together, placing a tendon autograft; (2) mechanical stimulation during healing; and (3) application of biologic healing agents such as corticosteroids, hyaluronic acid, and others that reduce scar formation, tissue engineering also has the potential to enhance healing. Some examples of commercially available engineered tendon tissue grafts are listed in Table 11.4 and can consist of acellularized allogeneic tendon that has been repopulated with tenocytes or stem cells. Rotator cuff injuries have been treated by biologic scaffolds that are intended to strengthen the suture, and suture fixation strength has been shown to increase following these augmentation procedures [14].

Skeletal muscles are made up of bundles of oriented and dense muscle fibers that were derived from cells called "myoblasts." There are two types of fiber types, with different reaction times (so-called fast-twitch and slow-twitch fibers), different sizes, different resistance to fatigue, and different force production capability. After injury, just as with other tissue types, macrophages are recruited to remove dead muscle cells. New muscle cells are regenerated by special cells called "satellite cells"; these cells only account for 1–5 % of the total muscle cell population, and the exact amount varies with age (lower for older muscle). Satellite cells can also migrate to the damaged muscle site and form scar tissue, causing a loss of functionality at that location.

If large amounts of muscle tissue are lost as the result of conventional trauma or during wartime, any successful regeneration of the lost mass must conclude with a tissue that contains aligned myofibrils with the proper receptors and components that can produce direct forces, blood vessels, and sensory and motor nerves. The two strategies that have been investigated for tissue engineering of skeletal muscle are to (1) biopsy the patient's muscle, expand the satellite cell population in tissue culture on a biocompatible three-dimensional matrix allowing cell differentiation, and implant the mature construct into the patient and (2) biopsy the patient's muscle, expand the satellite cell population, and implant the satellite cells on a transport matrix into the patient where the satellite cells are encouraged to differentiate.

A difficulty with satellite cell culture strategies is that apparently, satellite cells are all slightly different depending on their original source. In other words, satellite cells from the biceps are different than satellite cells obtained from one of the 23 facial muscles. This finding means that in order to engineer a bicep, a bicep biopsy is needed; to engineer the quadriceps, a quadriceps biopsy is needed, and so on. In addition, it is not particularly easy to stimulate differentiation of the satellite cells. The growth and signaling factors that are relevant for muscle tissue are at least partially known, but the knowledge when they should be active is not yet available.

The scaffolds used in tissue culture of satellite cells may be made either from natural or synthetic materials. The synthetic polymers include polylactic-co-glycolic acid, silicones (nonbiodegradable), and polyisopropylacrylamide; the latter is used in two-dimensional culture, producing sheets of tissue which may be layered to create desirable thicknesses. Natural and degradable materials used as scaffolds include collagen, fibrin, fibronectin, and acellular autologous muscle. If the scaffolds have nanoscale roughness or features that are aligned, the assembly of myoblasts into aligned myotubes is enhanced. This is an advantage of synthetic polymer scaffolds, while fibrin (a tough protein involved in the clotting of blood) enhances cell proliferation, and the cell sheet method offers control of construct architecture.

In order for muscle tissue to function, each individual muscle fiber must be connected with a motor neuron. This is achieved during myoblast formation when a specific receptor molecule called acetylcholine is expressed on the cell surface; when a motor neuron comes into the vicinity of a site where the receptor is found, a connection can be made. Application of electrical stimulation during cell culture assists in the development of the neuron–myoblast connection, and mechanical stressing during cell culture helps to align the cells and enlarge the thickness of myofibers.

A final requirement of engineered muscle tissue is establishment of a network of blood vessels, as the myoblasts need to be within 150 μm of a source of nutrients and oxygen. This is currently a major hurdle in the development of the technology for growing muscle and has limited success to small constructs implanted over several surgical procedures, with the time between procedures being used for in vivo vascularization. An optimal means of achieving a vascularized muscle construct has not yet been identified.

Muscle tissue engineering is not considered to be a standard method of care for replacing tissue lost through trauma or cancer surgery or as therapy for genetic muscle diseases such as Duchenne muscular dystrophy. One clinical approach has focused either on transplanting large numbers of myoblasts into the site where muscle tissue is needed, but this technique is somewhat limited because of the very large number (billions) of cells needed and multiple sites for injection. Another approach, as described previously, expands the myoblast population in vitro and then relies on a matrix to help transfer the cells to the implant site. Still a third approach has been reported, one which utilized implantation of decellularized pig urinary bladder into a site with a muscular deficit and attachment of the "scaffold" onto existing muscle, ensuring that the scaffold will experience normal mechanical loading. In a mild immune system reaction, the patient's body began to break down the xenograft and, in the process, stimulated native satellite cells to proliferate and grow new muscle [15]. Not all the missing muscle has been replaced, but the patient has regained much of his earlier movement ability.

Although this discussion has focused on developing muscle tissue culture for therapeutic purposes, we should not forget that animal muscle tissue is what humans generally regard as food. The most common cuts of beef, chicken, pork, etc. are all composed of muscle. Because of ethical concerns about breeding animals to be slaughtered for food, some groups (e.g., New Harvest) are suggesting that tissue culture could be a way to grow animal protein for consumption by humans. Another potential advantage of this method would be that the land resources needed now for grazing would not be required, and the waste generated by herds of animals would not exist. It's interesting to consider that as population pressures in the world increase demand for food, it may be someday possible and indeed necessary to grow food in underground laboratory warehouses.

11.4.3 Tissue Engineering the Heart

There is a great deal of interest in regenerating a specific type of muscle tissue, heart muscle. As of 2013, there are no FDA-approved products available for regenerating cardiac muscle. Nevertheless, there have been many reports of research focusing on transplantation of muscle "satellite" cells, as discussed in the previous section. The experimental work that has been done included expanding cells harvested from ten patients who had suffered several heart attacks, then injecting approximately 800 million cells into the sites where the heart muscle was damaged [16]. At 11 months follow-up, heart function had modestly improved for several patients.

When grown in a laboratory setting, heart muscle cells need to become organized and develop the ability to contract in a coordinated manner. During culture, it is also necessary to ensure the cells have access to adequate nutrient medium, so the tissue engineering scaffold may be made porous or designed with channels, and electrical stimulation of the cells has been found to aid the organization of the cells [17]. Tissue engineering or regeneration of the heart requires not only cardiomyocytes (heart muscle cells), but other cells too, for example, endothelial and smooth muscle cells, needed to build blood vessels. All these cells are found in the normal heart and are derived from progenitor cells which differentiate into different cell lineages under the influence of many growth factors. While the long-term goal of regenerative medicine is to acquire the knowledge and technology to grow an entire heart, at the present time no whole-organ constructs have been used in vivo on animals or humans. The current focus on regenerating heart tissue is on developing a tissue-engineered heart muscle graft or "heart patch" to replace the approximately 50 g of cardiac muscle that die from lack of oxygen during a heart attack and on tissue-engineered heart valves.

Several approaches have been used in developing a heart muscle graft. In one, cardiac myocytes are grown as sheets of cells on polymer membranes that are chemically designed to allow easy detachment of the cells when these are needed. Several layers of these cells are placed on top of each other, where they develop the ability to contract and propagate electrical signals, and are eventually implanted in the heart where the damaged muscle requires replacement. This procedure is currently confined to animal models. In another approach, a decellularized rat cell repopulated by cardiac myocytes and endothelial cells exhibited contraction, but at an activity level of only 2 %. Thinking along the lines of this approach, it may be worthwhile to regenerate hearts but only use portions of the new tissue for grafts or to use the decellularized matrix as a scaffold in vivo to repair a damaged heart while it is still in the patient [3]. Human hearts would be widely available for the purpose of providing allogeneic decellularized matrix, because non-vital hearts could be used as a source, and cells to seed the matrix could invade from the patient's own heart or be injected in a protective hydrogel suspension. Hydrogels used as scaffolds for heart muscle cells enable the cells to be mechanically stimulated, helping the cultured cells to mature and develop the ability to contract, resulting in constructs that functioned well when placed in rats.

Several key technological advances are still needed before a reasonable prospect of heart tissue repair can be expected. First, the shape of the heart is complex, and tissue engineering a graft that would meet the "architectural" requirements is not easy. Second, surgically placing a graft will lead to formation of scar tissue, which will interfere with growth of blood vessels that are essential to maintain the vitality of the new patch; the term for blood vessel growth is "angiogenesis," and it is a critical requirement of tissue-engineered heart tissue. So not only heart muscle cells need to be provided, but the smooth muscle and endothelial cells that comprise blood vessels need to be available and become organized. Third, it is not currently known what developmental stage is ideal for the cells that are used to seed the graft scaffold. Should the cells be fully mature so that they can immediately begin contracting, or should they be progenitor cells that will mature after implantation? Some scientists are taking an alternative path: instead of worrying how to coax cardiac progenitor cells into maturing in vitro, they prefer to use growth factors and other chemical cues that when injected into a damaged heart will enable the heart's own cells to repair any damage [18]. Fourth, the engineered heart patch will have already started to contract and generate electrical signals if the cells were permitted to reach a certain level of maturation; if that patch is implanted into a beating heart, it's not obvious how the two sets of myocytes will coordinate their rhythms. Fifth, much of the research is now being conducted in animals; there is no perfect animal model because of the differences in electrical properties between human hearts and those from sheep, pigs, dogs, and rats [17].

Over 100,000 patients need heart valves replaced each year in the USA and worldwide; it was estimated that the market for heart valves exceeded $1 billion in 2005 [19]. Synthetic heart valves, made from a pyrolytic carbon leaflet and a metal ring covered with a polyester fabric for suturing the valve to the heart, cannot respond to growth or physiological forces in the way a natural, biologic valve can. Also, the risk of developing a blood clot is estimated at 4 % per patient year with entirely synthetic valves. However, the development of prosthetic valves based on biologic components has provided the patients and surgeons with a choice of intact pig valves stabilized with an integrated suture sewing cuff, valves made from pieces of cow pericardium (a tough membrane that covers the heart), or allograft human valves, all of which may be used for adult surgeries. The risk of surgery-related mortality is low, and the lifespan of some of the bioprosthetic valves ranges from 15 to 20 years. There is therefore no overwhelming demand for developing a tissue-engineered valve for adults.

Children, however, do not tolerate prosthetic valves well, and their valves are usually reconstructed in an entirely surgical manner, relying on pieces of pericardium (the sac containing the heart) to reconstruct valves [19]. Therefore, the demand for tissue-engineered heart valves is primarily for pediatric cases. There have been several approaches taken in tissue engineering heart valves. The first relies on using an acellular matrix derived from a pig valve and assumes that decellularization removes all matter responsible for provoking an immune response in the new host. The process of removing cells may also be traumatic to the matrix, however. Cells may be seeded onto the matrix prior to surgery, or they will self-seed after the matrix is implanted. The latter strategy, however, has not proven to work in clinical cases. The cells which seed the matrix remodel it, create fibrous tissue, and cause the valve to contract (shrink) [19].

The second approach to valve tissue engineering utilizes a bioresorbable scaffold made of a synthetic polymer which is seeded with cells prior to implantation (Fig. 11.18). These valves are used in less stressful positions such as the pulmonary position (rather than the aortic valve which must absorb the pressures of blood arriving from the ventricle) because the valve is weak when the scaffold begins to degrade. The long-term performance of these valves is unknown.

Yet another approach involves cells seeded in a collagen gel. The cells interact with the collagen and organize collagen fibrils into an aligned and compact mass. Casting the gel into a mold allows fabrication of a construct resembling a heart valve leaflet. These constructs, and others made using other natural gel materials, are in preparation for testing in animals [19].

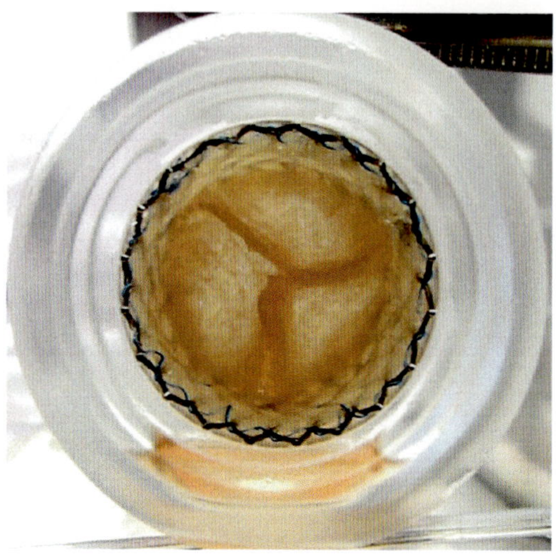

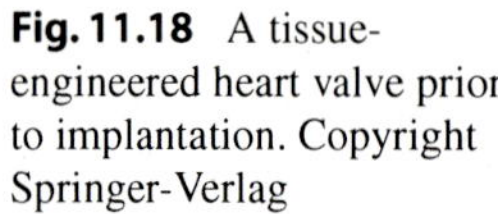

Fig. 11.18 A tissue-engineered heart valve prior to implantation. Copyright Springer-Verlag

In summary, there is not a likely prospect for tissue-engineered heart valves to be available any time soon because the bar set by current bioprosthetic valves is quite high (15–20 year lifetime).

11.4.4 Tissue Engineering the Kidney and Bladder

The tissue engineering of tissue is usually more easily accomplished than the tissue engineering of a complex organ. The more "simple" hollow or tubular organs, even those that have a multilayer architecture, such as blood vessels, trachea, and bladder, have in principle been demonstrated in the laboratory and in selected clinical cases. Large solid organs such as the kidney present a challenge, with more than 20 different cell types comprising the organ and a complex organizational structure needed for the kidney's function of filtering electrolytes from blood. The demand for novel kidney treatment is high (think of all the patients on dialysis), with some 19 million individuals suffering from chronic kidney disease in the USA alone; approximately 5–7 % of people worldwide are affected. Some success in creating kidney tissue to augment kidney function has been achieved in animal models when kidney cells were cultured in three dimensions using a gelatin matrix [20]. The constructs were injected into rats, and results indicate that there is potential for the biomaterial–cell combination being capable of enhancing the regeneration of the native kidney. Interestingly, the response of the native organ was highly dependent on the matrix that was used to culture kidney cells; gelatin proved to yield better results than matrices made from hyaluronic acid, polycaprolactone, and polylactic-co-glycolic acid [20].

Another group of scientists has recently reported success growing a kidney-like organ in vitro [21]. First, fetal mouse kidney cells were extracted and cultured for approximately 1 week and were observed to aggregate into what were called "organoids" that showed organization into nephrons. Then, the organoids were immersed into a bath of vascular endothelial growth factor (VEGF) in order to stimulate the formation of blood vessels. Additional VEGF was injected into the implantation site (a host kidney in a rat), and VEGF was also given intravenously for an additional 3 weeks. Experiments showed that the kidney grafts were able to filter proteins from rat blood, indicating that they were functional. Further work on developing a duct system into the kidney grafts, so that they may siphon urine to the bladder, is currently underway. Although use of fetal kidney cells from human donors is not a likely prospect, it may be feasible to someday use stem cells to accomplish kidney regeneration.

Treatment of damage sustained by bladder tissues as the result of cancer or trauma has relied on reconstruction using native non-urologic tissues such as gastrointestinal segments. In an ironic twist, that tissue is designed to absorb specific substances from digested matter, whereas urologic tissue is designed to excrete some of those very same substances [22]. This discrepancy in function may lead to postsurgical complications, and so there is a rationale for identifying alternative materials. Replacement of bladder tissue using only synthetic materials such as Teflon, silicone, or polyurethane has sometimes led to urinary stone formation.

Tissue engineering urinary tissues has been accomplished using synthetic polymers such as polylactic or polyglycolic acids, natural polymers such as collagen or alginate, and acellular matrix materials from a bladder or small intestine submucosa (one of the several tissue types found in the intestine) [22]. These materials have been discussed in this chapter previously and indeed are used in the tissue engineering of many tissues.

Cells used for bladder tissue regeneration may be sourced from autologous tissue remaining after surgery, expanded and used in with one of the scaffold materials to create a construct. The co-development and organization of multiple cell types to produce an endothelial cell lining and a muscle tissue component to engineered bladder replacement remain a challenge. However, numerous animal and some experimental treatments with humans indicate that the use of cell-seeded matrices yields better results than implantation of matrix alone (and counting on local cells to invade the matrix and proliferate). The Tengion company is conducting Phase I trials of a neo-urinary conduit for patients requiring removal of a cancerous bladder. In the process, a biopsy of fatty tissue is taken from the patient, and smooth muscle cells are isolated and allowed to proliferate. A tubelike scaffold made of biodegradable polymer fibers is seeded with the smooth muscle cells, placed in a bioreactor, and 4 weeks later the scaffold is ready for implantation. The patient's body will eventually convert the construct into a more complex collection of tissues, and the scaffold will disappear. Costs for the procedure are estimated at $300,000.

11.4.5 Tissue Engineering the Liver

The liver is another complex organ that performs a number of different functions, including protein synthesis, filtering toxins from blood, and producing substances needed to process food such as bile which is used to digest fats in the small intestine. Most of the liver is composed of cells called hepatocytes; other cells found in the liver include endothelial and Kupffer cells, which are involved in clearing pathogens from blood. In developed countries, drug toxicity and alcoholic liver disease are the principal causes of liver failure, while in developing countries hepatitis is the major concern. The World Health Organization reported in 2001 that 2.5 % of total deaths in the world were caused by liver disease. Death is often due to multiorgan failure, because liver disease can lead to problems with kidneys, neurologic impairment, and metabolic abnormalities.

Although the liver is capable of regenerating itself (it can recover from a loss of 70 % of its mass!), the only current cure for patients with end-stage liver cirrhosis, liver cancer, or chronic liver failure is a liver transplant. As with all other transplanted organs, there are complications due to the immune response and a shortage of viable organs. Partial liver grafts can potentially solve the shortage of donated organs, but immunological complications still remain. Tissue-engineered liver tissue may be a potential solution to donor tissue shortages with a possible decrease in the intensity of the immune response.

There are three approaches being taken to support a diseased liver. First, a liver support device that is meant to remain outside the patient's body can be used as a "bridge" therapy in patients waiting for a liver transplant. These bio-artificial livers contain hepatocytes, but there are numerous challenges and difficulties that limit their usefulness, including the difficulty of obtaining the large number of hepatocytes needed, the limited volume of blood that can be processed, and maintaining an adequate oxygen supply to the cells.

Second, transplantation of liver cells (in contrast to transplantation of the entire organ) has been found beneficial in animal and human trials. The advantages of this treatment include the ability to treat several patients with one donor organ, its minimally invasive nature, its low cost, and repeated administration if necessary. Difficulties associated with finding cells for transplantation are a major limitation of this technology (cryopreserved cells do not engraft efficiently, meaning that only about 30 % survive). Third, implantable devices in the form of microcarriers or biodegradable scaffolds are being developed, along with other means of encapsulating cells in order to enhance their survivability in the new host.

Successful liver tissue engineering begins with selection of cells. Primary hepatocytes would be the preferred cell type, but they do not maintain well in cryopreservation and lose phenotype. As we will see later, in order to develop a successful product, it is necessary to be able to store cells or constructs that are thawed when needed. Pig hepatocytes have been used in bio-artificial livers and in implantable devices.

Stem cells have also been considered to be a viable source for liver tissue engineering; adult, embryonic, and induced stem cells have been found to regenerate liver in animal models and proliferate just as normal hepatocytes do. Adult stem cells are more easily differentiated into hepatic lineages than embryonic and induced pluripotent stem cells, but there are difficulties associated with differentiating large quantities of cells.

Fetal hepatic progenitor cells (hepatoblasts) can proliferate extensively in vitro, and in animal models these cell integrate with injured liver and provoke only a minimal immune response. A clinical trial involving 25 patients with end-stage cirrhosis who were injected with fetal liver progenitor cells reported clinical improvements 6 months after implantation [23].

Maintaining any of the cell types successfully in culture is problematic, and there are indications that cell–cell interactions are key for preserving cell phenotype and function. Three-dimensional porous scaffolds made of synthetic polymers such as polylactic-co-glycolic acid, polyamide nanofibers, and polycaprolactone have been used as supports for hepatocytes and for stem cells. Natural polymer scaffolds made of alginate, hyaluronate, and chitosan have been used with hepatocytes, fetal liver progenitor cells, and adult stem cells. Decellularized liver matrix is also of interest, as there is evidence that not only is the architecture of liver best approximated using that ECM, but also that important growth factors and signaling molecules are preserved after proper decellularization. These matrices also induce rapid differentiation of stem cells into hepatic cells. In addition, the possibility of using decellularized matrix with a preserved vascular structure could eliminate one of the more difficult problems associated with tissue engineering, i.e., vascularization.

If decellularized matrix is not used as a scaffold, then it is necessary to provide appropriate growth factors such as VEGF or hepatocyte growth factor (HGF) either into the tissue culture environment, or in vivo by implantation into the liver, or subcutaneously to enable stem cell differentiation and development of a vascular network. The growth factors are delivered using collagen gel, polyethylene glycol gel, or polylactic-co-glycolic acid microspheres.

11.4.6 Neural Tissue

Tissue engineering and regeneration of nerve tissue lags behind developments in connective, liver and kidney tissues. And yet, the loss of the senses or total paralysis has dramatic effects on patient quality of life and significant implications for the care of such patients. The nerves present in the eye, ear, spinal cord, brain, and peripheral nervous system inhabit different environments, and so the complexity of engineering replacement tissues is high. Fortunately, the early beliefs that nerves cannot regenerate have been proved false, and laboratory studies have successfully reported "growing" nervous tissue. However, tissue engineering of nerve tissue is currently done in vivo which requires that the "bioreactor," scaffold, and growth factors must be provided at the site of injury, not outside the body in a laboratory.

Peripheral nerves (PNS) are what we commonly consider to be "nerves"; they are located outside the brain and the spinal cord where they normally have no mechanical protection and are responsible for sensing and for transmitting impulses to muscles. The structure of peripheral nerves resembles a conduit filled with sensory and motor axons (the long structures protruding out of a neuron or nerve cell) and structural support cells. Axons can be quite long; the longest (the sciatic nerve) runs from the base of the spine to the end of the big toe. Axons may be covered with a fatty substance called "myelin," and it is the loss of myelin that accompanies the disease multiple sclerosis. The entire peripheral nerve is covered by a thin protective membrane. Some peripheral nerves originate at the spinal cord, while others originate from the brain.

After an injury to a peripheral nerve, success of repair depends on the continued survival of the detached tissue. The closer the injury is to the spinal cord, the more doubtful it is that the nerve will be regenerated. Treatment can consist of suturing the two ends of the nerve together or utilizing an autologous graft obtained from another part of the patient's body. Small injury gaps of a few millimeters may be treated by placing a hollow tube made of silicone or degradable collagen called a "nerve guide" that allows the two nerve ends to be brought closely together and serves as a guide for the formation of a clot followed by regeneration of the nerve. The size of the gap that can be bridged by a regenerating nerve is called the "critical gap length," and for primates it can be approximately 30 mm. The critical gap length increases if the nerve guides are filled with matrices of hydrogels or collagen, if the matrices have been aligned by application of a magnetic field, or if a scaffold is present in the guide [24]. As with most other cell types, introduction of specific growth factors also enables regeneration.

11.4.7 Case Study 1: Peripheral Nerve Regrowth in the Thumb Using a Collagen Nerve Guide

A 24-year-old male presented to the emergency room following an accident occurring while doing plumbing work. The patient's fingers were profusely bleeding. He had severed a common digital nerve to the index finger on his dominant hand, with a 15 mm gap between nerve ends. To repair the nerve injury (segmental nerve loss), the patient was offered a choice of either a collagen nerve guide or autograft. The patient opted for repair using a tubular collagen guide. A collagen conduit is made of type 1 collagen and is resorbable and semipermeable. Nerve guides are designed to create a protective environment for axonal growth across a nerve gap or segmental nerve loss and allow for nutrient exchange and accessibility by neurotrophic growth factors. The surgery was performed by an experienced hand surgeon using delicate microsurgical instruments. After the repair, the patient had successful physiological recovery. This was ascertained using motor and sensory evaluation which included tests to determine grip strength, cold, and pain tolerance.

Injury to the spinal cord is usually a serious problem because it is often accompanied by immediate nerve cell death and disruption of the blood supply to the injury site. In addition, a scar forms that is quite effective in inhibiting future regeneration. Treatment can involve transplanting cells such as peripheral nerves, Schwann cells (a type of cell that keeps nerve fibers alive), stem cells, or genetically modified cells to the site to act as a "bridge" and aid spinal cord regeneration. A nerve guide filled with a scaffold consisting of fibrin, methylcellulose or Matrigel™ (a jellylike protein mixture used as for cell culture) will normally assist spinal cord repair. Unfortunately, however, there is no reproducible technique for spinal cord therapy, and challenges in dealing with scar tissue, increasing the number of axons that regenerate, and facilitating the formation of myelin sheaths still remain.

Treating damage to white or gray matter in the brain poses its own set of challenges. The injury likely causes neuron cell death and other phenomena that are common to peripheral nerve cells and the spinal cord damage, and cell replacement or provision of an environment that encourages regeneration is needed. Many strategies have been pursued in treating victims of stroke or trauma, including transplanting fetal and genetically modified cells, neural precursor cells, and stem cells. As with spinal cord injury, no individual tissue engineering treatment is currently considered to be standard. Therapy of degenerative diseases such as Parkinson's or Alzheimer's does not conform to the usual definition of tissue engineering, as it is primarily attempted (in the case of Parkinson's) by injecting stem cells into the brain. Results of such interventions vary widely.

11.5 The Market for Tissue-Engineered Products: Has the Promise Been Fulfilled?

While tissue engineering has truly energized a large portion of the bioengineering research community, how has this field fared in the financial markets? Almost all analysts agree that there is great potential for the technology; the projected compounded growth rate over the period 2009–2018 for the tissue-engineered and cell therapy global market is projected to increase from a low of 14 % for skin products to slightly over 20 % for treating patients with cancer or heart disease and peaking at slightly over 40 % for organ replacement or transplant [25].

In 2008, there were four FDA-approved tissue-engineered skin products available that primarily served a market composed of patients requiring treatment for severe burns, war-inflicted wounds, or some other trauma; at that same time, there were five FDA-approved cellular or tissue-based products for musculoskeletal applications, serving a market consisting primarily of arthritis, spine surgery, long bone non-unions, and periodontal-disease-related jawbone defect patients (the jawbone resorbed because of a bone infection caused by oral bacteria) [26]. Today, in 2013, these numbers have not changed significantly. There is still only one FDA-approved cartilage replacement (Carticel™), although approximately nine other scaffold/cartilage cell products are in Phase II or Phase III clinical trials. As far as wound healing products go, as of January 15, 2013, there were approximately seven products that the Blue Cross Blue Shield insurance companies considered to be a normal standard of care and would therefore reimburse their use. At the same time, there are approximately 64 products considered to be at the experimental stage. Why has the enthusiasm about tissue engineering and regenerative medicine technology not yet yielded a larger variety of products for a number of different applications?

Successfully processing a tissue-engineered bone, piece of cartilage, or heart muscle in a research laboratory is obviously a far cry from how a successful business needs to operate; the process for bringing a product to market is long and complex (Fig. 11.19). First, the inexpensive student labor in a research setting cannot be replicated in a commercial setting, where expensive skilled full-time technical workers are needed.

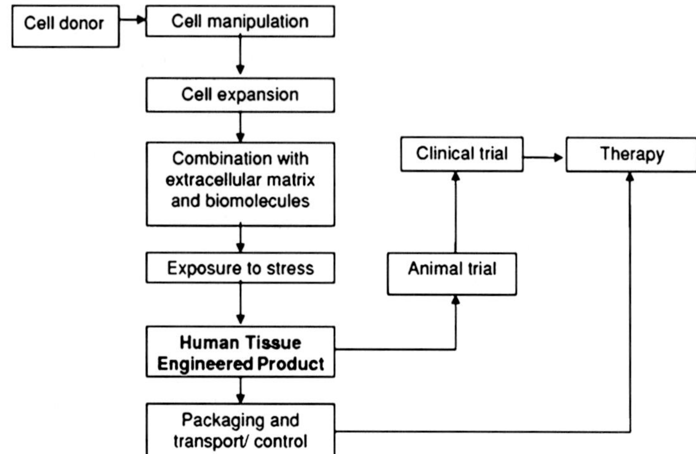

Fig. 11.19 The process for developing a therapeutic product based on tissue engineering principles is long; technical, regulatory, and marketing challenges conspire to delay translation of research discoveries into bedside therapies. Copyright Springer Science + Business Media B.V.

Second, the mistakes commonly made by student workers cannot be allowed to occur in business; for that reason, there are extensive (and expensive) quality-control measures that have to be implemented. Documentation is even more critical than in a research lab and may be requested by the FDA to verify "good manufacturing practices" at the industrial site. Every step in the process of creating a tissue-engineered product follows a strict protocol, and any deviation must be recorded and explained.

Third, scaling-up production from a research laboratory setting, where a few constructs may be cultured at any given time, is dissimilar from the industrial setting where hundreds to thousands of individual tissue constructs are incubated simultaneously. The maintenance of sterile conditions (asepsis) on that scale entails high costs.

Fourth, shelf life is important; a commercial product is usually not developed on a customized basis. Most products are manufactured and then stored, ready for use when needed. Therefore, an effective storage system must be developed and maintained.

Fifth, no product will be sold unless it receives FDA approval. Tissue-engineered products lie on the borders of various agency jurisdictions; products that are composed of or intended to contain intact cells lie within the jurisdiction of the Center for Biologics Evaluation and Research. Hybrid products where the cell is the primary mode of action will be regulated as biologics, but products where the matrix produced by the cell is the primary mode of action are regulated as devices or as biologics. The uncertainty and potential need to satisfy multiple centers within the FDA contributes to development costs.

Sixth, someone has to pay for a product. A physician or a surgeon needs to be able to write a diagnostic code acceptable to health insurance carriers, and the carrier has to agree to pay. If the tissue engineering treatment is considered to be experimental and not a currently accepted standard of care, the insurer will probably not pay for the treatment, and therefore the physician will not prescribe a tissue engineering treatment.

Of course, there are other expenses that do not occur in a laboratory setting such as legal fees, marketing, and promotional costs. All these items constitute significant barriers to the introduction of any new biomedical technology to the market, but tissue engineering is still new enough that some of the regulatory issues have not yet been worked out.

Knowing all this, the clever entrepreneur or tissue engineering startup company will seek to develop products that require as little as possible in the way of human labor and which can be stored indefinitely. The example of Dermagraft™, a skin implant that was developed in the 1990s, illustrates the benefits of planning ahead [27].

Dermagraft was envisioned from the very beginning as an allogeneic product that was to have a shelf life of 6 months. The cells for the product were taken from a single donor and passaged eight times over a period of a little more than a year. In that short time, the initial sample proliferated enough to provide enough cells for 15–20 years of production. One advantage to using only a single cell line is that the cells have been thoroughly characterized and tested, an expensive process that only needs to be done a single time.

Because bioreactors are themselves expensive and because inserting and removing the construct from a bioreactor could compromise sterility, the company decided to have the bioreactor also function as the packaging for the final product. In this way, it would need to be sterilized only once. The bioreactor in this case was a polymer bag made from ethylene vinyl acetate (Fig. 11.20); each bag was divided into eight compartments, each containing a knitted mesh of polylactide–polyglycolide polymer which served as the scaffold. Twelve bags were all connected to a single system that provided nutrients to the cells, for a total of 96 constructs incubated at the same time. After the cells had proliferated to the desired amount, the cell culture medium was emptied, and a cryopreservative solution was added to each bag and each cavity. The cavities were each heat-sealed, cut out of the bag, put into additional packaging, and deep-frozen until needed for implantation.

It is also extremely fortunate for the Smith and Nephew company, who manufacture Dermagraft, that even though the product is allogeneic, it does not appear to cause an immune response. As of 2006, approximately 90,000 implants had been placed in 25,000 patients without a single record of an immune reaction [27]. It is believed that the reason for this behavior is that the product does not contain any antigen-presenting cells such as macrophages.

11.6 Summary

It is generally agreed that the potential for the tissue engineering approach tosolving the problem of inadequate supply of organs for transplant and for tissue needed in reconstructive surgery is great and will provide a significant health benefit for many thousands or patients who cannot survive without transplants.

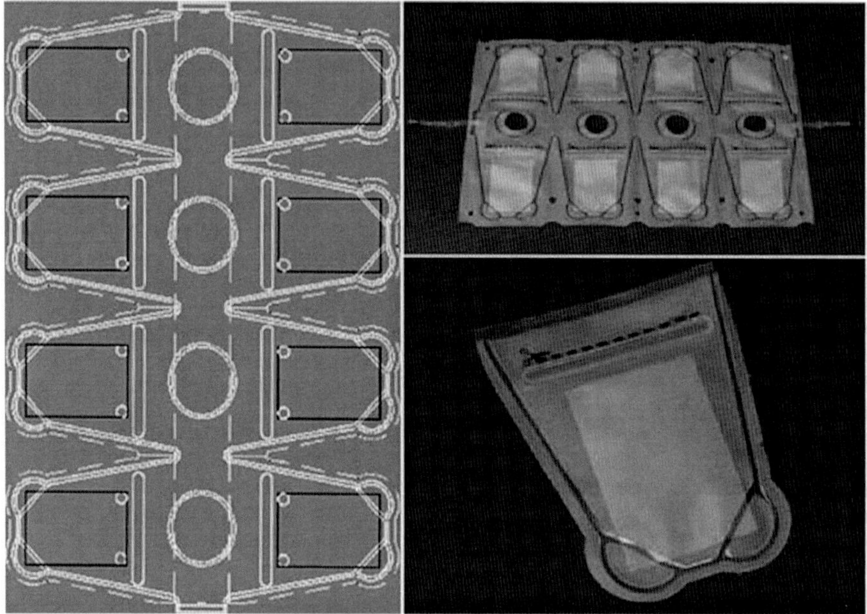

Fig. 11.20 The Dermagraft bioreactor design. On the *left*, the *black rectangles* represent knitted polylactide-co-glycolide scaffolds. The *white lines* are where the two pieces of ethylene vinyl acetate were welded together by heat, and the *broken white lines* are where cuts will be made to separate the individual skin grafts. In the *upper image* on the *right* is the complete bioreactor with inlet and outlet ports. In the *lower image* on the *right* is a separated individual piece of Dermagraft. Copyright Springer Berlin Heidelberg

The technology is complex and poses challenges involving the immune system, as well as needing additional knowledge about the regulatory mechanisms of cells in order to optimize cell growth, proliferation, and organization into suitable tissue. It is likely that many tissue products will be available long before organ products enter the market. There is also a risk that tissue engineering has become so "over-hyped" that the lack of progress in bringing discoveries from the bench to the bedside will eventually reduce the enthusiasm of investors who will sour on the potential of the technology.

There are also a number of nonscience issues that will affect the rate at which tissue engineering and regenerative technologies develop. One is of course the funding issue; given the economic climate in the world today, how likely is it that governments, which are the only bodies with sufficient resources to finance such large-scale projects, will continue to provide research funding at historic levels? Some scientists have suggested that the USA funds a special national initiative to develop a tissue-engineered heart, in a way similar to the mission to put a man on the moon in the 1960s. Other concerns include the regulation of tissue-engineered constructs and the eventual costs to patients and insurers. Nevertheless, this technology has captured the imagination of the public and is unlikely to fade away.

11.7 Foundational Concepts

- Tissue engineering and regenerative medicine is a technology that seeks to find methods of inducing damaged tissue to heal itself or growing replacement tissues and organs in vitro (in the laboratory). The components typically necessary for this process to occur successfully include an appropriate cell or cells, a scaffold or matrix that provides support for the cells while they proliferate, growth factors to stimulate proliferation and differentiation of cells into the desirable phenotype, and a means of delivering the tissue or organ to its site in the body.
- Cells used in tissue engineering are either primary cells (e.g., chondrocytes for cartilage, myoblasts for muscle, hepatocytes for the liver) or stem cells (e.g., embryonic stem cells, induced pluripotent adult stem cells, or mesenchymal adult stem cells). The scaffold materials can be synthetic polymers such as the biodegrading polylactic acid and polycaprolactone or natural materials such as collagen, chitosan, or alginate. More recently, researchers have experimented with decellularized tissues. The extracellular matrix that remains after cells are removed provokes a minimal immune response and provides important morphologic and biochemical cues for cells that enable their proper function.
- Tissue engineering principles have been used to successfully produce cartilage and skin replacement materials that are presently on the market.

References

1. Langer, R., & Vacanti, J. (1993). Tissue engineering. *Science, 280*, 920–926.
2. Center for Disease Control and Prevention. (2013). *Leading causes of death.* http://www.cdc.gov/nchs/fastats/lcod.htm.
3. Badylak, S., Taylor, D., & Uygun, K. (2011). Whole-organ tissue engineering: Decellularization and recellularization of three-dimensional matrix scaffolds. *Annual Review of Biomedical Engineering, 13*, 27–53.
4. Committee on the Biological and Biomedical Applications of Stem Cells. (2002). *Stem cells and the future of regenerative medicine.* Washington, DC: National Academy Press.
5. Wilson, J., & Chaikof, E. (2008). Challenges and emerging technologies in the immunoisolation of cells and tissues. *Advanced Drug Delivery Reviews, 14*, 124–145.
6. Ikada, Y. (2006). Challenges in tissue engineering. *Journal of the Royal Society, Interface, 3*, 589–601.
7. Kaully, T., Kaufman-Francis, K., Lesman, A. & Levenberg, S. et al. (2010). Vascularization: The conduit to viable engineered tissues. In P. Johnson & A. Mikos (Eds.), *Advances in tissue engineering: Angiogenesis.* New Rochelle, NY: Mary Ann Liebert.
8. Mikos, A., Bao, Y., Cima, L., Ingber, D., Vacanti, J. & Langer, R. et al. (1993). Preparation of poly(glycolic acid) bonded fiber structures for cell attachment and transplantation. *Journal of Biomedical Materials Research, 27*, 183–189. http://www.cdc.gov/nchs/fastats/lcod.htm.
9. Lee, K., Silva, E., & Mooney, D. (2011). Growth factor delivery-based tissue engineering: General approaches and a review of recent developments. *Journal of the Royal Society, Interface, 8*, 153–170.

10. Korossis, S., Bolland, F., Kearney, J., Fisher, J. & Ingham, E. et al. (2005). Bioreactors in tissue engineering. In N. Ashammakhi & R. Reis (Eds.), *Topics in tissue engineering* (Vol. 2). EXPERTISSUES e-book.
11. Benders, K., van Weeren, P., Badylak, S., Saris, D., Dhert, W. & Malda, J. et al. (2013). Extracellular matrix scaffolds for cartilage and bone regeneration. *Trends in Biotechnology, 31*, 169–176.
12. Ikeda, E., Morita, R., Nakao, K., Ishida, K., Nakamura, T. & Takano-Yamamoto, T. et al. (2009). Fully functional bioengineered tooth replacement as an organ replacement therapy. *Proceedings of the National Academy of Sciences, 106*, 13145–13146.
13. Gaida, J., Alfredson, H., Kiss, Z., Bass, S. & Cook, J. et al. (2010). Asymptomatic Achilles tendon pathology is associated with a central fat distribution in men and a peripheral fat distribution in women: A cross-sectional study of 298 individuals. *BMC Musculoskeletal Disorders, 11*, 41.
14. Derwin, K., Baker, E., Spragg, R., Leigh, D. & Iannotti, J. et al. (2006). Commercial extracellular matrix scaffolds for rotator cuff tendon repair. Biomechanical, biochemical, and cellular properties. *Journal of Bone and Joint Surgery. American volume, 88*, 2665–2672.
15. Fountain, H. (2012, September 15). A first: Organs tailor-made with body's own cells. *The New York Times*, New York.
16. Menasche, P., Hagege, A., Vilquin, J-T., Desnos, M., Abergel, E. & Pouzet, B. et al. (2003). Autologous skeletal myoblast transplantation for severe postinfarction left ventricular dysfunction. *Journal of the American College of Cardiology, 41*, 1078–1083.
17. Vunjak-Novakovic, G., Lui, K., Tandon, N. & Chien, K. et al. (2011). Bioengineering heart muscle: A paradigm for regenerative medicine. *Annual Review of Biomedical Engineering, 13*, 245–267.
18. Jha, A. (2013, January 29). Cell researchers take new route to heart repair. *The Guardian*, London.
19. Vesely, I. (2005). Heart valve tissue engineering. *Circulation Research, 97*, 743–755.
20. Basu, J., Genheimer, C., Rivera, E., Payne, R., Mihalko, K. & Guthrie, K., et al. (2011). Functional evaluation of primary cell/biomaterial neo-kidney augment prototypes for renal tissue engineering. *Cell Transplantation, 20*, 1771–1790.
21. Xinaris, C., Benedetti, V., Rizzo, P., Abbate, M., Corna, D. & Azzollini, N. et al. (2012). In vivo maturation of functional renal organoids formed from embryonic cell suspensions. *Journal of the American Society of Nephrology, 23*, 1857–1868.
22. Atala, A. (2011). Tissue engineering of human bladder. *British Medical Bulletin, 97*, 81–104.
23. Khan, A., Shaik, M., Parveen, N., Rajendraprasad, A., Aleem, M. & Habeeb, M. et al. (2010). Human fetal-derived stem cell transplantation as supportive modality in the management of end-stage decompensated liver cirrhosis. *Cell Transplantation, 19*, 409–418.
24. Dalton, P., Harvey, A., Oudega, M. & Plant, G. et al. (2008). Tissue engineering of the nervous system. In C. Van Blitterswijk et al. (Eds.), *Tissue engineering* (pp. 611–647). New York, NY: Academic.
25. MedMarket Dilligence LLC. (2010). Tissue engineering, cell therapy and transplantation: products, technologies, and market opportunities, worldwide, 2009–2018. http://www.mediligence.com/rpt/rpt-s520.htm.
26. Hellman, K. (2008). Tissue engineering: Translating science to product. In N. Ashammakhi, R. Reis, & F. Chiellini, (Eds.), *Topics in tissue engineering*. http://www.oulu.fi/spareparts/ebook_topics_in_t_e_vol4/index.html
27. Mansbridge, J. (2006). Commercial considerations in tissue engineering. *Journal of Anatomy, 209*, 527–532.

Genetic Engineering 12

> *"We used to think that our fate was in our stars, but now we know that, in large measure, our fate is in our genes."*
>
> James Watson

Biologists once could only study plants and animals at a macroscopic level, whatever was visible with the naked eye. The development of optical microscopes made it possible to discover and view cells, the fundamental building blocks of living tissue. When microscopes became even more powerful, it became evident that cells were highly complex structures containing components having discrete functions. The introduction of biochemical technologies capable of manipulating reactions occurring in biological systems enabled a quantum leap in "visualizing" biological molecules and gave birth to the field of molecular biology. Within this field, genetics have become a focus area of study, and the understanding of how genes affect growth and development has led to efforts to control these processes by "genetic engineering."

In this chapter, we will begin by discussing the molecules at the center of genetic engineering (DNA, RNA), then explain how genetic information may be altered, provide examples of targets of genetic engineering, and show how "personalized medicine" can eventually be realized through an understanding of a person's genome.

12.1 Introduction: What Is Genetic Engineering?

The US Food and Drug Administration (FDA) defines genetic engineering as "a process in which recombinant DNA (DNA which has been "combined" in the laboratory from various sequences into a product not found in nature) technology is used to introduce desirable traits into organisms." Over the last three decades, the methods developed while pursuing genetic engineering, such as gene manipulation, gene

G.R. Baran et al., *Healthcare and Biomedical Technology in the 21st Century: An Introduction for Non-Science Majors*, DOI 10.1007/978-1-4614-8541-4_12,

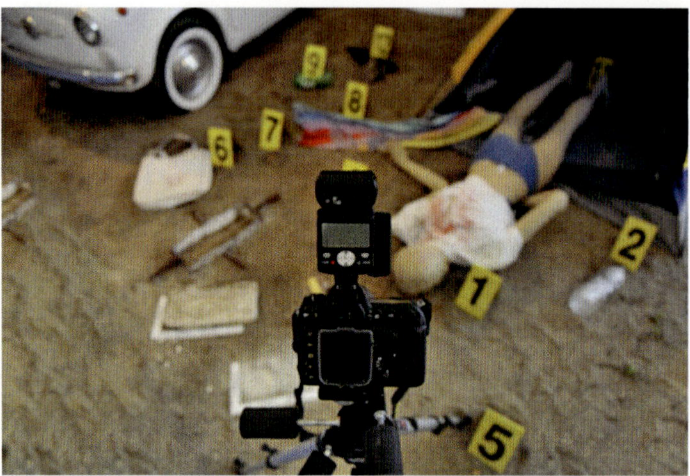

Fig. 12.1 Genetic testing is now done during criminal investigations as portrayed on popular television programs

cloning, recombinant DNA technology, and genetic modification, and mapping and sequencing have found applications in drug discovery, study of the molecular bases for diseases, and prediction of hereditary traits in humans including risks of developing particular illnesses, personal identification (Fig. 12.1), and agriculture.

12.2 The Biochemistry Basis of Genetic Engineering

The hereditary information of organisms is transferred to their offspring via information that is encoded in deoxyribonucleic acid (DNA). DNA stores all the genetic information used for the development and functioning of an organism. The DNA molecule itself is about 2.5 nm thick, but its length has been measured as ranging from 1 to 3 m (Fig. 12.2).

Considering that each cell in our body contains DNA, the DNA molecule must be tightly wound; in its tightly packaged form, it is called the chromosome and contains segments of DNA called genes that direct synthesis of proteins.

Because cells multiply by dividing, each new cell must also contain its own DNA, so it is necessary that the entire DNA molecule be able to copy itself. Because the instructions for making all the necessary proteins an organism needs are also found in the DNA molecule, a mechanism is required by which only portions of the DNA molecule can be copied. The structure of DNA, the "double helix" (resembling a twisted ladder), provides a means for self-replication of both the entire molecule and of only short portions of the molecule.

As an aside, all the reactions involving DNA and RNA described throughout this chapter have been animated in short narrated video clips, which may be found online on a variety of sites, including www.dnatube.com with many interesting movies on a variety of science

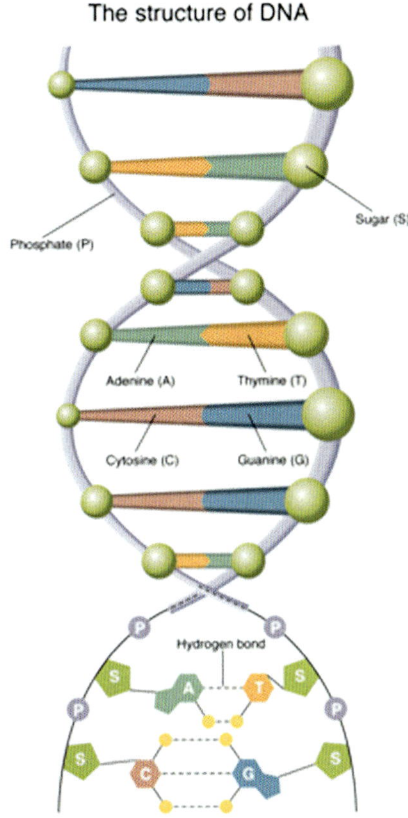

Fig. 12.2 DNA molecule with bases labeled, showing the twisted double-helix structure, and (hydrogen) bonding between bases

topics, and on www.dnalc.org/resources, a site sponsored by the research group at Cold Spring Harbor Laboratory. We suggest that after reading the text, you watch some of these video clips, and then reread the text to obtain a better understanding of these biochemical processes.

Imagine the DNA molecule as a zipper, with each side of the zipper called a "nucleotide." Each of the two nucleotides has a chain-like pattern with links consisting of one sugar group, followed by one phosphate group, and followed by one of four bases: adenine (A), guanine (G), cytosine (C), and thymine (T); this three-link pattern is repeated approximately 1–2 billion times in a DNA strand. The bases on one chain are paired with bases of the other chain on the opposing side of the double helix (the other half of the zipper) by pairing either A with T or G with C when the DNA molecule is "zipped up." Genetic information is determined by the order in which the bases are arranged. For example, a base sequence like TTAGGT might be the way the molecule codes for a cleft chin; TTCGAT might be the way the DNA molecule codes for freckles. Many other traits, e.g., naturally curly hair, left or right handedness, the ability to curl the sides of the tongue upwards, attached or unattached earlobes, as well as the likelihood of developing certain illnesses, are the results of several genes acting together.

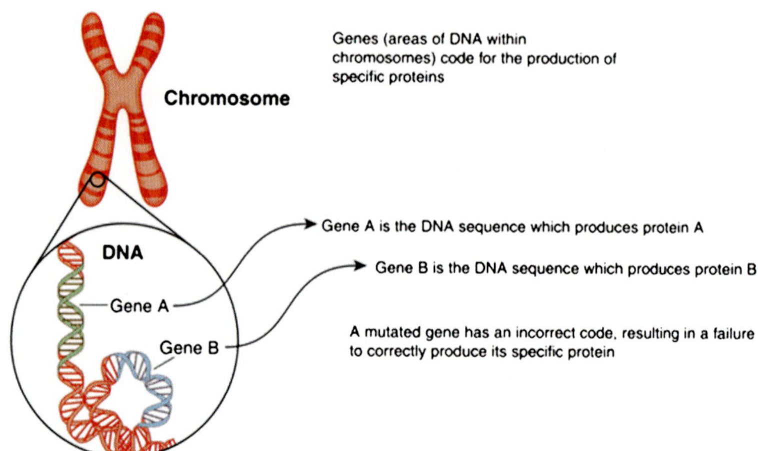

Fig. 12.3 Genes are located in the chromosome. Each human has 23 pairs of chromosomes. The genes contain code for producing specific proteins, and the proteins are used to construct the human body and to carry out various tasks that enable life

The segments of a DNA molecule that contain the instructions for constructing and controlling various components of cells are called genes (Fig. 12.3). There are 23 pairs of chromosomes in humans, with each chromosome containing many genes. Humans normally have two copies of each chromosome with one copy from the father and another from the mother, obtained during conception. Chromosomes are located in the nucleus of each cell and in humans contain approximately 21,000 genes (the exact number of genes in humans is still being investigated!).

The way that DNA encodes the complete characteristics of an organism as complex as the human being is remarkable; the efficiency of this method is unsurpassed, particularly when it has been estimated that only 750 MB would be needed to store an entire human genome on a computer, in contrast with Microsoft's Windows XP operating system, which requires 1,500 MB! Interestingly, there appears to be no correlation between the complexity of an organism and the size of its genome; several simple creatures like the amoeba have genomes significantly larger than that of a human.

Genes deliver their encoded genetic information via proteins through the process of gene "expression," which consists of two steps: transcription and translation (Fig. 12.4). Transcription, which may be thought of as the process of reading or imaging the DNA molecule, begins with separation of the DNA nucleotides by an enzyme acting like the slider on a zipper, i.e., portions of the DNA molecule are unzipped. Then, another enzyme pairs free bases that complement the exposed DNA bases in order to build a molecule of messenger ribonucleic acid (mRNA). The mRNA molecule that is assembled, using one of the DNA nucleotides as a template, is a copy of the non-template DNA strand. The nucleotide that serves as the template is called the antisense strand, while the nucleotide that is transcribed is called the sense strand.

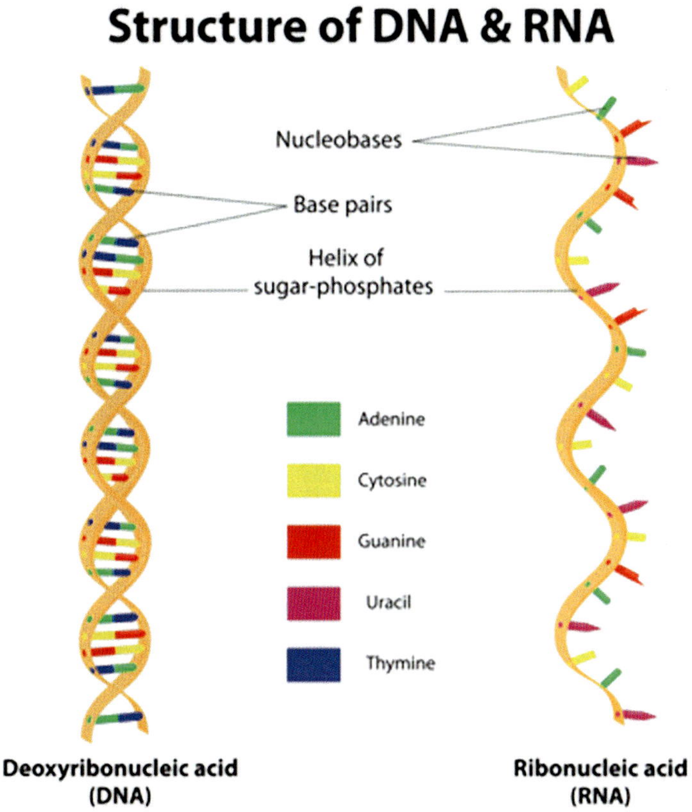

Fig. 12.4 Structures of DNA and RNA. After the DNA molecule separates, unbound bases found in the vicinity of the molecule pair with the exposed portion of the DNA molecule and build a RNA molecule that carries information (the message) about the specific DNA that participated in its synthesis

When the mRNA is completed on a segment of DNA, the mRNA nucleotide breaks free. This RNA molecule has a structure that is very similar to DNA, except that it is a single-strand molecule. It also consists of four bases: adenine (A), guanine (G), cytosine (C), and uracil (U) instead of thymine (T). The messenger RNA produced by transcription has the same sequence (is a copy) as the non-template strand coding in the DNA, except for U being substituted for T. In this way, the mRNA is now a copy of a portion of the genetic information in the DNA.

The process of translation produces proteins from the genetic information stored in the messenger RNA after it reaches the cytoplasm of the cell. In this process, matching genetic codes from the messenger RNA are used to synthesize various proteins from chains of the approximately 20 available amino acids (Fig. 12.5). Proteins, produced as the result of gene expression, determine cell and body function and structure. The gene expression process is highly regulated so that the right amounts of gene products, i.e., proteins, can be produced at the right time

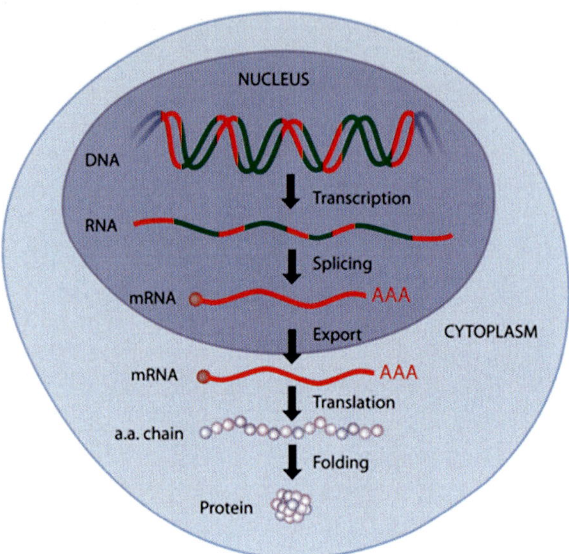

Fig. 12.5 A summary of protein synthesis. DNA is transcribed onto a messenger RNA molecule, which undergoes additional chemical processing before being exported out of the nucleus and into the cell cytoplasm. The modified mRNA is translated in the cytoplasm by the ribosomes into a chain of amino acids that when free, fold, and form a protein

(e.g., regulation of insulin gene expression in response to increases in blood-glucose levels is essential for maintaining normal glucose levels, but this process is disrupted in diabetic patients). After transcription, the messenger RNA has to travel out of the nucleus a relatively long distance to the cytoplasm to start the translation process. Therefore, translational regulation involves the control over the export of RNA and the protection of the RNA from degradation.

Not all the genes in the human genome are used in the same way. Some are needed in every cell for the basic survival of the cell and are called "housekeeping genes." Other specialized genes, for example, those that encode for calcium deposition, are found in bone cells. So not all genes are needed in the same quantity at the same time and a regulatory or control system is needed to police which genes are expressed. Specialized proteins called transcription factors determine which genes are expressed, i.e., which proteins will be produced. Protein expression can also be controlled during translation by proteins that are involved in repressing the translation process. The "cross talk" among these cell regulatory systems, along with environmental and developmental conditions, further complicates the system. Therefore, one gene may significantly influence more than one characteristic or function of the organism, and two organisms with even the same genetic instructions (genotype) do not necessarily have the same functions and appearances (phenotype). Identical twins, for example, have the same genotype but do not have all identical characteristics (phenotype) and in many cases even look different from each other.

Because the regulatory process involves proteins, which are themselves coded by genes, you can easily imagine how any mistake or abnormality in this process can lead to significant consequences. Scientists have learned that several diseases are the result from the absence of transcription factors or mistakes made during translation. By analyzing a patient's genome, it is possible to determine which errors are being made in the regulatory process. This insight provides the reason why medical scientists believe that genetic engineering can be a significant weapon in curing or preventing genetically linked diseases.

The DNA "story" is a fascinating tale of scientific progress, in which the discoveries made by scientists are used as springboards for the next set of experiments and which illustrate portions of the scientific method. Considering how important and far reaching are the implications of the discovery of DNA, its structure, and eventually its manipulation, it is well-worth reading.

The substance which was eventually to be named DNA was first isolated in 1869 by a Swiss biochemist named Friedrich Miescher, who called it "nuclein" because he had obtained it from the nuclei of white blood cells. Subsequent analysis showed the substance to be an acid, and so the substance got a new name, nucleic acid. At about the same time, advances in other technologies, particularly microscopy, were providing insights about the structure of cells. It was possible to identify chromosomes using new dyes and to observe the cell in various stages of replication (division), so that it became obvious that chromosomes were important participants in cell division. Oskar Hertwig, a German researcher, realizing that chromosomes also contained nucleic acid, theorized that nuclein was involved in the transmission of hereditary information.

Further chemical analyses of nucleic acid had revealed it to contain the sugar, phosphate, and four bases described earlier, and Phoebus Levene in New York was able to show the order in which these components occurred in the molecule. He was certain that all molecules of nuclein contained the same amounts of the four bases and that the length of this molecule was considerably underestimated. Many scientists thought that because of the regularity of the molecular composition, nuclein was more likely made of proteins, because of their rich variety of compositions and lengths, and that it must be involved in the transmission of genetic data. A fortunate discovery came about when Fred Griffith, an English microbiologist, found that mixing two variants of bacteria allowed the transmission of shape characteristics from one species to another; follow-up work by another group of scientists led by Oswald Avery showed that nucleic acid, not proteins, was the substance carrying hereditary information.

A theoretical argument suggesting the substance (whatever it would be) that carried complex genetic information had to be a molecule with features allowing for great diversity was provided by a physicist, Erwin Schrödinger, who pointed out that simple crystal-like molecular structures arranged in periodic patterns could not carry the amount of complex information needed to transmit familial characteristics from a parent to offspring. This hypothesis, together with the results produced by Avery's team, further solidified the central role of nucleic acid.

A biochemist, Erwin Chargaff working at Columbia University in the 1940s, focused on analysis of nucleic acid and published what were called Chargaff's rules. He discovered that the amount of the base guanine (G) equaled the amount of the base cytosine (C) and that the amount of the base adenine (A) equaled the amount of the base thymine (T). This finding strongly suggested that those bases were paired in the nucleic acid structure. Chargaff discussed his findings with

Frances Crick and James Watson in 1952, who were both working in Cambridge England on determining nucleic acid structure. The structure of the molecule was seen as a crucial piece of knowledge worth pursuing, as it could explain how the molecule could transmit the genetic code. As a side note, Chargaff became increasingly disillusioned with the new field of molecular biology (his area of research!) and was quoted as saying that "the technology of genetic engineering poses a greater threat to the world than the advent of nuclear technology."

At about the same time, another group consisting of Maurice Wilkins and Rosalind Franklin at King's College in London were using a technique called X-ray crystallography to puzzle together the structure of DNA. This technique relies on a beam of X-rays being scattered from periodic structures (like crystals or DNA) and forming patterns on photographic film. Analysis of the pattern provided insight about the structure of the scattering molecule. Wilkins believed that nucleic acid had a periodic structure because of the way in which he could pull long strands of the substance from solutions. Because the X-rays are scattered in distinct ways that depend on the spacing between atoms within a molecule, it is possible to calculate where atoms are placed with respect to each other in the molecule or crystal. This information is combined with chemical analysis, which identifies which types of atoms are present (e.g., nitrogen (N), oxygen (O), and carbon (C)), and with chromatographic and other analyses, which identify the subgroups of atoms found in the molecule (e.g., PO_4, NH_2, COOH), to construct a model of the molecule's structure. Then, if the molecule behaves as the structure implies (e.g., it has a certain length or it breaks apart easily in certain locations), confidence in the model grows. In any case, Rosalind Franklin had the idea that nucleic acid had a helical shape, and it was work by Frances Crick at Cambridge and Alex Stokes at King's College (both men were physicists) that solved the mathematical equations showing what sort of X-ray diffraction pattern would be given by a helical structure; without that contribution, it would have been impossible to interpret the X-ray diffraction data.

Also at about the same time, the American chemist Linus Pauling, who had already showed that some proteins had a helical structure, started developing a helical model for nucleic acid. The race to discover the structure was on! The three main teams consisted of Francis Crick and James Watson working together at Cambridge university, Linus Pauling in California, and Maurice Wilkins and Rosalind Franklin at King's College in London. Unfortunately, issues related to working assignments in King's College led to a disagreement between Wilkins and Franklin, and their collaboration became difficult. Franklin began preparing manuscripts for publication that included a helical structure for nucleic acid. In their turn, Crick and Watson believed nucleic acid must have a structure allowing it to copy itself, and that was the way genetic information was transmitted from parent to offspring and during cell division.

In January 1953, Linus Pauling submitted a manuscript for publication that showed a helical structure for nucleic acid (DNA). However, in his model, the phosphate groups were located on the inside of the helix. The British researchers knew this was a mistake and decided to move quickly before Pauling could spot his own

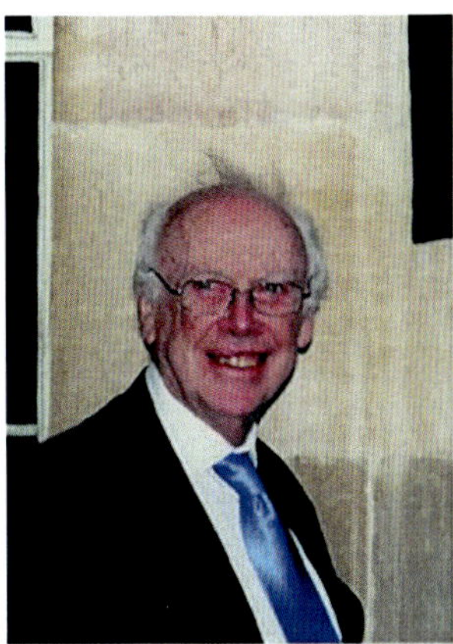
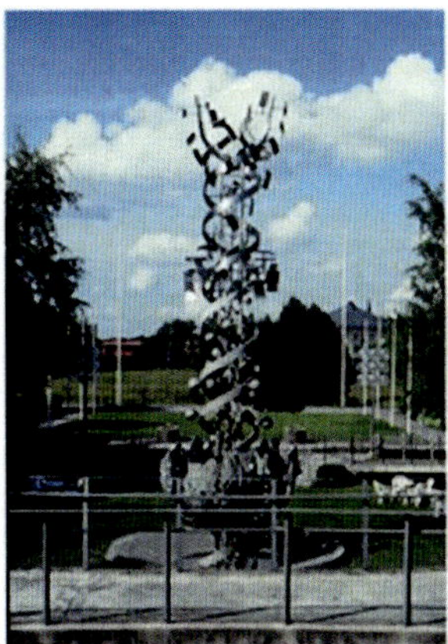
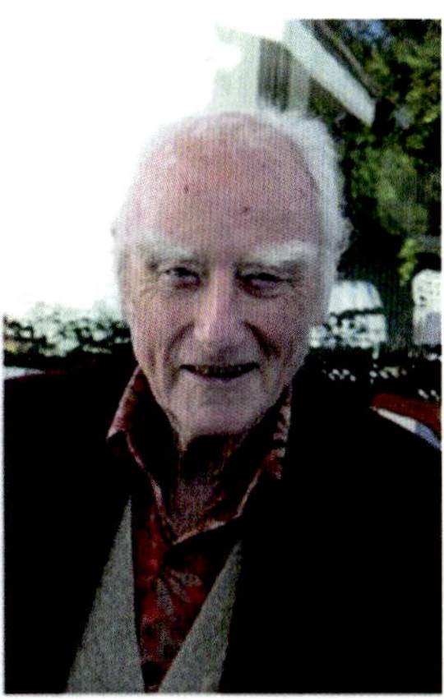

Fig. 12.6 James Watson (*left*) and Francis Crick (*right*) with a statue of the DNA molecule structure. Copyrighted by Springer Science+Business Media B.V.

error. Watson traveled to London to meet with Wilkins, who tried to involve Franklin in the discussions, but she was not interested, even though she had known that the phosphate groups properly belonged on the outside of the helix. Her research strategy was to gather more data before attempting to build a model, while the others were motivated by the race to be first to publish. Also, she was in the process of changing jobs and would be working on another project at the new location. Wilkins, without asking Franklin's permission, decided to show Watson X-ray patterns of a hydrated (water-exposed) form of DNA, providing him with an essential bit of information; the X-ray patterns were much clearer and more revealing than the patterns he had seen before of a dry form of DNA. He returned to Cambridge, and he and Crick furiously began building a physical model using metal plates and rods. They were visited by an American chemist, Jerry Donahue, who told them that a type of chemical bond called a hydrogen bond would explain the pairing of the bases A to T and C to G.

Watson and Crick finished building their model on March 7, 1953. Wilkins came to see it the next day, and after returning to London, Franklin was told of Watson and Crick's work. On March 6, Franklin's two manuscripts on the dry form of DNA reached the editor of Acta Crystallographica, a scientific journal dedicated to the publication of research on crystal structure. Franklin prepared another manuscript on March 17 1953 describing the hydrated form of DNA, but it is unclear how much of that paper was influenced by what she had heard about Watson and Crick's model.

The paper credited as being first to describe the structure of DNA was published by Watson and Crick (Fig. 12.6) in the journal Nature on April 25 1953. In it, they placed a footnote acknowledging "having been stimulated by a general knowledge" of the work by Wilkins and Franklin. Two papers by Wilkins and Franklin describing their X-ray work were published in the same issue of Nature, second and third behind the Watson and Crick paper.

In one of science's great understatements, Watson and Crick wrote "It has not escaped our notice that the specific pairing we have postulated suggests a possible copying mechanism for the genetic material." This of course was exactly correct, and the insight led not only to the field of genetic engineering, but has also contributed to an explosion of new knowledge developed using the techniques of molecular biology.

Watson and Crick won the race to discover the structure of DNA and were joined by Wilkins in receiving the Nobel Prize in 1962. Tragically, Franklin died of ovarian cancer in 1958 at the age of 37; perhaps the X-ray work she did had contributed to the onset of that disease. She was not a co-recipient of the Nobel, and many believe that her contributions have never been properly credited—perhaps an example of sexism in science.

One point to this story is that it demonstrates how science works in the "real world." New knowledge is assembled from contributions by many researchers. Sometimes, mistakes are made. Scientists have egos and burn with the desire to be the first to make a discovery; unfortunately, they are also human and occasionally tend to minimize the contributions of others.

12.3 How to Introduce Foreign DNA into a Cell: Vectors for Genetic Engineering

We have just discussed (in a quite abbreviated manner) one of the most important biochemical processes occurring in living things: the way in which genetic information is replicated. We have also shown how genetic information is responsible for the synthesis of proteins and suggested how mistakes in genetic coding could be responsible for the onset of diseases. These insights can be used to manipulate genetic code, making it possible to modify the expected characteristics of offspring, or in adults, to potentially cure hereditary diseases. The discussions that follow in Sect. 12.3 of this chapter should be understood to be pertinent for human cells in particular; plants and other life forms may also be genetically engineered, but the techniques used would differ.

It should be appreciated that this topic is worthy of its own textbook or textbooks. The formidable background in biology and biochemistry needed to fully understand the techniques of recombinant DNA technology, and the continual rapid evolution of the state of the art, is guaranteed to ensure that this short section can only contain an abbreviated telling of the story.

A primary goal of genetic engineering is to modify the genotype in order to change the phenotype of an organism by manipulating the structure and characteristics of its genes [1]. The first step in gene manipulation is to obtain a source of nucleic acid, e.g., DNA or RNA, by opening cells to expose, extract, and purify nucleic acids. The extracted nucleic acids may then be modified by deletion of gene sequences or by insertion of DNA prepared elsewhere into the host DNA in a process called hybridization. The new, not naturally occurring DNA is called recombinant DNA.

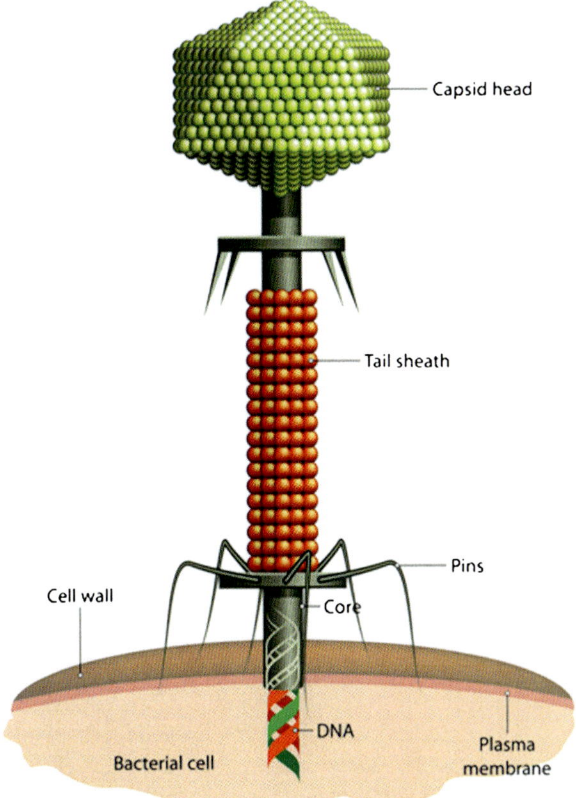

Fig. 12.7 A bacteriophage, a type of virus in the process of infecting (transferring DNA) into a host bacterial cell. It attaches to receptors on the cell membrane and injects its generic material into the host. Similar mechanisms exist in mammalian cells

Recombinant DNA technology was first shown to work in 1972–1974 based on an idea by a graduate student (Peter Lobban) and his mentor (A. Dale Kaiser) at Stanford University. Later work by three other researchers (Werner Arber, Daniel Nathans, and Hamilton Smith), who developed the chemistry that enabled the technology, earned them the Nobel Prize in Medicine in 1978. The first transgenic animal (a mouse) was created in 1974, and the first genetic engineering company (Genentech) was formed in 1976 and announced production of genetically engineered human insulin in 1978. Interestingly, several biological substances of interest to humans, e.g., insulin, are made by bacteria whose DNA has been modified!

The desired DNA molecules must be amplified or copied many millions of times if they are to have any utility for therapeutic purposes. In this case, the rapid growth and replication of bacterial cells can be exploited; a liter of bacterial cells can produce ten times as much of the desired DNA as all the cells in a human body. The desired DNA sequence is linked to the DNA of a carrier called a vector for transport into bacterial cells that have been treated to receive the vector. A common vector that can be used to transport human DNA into a bacterial cell is called a bacteriophage, which is essentially a bacterial virus (Fig. 12.7). Plasmids are circular DNA molecules that can self-replicate and be delivered to the bacterial cell host.

In some instances it is preferred to express the desired gene sequence directly in a human cell, rather than in a bacterial cell. When the inserted gene sequence directs synthesis of a protein, that protein has the opportunity to be modified by carbohydrates and lipids in a normal fashion. Since viruses are very efficient in infecting and replicating their genetic materials in living cells, they can also be used as effective vectors for delivery of recombinant DNA into cells. Viruses used for genetic engineering, e.g., the common cold virus, are modified to minimize their risk by either completely or partially deleting their genetic materials. Viral vectors have three main structures: the genetic materials (DNA or RNA), a protein shell called a capsid that protects these genetic materials from being degraded by the host where it is injected, and in some cases a protein tail that can attach to the host cells and then inject the viral genetic materials into the cells. The desired recombinant DNA is placed in the capsid or inserted into the remaining genetic materials in the capsid. Lipids, peptides, or polymers may also be used as gene delivery vehicles to protect genes from being degraded in the body and to deliver genes to targeted cells.

Viral vectors are far more efficient than plasmids in delivering genetic material to human cells, but they tend to be more complex, can induce a strong immune response by the host, and could potentially be toxic for the body. Nonviral vectors are less efficient and tend to have mostly transient effects but are generally less toxic and very simple, but they too may induce a moderate immune response.

Transfecting bacterial cells using phages or animal cells using a virus, plasmid, or a synthetic vector are examples of DNA amplification using living, in vivo methods. Another way to replicate desired DNA sequences is the polymerase chain reaction, often referred to by its acronym PCR. This method is done in vitro, i.e., in a laboratory setting using special reactors and an enzyme called *taq* polymerase (obtained from a bacterium that lives in hot springs at temperatures of 75 °C). This process, developed in 1988, consists of first heating DNA to 95 °C, causing the strands of DNA to separate. Then, primer molecules are added at a temperature of 55 °C; these primers are specially made to bind to the portions of the DNA molecule of interest. In the final step, the polymerase is added and the temperature increased to 73 °C, and the synthesis of a complementary strand to each template occurs. In this process then, two new DNA molecules are synthesized from one template molecule. The heating and cooling cycles are repeated many times over and can be automatically programmed.

12.4 Genetic Engineering in Plants and Animals

Genetic engineering has been used in agricultural applications for some time. Genetically modified plants (also known as GM crops) have been designed to have high yield, resistance to insects, bacterial or fungal infections, tolerance of harsh environmental conditions, improvements in product shelf life, and/or increased nutritional value. While crops with some of these characteristics have been successfully developed, concerns over possible ecological side effects have limited their widespread use. For example, the gene for toxin production has been inserted into plants such as corn, cotton, and potato to obtain insect-resistant seeds. Although

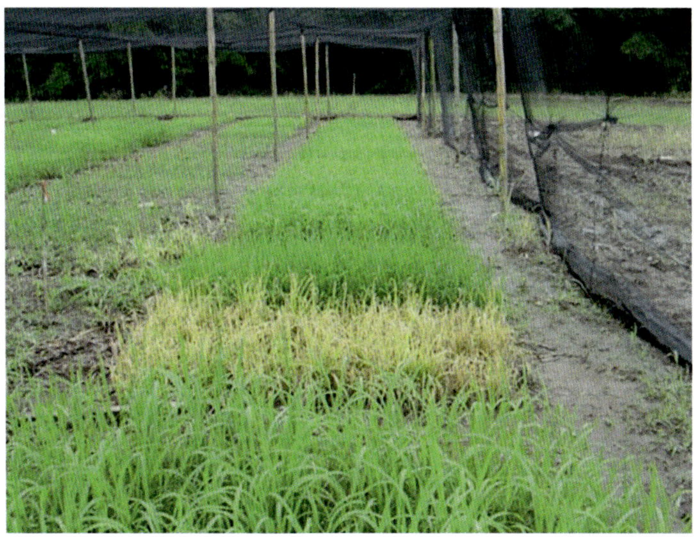

Fig. 12.8 The *green rice* has been genetically modified to resist herbicides, while the *yellow-looking rice* plants are "natural," unmodified rice. Copyrighted by Springer Science + Business Media B.V.

there were some early concerns that modified pollen from such plants could hurt the Monarch butterfly population, a report in the Proceedings of the National Academy of Sciences in 2001 suggests that the potential risk to these insects is negligible.

Other examples of genetically modified crops include pesticide-spray-resistant rapeseeds (rape is a plant widely grown for the canola oil that can be extracted from its seeds), vitamin A-enriched rice, herbicide-tolerant rice (Fig. 12.8), and longer-lasting tomatoes (www.bionetonline.org). The potential advantages of these modified crops are obvious: reduced need to spray pesticide and therefore contaminate the surrounding environment, larger crop yields, and enriching the diet of poor people whose principal food may be rice and who have little access to balanced nutrition.

However, often "it's not nice to fool Mother Nature." What might be some of the undesirable consequences? For example, what about possible "cross-pollination" between plants? GM plants could pollinate neighboring weeds, and the gene responsible for conferring pesticide resistance could then enter the genome of the weeds making them also resistant to pesticides. And, as is the case with bacteria that have become tolerant to antibiotics, the pests that survive feeding on genetically modified plants will become tolerant to pesticides that are normally used in other agricultural applications.

Rice genetically modified to contain elevated levels of vitamin A is sterile, meaning it cannot self-reproduce. In part, this is a safeguard to prevent the uncontrolled spread of a genetically modified crop. However, this characteristic also forces the rice farmer to buy rice seed every planting season and contributes to the yearly profit of the large agribusinesses that tend to be from the West. There is a concern that the poor in undeveloped countries will become overly dependent on the Western world, increasing resentment against the West.

As you may imagine, the idea of genetically modified foods often arouses strong feelings, and sometimes it is not easy to have a rational debate between parties who call it all "Frankenfood" and those who claim it to be without any potential harm. However, we should remember that since the dawn of civilization farmers have been modifying the genome of their crops by only replanting those crops with desirable phenotypes, e.g., replanting seeds of large zucchinis. The difference, of course, is that with genetic engineering, we are modifying the genome of our plants at a much more rapid rate and in a more systematic manner, which may not give us enough time to evaluate the environmental and health consequences of these manipulations. Perhaps the safest course is to institute strong regulatory and review processes. In the USA, the FDA evaluates GM animals as strictly as it evaluates drugs. It published a guidance document in January 2009 for industry that outlined the procedures to be followed in order to obtain FDA approval. In the European Union, several member countries (Denmark, Spain, the UK) appear to be in favor of permitting GM crops, while others resist. These debates, often about the danger of contaminating non-GM seed stock with GM seeds, frequently take on political overtones, with the USA, Canada, and Argentina strongly pressuring the EU to permit importation and sale of GM foods. In 2011, with support from the government of the UK, the EU has permitted the importation of GM crops as animal feed. More information about the regulatory process in the EU, as well as a timeline of various related actions, may be found on the website www.genewatch.org.

What do you think: how much testing would be needed before you felt comfortable with large-scale planting of GM grasses or food plants?

The creation of genetically altered animals is far more complicated in terms of both technical difficulty and ethical implications. Genetic engineering can be used to produce transgenic animals that exhibit human diseases (e.g., sickle-cell anemia). Genetically altered animal models can also be used to perform phenotypic tests with genes whose function is unknown (change the genome and see what happens). However, as discussed below, the genetic engineering of animals has important and significant ethical implications, especially as it relates to applications in humans.

Genetic engineering can be used to generate several different classes of genetically modified organisms:

Transgenic organisms in which a gene or genes are transferred from a different species (e.g., cows that produce insulin in their milk)

Knockout organisms (Fig. 12.9) in which one or more genes of a mouse are selectively turned off (e.g., p53 knockout mice with high incidence of cancer)

Knockin organisms in which a gene is replaced by another to determine if the two genes are functionally equivalent (e.g., a knockin cell line for studies of fungal infections)

Chimera animals that are formed from two or more different populations of genetically distinct cells that originated in different fertilized cells (e.g., a chimeric "geep," mixture of goat and sheep, to study fetus development)

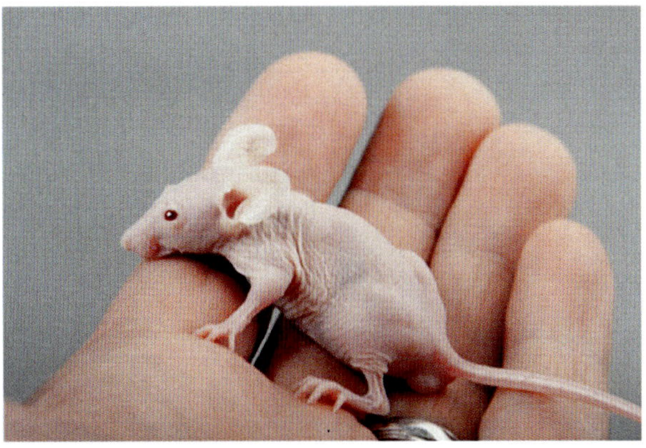

Fig. 12.9 A genetically modified (hairless) mouse

These examples pertain mostly to animals bred for health-related research, pharmaceutical development, or more exotic reasons. For example, researchers are breeding mice that will sniff out bombs! Mice have about ten million neurons devoted to smell; each has just one odor receptor, and each receptor is controlled by a gene. By finding the gene that controls the receptor for a chemical compound similar to TNT (bomb explosive), the scientists hope to tune 10 % of all the neurons to the explosive chemical [2]. Of course, most of us do not come into contact with these modified species. However, the development of GM animals for consumption by humans or for human public health purposes poses a different scenario, because a considerably larger human population is potentially affected, including some who may be unaware of their contact with GM foods or animals.

For example, the UK company Oxitec breeds GM mosquitoes and has sold them to Brazil, where they have been released beginning in February 2011. The reason for developing these mosquitoes is a good one: to control the population of wild mosquitoes, thereby reducing the proliferation of diseases such as dengue fever which is spread by mosquito bites. The Oxitec mosquito breeds with wild mosquito females, competing with the wild males. If mating with the Oxitec mosquito produces larvae, only 3–4 % of the offspring are expected to survive due to the presence of a gene fragment for the herpes virus. It turns out, however, that mosquitoes that come into contact with antibiotics, for example, by feeding on antibiotic-fortified animal feed, could pass on greater hardiness to their offspring. Similarly, no one knows what could eventually happen if these genetically modified mosquitoes bite humans, even though there is no reason to suspect any potential harm.

GM animals grown for food include cows and salmon. While it is true that most research done on such animals is funded by for-profit industry, and the public tends to suspect their motives and question assurances of safety, the US government appears to be quite shy when it comes to funding such research. Since 1999, fewer than 0.1 % of research grants funded by the US Department of Agriculture have been awarded for work on genetically engineered food animals [3]. Examples of proposals submitted include developing salmon that grow to market size more quickly than conventional salmon, pigs that produce more milk to nurse healthier young or to more efficiently digest plant phosphorus resulting in a reduction of

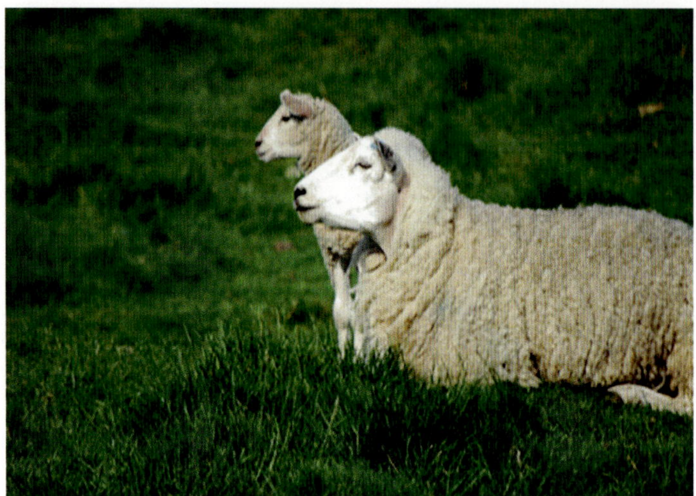

Fig. 12.10 Dolly, the name of the first cloned sheep

pollution from animal waste, goats engineered to produce milk containing human lysozymes (an enzyme naturally found in tears, saliva, human milk, and mucus that destroys bacteria) to combat diarrhea, and cows, sheep, goats, and pigs with increased muscle mass (edible meat) without a reduction in fertility.

Political and economic concerns are sometimes involved. A company called AquaBounty has been attempting to obtain FDA approval for a breed of GM salmon. However, representatives of salmon-exporting states such as Alaska, Washington, and Oregon have introduced legislation in the US Congress to ban the sale of GM salmon. As of January 2013, the FDA has issued a finding that it has no evidence that GM salmon would cause environmental harm.

Animals may also be cloned (Fig. 12.10). Cloned offspring are exact genetic copies of their parents, and contain no recombinant DNA, only the original "natural" DNA. In the USA, the FDA has also addressed this issue in a public risk assessment document issued in January 2008. The FDA has found there to be no potential harm in consuming cloned animal products, and no potential harm in animals consuming feed containing cloned animal tissue. As a result, the FDA does not require cloned animal products to be labeled as such. The lack of a "cloned animal product" label disturbs those who believe that the public has a right to know the source of the food it consumes, but because there has been no finding of risk, the manufacturers are left with the freedom to decide how they wish to label such food products. In focus groups organized by the FDA, approximately one-third of the participants stated that they would not consume such products under any circumstances. Of course, there currently is no easy way for the public to differentiate cloned animals from original animals, so unless there is a public outcry demanding labels, it is likely that consumers will never know if the milk or beef they are consuming came from a cloned animal.

What do you think: would you consume genetically modified foods if there were some benefit such as extra protein or a longer refrigerator life?

12.5 Genetic Testing: Genomics, Proteomics, and Metabolomics

In the previous sections we have discussed the structure of the DNA molecule and how genetic information is replicated. Knowing which genes are responsible for specific traits in plants permits scientists to engineer plant DNA to endow the offspring with resistance to toxins and pests and improve hardiness in times of drought. There is also a great deal of interest in manipulating the DNA of animals used for food in the hope of reducing animal susceptibility to disease and increasing yields of animal products such as milk. The process of introducing GM crops and animals is a slow one, with agencies such as the FDA and USDA requiring considerable proof that the genetically modified plant or animal cannot cause harm to the environment or to consumers. There is also some concern and fear on the part of the public.

Analysis of plant DNA or of snippets of animal DNA is relatively simple when compared with analysis of human DNA. And yet, because every person has one or more genes which can lead to predispositions to various diseases, there is a huge potential payoff if it proved possible to inactivate disease-causing genes. Even acquired conditions, such as trauma and burns, may have genetic components that modulate (affect) their progression. If these genetic defects can be identified, it may be possible to treat the patient by replacing a defective gene with a gene that functions and expresses proteins normally. Of course, this is not at all simple, because most genetic diseases are caused by malfunctions in several genes and replacing all defective genes is not only technically difficult, but may have unknown undesirable consequences. There are very few monogenic diseases, i.e., diseases that are caused by malfunctions in a single gene; examples include cystic fibrosis, muscular dystrophy, and hemophilia. Most genetic abnormalities are, in fact, polygenic, i.e., caused by the combined action of more than one gene (e.g., hypertension, coronary heart disease, diabetes).

While many people tend to think of genetic diseases as those that appear at birth or in early childhood, a large proportion of diseases appearing in later life also have strong genetic components. For example, females with the BRCA1 and BRCA2 genes may be at a much higher risk of developing breast cancer; genetic predisposition may even play a role in the susceptibility to drug addictions. It is exciting to think that it could be possible to change a person's genome and reduce their likelihood of contracting disease; this is the promise of gene therapy;

In gene therapy, treatment or cure can in principle be achieved, but only if the proper or normal gene sequence can be introduced into the patient's DNA. In the late 1980s, it was proposed that the human genome be sequenced and deciphered. The genome is an organisms complete set of DNA including all of its genes. In other words, the order in which the base pairs occurred would be determined; in humans, there are more than three billion base pairs. At the time the idea was suggested, it was unclear what the potential payoff could be, and interest was not unanimous in the scientific community. However, the idea captured the attention of an administrator at the US Department of Energy, who thought the information would be useful in predicting the effects of nuclear radiation on humans.

Also, the project was big enough so that it would keep many of the scientists at the laboratories funded by the Department of Energy busy; there was less and less work needed on nuclear bomb making. Some of the world's most prominent scientists, Nobel Prize winners like James Watson, also became enthusiastic; other scientists wondered why the Department of Energy should be involved in what was essentially a biological project.

As momentum gathered, in 1988 a National Research Council committee gave the idea a thumbs-up; it also recommended that before tackling the human genome, the genetic data for simpler organisms such as yeast, *E. coli*, and the mouse should be determined. That seemed to turn the tide, as even most of the skeptical scientists were convinced of the value of developing genome sequencing technology, and the National Institutes of Health, which had previously not been involved, jumped into the thick of things by naming James Watson to head an office of genetic research. With that move, in effect the NIH had taken over. The work would be conducted in a number of laboratories at various universities and at the NIH, but the NIH would coordinate and fund the project.

Watson began by pushing for identification of portions of the human chromosomes, arguing (partly in jest) that if NIH scientists could find the gene responsible for Alzheimer's disease, members of Congress would be motivated to maintain funding for the project. Progress soon was made; then, in 1991, Craig Venter, a scientist at the NIH, made waves by arguing that sequencing the entire genetic code was a waste of time and that the focus ought to be the genes that cause disease. Also, he and his group at the NIH began patenting genes they had identified, even though they did not know the exact function of those genes. Watson was furious, saying that no one could have the right to patent human DNA; he lost his job at the NIH, and Venter quit too, leaving to form a private industrial group called the Institute for Genomic Research.

Francis Collins was picked to head the effort at the NIH. Both the NIH and Venter's company continued to identify genes, but sequencing the entire genome remained difficult, because the technology needed to do that was not evolving sufficiently rapidly. Nevertheless, the genome of yeast was completed in 1996, and it seemed that the human genome was just a matter of time. The NIH continued to prefer a methodical, organized approach; but that was not Venter's style. In 1998, he announced that he had formed another new company, Celera Genomics, and that they would complete sequencing the human genome in 3 years using new technology and supercomputers, then give the information away. They would make their money by selling analytical expertise to subscribers.

NIH scientists were stunned; what if Congress believed Venter and cut funding for the project to NIH? They were mobilized to intensify their efforts and also launched a campaign to ensure that everyone understood that Venter was able to proceed only because he had had access to NIH data. The race was on, and eventually, even though there were many arguments and recriminations, both the NIH and Venter published human genome data at the same time in 2003—though in different journals. The project ended up costing nearly three billion dollars.

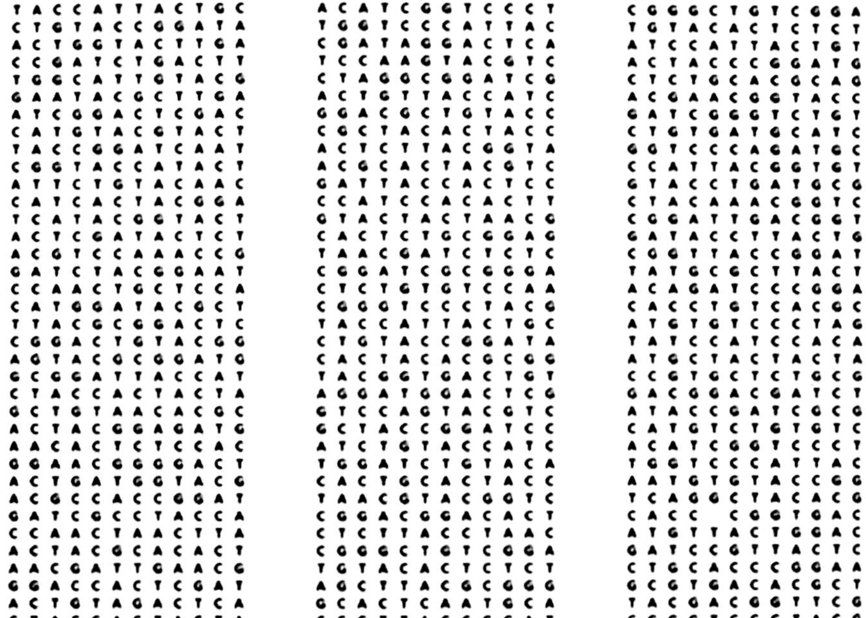

Fig. 12.11 The result of gene sequencing is a depiction of the genome; a small fraction is represented here by a list of the bases in the order they occur

12.5.1 Determining the Genome: Genomics

It should be clear from the history of the Human Genome Project that technology is heavily involved in the analysis of the genome. What is actually done in such a project? How is a human genome determined? The process is called genome sequencing, which involves determining the exact order of the three billion chemical building blocks called bases that make up the DNA of the 24 different human chromosomes (Fig. 12.11). Although there are only four different bases, the DNA molecule is three billion bases long. Human DNA is approximately 2.5 nm thick, but 1–3 m long if stretched out!

One of the first methods used for sequencing, developed by Frederick Sanger in 1977, was used until approximately 2004, though throughout that period it changed and became more reliant on automation. In the Sanger method, each chromosome, containing between 50 and 250 million bases, is first broken into small pieces using heat and chemical methods in a process called subcloning. Then, each of the small pieces is used as a template to generate fragments that differ from each other only slightly, by the presence of a single base. The fragments are also tagged by a fluorescent dye, so that each fragment will glow with a color characteristic of the single base that makes one of its ends chemically different. Many copies of short pieces of the DNA we wish to sequence are made in bacterial culture, because the light signal will only be detectable if large amounts of the target DNA are available.

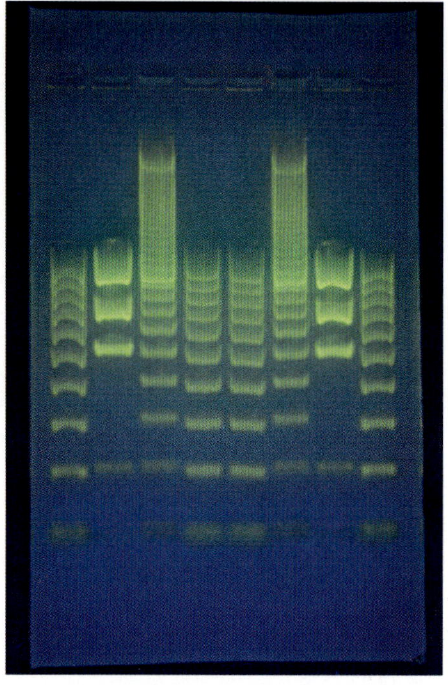

Fig. 12.12 Gel electrophoresis. Agarose gels are first loaded with DNA in solution. Under the influence of an electric field, the DNA molecule fragments move from one end of the gel column to the other. The speed with which they travel depends on the size of the fragment

Then, all the small fragments are separated out by flowing them through a gel packed into a slablike container. The fragments will travel through the gel at a speed proportional to their length. When they come out the other end, an ultraviolet laser is focused on the gel and causes the dye tags to fluoresce (Fig. 12.12). In this way, it is possible to classify fragments of different lengths by their characteristic base.

This methodology, the Sanger method, was overtaken by the development of second generation sequencing methods; these avoid cloning DNA fragments in bacteria and are considerably more efficient. While the first human genome took 10 years to sequence and an additional 3 years for analysis, today it is possible to sequence five human genomes in a single analytical run, producing data in about a week!

Human genome sequencing is not to be confused with DNA profiling, as is done in criminal cases or when testing for paternity. Profiling, first described in 1984 and made commercially available in 1987, relies on analyzing only short segments of DNA (called "short tandem repeats" or STR) that are known to be highly variable between different individuals. That means that the likelihood of a match between two samples of DNA is extremely unlikely, unless they come from the same individual or from monozygotic (identical) twins. If no identical twins are involved, the theoretical possibility of a match is on the order of 1 in 100 billion. Certain portions of the STRs are known to derive from the father and others from the mother, and so parentage may also be evaluated by focusing on those portions.

Automation and sophisticated computer methods (bioinformatics) are now applied to analyzing the DNA molecule. It should be possible to sequence the DNA of any individual who wishes to have that information; several for-profit companies now offer direct-to-consumer genetic testing. All that is necessary is that an individual provides a sample of saliva, pays the required fee ($4,995 as of Fall 2012), and sends the saliva off to be tested. The company will provide a complete analysis of each subscriber's DNA and can indicate which aspects of the DNA may be predictive of developing a particular disease. The information can be useful in some cases; for example, if you are a female whose mother and aunt developed breast cancer, perhaps you would wish to know if your DNA indicates an increased chance of developing that disease yourself. Perhaps the first application of genetic testing in humans occurred in 1969, when Ashkenazi Jews were tested to see if they were carriers of Tay–Sachs, a genetic disease which has a 25 % chance of striking a child whose both parents are carriers. Until testing began, no one could know if they would be likely to conceive a child who was sure to die from the disease.

Genetic testing is no longer the stuff of science fiction; the state of New York, for example, mandates the screening of infant genetic data for 40 different diseases and disorders. The disease called phenylketonuria (PKU), which causes delayed development, mental retardation, and other problems, only becomes apparent later in life. Knowing if a newborn carries the genetic signature for PKU could, for example, enable the parents to ensure that their child followed a strict diet avoiding eggs, milk, and some other foods and thereby avoid development of symptoms in the child. The test for PKY involves detection of a specific enzyme that is produced by the child's genes which is different from the type of testing used for the HEXA gene responsible for Tay–Sachs, which directly looks for the presence of that gene.

Today, genetic tests for specific diseases can also be ordered online for fees below $1,000. Participants in such testing may be asked if they are willing to provide additional information about their phenotype (medical history, traits such as nose and ear shape, etc.). This information can potentially be analyzed to search for correlations between genetic data and medical conditions and outcomes. It turns out that there are about ten million locations in the human genome where the genetic sequence can vary from one individual to another. Sampling those locations and determining if mutations are present that correlate with specific medical diseases or conditions is the approach taken by many commercial entities in this field. Of course, we are not currently able to sample all ten million locations, and a correlation is not causative; the presence of a mutation may increase the likelihood of a particular disease condition, but not in all cases. That is why it should be understood that the interpretation of genomic testing results requires a considerable degree of sophistication and cannot always be done with absolute certainty.

What do you think: would you want to know which diseases you are more likely to develop as a result of your genetic makeup? How about knowing this about your children? Right now, you need to get tested for sexually transmitted diseases before obtaining a marriage license; should you and your future partner voluntarily submit to genetic testing? Would you be willing to marry a person who is healthy now but is likely to develop a serious debilitating disease in a few years?

Perhaps for this reason, professional organizations such as the American Medical Association have called for legislation to force these companies to disclose the results of genetic testing to patients' physicians, rather than directly to the patients themselves. You may decide for yourself if the AMA is more motivated by its concern for patients or by the wishes of its members to control information and even potentially financially benefit from this type of testing.

If you do decide to go ahead with genetic testing, can you be sure that the testing lab won't make any mistakes? After all, if you receive notice that you are carrying genetic code for developing Parkinson's disease, it's not as if you would make any life changes, or would you?

Well, it turns out that mistakes do happen. A report by the United States Government Accountability Office (GAO) issued in July 2010 stated consumers utilizing direct-to-consumer genetic testing received test results that were often misleading, of little or no practical use, and disease predictions that varied widely among companies. Some companies tried to use the test results to market diet supplements to consumers, claiming that the supplements could "repair damaged DNA" even though experts have stated that there is no basis for such claims. Furthermore, sample mixups have occurred with consumers obtaining incorrect information.

Let's assume that you have had genetic testing done, and it was done properly at a reputable laboratory, and the results are valid. What now? Is your information private and will it always be protected? Is there a chance that you might suffer discrimination as a result of your genetic makeup? Furthermore, if you are a woman who has tested positive for predisposition to a familial form of breast cancer, the chances are that your close female relatives (e.g., mother, sister) are also very likely to be predisposed to breast cancer. But did your sister or mother consent to such testing and did they want you to know such information about them? These are of course difficult questions for which we do not have reasonable answers at this time and most likely require that we develop new laws and social frameworks for addressing them.

In 2008, the US Congress passed the Genetic Information Nondiscrimination Act (GINA), which prohibits using genetic information for determining health insurance rates or employment. However, the act does not prohibit the information from being used to determine rates for long-term care insurance or life insurance. So, women who carry the genetic code for breast cancer and men who carry the code for prostate cancer, for example, can't be denied jobs, but they can be denied life insurance.

Regarding privacy, it's important to know that private medical information may not remain confidential forever. In 2009, several parents sued the Texas Health Department and Texas A&M University because they learned that the screening blood collected from their newborns had been kept on file and eventually distributed to scientists for further study. Because the blood samples were collected more than 10 years earlier, when no one would have even dreamed of asking consent for genetic testing, the parents won and the case was settled out of court.

As a result of concerns associated with genetic testing regarding privacy, potential effects on various forms of insurance, potential for mis- or over-interpretation, etc., many people are hesitant to take advantage of this powerful technology to enhance their healthcare. Nevertheless, it is also a fact that progress in predicting and understanding the genetic basis for disease may be critical for developing preventative therapies, for better planning of the life cycle, and for development of new drug strategies for curing disease. For example, sampling the research scientific literature for 2010 and 2011 reveals these genetic-test-related advances: specific gene variants were tied to poor outcomes for patients on an anticlotting drug therapy for heart disease; a patient's whole genome revealed disease and medication risks; three genes were identified that were linked to stuttering in some patients; another three genes were tied to age-related macular degeneration, degeneration, and a blinding eye disease; a new type of blood test for "foreign" DNA appeared to predict the likelihood of transplant failure; and interestingly enough, people with one or two copies of a variant gene called OXTR were found to be less optimistic and with lower self-esteem than people with two copies of a different variant of OXTR.

The likelihood that these types of studies can be useful is markedly increased as more patients prove willing to provide genetic information for research and testing.

12.5.2 Proteomics

A similar current field of research that is likely to have applications in understanding the progress of various diseases is called proteomics. Whereas in genomics we seek to sequence the DNA of an individual, in proteomics we seek to analyze and identify the proteins synthesized by cells. The proteome is extremely dynamic and reflects the state of the cell or tissue as well as environmental stimuli. Therefore, the important goal of proteomics is to systematically study the diverse cellular states and the molecular mechanisms which control them, thus providing an understanding of fundamental biological processes. Because proteomics is the link between genes, proteins, and disease, it complements the information contained in a genome by providing information relevant to drug discovery, diagnostics (biomarkers), and molecular medicine. Advances in proteomics may help scientists design medications that are "personalized" for different individuals and therefore would be more effective with fewer side effects.

This obviously could have important consequences, as, for example, Alzheimer's disease is the result of abnormal deposition of certain proteins in the brain. Many of the best-selling drugs target proteins or are proteins themselves. The task of identifying proteins is complicated by their immense number; in April 2012, the National Human Genome Research Institute of the National Institutes of Health was quoted as saying that humans have approximately 21,000 genes. Earlier, it was thought that there were many more, with each gene producing a single protein, but now, we know that single genes can be responsible for coding more than one type of protein, and fewer genes are needed than the approximately 90,000 proteins found in the human body. While DNA is the same in each cell from a given individual, different cell types produce different proteins, and they can also vary with time and cell condition. Although proteomics has the potential of providing more relevant information than genomics, the problem of analyzing so many proteins under different conditions, and after they are modified by enzymes, is complex and not yet solved.

Some of the technology used in proteomics is somewhat similar to that used in human genome studies. A key issue is to obtain proteins of interest, so, for example, if we were to study protein expression in a specific type of cell, or in a specific cell found in a sample of human tissue, we would need to ensure that the individual cell type was isolated and dissected out. Laser capture dissection functions by melting a sensitive plastic film onto the region of interest, and then the film with the adherent tissue is moved to another instrument for protein analysis.

Proteins are separated using the same approach as in human genome studies; the proteins or protein fragments flow through a gel, and the speed of their flow depends on their size. Once the proteins are separated, they have to be indentified and quantitated. The levels of a protein also determine its reactivity with other biochemical compounds such as drugs or enzymes, and so differences in amounts could provide clues for disease diagnosis. The most comprehensive and versatile tool in proteomics is mass spectroscopy, a technique which provides information about the masses (size, molecular weight) of the molecules in the sample being studied. The implementation of sophisticated software to analyze the data provided by mass spectroscopy is essential.

12.5.3 Metabolomics

The focus of the post-genomic era is to understand functions and interactions within a complex biological system. Genomics has fueled the growth of other "omic" sciences like transcriptomics and proteomics, which, together with the rapid development of instrumentation and bioinformatics, have lead to technology platforms that can now be used in medicine and industry. One of the relatively new "omic" sciences is the field of metabolomics. Metabolomics has been viewed as a vital piece of the "Rosetta stone" for deciphering the puzzle of complex systems. Metabolomics encompasses the study of metabolites and their changes over time as a consequence of stimuli. The concentrations of the metabolites are regulated by enzymes, which are the components of the proteome. Hence, metabolomics studies are complementary to genomics and proteomics studies. More importantly, metabolomics is downstream of the other two "omics," placing it close to the cell's physiologic state.

Information at the level of the metabolome is critical to understanding the function of physiologic pathways to define clinical questions in health and disease. Standard gene analysis technology cannot provide an accurate assessment of metabolites or detect the flux that modifies protein function; this information can be obtained using newly developed metabolomics technologies. In concert with genomics and proteomics, metabolomics can provide a holistic understanding of the physiologic pathways, molecular interactions, and regulatory signals underlying the disease processes. Because metabolome analysis can provide valuable information on drug mechanisms and individual response (or lack of response) to drug treatment, it is also an integral part of drug discovery and the emerging concept of "personalized medicine."

The following quote from an article in the scientific journal Nature regarding the vision of research in the future makes an important point:

> By 2020, personalized health care could involve doctors monitoring the metabolic activities of a patient's gut microbes and, possibly, modulating them therapeutically. The use of mathematical models to interpret metabolic data obtained using Nuclear Magnetic Resonance (NMR) and mass spectroscopy will help us understand the changing patterns of human disease on a global scale, and generate targets for drug or nutritional interventions.

Metabolomics investigations can define underlying changes in human physiology associated with noncommunicable diseases and thereby support development of drugs and other interventions to manage cardiovascular disease, chronic respiratory disease, diabetes, cancer, and miscellaneous chronic diseases. Such data can also support new approaches to morbid conditions that lead to these diseases such as obesity, hypertension, and liver–kidney malfunction. Metabolomics data can help define pathogen physiology and host–pathogen interactions to support drug discovery and development leading to new treatments for infectious diseases such as hepatitis (especially HCV), TB, and AIDS. Because metabolomics methodologies are at the cutting edge of drug targeting and diagnostics, they will be a critical part of research in all universities.

The core of metabolomics is the application of tools from analytical chemistry to profile the maximum number of metabolites found within an organism, tissue, cell, or biofluid. More specifically, metabolomics studies measure multiple (10's to 100's) of metabolites at once and generate metabolic profiles or "fingerprints." In order to perform these studies, a database of all the metabolites in a cell is needed. Fortunately, the Human Metabolome Project is currently underway. The central aim of this project is to identify, quantify, catalog, and store data on all metabolites that can potentially be found in human tissues and biofluids at concentrations >1 μM. Over 6,500 metabolites have already been identified. This database can now be used similarly to gene and proteomics studies to identify metabolites in comparative studies. For example, it was recently reported that the metabolite glycine was found in higher than normal amounts in cancer cells. So, by interfering with the metabolic pathways that involve glycine, it may be possible to reduce tumor growth.

Interestingly enough, it has also been found that many metabolites are found in saliva, and they include some that are not related to oral diseases. Salivary biomarkers have been identified for breast, pancreatic, lung, ovarian, and gastric cancer; potentially, testing saliva could provide important diagnostic information for those diseases.

The "-omics" sciences offer the promise of developing a personalized medicine. This possible future of medicine, introduced by Dr. Collins of the NIH in 2005, recognizes that "one size does not fit all." The same medications administered to patients with different genes may yield different effects. Currently, in 2012, several "pharmacogenetic" tests (tests that establish how genetic variations affect the response to drugs) are available and are being used to design better treatments for patients with childhood leukemia, breast cancer, and heart disease. For an example of the power of this approach, imagine that you or a loved one is found to carry the BRCA1 and BRCA2 genes and so is predisposed to develop breast cancer. One "treatment" pursued by such women is a radical mastectomy. Would it not be desirable to learn how your genetic makeup influences specifically your likelihood of developing breast cancer before taking the more radical approach of mastectomy?

Other advantages of personalized medicine include more accurate dosing and an increase in the availability of new drugs: companies could develop drugs for patients with specific genetic profiles, and evaluating the drug on a population of only such individuals could streamline clinical trials and speed the advancement of a drug to market.

12.6 Case Studies Involving Gene Therapy

Due to the tight regulations surrounding genetically modified animals and their great potential in treating diseases, the concerns expressed over their possible impact on the environment and human health are not as critical. Nevertheless, serious and even deadly side effects of gene therapy for treating human diseases have been observed in a few clinical studies and a more in-depth understanding of the process by which gene therapy may impact the human body is required before the full potential of these powerful therapies can be realized. While the scientific community which discovers and develops these powerful technologies must make sure that they are applied responsibly, the ultimate oversight is and must remain with the society at large and their governmental representatives who regulate this field.

There are essentially three different strategies for gene therapy. In the first, called gene replacement therapy, the physicians must know which defective protein is responsible for disease. With the selection of an appropriate vector, it is possible to deliver genetic material to cells that will cause them to make the normal protein. The second strategy is called therapeutic gene therapy. In this approach, genes are delivered to cells to help them make proteins that treat the disease. An example includes delivering a gene to cancer cells causing them to produce a protein with anticancer properties. Finally, in the third strategy called gene knockdown therapy, genes may be delivered to cells to provide the code to inactivate some genes that are being expressed in the patient. Discoveries associated with this approach have won Nobel Prizes! Control of viral infections like influenza or inactivating blood vessel formation in order to "starve" tumors is possible with this therapy.

12.6.1 Cystic Fibrosis

Cystic fibrosis is a disease passed on by heredity in which heavy secretions of mucus in the lungs make breathing difficult, lead to poor respiration, and contribute to infections. If left untreated, most patients suffering from cystic fibrosis will die by the age of 30. The cause of the disease is a mutated gene, in which ONLY 3 BASE PAIRS of the DNA are missing! As a result, the protein coded by this stretch of DNA is also defective and cannot properly fulfill its role of maintaining the necessary ion balance across the cell membrane. The effect is that the mucus produced by cells in the lungs, pancreas, and small intestine does not contain enough water and is too thick for cilia (small hair-like projections from cells) to move and dispose of potentially infectious particles we breathe in.

Because we know the exact defect and its location in a specific gene responsible for the disease, and because it appears that only one gene is involved, it may be possible to deliver a normal version of this gene into the cells, particularly those lining the lungs as they are accessible using inhaler technology. Knowing the characteristics of the specific cells involved, researchers have used a virus as a vector for delivering the normal gene. Clinical trials began in 1993 and are continuing as adjustments are made to the vector and delivery method, but at the present time, the methods are inefficient and cannot deliver adequate amounts of normal genes to the cells.

12.6.2 ADA-SCID

Adenosine deaminase (ADA) deficiency is an inherited disorder that damages the immune system and causes severe combined immunodeficiency (SCID). Severe combined immunodeficiency caused by the lack of the enzyme adenosine deaminase (ADA) is the so-called bubble-boy disease. Patients who lack the enzyme cannot rid themselves of a natural toxin called "deoxyadenosine," which destroys the body's immune system as it builds up. As a result, the patients have no natural defense mechanisms, and, unless they are protected from the outside world, will always develop infections and never improve. Adenosine deaminase deficiency is very rare and is estimated to occur in approximately 1 in 200,000–1,000,000 newborns worldwide. Treatment options include bone marrow transplants, but these also require medications that inhibit the immune system, or injections of ADA derived from cattle, which carries the risk that the patient will develop antibodies to the drug. This is a rare disease, meaning that the potential market is small and pharmaceutical companies will only participate in developing treatment under the orphan drug program.

The disease derives from a mutation in a single gene, so it is a good candidate for a gene therapy approach. Researchers led by Fabio Candotti at the National Institutes of Health had already developed a way to introduce normal genes into a mouse model of SCID and adopted their approach for treating Katlyn Demerchant, a 2-year-old girl who came to them in 2007. They extracted some of Katlyn's bone marrow stem cells, inoculated them with an engineered retrovirus, and injected the engineered cells back into Katlyn. Six months after the procedure, Katlyn returned home not needing to be isolated any more.

12.6.3 Ornithine Transcarbamylase Deficiency

Ornithine transcarbamylase (OTC) is an enzyme responsible for breaking down nitrogen in the brain; without it, ammonia can build up and poison the brain. James

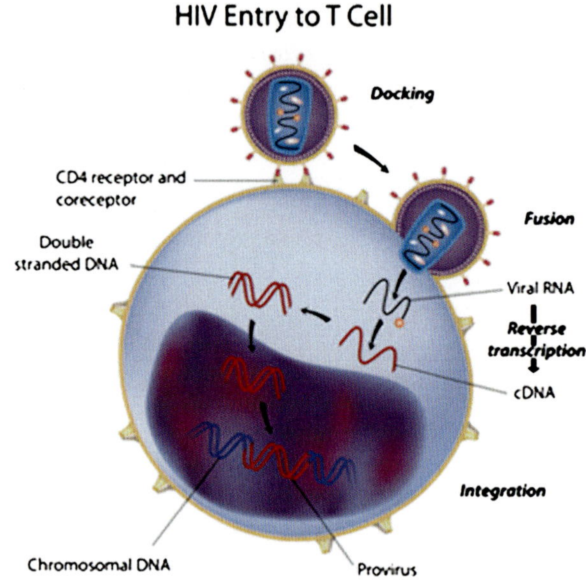

Fig. 12.13 Process of HIV infection. Proteins on the surface of the virus (*red-tipped features*) attach to CD4 receptors (*small yellow protrusions*) on the T-cell surface. This is the docking process and is followed by fusion, when the virus infects the cell by releasing its RNA and some enzymes into the cell. The RNA is translated into viral DNA, which is incorporated into the cell's native DNA. The cell proliferates and makes copies of the altered DNA. Medications called entry inhibitors seek to disrupt the docking and fusion processes

Wilson at the University of Pennsylvania developed a vector based on the adenovirus that causes the common cold which could easily transfer genes from one cell to another and which appeared to be ideal for this purpose. In 1999, Wilson received approval for a Phase I study comprising 18 patients, into whom he injected normally functioning OTC gene using the adenovirus vector. However, the results were tragic in one case, with 18-year-old participant Jesse Gelsinger suffering from massive organ failure and dying 3 days after treatment. It turned out that the virus caused a powerful immune reaction, and to this day, the investigators do not know exactly why Jesse had such a negative reaction to the virus.

Jesse's death almost caused all gene therapy research to stop; researchers were afraid to take any chances. However, this unfortunate event did lead to a better understanding of the role of the vector, and care is now taken to use less immunogenic vectors.

12.6.4 HIV

In 2010, the first gene successful therapy-based treatment of a patient with HIV was reported, in that the patient now appears to be fully cured of his infection without the need to continue antiretroviral drugs (drugs intended for use against retroviruses, which are viruses consisting of RNA, not DNA; HIV is the best known retrovirus). In this case and with other similar patients, the strategy used by researchers was to alter the patients' T cells, which are the immune cells the HIV virus attaches to and uses to replicate itself (Fig. 12.13). You will remember from our discussion of cell surfaces that virus particles and proteins communicate with cells through receptors and that receptors are typically highly specific, responding to and binding a select group of ligands. So, now the researchers' strategy becomes clearer: damage or inactivate the T-cell receptor that HIV binds to! And that's exactly what they did.

The patients first had their T cells removed and modified in the laboratory by exposure to an enzyme called a "zinc finger nuclease" which disables the gene coding for the specific receptor (CCR5) used by HIV. Approximately ten billion cells were reinjected into each patient's body, and studies showed that the modified cells persisted for approximately 6 months. Although this does not represent a final cure for HIV, scientists hope that the treatment can strengthen patients so that they can maintain their disease in equilibrium, i.e., not get any worse.

12.6.5 Parkinson's Disease

There is currently no cure for Parkinson's disease, although there are ameliorating treatments (treatments reducing the intensity of symptoms) ranging from drugs to brain stimulation. As the disease progresses, the patient's tremors worsen because of an overactive brain region, the subthalamic nucleus. The gene therapy approach for treating this disease is to use an associated adenovirus vector containing a gene that codes for glutamic acid decarboxylase (GAD) that helps synthesize a neurotransmitter called GABA and could control tremors. Preliminary studies have shown that the motor skills of patients undergoing gene therapy improved by 23 % as compared with a placebo group's improvement of 12 % [4]. Unfortunately, the improvement is not as great as that which follows brain stimulation, although there is cause for optimism [5].

12.6.6 Rheumatoid Arthritis

Rheumatoid arthritis is an autoimmune disease (the body mistakenly attacks its own tissues) afflicting approximately 1 % of the population, with women being three times more likely to develop it than men. It is characterized by inflammation of the joints, eventual destruction of cartilage in the joints, disfigurement of the joints, and fusion of the joints. The cause of the disease is unknown, and currently accepted treatment options include analgesics for pain, anti-inflammatory drugs, and physical therapy. Because arthritis is not a life-threatening disease, the push for a gene therapy approach has not been as strong as with other diseases. However, current approaches utilize the associated adenovirus vector used for some cases to deliver a gene for a knockdown strategy to suppress the release of inflammatory compounds called cytokines, such as IL1β and TNF-α. IL1β increases cartilage destruction, and it has been the target of more standard medication as well. The vector containing a gene encoding an IL1β agonist (a substance that initiates a response when bound to a receptor) is typically injected into affected joints, in animal models such as rabbits and mice. Inhibiting TNF-α seems to be meeting with more success, with injections of standard medications every 2 or 8 weeks. It is hoped that gene transfer could result in longer-term control and be provided locally (at the site of the disease) rather than systemically as with standard means of dosing. A variety of vectors have been used, including plasmids, adenovirus, retrovirus, lentivirus, and associated adenovirus (AAV), but AAV appears to have the inside track based on its safety, efficacy, and level and length of expression of the desired gene product [6]. However, an interesting recent report had researchers using polymer particles coated with DNA injected into the arthritic site such as a joint and finding that expression of an anti-inflammatory compound called IDO resulted in significant reduction of swelling in an animal model [7]. There are also a number of other molecules that are being explored as targets for gene transfer therapy [6].

Development of more effective approaches could benefit from recent discoveries in the field of "epigenetics," which focuses on ways of discovering the modifications in genes that help determine if someone with a gene that increases the risk of developing a disease actually gets that disease. Recently, researchers have found four chemical tags that appear to be truly linked with the risk of developing rheumatoid arthritis, and all four were in a single gene [8].

12.6.7 Cancer

To date, most gene therapies are used to treat different cancers. Researchers replace missing or altered genes such as p53 (protein 53, a substance that is crucial in regulating the cell cycle and preventing cancer; if the gene encoding this protein is damaged or altered, the synthesis of p53 will be affected and the cell may lose its anticancer "guardian") in attempts to return a natural cancer-fighting ability to the body's cells [9, 10]. Studies are underway to strengthen our own natural immune response, where the thinking is that if our body recognizes a cancer as a foreign body, its strengthened immune system can combat the cancer. The technique involves inserting a gene into white blood cells that will cause expression of a T-cell receptor; in its position on the cell surface, the receptor binds molecules on the surfaces of cancer cells, and the binding event activates the white blood cells to kill the tumor cells.

Because tumors need a food and oxygen source just as normal cells do, they can only survive if they are fed through a network of blood vessels. One gene therapeutic target is prevention of the development of blood vessels in tumors (so-called antiangiogenic therapy, Fig. 12.14), because in order for tumors to grow larger, they require a nutrient supply. Disrupting blood vessel formation by interfering with the action of growth factors (compounds such as vascular endothelial growth factor VEGF and angiopoietin) could in turn interfere with tumor growth. In other attempts to weaken cancer cells, genes are inserted into the cells to make them more susceptible to radiation or chemotherapy. Alternatively, it may be also possible to insert genes into normal cells that will make them more resistant to the side effects of systemic cancer therapies.

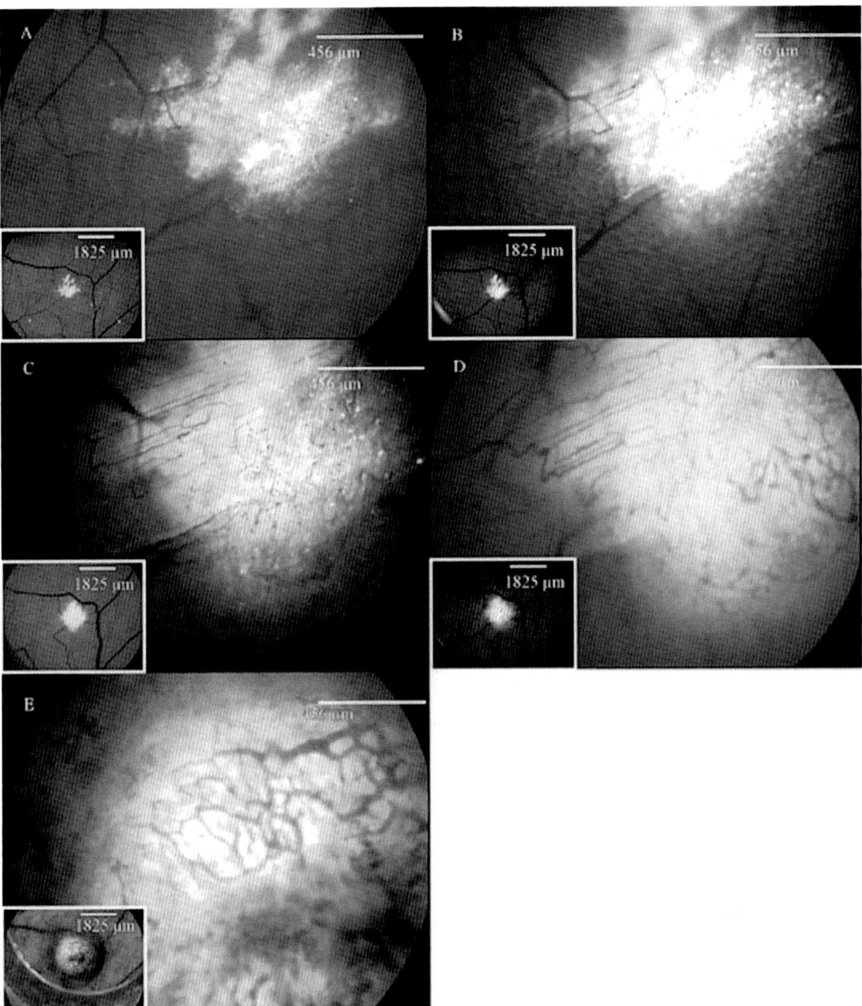

Fig. 12.14 This set of images depict the progress of blood vessel formation (angiogenesis) in an animal infected with a tumor. On day 1 (**a**), no blood vessels are seen in the white tumor area. On day 3 (**b**), the tumor is enlarged, though there is still no evidence of angiogenesis. On day 5 (**c**), tumor growth continues and some twisted blood vessels are seen. The number and size of the vessels continue to increase on day 7 (**d**) and day 10 (**e**). Copyrighted by Springer-Verlag

There are several reports of success using gene therapy for treating cancer. In one such study, melanoma was successfully treated [11]. Drugs are being developed by GlaxoSmithKline that target the communications systems in cancer cells, and in large studies (approximately 300 participants with advanced melanoma) patients experienced a doubling of progression-free survival. Although this cannot yet be considered a cure, it certainly is a step forward in the search for a cure. In another clinical trial, patients suffering from head and neck cancer were treated with an adenovirus vector containing a gene segment that encoded p53, and when the patients were also treated with conventional chemotherapy, tumors shrank for 25 of 30 patients. As was mentioned previously, gene therapy works best if the defective gene is known; then, a replacement healthy gene can be implanted. Leukemia has also been treated; though it was a small study involving only three patients with chronic lymphocytic leukemia who were near death, the results suggested a promising route for treatment [12]. The T cells (white blood cells maturing in the thymus gland that are involved in the immune system) of the patients were removed and modified to express a receptor for B cells (white blood cells whose primary function is to make antibodies). When the modified T cells were reinjected into the patients, they hunted down, bound to, and killed almost all the B cells, cancerous and healthy. This process produced kidney distress and high fevers in the patients, but the three patients have been in remission for at least a year. A benefit with this approach is that altered T cells remain in circulation for years.

Obviously, and as the name suggests, in order to treat cancer by gene therapy, it is important to understand the genetic background of the patient and their particular cancer. We have alluded previously to the concept of personalized medicine, and in that scenario, patients would have their cancers analyzed in order to determine which genetic abnormality or mutation had caused their cancer. With that information, physicians could (in principle) be able to customize a gene therapy targeting that specific patient's cancer. Much more research and data analysis are needed before medical technology reaches that stage. In the meantime, to help identify all the genetic mutations causing cancer, an organization called the International Cancer Genome Consortium (www.icgc.org) collects and publishes data from studies that have identified successes or failures with treatments targeting specific genes. Those data will be vital pieces of information that will assist in the progress of gene therapy.

12.6.8 Homozygous Familial Hypercholesterolemia

Homozygous Familial Hypercholesterolemia (HoFH) is an inherited disease characterized by the patient having extremely high cholesterol levels that lead to heart attacks; the typical life span for these patients is 33 years. The F.D.A. has recently (2013) approved two drugs, Kynamro and Juxtapid, which work by interfering with the messenger RNA responsible for stimulating production of a protein that forms the particles carrying LDL cholesterol in the blood [13]. There are serious side effects associated with at least one of these drugs (Kynamro), and the costs average approximately $250,000/year.

12.7 Summary

The idea of manipulating the DNA of plants and animals can provoke powerful emotions and fears. Imagine how frightening is the prospect of manipulating human DNA, particularly if it were to take place in the embryo. Although it is possible that the manipulation can be carried out for noble purposes (to cure a hereditary disease before the child is born), the technique could also be used for less "noble" reasons. For example, scientists, in principle, could use genetic engineering to enhance appearance, athletic performance, or a work-related characteristic. Now that the technology is out there and being better understood, it is likely that someone, somewhere is likely to try to abuse it. Preventing such a scenario requires that the public remain involved, interested, and, most of all, educated about the potential benefits and harmful side effects of this emerging field.

12.8 Foundational Concepts

- DNA contains the hereditary information of an organism and instructions how to make the proteins that compose the organism. The molecule has the structure of a double helix (similar to a twisted ladder or a twisted zipper), with each side of the zipper called a "nucleotide," and each nucleotide consisting of a repeated three-group link of a sugar, a phosphate, and one of four nucleic acid bases. The order of the bases determines the genetic information, and sequences of bases are called a "gene." The bases on one nucleotide are bonded to the bases on the other nucleotide.
- Gene expression is a process in which (1) the nucleotides are separated by an enzyme, (2) the nucleotides are a template onto which other amino acids congregate to form messenger RNA, and (3) the messenger RNA is released from the DNA and goes on to produce proteins. Not all genes are active in each cell, and not all genes are active all the time, meaning that different proteins may be produced by different cells and at different times.
- Transfection is a means of incorporating DNA into a cell using a vector (carrier) in an effort to stimulate the cell to perform a certain function, such as producing a protein it normally does not produce or to stop it from producing a protein. This technique is used to produce cells that do not usually occur in nature and is the way in which genetically modified crops and animals are made.
- Genetically modified animals may be given genes from other species (they are then called "transgenic"), or the activity of some naturally occurring genes may be turned off (knockout animal varieties), or they may be cloned (no gene manipulation involved).
- It is now possible for humans to have their entire genome (all genetic information) analyzed and to estimate the likelihood of eventually succumbing to a heredity-linked disease such as breast or prostate cancer or Tay–Sachs. However, there is a danger of oversimplistic interpretation of such analyses.
- Gene therapy can follow different strategies: (1) gene replacement (if it is known exactly which gene is missing, the gene may be replaced), (2) therapeutic gene therapy (if the disease is caused by a missing protein, the gene for encoding that protein may be inserted), and (3) gene knockdown therapy (if a gene is being overexpressed, the gene can be inactivated).

– Knowledge of an individual's genome, and a better understanding of how different diseases and drugs interact with proteins, may lead to development of "personalized medicine," where it will be possible to predict exactly which drugs and which concentrations are most likely to aid a specific patient in the treatment of their disease.

References

1. Nicholl, D. (2004). *An introduction to genetic engineering* (3rd ed.). Cambridge, UK: Cambridge University Press.
2. Hotz, R. (2013, March 9). Sniffing out a more-efficient mine sweeper. *The Wall Street Journal*, New York.
3. Maxmen, A. (2012). Politics holds back animal engineers. *Nature, 490*(7420), 318–319.
4. Morgan, P. (2011). *Gene therapy, successful against Parkinson's, continues on the road to redemption.* Discover http://blogs.discovermagazine.com/80beats/2011/03/17/gene-therapy-continues-on-the-road-to-redemption/#.UOcN-qXzbHh
5. Sheridan, C. (2007). Positive clinical data in Parkinson's and ischemia buoy gene therapy. *Nature Biotechnology, 25*, 823–824.
6. Traister, R., & Hirsch, R. (2008). Gene therapy for arthritis. *Modern Rheumatology, 18*, 2–14.
7. Huang, L., Lemos, H., Li, L., Li, M., Chandler, P. & Baban, B. et al. (2012). Engineering DNA nanoparticles as immunomodulatory reagents that activate regulatory T cell. *The Journal of Immunology, 188*, 4913.
8. Kolata, G. (2013, January 20). Study finds how genes that cause illness work. *The New York Times*, New York.
9. Roth, J. (1996). Adenovirus-mediated p53 gene transfer to tumors of patients with lung cancer. *Nature Medicine, 2*, 985–991.
10. Roth, J., Swisher, S., & Meyn, R. (1999). p53 tumor suppressor gene therapy for cancer. *Oncology, 13*, 148–154.
11. Morgan, R., Dudley, M., Wunderlich, J., Hughes, M., Yang, J. & Sherry, R. et al. (2006). Cancer regression in patients after transfer of genetically engineered lymphocytes. *Science, 314*, 126–129.
12. Porter, D., Levine, B., Kalos, M., Bagg, A. & June, C. et al. (2011). Chimeric antigen-receptor-modified T cells in chronic lymphoid leukemia. *New England Journal of Medicine, 365*, 725–733.
13. Pollack, A. (2013, January 29). F.D.A. approves genetic drug to treat rare disease. *The New York Times*, New York.

A Trip to the Dentist 13

Every tooth in a man's head is more valuable than a diamond.

Miguel de Cervantes, *Don Quixote,* 1605

The fluoridation of water in many US communities is estimated to have saved between $16 and $19 per person per year [1]. The cumulative effects of these savings, measured against an average per person annual cost of $0.50 per person, are enormous. And yet, in the past few years, several communities are discontinuing water fluoridation, with some politicians arguing that the introduction of fluoride should be a personal and individual decision, not one made by government [2]. Now, fluoridation has joined other hot-button topics in the debate about government's role in healthcare policy.

Although the incidence of tooth decay has markedly decreased since the adoption of drinking water fluoridation, occasional visits to the dentist are still needed for treatment of gum disease and malocclusion (requiring orthodontic treatment). In this chapter, we will explain many of the common procedures and enabling technologies that a dentist uses to treat oral disease.

13.1 Introduction

Have you ever noticed that, for some reason, most health insurance policies readily pay for visits to a physician, but not for dental care? Granted, dental problems are not usually life threatening, but neither is the common cold. Perhaps this discrepancy in payment options explains why most folks reserve trips to the dentist for cases of real need: the pain of a toothache.

Other than treating painful teeth, however, the dentist can take advantage of several technologies to treat a variety of other oral health problems, including improved mastication (chewing) and esthetics. It's doubtful that dental patients get many

G.R. Baran et al., *Healthcare and Biomedical Technology in the 21st Century: An Introduction for Non-Science Majors*, DOI 10.1007/978-1-4614-8541-4_13,

opportunities to ask questions of a dentist; often their mouths are packed full of suction devices, irrigation devices, gauze rolls, and the fingers of the dentist. Here, we will discuss several dental technologies, note areas where advancement has been made, remove some of the mystery surrounding a visit to the dentist, and try to reduce some of the phobias that accompany dental treatment.

13.2 Tooth Structure

Figure 13.1 is a schematic diagram of a tooth. Although this is a molar (a back tooth or a posterior tooth), all teeth have certain common characteristics. The external surface is composed of dental enamel, a hard and brittle material. Underneath the enamel lies the dentin, which contains less mineral and is not as hard. They are connected together through an interface called the "dentinoenamel junction." The tooth is an extremely well-evolved structure [3]. The external hard shell of enamel is wear resistant to enable chewing, and the interior dentin is softer and less rigid, allowing it to serve as a shock absorber when the tooth is subjected to force (chewing or trauma). Located within the dentin is the pulpal chamber, which is composed of soft tissue that includes a nerve and blood vessels. The nerve and blood vessels pass from the pulp through the roots and out the tip of the tooth (apex) and connect to the external body. The nerve allows you to feel pain if the tooth is damaged, and the

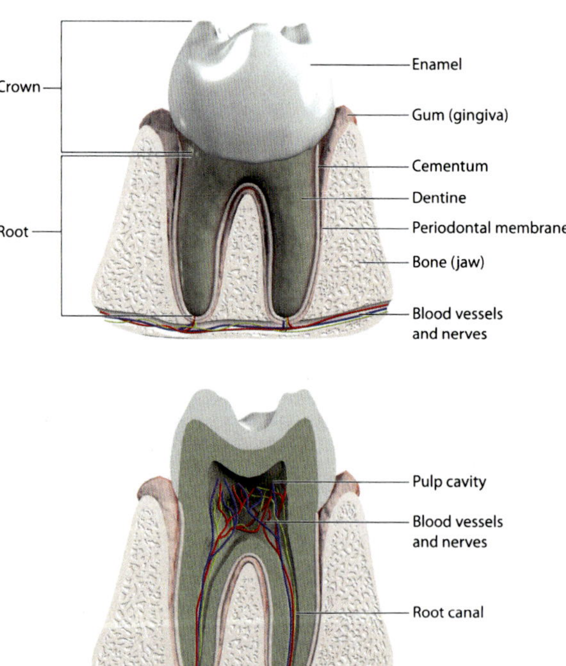

Fig. 13.1 A schematic diagram of a posterior tooth (molar)

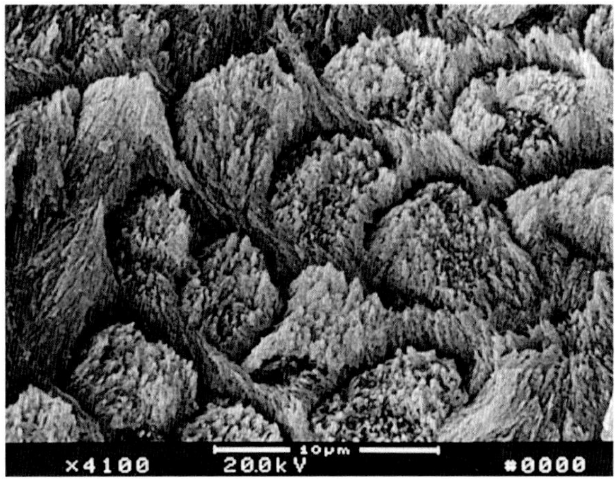

Fig. 13.2 High-magnification scanning electron microscope image depicting acid-treated dental enamel

blood vessels provide nutrients to the living cells lining the surface of the pulp chamber (odontoblasts). The cementum, a calcified layer, covers the tooth roots.

The tooth enamel consists of rods of hydroxyapatite mineral arranged with the long axis perpendicular to the surface. Enamel is the most highly mineralized tissue in the human body, consisting of 96 % by weight of hydroxyapatite; the remaining 4 % consists of proteins and some water. The mineral density is not constant across the enamel prism, with the result that enamel exposed to an acidic solution will not dissolve uniformly, revealing a regularly pitted surface when viewed at high magnification (Fig. 13.2).

13.3 The Dental Exam

13.3.1 Looking for Decay

The beginning of a visit to the dentist is similar to a visit with a physician. For new patients, a health history is obtained, and for returning patients the health history is updated. It's important for the dentist to know if the patient is on medication for some other condition, or if there is a history of heart trouble or reaction to anesthesia. If the visit is a regularly scheduled checkup, the dentist will closely examine the teeth, especially the narrow pits and fissures found on the occlusal surfaces of back teeth (the surfaces that are involved in chewing; Fig. 13.3). The dentist is looking for discoloration in the pits and fissures and any evidence of enamel breakdown and softening.

The dentist may use an instrument with a curved and pointed tip called an explorer to probe the occlusal surfaces of the teeth, searching on those surfaces for a "catch" of the explorer's tip: a place where the tip gets caught in a pit or fissure. Should that happen, the dentist will examine that area more closely, because decay is more likely to occur in a pit than on a smooth surface. The dentist will also probe

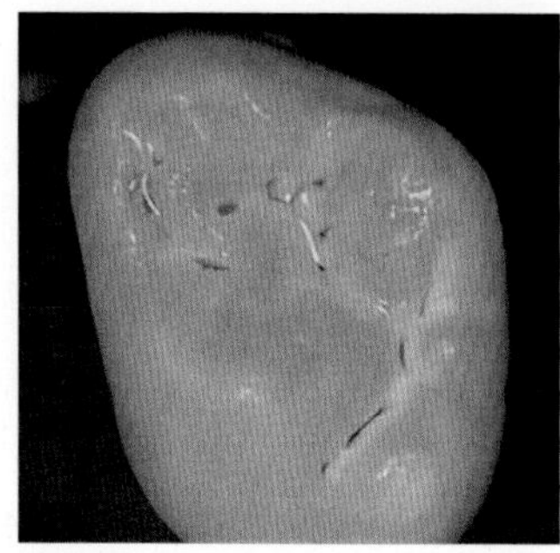

Fig. 13.3 View of the occlusal surface of a molar (rear tooth) showing discolored pits and fissures. Image courtesy of Dr. Kenneth Boberick

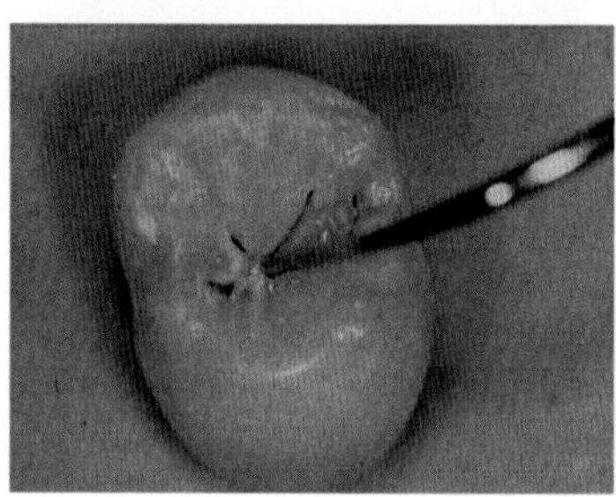

Fig. 13.4 Use of an explorer to probe the pits and fissures where tooth decay often begins. Image courtesy of Dr. Kenneth Boberick

to find an area that is soft, because decaying tooth structure is softer than healthy tooth structure (Fig. 13.4). Routine use of an explorer is gradually being replaced with a more visual, less invasive, determination of dental decay based on evaluation of the color and opacity of the enamel surrounding the pits and fissures. Discolored fissures with areas of opacity (white) radiating up the inclines, as shown in Fig. 13.3, would be considered suspicious and require further evaluation, possibly by X-rays.

About once a year, the dentist will obtain X-rays of the patient's teeth, in particular of the molars and premolars, which are located in the back of the mouth. They have many naturally occurring pits and fissures and are difficult to clean because of their location, and so it is possible that they will begin to decay before teeth at the front of the mouth. The X-rays will also help the dentist to identify decay that may be occurring under existing restorations or between the teeth, areas not easily visualized during the oral exam. The X-ray images are called "bitewings" (Fig. 13.5).

If one compares the diagram (Fig. 13.1) with the bitewing X-ray (Fig. 13.5), one can perceive how the different materials in a tooth are visualized on an X-ray, as different portions of the tooth have different X-ray attenuation coefficients. On a healthy tooth, the mineralized enamel on the outside of the tooth absorbs more of the X-ray than the less mineralized dentin found just underneath the enamel. The enamel contains more hydroxyapatite mineral (96 %) than the dentin (70 %); the portion of the tooth on the X-ray in Fig. 13.5 that shows up as bright white is a silver filling, a dental amalgam. Because it is metallic, it has a higher attenuation coefficient for X-rays than the enamel. Between two of the teeth, and highlighted by a circle, is a zone of enamel and dentin that appears to be a weak absorber; it is said to be more "radiolucent." This zone, particularly when it is compared with other

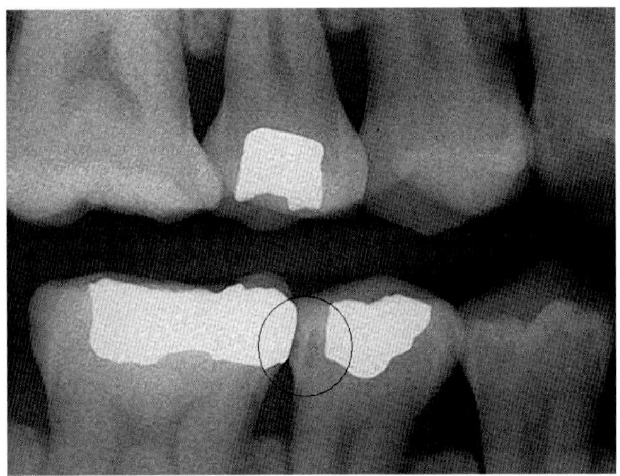

Fig. 13.5 A bitewing X-ray picture of posterior teeth. Inside the circle is an area of decay, which is less mineralized and shows up as a dark (radiolucent) area. The pulp tissue (nerves and blood vessels) in these teeth is clearly visible as a dark radiolucent area at the center of the tooth extending from the top of each tooth (the crown portion) down the root into the jaw bone. Image courtesy of Dr. Kenneth Boberick

areas of normal dentin, will indicate to the dentist that tooth decay is in progress between the teeth. It was mentioned earlier that decaying tooth structure was softer than healthy structure; that's because decay causes a loss of hydroxyapatite mineral as it is dissolved by acid produced by bacteria. For the same reason (i.e., loss of mineral), the decayed zone is more radiolucent than healthy tooth structure. In cases like this where decay is between the teeth or under an existing restoration, X-ray imaging is crucial if decay is to be detected, because the location of the decay makes it difficult to see during a dental examination. It is likely, however, that the patient was experiencing some sensation in that tooth, perhaps to temperature extremes, e.g., cold or hot foods or liquids.

13.3.2 Other Oral Issues

The dentist will look for other signs of oral health problems, including signs that patients do not brush properly, evidenced by a particular wear pattern on the teeth (Fig. 13.6).

This missing tooth structure is difficult to replace, because preparation of the tooth for a filling (drilling with a bur) is contraindicated when there is no decay present; and if a preparation is attempted, healthy tooth structure will be removed.

The soft tissues in the mouth are also susceptible to disease. There are several billion bacteria happily residing in your mouth (yes, humans have filthy mouths), and scientists have identified approximately 700 different kinds. Many of these bacterial species are capable of adhering to a tooth surface, forming a biofilm that traps food debris, and forming a bioactive layer on the tooth called "plaque" (Fig. 13.7). The soft bioactive plaque layer is what should be removed when brushing and flossing the teeth. Bacteria require at least 24 h to mature and begin colonizing the surface of a tooth, and that is why daily brushing and flossing are important. If it is not removed, plaque eventually turns into a hard substance called "tartar" (Fig. 13.8),

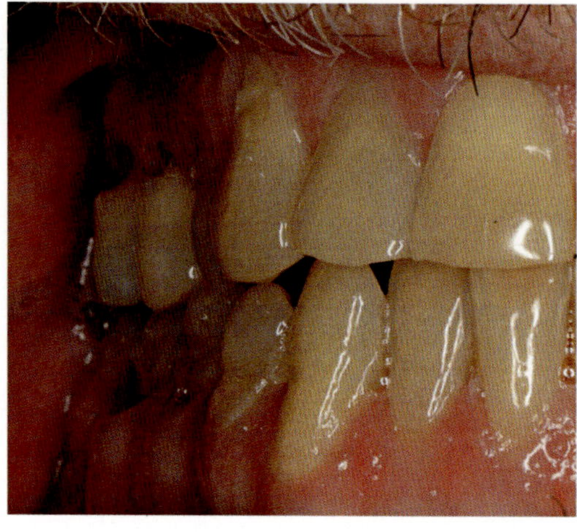

Fig. 13.6 Loss of tooth structure near the gum because of heavy occlusion combined with vigorous and improper tooth brushing. Image courtesy of Dr. Kenneth Boberick

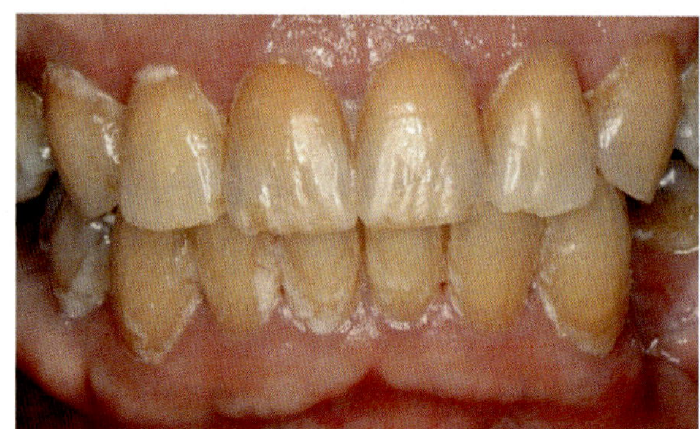

Fig. 13.7 Accumulation of soft plaque resulting in gingivitis. Note deposits on the teeth. Image courtesy of Dr. Kenneth Boberick

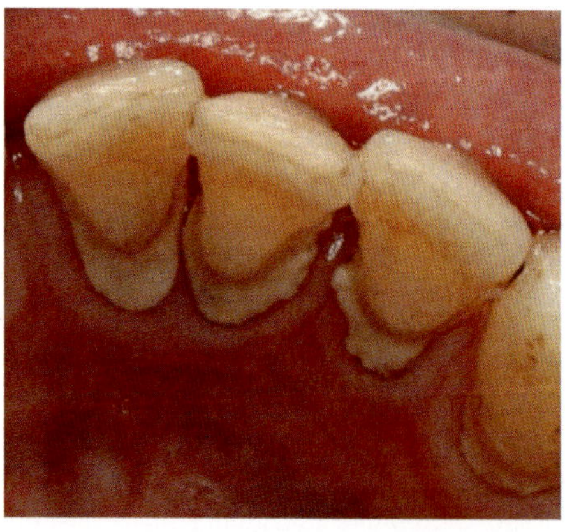

Fig. 13.8 Calcified plaque, called tartar (the white material), near the gum line. Image courtesy of Dr. Kenneth Boberick

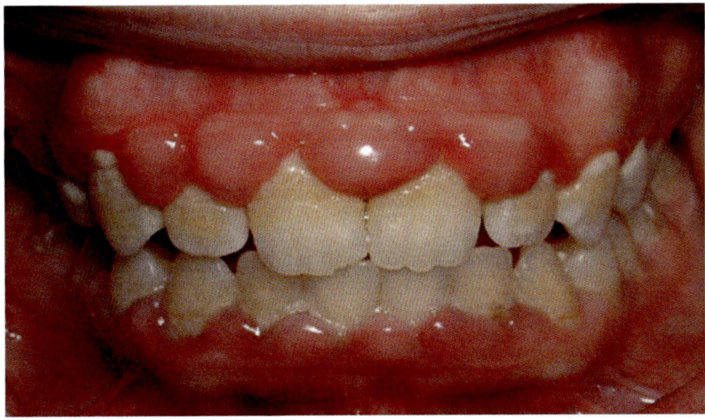

Fig. 13.9 Advanced periodontitis. Note inflammation and swelling of gum tissue. Image courtesy of Dr. Susan Chialastri

which can only be removed at the dentist's office during a tooth cleaning procedure, when the tooth surfaces are scraped with an instrument called a "scaler." If the tartar is not removed, gingivitis (inflammation or reddening and swelling of the gums) may progress to a disease state called "periodontitis," a more serious condition characterized by loss of bone in which the teeth are anchored [4].

Figure 13.9 shows an advanced state of periodontitis, where gum tissue has become swollen and inflamed, has detached from the tooth, and formed a "pocket" next to the tooth. The pocket collects bacteria and food debris, all the necessary ingredients for an infectious site. Sometimes, a dentist specializing in diseases of the gum (a "periodontist"), will perform surgery, cutting away portions of the gum to reduce the size of the periodontal pocket. Surgery can expose the root surface of the tooth resulting in sensitivity to temperature with patients reporting pain after eating cold ice cream or drinking hot coffee. Replacement of missing bone and gum is not always possible and eventually the tooth may be lost. Preservation of gum tissue is important, particularly as we age, because gums recede naturally as part of the aging process and will therefore expose more of the tooth root. The expression "long in the tooth," sometimes used to refer to an older individual, comes from the shrinkage of the gums that occurs in old age.

A patient complaining of neck pain or a sore jaw will have the occlusal surfaces of their teeth examined for evidence of wear; bruxing is the habit of grinding teeth while asleep and which may cause not only pain but also extreme occlusal wear and possibly cracks to form in the tooth structure. Figure 13.10 shows the occlusal surfaces of a typical bruxing patient. The most common cause of bruxism is stress, and the best treatment is prevention either through behavioral modification to reduce stress or the fabrication of an occlusal guard. The occlusal guard is made from a polymer called acrylic and is worn at night providing separation of the teeth preventing tooth-to-tooth contact and resultant wear (Fig. 13.10).

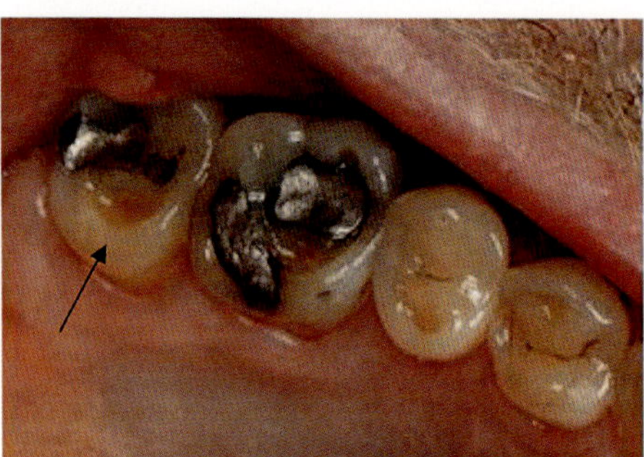

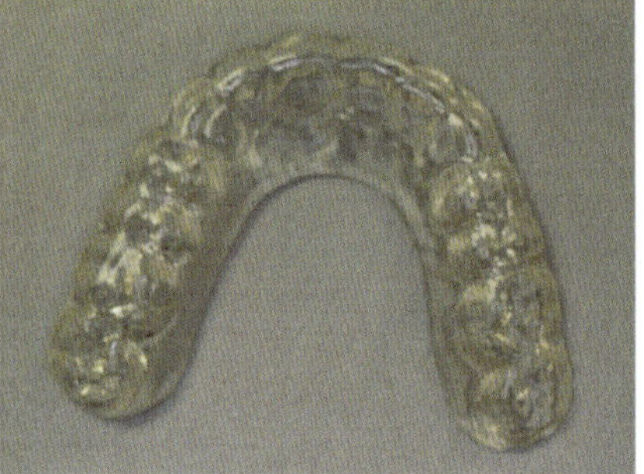

Fig. 13.10 (*Left*) Occlusal wear from bruxism. (*Right*) An occlusal nightguard made from polymer acrylic that is worn over the upper teeth and prevents wear caused by tooth to tooth contact. Image courtesy of Dr. Kenneth Boberick

A dentist will pay particular attention to the way a young patient's teeth are growing in (erupting) and what the patient's "bite" (occlusion) is like. If the teeth are found to be crowded or growing at improper angles, either orthodontic treatment with possible extraction of teeth to provide adequate space for the neighboring teeth (for mild malocclusion) or orthognathic surgery (for severe malocclusion) will be indicated.

13.4 Dental Treatments with No Tooth Preparation

The desire to improve body image and facial esthetics is a motivating factor for many patients to visit the dentist. As a result, procedures and materials have been developed that allow the dentist to improve the esthetics of a patient's oral appearance. For example, tooth whitening has become popular with patients looking for a brighter smile.

13.4.1 Tooth Bleaching

The determination of tooth color or shade is largely a factor of the interaction of light as it passes through the outer layer of enamel and is reflected back by the underlying dentin. Some people have naturally whiter enamel and teeth, but that whiter shade can become discolored for a variety of reasons. A lifestyle that includes either heavy tea or black coffee consumption, or smoking, will cause teeth to darken. These stains are on the surface of the teeth (extrinsic) and can usually be removed with regular cleanings. The teeth of older patients are naturally more yellow than those of younger patients because the enamel has worn away allowing the darker dentin to show through. Some medications (tetracycline given in early childhood) can discolor teeth, but this only occurs during the development period of the tooth; tetracycline consumption will not affect the tooth color after it has erupted into the mouth. Tetracycline stains are inside the tooth (intrinsic) and cannot be removed by cleaning.

If a patient is unsatisfied with the color or brightness of their teeth, the dentist can proceed with a tooth bleaching procedure. This process utilizes a chemical called carbamide peroxide, which decomposes in the presence of water to form hydrogen peroxide; it is the hydrogen peroxide that is responsible for whitening the teeth. The carbamide peroxide is suspended in a gel to prevent it from easily flowing away from the tooth, and a custom-made tray, like a mouthguard, is used to contain the gel. The tray is filled with the gel and placed into the patient's mouth so that the tray surrounds the teeth. It remains there for a period of time (approximately 30 min) and is then removed. The treatment is repeated several times over the course of many days until an acceptable shade or color is achieved. There are also home kit versions available, but they may not contain the same strength of peroxide as is available at the dentist's office, so that home treatments generally take a longer time to show an effect.

There is a lack of agreement as to the exact mechanism of tooth bleaching, but it is believed that the peroxide penetrates into the enamel and eventually into the dentin, where it bleaches some of the naturally present organic compounds. Bleaching is a procedure that requires periodic maintenance, meaning the effects of bleaching treatments are not permanent, and for many patients there may be a bounce-back effect, with some of the bleached-out color returning, requiring re-bleaching. Bleaching with a strong concentration of carbamide peroxide, bleaching for a longer duration than recommended, or bleaching exposed root surfaces (with no enamel cover) can cause tooth sensitivity. This sensitivity usually decreases and disappears over time after the bleaching has stopped.

13.4.2 Tooth Sealants

"An ounce of prevention is worth a pound of cure" is a phrase we've all heard; no truer words could be spoken when it comes to dental care. The anxiety associated with dental treatment usually is related to a need to repair a decayed or missing tooth. Thankfully, due to improvements in preventive care, the incidence of dental decay continues to decrease in the USA. We have already discussed the pits and fissures present on tooth surfaces (Figs. 13.2 and 13.3), and these are often the sites where decay can start. It makes sense, therefore, to seal the openings of the pits and fissures, thereby ensuring that bacterial and food debris cannot get trapped inside. In fact, this has been proven to be an effective preventive procedure and is commonly done to the teeth of children, because young teeth are most susceptible to the development of tooth decay (called "caries") because of poor oral hygiene and a high-sugar diet. Take another look at Fig. 13.2; there, you will note the rough surface of enamel exposed to an acid solution for approximately 40 s. On a microscopic level, the surface appears rough, and it is this roughness that provides the micromechanical retention necessary for bonding a protective coating of polymer. In the tooth sealing procedure, the dentist will first clean the occlusal (the top, flatter surface) portion of the tooth, then expose it briefly to a solution of phosphoric acid, rinse the acid solution off, and finally dry the tooth surface. Then, a very small amount of an epoxy-like resin is painted onto the etched surface and exposed to an

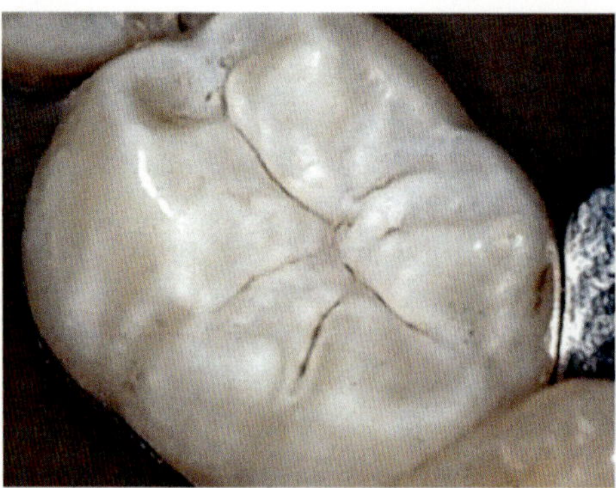
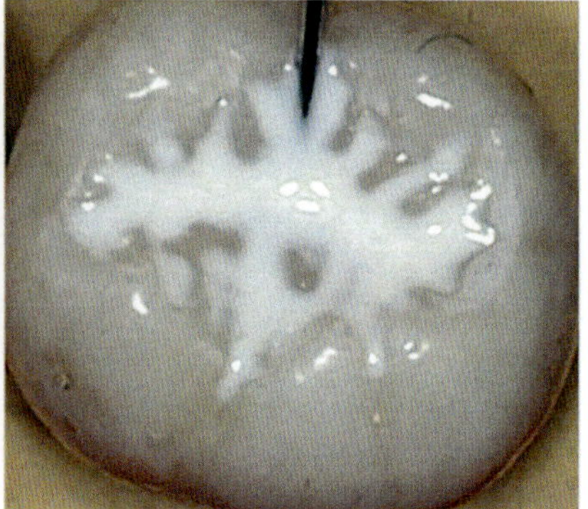

Fig. 13.11 (*Left*) Drying a tooth that has been acid etched produces the characteristic "frosty" appearance shown. (*Right*) The sealant material located in the tooth fissures contains a coloring agent that will permit the dentist to ascertain if the sealant has remained in place during subsequent appointments. Image courtesy of Dr. Kenneth Boberick

intense white light. Recall that some thermosetting polymers harden (cure or polymerize) through the action of heat or mixing together of two components, one containing a catalyst and the other containing an accelerator, while others contain a catalyst that is activated by irradiation with light. The dental resins are the latter type of polymer; exposure to the light for approximately 30 s will harden the resin on the tooth surface. Before it hardens, the liquid resin will flow around and penetrate the microporosity on the acid-etched surface of the tooth enamel. After hardening, the resin will be mechanically locked in place. The dentist knows the acid etching of the enamel was successful when drying the tooth produces the frosty appearance shown in Fig. 13.11. Eventually, the sealant will be worn away through chewing and may be reapplied if in the judgment of the dentist the patient is still in the high-risk category of developing dental caries. This is a low-cost yet effective method to reduce the chances of developing decay on the occlusal surfaces of teeth; note that sealant is not used between teeth (interproximally), the other area where decay often occurs, because there are no pits or fissures there, and application of etchant and sealant is difficult in this relatively inaccessible area. Figure 13.11 shows a sealant material applied to the pits and fissures of a molar tooth.

13.5 Restoration of Decayed Teeth

Perhaps no other sound is as distressing to the dental patient as the high-pitched whine of the dental drill (called a "handpiece"). These highly engineered devices are essential in the preparation of teeth requiring reconstruction. There are two types of handpieces: high-speed running at speeds up to 400,000 revolutions/minute (rpm) and low-speed running at speeds between 5,000 and 25,000 rpm. The engine driving these handpieces is a small air turbine. An air hose connected to the rear of the handpiece conducts pressurized air into the handpiece, past and through the vanes of a turbine, making it spin.

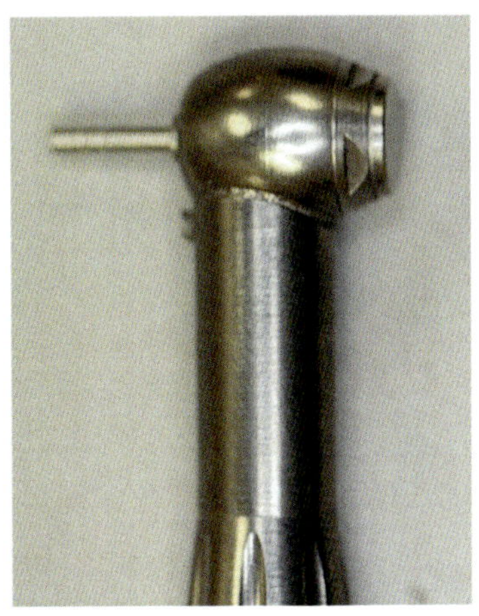

Fig. 13.12 Close-up of the head of a dental handpiece with a dental "bur" (a cutting tool, usually coated with fine diamond powder) attached in the chuck. Image courtesy of Dr. Kenneth Boberick

The head of the handpiece (Fig. 13.12) is designed to hold the bit, the part that actually contacts the tooth and grinds it away. The bit used in dentistry is called a "bur," and is made typically with a stainless steel shaft, and coated with extremely hard carbide or with diamond particles. The coating needs to be harder than the tooth enamel in order for the bur to cut effectively through enamel. Most burs are one-time use only, but some burs are reusable and are cleaned and sterilized (as are the handpieces) after having been used with a patient. In order to minimize damage to the pulp tissue (nerve) and to improve cutting efficiency, the handpiece head also contains outlets through which a water spray is directed onto the site where cutting is being done. The water spray cools the bur and the tooth structure and carries away particles of tooth debris. That is why this procedure is accompanied by the presence of a water suction tube inserted into the patient's mouth, to carry away the cooling water. Some dental handpieces also have fiber optics built into the handpiece head, directing light where the cutting is being done so that the dentist has a better view of the work site.

Because of its high mineral content, dental enamel is quite hard; high-speed handpieces are used to cut away this portion of tooth structure. However, dental caries usually progresses beyond enamel and into the dentin. This tissue has a much lower mineral content, and decay advances much more quickly in dentin than in enamel. Because of its relative softness, and because the dental pulp is close, the dentist will typically change to a low-speed handpiece when cutting dentin. This handpiece cuts more slowly giving the dentist more control, lessening the danger of accidental penetration into the pulp.

When preparing a tooth for restoration, it is essential to remove all traces of tooth decay. Although decay has a different color than healthy tooth material, the dentist may also use a special dye that only binds to decayed tooth material, allowing him to see if any decay remains. After removal of the decay, the completion of tooth preparation depends on the type of material that will be used: dental amalgam (silver filling material) or dental composite (a white, toothlike material).

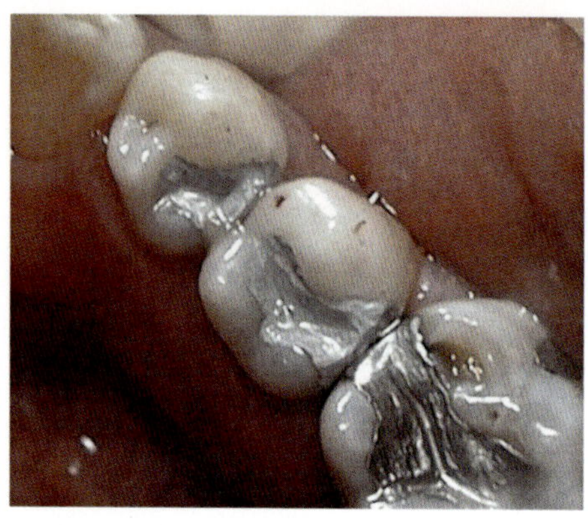

Fig. 13.13 Two recently placed amalgams (*upper left* and *middle*) and one older, slightly discolored amalgam restoration. Image courtesy of Dr. Kenneth Boberick

13.5.1 Restoring Teeth Using Dental Amalgam

Dental amalgam has been part of dental technology for over a century [5]. The material consists of two components: liquid mercury and an alloy of silver, tin, copper, and a bit of zinc. The alloy is prepared separately by first melting the various metals together, then spraying the molten mixture through a special nozzle, so that as the alloy cools and freezes, it forms small particles approximately 30 μm in size. The phase that forms has the chemical formula Ag_3Sn and contains dissolved copper and zinc. Some alloys, those containing higher amounts of copper, will consist of Ag_3Sn and Ag_3Cu_2.

The powdered alloy and liquid mercury are packaged in a way that keeps them separated until ready for use. Then, the dentist's assistant will take the capsule containing the two components and place it into a machine that rapidly shakes the capsule, allowing the mercury and alloy powder to combine. After 10–15 s of mixing, the amalgam is ready to be inserted into the prepared tooth, as it begins to harden after mixing. A chemical reaction occurs between the mercury and alloy, causing the mercury to combine with silver, tin, and copper to form new compounds. The dentist will adapt the moldable mixture into the prepared tooth, carving the excess before it hardens. After the material hardens, additional shaping of the filling (restoration) can be done with a bur and a low-speed handpiece.

Typical amalgam restorations are shown in Fig. 13.13. Apparently, these teeth had decay both in the fissures and between the teeth. The two smaller premolar teeth have recently placed amalgam restorations that still need to be polished. Polishing improves the properties of the amalgam and helps to make the junction between tooth and filling smooth so additional (recurrent) decay does not occur. You will note that the restoration is not at all toothlike in appearance, and as the amalgam ages, it will turn dark gray in color as seen in the older filling in the larger molar tooth. Many patients prefer not to have amalgam in their mouths, as it is not esthetically pleasing in appearance. Also, the presence of mercury is a concern for some.

Mercury is toxic when it is in an elemental state or after it has reacted with some organic compounds to form a mercury carbonyl. Although there are periodic health-scare stories about the danger of mercury-containing restorations, there has never been peer-reviewed evidence published linking dental amalgam to the onset of disease. There is a greater likelihood of ingesting excessive mercury from eating fish than from an amalgam restoration. There are, however, environmental concerns associated with the leftover scraps of excess amalgam. Although a dentist can turn in amalgam leftover from restoring teeth to a refiner and be paid for the silver content, the amalgam pieces that are removed by the suction device are not as easily handled. These scrap pieces can be captured using special filtering devices installed in the dental office, and many municipalities have instituted laws requiring the capture of this waste material before it enters the sewer system. Until the management of this material is mandated nationwide, it will continue to enter the sewer system and ultimately pose a danger to the environment. Nonetheless, it should be noted that the quantity of mercury released into the environment through dental amalgam is minor in comparison to the mercury released during mining operations, the mercury found in discarded cathode ray tubes (old TV and computer screens), and other electrical components.

Dental amalgam restorations can last for quite a long time. Figure 13.10 showed amalgam restorations that have been in service for over 35 years. Failures are associated with fracture of the amalgam (if the restoration is not thick enough to sustain chewing forces), fracture of the tooth due to over-preparation or by the development of recurrent decay (so-called secondary caries). Amalgam does not bond to tooth structure, so there is always a small gap (approximately 50 μm) between the amalgam and the walls of the tooth. You will note in Fig. 13.13 that there is evidence of fractures along the edge of the older amalgam in the larger molar restoration. The edges of the older amalgam are not as smooth as the recently placed restorations in the premolars. Depending on the size of these marginal failures, food debris and bacteria may get trapped in the small crevice, and decay can proceed along the amalgam–tooth gap.

As the newer tooth-colored materials (see the following section) and bonding agents improve in quality, it is likely that amalgam may be phased out as a restorative material, even though the properties of the amalgam make it user-friendly for the dentist (i.e., it can be placed in areas of the mouth not ideally suited to the tooth-colored materials). Tooth-colored materials need a dry environment for proper placement, a requirement not readily available in the back of the mouth. The Scandinavian countries have limited the use of amalgam; Germany has also not permitted one brand of amalgam to be sold. A large German manufacturer (Degussa) has pulled out of the amalgam business, and so it will not be surprising if eventually the USA also bans or heavily regulates dental amalgam.

In any event, the fact that amalgam does not adhere or bond to tooth structure means that the tooth being restored must be prepared in such a way as to make mechanical retention possible. An illustration of such a preparation is shown in Fig. 13.14. There, it is seen that the walls of the cavity prepared by the dentist taper so that the amalgam restoration will stay in place. Otherwise, it would be easy for the amalgam to simply be removed if a particularly sticky substance such as chewing gum were to adhere to it. Because of the need to provide the taper and the need

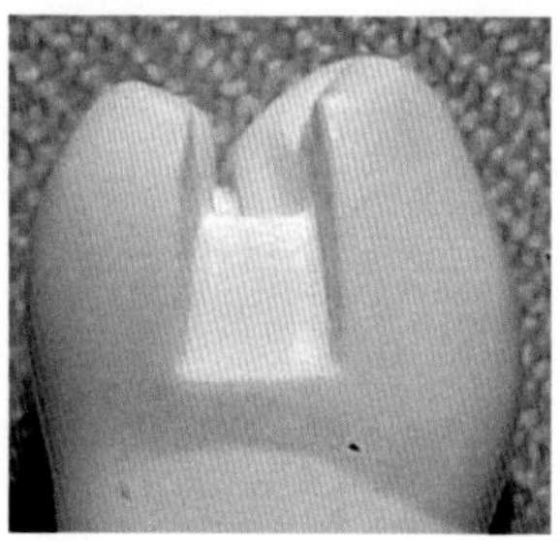

Fig. 13.14 The outline of an amalgam restoration on a model of a tooth, showing the tapered walls of the preparation, designed so the amalgam is retained within the tooth. Image courtesy of Dr. Kenneth Boberick

for a certain thickness of amalgam material to provide strength, the dentist must often remove healthy tooth structure as well as decayed tissue, and so amalgam restorations are not viewed as being particularly "conservative."

13.5.2 Restoring Teeth Using Dental Composite

Recall from Chap. 7 that a composite is a material consisting of two or more distinct materials that retain their individual identity after being combined together; i.e., there is no chemical reaction between them. Composites are designed in order to yield a material that takes advantage of the desirable properties of the components, while the undesirable properties are minimized through the presence of the other components.

Dental composites were introduced in the 1960s primarily as an esthetically pleasing alternative to dental amalgam; the images of dental amalgam restorations shown throughout this chapter leave no doubt about their lack of a natural appearance. The two main components of a dental composite are an organic polymer phase, which serves as the matrix or mortar that holds everything together, and an inorganic ceramic filler phase, which provides strength to the composite. The polymer matrix is similar in chemical composition to the dental sealants discussed earlier, both having been derived from epoxies. Other compounds suspended in the matrix include coloring agents, as the manufacturers seek to provide composites with shades of color that will closely match the majority of patients' teeth. Even a fluorescing additive is included, so that if a patient walks into a club where there is ultraviolet (black) light, the restored tooth will exhibit the same kind of fluorescence as the neighboring natural teeth. Sunlight also contains an ultraviolet light component, so the additives add to the pleasing appearance of the restoration in daylight too.

The catalyst that begins the polymerization of the matrix is dissolved in the matrix phase and, in contemporary dental composites, is activated by intense light. The prepared composite is thus kept stored in light-tight containers until ready for use.

The inorganic filler consists of a specially compounded glass or of quartz (a form of silicon dioxide, SiO_2). The glass contains additives of heavy-metal oxides such as barium oxide, which contributes a high attenuation coefficient to the glass filler particles and therefore, to the composite as well, rendering it visible on an X-ray image. Otherwise, because the organic polymer matrix does not absorb X-rays, the restoration could not be seen in a bitewing and could be mistaken for tooth decay. The filler material is milled into a fine powder, typically until the average particle diameter is less than 2 μm. Early in the development of composites, the filler particles were spherical in shape and larger, but it was found that they became easily dislodged from the matrix, and a rough composite restoration surface would result. Now, most filler particles are irregular in shape and range in size from 2 μm to nano-sized. Mixtures of different sizes of particles produce "hybrid" composites, which are the predominant kind of composite material used today.

You may remember from the surface chemistry discussion that hydrophobic materials and hydrophilic materials are not generally compatible. In dental composites, the organic matrix is hydrophobic, and the filler is hydrophilic. When mixed together, the filler particles tend to clump together rather than being evenly dispersed throughout the matrix; this prevents the development of optimum properties. So, in an effort to improve mixing and also to strengthen the bond between filler particles and the matrix (remember the spherical particles that were being lost?), manufacturers coat the filler with a compound called a silane. This chemical has a molecule whose one end bonds to the glass or quartz surface, and the other end is capable of bonding with the matrix.

After the dentist has finished preparing the tooth, several steps may be taken to help "bond" the composite to the tooth structure [6]. Because the dentin has just been cut using a bur, there is a "smear layer" covering it composed of inorganic hydroxyapatite debris and smeared collagen. This layer needs to be removed or modified, and just as is done with enamel, dentin is also etched. Acid etching removes the smear layer and modifies (demineralizes) the intertubular dentin between the tubules allowing for the liquid bonding agent to penetrate between the individual collagen fibers and create a hybrid layer of polymer and collagen which provides much of the retention required to hold the composite restoration in place. Imagine the dentin is like a sponge with many spaces that can be filled if the sponge is exposed to liquid (bonding agent). Many times the etching will expose the dentin "tubules" that travel down toward the tooth pulp (Fig. 13.15).

If these tubules are left open, inflammation and pain can occur because of the movement of pulpal fluid or the penetration of toxins from bacteria toward the pulp, causing it to become infected. Sealing these tubules with polymer resin provides an opportunity to prevent tooth sensitivity and achieve additional retention. Acid etching demineralizes dentin producing the spongelike intertubular dentin described earlier, and it is these open tubules that provide the opportunity to achieve penetration into dentin by a resin bonding agent (containing no filler) painted onto the etched dentin before the composite is placed over the bonding agent (Fig. 13.16). The penetrating resin material is polymerized and forms tags that help hold it in place.

Because the dentin is hydrophilic (high water content) and the composite is hydrophobic, dentin bonding agents must contain molecules that are both hydrophilic and hydrophobic. The hydrophilic molecules are able to penetrate the moist

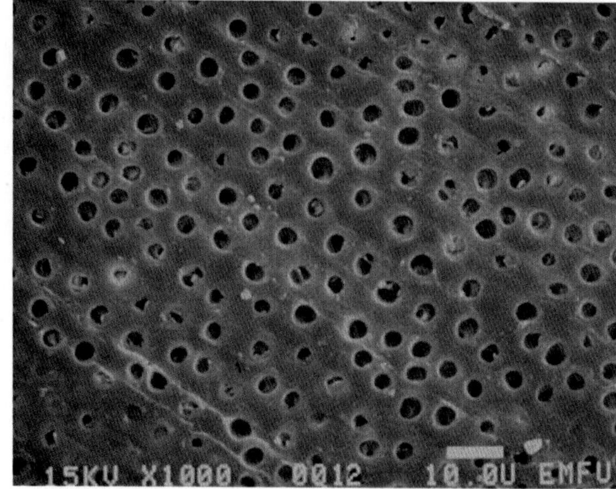

Fig. 13.15 Scanning electron microscope image of etched dentin, showing exposed dentinal tubules that may subsequently be filled with a polymer bonding agent that will help to mechanically retain a composite restoration. Image courtesy of Dr. James Drummond

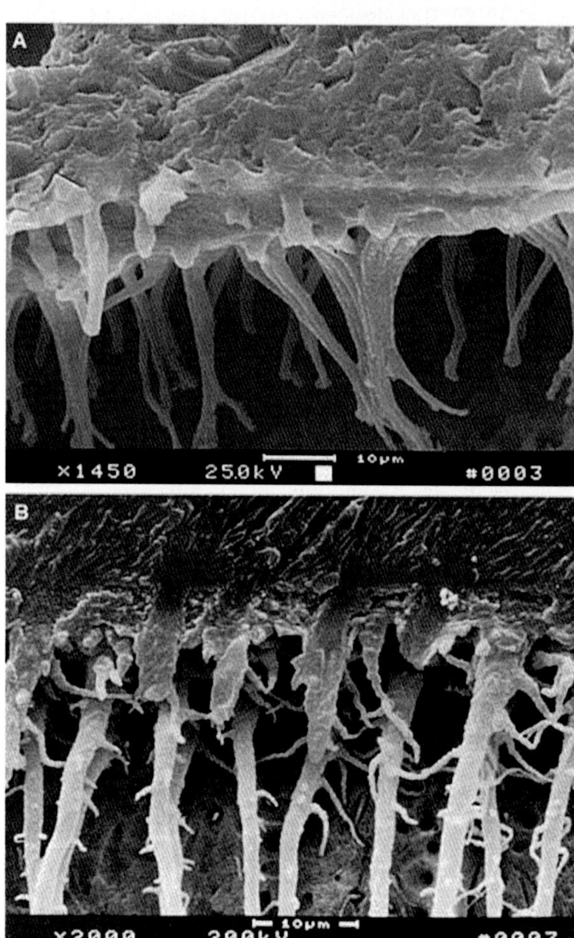

Fig. 13.16 Scanning electron microscope images of tags that protruded into the tubules of etched dentin. The dentin has been completely removed by acid in order to reveal the tags

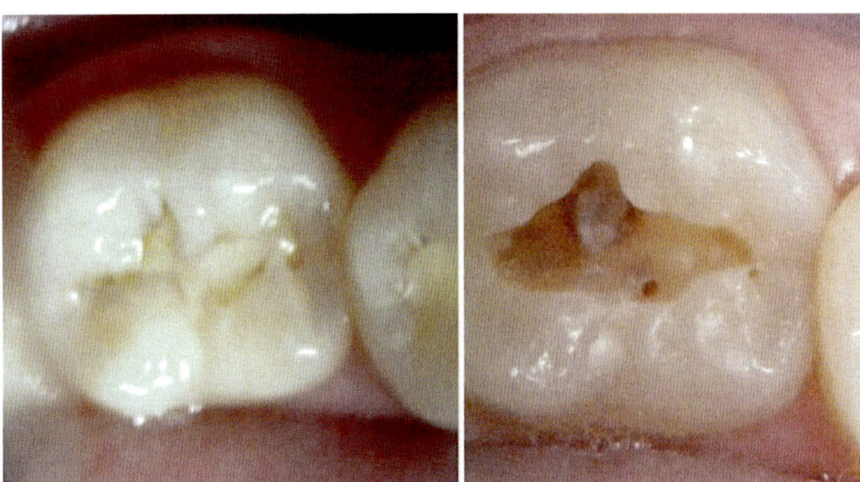

Fig. 13.17 (*Left*) Posterior tooth restored with composite. Note the staining at the interface between the tooth and filling indicating possible recurrent decay. (*Right*) Same tooth with recurrent decay visible after composite removal. Image courtesy of Dr. Kenneth Boberick

dentin interlocking with the exposed collagen fibers, while the hydrophobic molecules remain on the dentin surface and are able to bond to the composite. Dentin bonding is highly technique sensitive and requires the dentist to pay meticulous attention to detail.

The increase in surface area of contact between dentin and bonding agent improves the adhesion of composite to dentin, and portions of the etched enamel infiltrated by bonding agent are responsible for retaining the composite on the enamel portion of the prepared tooth. So, another advantage of dental composites over amalgam is that they can bond to teeth, and therefore, the preparation of the tooth can be more conservative; healthy tooth structure does not have to be removed to design a keyed-in restoration. A finished composite restoration appears much more natural (Fig. 13.17) than does an amalgam restoration and is useful for restoring anterior (front) teeth, where amalgam would not have been considered.

Composites are not perfect restorative materials. Even though they contain approximately 80 % by weight of filler, they are weaker than dental amalgam. The polymerization (hardening) process is accompanied by a volume change; the composite shrinks. Because it is bonded to the tooth, the shrinkage causes a tensile stress at the interface that tends to pull the composite away from the tooth. Research is ongoing to develop materials and processes that do not cause development of tensile stresses at these weak points.

Although the bond between composite and tooth is strong, that interface remains a potential site of failure and is often where decay begins again. Decay is usually suspected if the interface develops a stain that cannot be removed during a routine cleaning. Replacement of the existing restoration is often the recommended treatment to remove recurrent decay.

13.6 Restoration of Badly Damaged or Missing Teeth

In some cases, so much of the tooth structure has had to be removed that there is no possibility of long-term repair with an amalgam or a composite, either because these materials are not sufficiently strong to be used for a major portion of the tooth or there is not enough remaining tooth to retain the restorative material over the long term. These badly damaged teeth require additional procedures designed to cover and strengthen the remaining tooth and restorative material. If a tooth has been lost, it is important that the space left by the tooth become occupied by a replacement for the missing tooth. There are a number of different methods that can be used to replace missing teeth, but we will first look at a procedure to restore a single tooth badly damaged by decay.

13.6.1 Single-Tooth Restoration

"Crowns," sometimes called caps, are a traditional way of restoring a badly damaged tooth that cannot be repaired with dental amalgam or composite. Crowns can be made of only metal, or from metal covered with porcelain for a more natural appearance, or they can be all ceramic (most lifelike). After the decay is removed, some of the missing tooth is "built up" with amalgam or composite with the goal of replacing the tooth structure lost to decay; but this is not a long-term solution because of the increased incidence of tooth fracture and recurrent decay. This "built-up" tooth is then prepared by the dentist to receive a crown or cap which covers and strengthens the remaining tooth structure. The preparation design removes a specific amount of material (tooth and filling), reducing its size so that there is adequate space for the restoration. Another critical preparation requirement is to carefully shape the margin, the area where the crown ends and unprepared tooth structure begins. These interface areas are as sensitive to secondary caries with crowns as they are with amalgam and composite. The margin should also provide a smooth transition from crown to tooth minimizing the accumulation of plaque and the possibility of recurrent decay. In past decades, and when the tooth requiring a restoration was in the posterior region where it was not usually seen, all-metal crowns made of a corrosion-resistant alloy would be used. Suitable materials include gold alloys, silver–palladium alloys, and nickel–chromium alloys; all have corrosion resistance and are biocompatible (unless the patient is allergic to nickel, in which case that alloy cannot be used). Figure 13.18 shows the typical preparation design for an all-metal crown, and Fig. 13.19 shows two gold crowns in a patient's mouth.

The dentist will begin by preparing the tooth (it would look similar to the preparation shown in Fig. 13.18), then make an impression of the mouth using a rubbery material that records the locations and shapes of the teeth, including the prepared tooth. Some patients with a strong gag reflex may have problems with this procedure. If a satisfactory impression is obtained, it is sent to a dental laboratory where a technician uses it to make a stone model of the patient's teeth and positions in the jaw. Figure 13.20 shows an elastomeric (rubbery) impression and poured stone model.

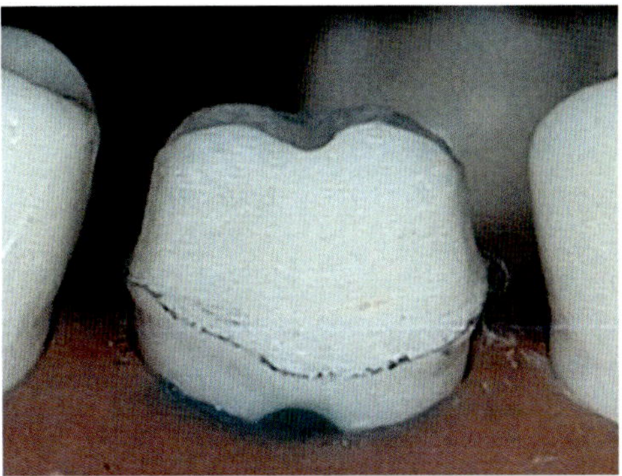

Fig. 13.18 Example of an all-metal crown preparation on a plastic tooth model. Note the large amount of tooth structure removed. The crown margin is highlighted in pencil. Image courtesy of Dr. Kenneth Boberick

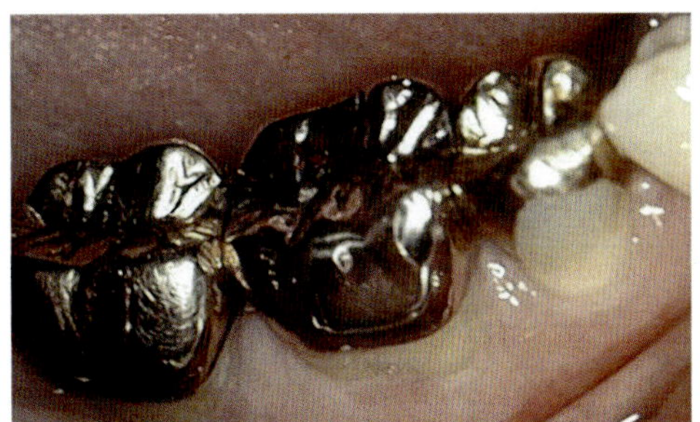

Fig. 13.19 Two gold crowns in service for 15 years. Image courtesy of Dr. Kenneth Boberick

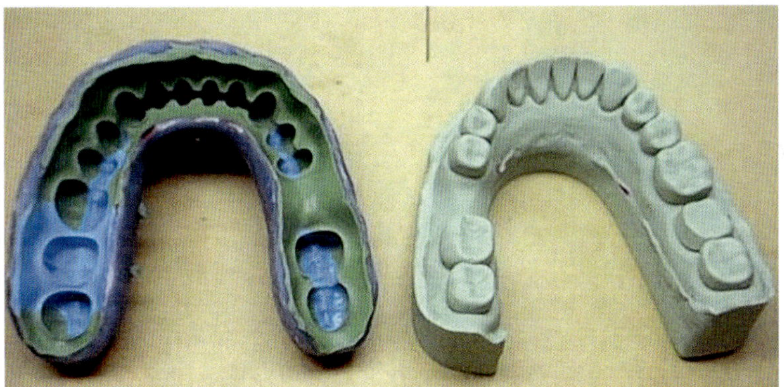

Fig. 13.20 On the *left* is an elastomeric impression of a patient's mouth. On the *right* is a stone (a type of plaster) model poured from the impression that is an exact replica of the patient. The wax pattern is fabricated on this model. Image courtesy of Dr. Kenneth Boberick

The laboratory technician then employs a centuries-old fabrication method used by jewelers and sculptors called the "lost wax" technique. The missing tooth structure is modeled in wax (Fig. 13.21); the wax pattern is carefully removed and invested (surrounded by a liquid refractory material that quickly hardens); the wax is melted

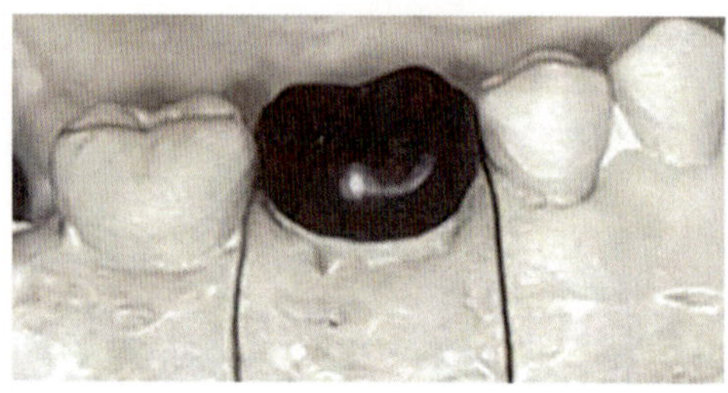

Fig. 13.21 Wax pattern of a crown on a stone model. Image courtesy of Dr. Kenneth Boberick

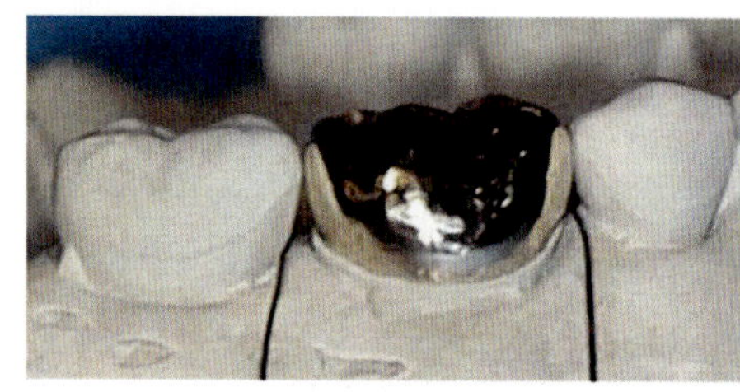

Fig. 13.22 Polished cast gold crown seated on stone model. Image courtesy of Dr. Kenneth Boberick

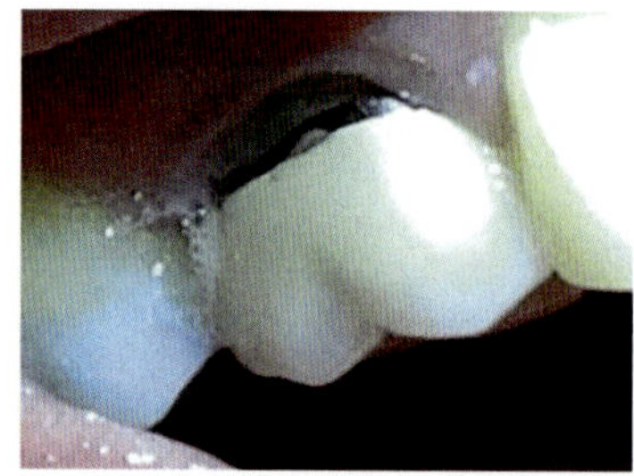

Fig. 13.23 A finished porcelain-fused-to-metal restoration showing a visible metal collar near the gum. Image courtesy of Dr. Kenneth Boberick

away in an oven leaving a hollow space that is filled with molten metal replicating the lost (melted) wax pattern. The metal casting is cleaned and fitted back on the stone model for adjustments (Fig. 13.22) before being eventually cemented onto the prepared tooth in the patient's mouth. It is here that the precision of this technique becomes important, because a crown that is too small will not be able to be fully seated and will remain "high." The patient will not be able to function properly, and the crown will have to be remade. If the crown is too large, then it is likely that a large area of the cement used to keep the crown in place will be exposed to oral fluids. Although a small cement line will always be visible at the margins, the cement is slightly soluble in saliva, and over many years of exposure, cement can wash out, the crown become loose, or decay will start under the crown.

Patients desiring a more lifelike restoration can request a porcelain-fused-to-metal crown. The procedure on the part of the dentist is the same as with a metal crown, except that more tooth structure has to be removed, because room is needed not only for the metal substructure, but for a porcelain coating as well. Although the crown is more natural looking, there will sometimes be a thin band of the supporting metal framework showing (Fig. 13.23), unless it can be hidden under the gum.

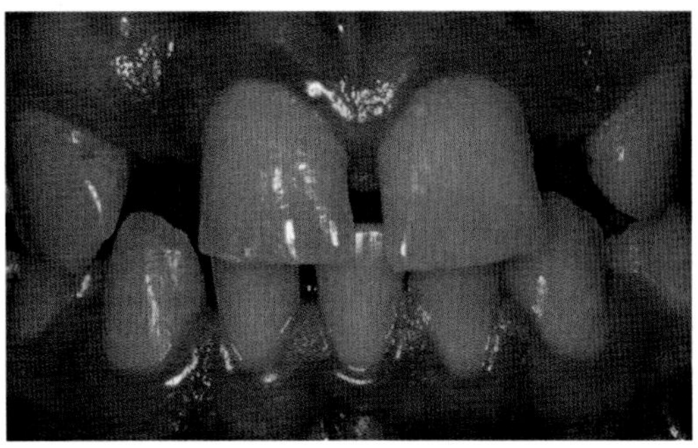

Fig. 13.24 An image of a dental patient with two missing anterior teeth. Image courtesy of Dr. Matthew Palermo

In Fig. 13.23, the metal crown margin was originally hidden below the gum, but after 30 years of service, the gum receded exposing the metal margin. Sometimes, the metal collar can be covered by porcelain, but the cement margin between tooth and crown will still be visible if it lies above the gum line (Fig. 13.26).

These restorations are extremely lifelike when made by a skilled technician, who introduces coloring and toothlike features into the porcelain; that is the clear advantage to this type of restoration. On the disadvantages' side, these restorations are more expensive because of the time involved, and the porcelain is brittle; if the crown has to be removed because the cement is breaking down, it is likely the porcelain will crack during removal, and a new restoration will be required.

The next generation of dental technologies is moving away from using metal toward the use of all-ceramic crowns. They can be made using a technique similar to the "lost wax technique" described earlier, but a new computer-controlled manufacturing process (computer-aided design–computer-aided manufacturing or CAD–CAM) is now widely available [7]. CAD–CAM can be used either at the dentist's office (for a crown that can be finished an hour after the tooth is prepared) or in a laboratory (if the crown is prepared in another location, it is not available as quickly, but many more customization options are available). Tooth preparation by the dentist is similar as for the all-metal or porcelain-fused-to-metal crowns, except that the thickness of the restorative material at the margins is planned to be somewhat greater. If the CAD–CAM device is present at the dentist's office, an elastomeric impression is not made; rather the dentist moves an electronic wand over the prepared tooth, with the wand having a sensor that records the size and shape of the preparation for use by a computer. This optical impression allows for the generation of a virtual 3-D computer image of the prepared tooth on which the finished crown can be "virtually" fabricated. Then, after review, the crown is machined from a single block of ceramic material. Advantages to this system include speed, and the ceramic that is used is stronger than ordinary dental porcelain. The primary disadvantage is that the crown will only have a single color, so this system is best suited for posterior teeth. If the CAD–CAM used is at a laboratory site, the dentist will take an impression, either elastomeric (as with all-metal or porcelain-fused-to-metal crowns) or optical, and send the impression to the laboratory, where a plaster model will be made and scanned by

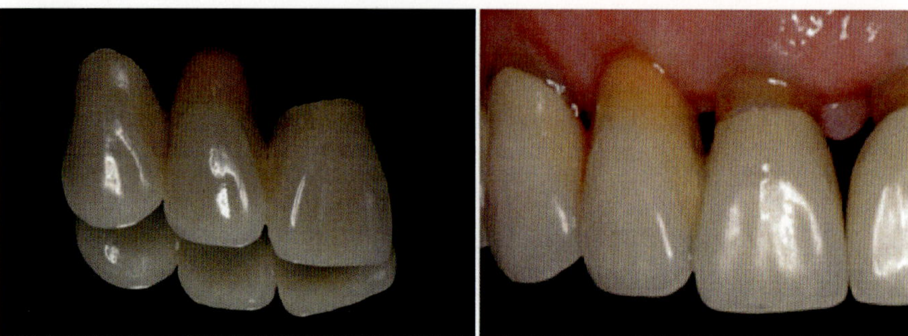

Fig. 13.26 On the *left* is a three-unit anterior bridge. On the *right* is the same bridge in a patient's mouth. Note the margin between tooth and crown is visible above the gum line. Image courtesy of Dr. Matthew Palermo

a visible light scanning machine. A core for the restoration will be machined by a controlling computer, and technicians are able to coat the core with a tinted porcelain to achieve a lifelike effect. This system is better suited for anterior teeth.

CAD–CAM crowns are all either entirely made from or have a core made from technologically advanced ceramics such as zirconia or alumina. These materials are some of the toughest (crack resistant) and strongest ceramics available. The only ceramics that are stronger, such as silicon carbide and silicon nitride, are black.

13.6.2 Restoration of Missing Teeth

Patients sometimes lose teeth; they either get knocked out in an accident or a contact sport or are extracted due to decay. Other patients may have congenitally missing teeth, meaning that a permanent tooth never formed and therefore did not erupt to fill the space left after a baby tooth is lost. If the missing tooth is an anterior tooth, then the visual impact is strong and consequently, there is a strong motivation to replace it (Fig. 13.24). If the missing tooth is a posterior tooth, the esthetic concerns may not be as strong, but there is a functional issue involved. Not only is chewing immediately compromised by the lost tooth, but the teeth on both sides of the missing tooth will gradually tilt into the available space, disrupting the harmony of the dental arch, further compromising chewing ability. Also, as they tilt in, they may lose contact with the opposing teeth (on the opposite jaw), and those teeth may begin to erupt out of their sockets and get loose. So, the optimal course of treatment is to replace the missing tooth or teeth.

There are a variety of options available for replacing missing teeth. First, a decision has to be made if the replacement is to be fixed (permanent) or removable [8]. Athletes who participate in sports with a high risk of tooth loss (hockey) may prefer the removable option until their playing days are over, while others may prefer a more permanent "fixed" solution. Removable replacements for missing teeth have a variety of names, but they are generically called removable partial dentures.

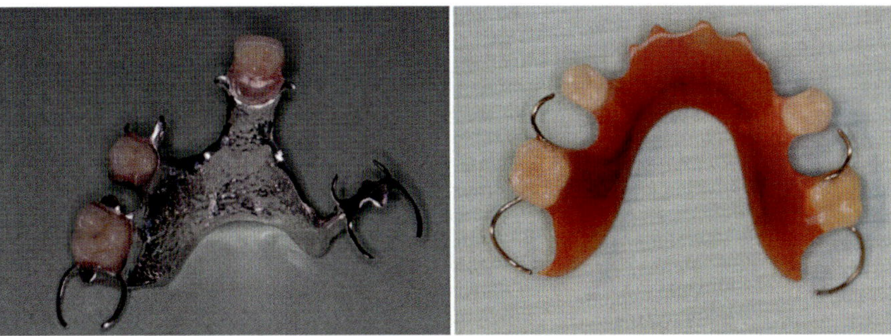

Fig. 13.25 Removable partial dentures for replacement of missing teeth. (*Left*) Cast metal framework with flesh-colored acrylic and teeth added. (*Right*) All-acrylic denture. Image courtesy of Dr. Matthew Palermo

They can be made entirely of acrylic polymer (flippers), but more commonly they consist of a metal framework onto which is attached flesh-colored acrylic polymer and natural-looking acrylic teeth. Removable partial dentures made entirely of acrylic polymer are usually prescribed when additional teeth may be lost in the short term. Additional teeth can be added more easily to an all-acrylic denture than dentures made of a metal framework. The metal structure is designed in such a way as to fit into the patient's mouth and lock into place around existing teeth, which serve as anchor points. The dentures must be taken out at night, cleaned, and stored for use the next day. Figure 13.25 shows an all-acrylic denture with wire clasps for retention and a cast metal framework partial denture.

This is a relatively low-cost solution, but it is not always comfortable, and patients with a low tolerance for inconvenience will simply stop wearing it. In addition, the pink areas that rest on the gum may cause irritation (sore spots), and food can get trapped between the denture and the gum causing pain. Eventual changes to the profile of the jaw will require that the denture be adjusted or remade to obtain a better fit.

The two "permanent" solutions for tooth replacement are implants or cemented bridges. A "bridge" can be made to fit over the space vacated by the missing teeth. The two teeth on both sides of the missing tooth are prepared for crowns (those two teeth are called "abutments," and the missing tooth is called the pontic), and a metal casting is made to replace both the missing tooth and the prepared tooth structure of the abutment teeth. The bridge is cemented onto the abutment teeth and may be made from metal only, from porcelain fused to metal, or be an all-ceramic bridge. Figure 13.26 shows an anterior three-unit bridge.

An advantage to this treatment option is that the missing tooth is replaced, and the technology is standard. Disadvantages are that bridges require support (abutments) on both sides of the missing tooth, and the abutment teeth require extensive preparation, sometimes removing healthy tooth structure. The longer the bridge, the thicker the bridge components must be to prevent flexing of the bridge during function, which could result in material fracture.

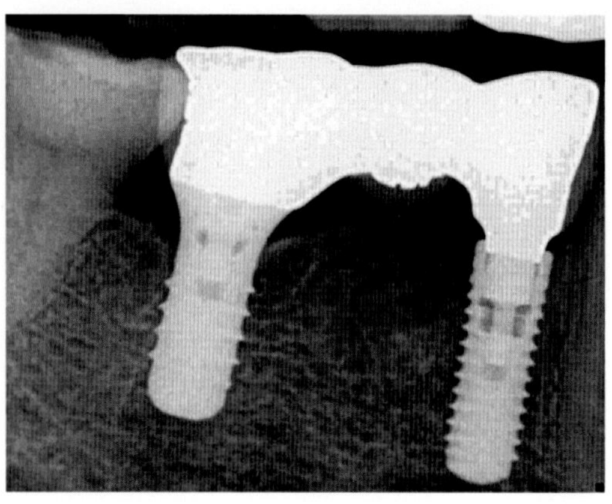

Fig. 13.27 An X-ray image of two implants supporting a three-unit bridge. Image courtesy of Dr. Kenneth Boberick

An alternative to fabricating fixed or removable partial dentures is to place a dental implant [9]. Dental implants are root form (meaning they resemble the root of a tooth) and usually made from titanium or a titanium-6 % aluminum-4 % vanadium alloy, though ceramic implants are also available. Figure 13.27 shows a radiographic image (X-ray) of two implants in a patient's mouth. The implants are supporting a three-unit porcelain-fused-to-metal bridge. If you look closely, you can see the outline of the screws that attach the bridge to the implants. The surface of the implant may be slightly roughened, covered with a sprayed-on titanium particle coating or coated with hydroxyapatite. The implant may also have screw threads machined on it. As mentioned previously, the reason for using titanium or titanium alloys is that they have the ability to osseointegrate (bond strongly with bone), so these implants will be securely positioned and not move while the patient is chewing. The great variety of implant surface treatments, finishes, and coatings is primarily due to the desire of the manufacturers to avoid patent infringement lawsuits. Implants are also available in different sizes: narrow implants for replacing anterior teeth and wider implants for posterior teeth.

The complete implant procedure takes longer than restoring the missing space with a fixed or removable partial denture, because surgery and healing time are needed. First, the dentist will make an incision through the gum, then use a drill to make a hole in the jawbone. The implant is screwed into the hole to obtain tight contact with the surrounding bone and improve osseointegration, and the gum is sewn up over the implant so that the implant is not visible. Then, the patient is sent home, and the bone is given approximately 3–6 months to heal and osseointegrate the implant. A root form implant is exactly that: it looks like the root of a tooth only, and additional steps are necessary to replace the portion of the missing tooth that lies above the gum. During the second visit, X-rays will be taken to ensure that the bone has healed, and the dentist will again cut the gum to expose the head of the implant. At that time, the second component, called the "abutment" or "coping," is added. This resembles the core of a tooth prepared for a crown and is screwed into the implant. After impressions are taken of all the teeth and the exposed coping or abutment, a crown is made and cemented onto the abutment at a third visit.

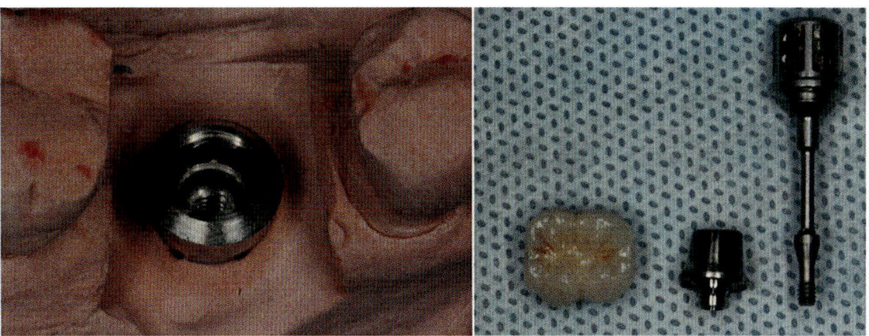

Fig. 13.28 On the *left* is the implant analog (replica of the implant in the patient's mouth) in a stone model. On the *right* are the components of an implant restoration–porcelain crown, abutment, and retaining screw (with screw driver). Image courtesy of Dr. Kenneth Boberick

Figure 13.28 shows the components of an implant, implant abutment, and implant crown as it would appear from the dental laboratory. A replica of the implant called an implant analog is embedded in a stone model (Fig. 13.28 left). This analog is a replica of the implant in the patient's mouth and provides the laboratory with a precise relationship of the implant to the surrounding and opposing teeth in the mouth. An abutment or core is fabricated to fit onto the implant. The abutment is retained in the implant by a screw and in this case, a porcelain-fused-to-metal crown was fabricated to fit over the abutment (Fig. 13.28 right).

Dental implants are designed to last for the life of the patient, and because they are multicomponent, in principle if the crown portion is damaged, it can be replaced. The critical issues for implant success include good bone support for the implant and rigid fixation of the implant in bone. If the implant is even slightly loose, the small amount of motion it experiences when the patient chews will contribute to more loosening and eventual implant failure. A second important factor is the degree to which the patient keeps the gums healthy. The implant is surrounded by gum tissue, and in contrast to the natural state where the tooth is connected to the soft tissue of the gum by a strong and well-organized network of fibers called the periodontal ligament, no such "ligament complex" exists between an implant and soft tissue. Any attachment that does form is fragile and susceptible to inflammation from bacterial plaque. The fragile attachment remains a potential source for problems due to bacterial colonization and possible migration of bacteria into the jaw bone; that's why it's so important for a patient to clean the implant neck thoroughly and to have the dentist closely monitor the state of bone health. Actually, it is very important to keep all the teeth clean as infections in other areas of the mouth can produce seed bacteria colonizing the implant. Infections of the bone are difficult to treat, and removal of a failing osseointegrated implant is a difficult procedure. Finally, the positioning of the implant with respect to the direction of chewing forces is important. These forces should be aligned as much as possible with the long axis of the implant so there is no tipping moment which could eventually cause the implant to fail.

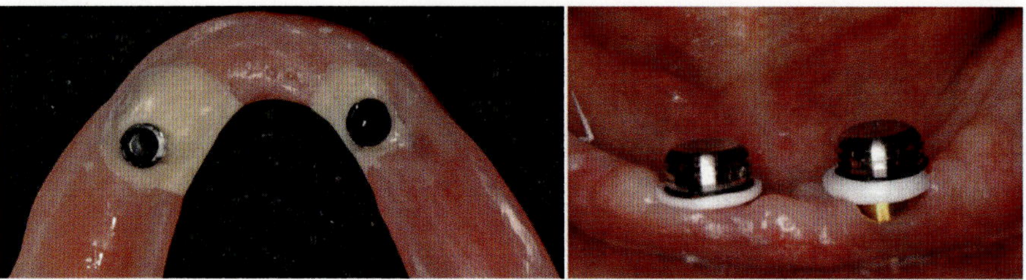

Fig. 13.29 (*Left*) Tissue side of an implant overdenture showing the implant attachments. (*Right*) Overdenture implants visible in a patient's mouth. Image courtesy of Dr. Matthew Palermo

Implants can be placed in many locations provided anatomic landmarks such as nerve trunks (a bundle of nerves) and sinus cavities are avoided. They can be used to replace single teeth, as abutments for bridges, with special attention paid to ensure that the two implants are oriented in the same direction, and as anchor points to aid in the retention of full dentures using specialty attachments inserted into the denture base. Figure 13.29 (left) shows the tissue side of an implant denture with the implant attachments visible; the implants in the mouth are shown in Fig. 13.29 (right). The denture attachments would fit over the implants providing support and retention.

13.7 Orthodontics

Although statistics vary widely, anywhere between 20 and 50 % of American children have malocclusion (a bad bite, where the teeth are not in their optimum positions; e.g., overbite, underbite, crossbite, crowding, excessive spacing), and the most common treatment for this condition is orthodontia, sometimes referred to as "getting braces." This procedure, which is carried out over a period of several years, begins with brackets being bonded onto the patient's teeth, and a wire is threaded through slots in the brackets and held in place by elastics (small rubber bands). A specialist, called an orthodontist, with the help of X-rays will analyze and treatment plan each case individually to correctly apply site-specific pressure to individual teeth moving them to more ideal positions.

The purpose of orthodontic treatment is to cause tooth movement to an "ideal" location with the goal of having all the teeth appear "normal," giving the patient a pleasant smile and ensuring that the teeth all occlude (fit into each other) in the proper way. In cases of malocclusion, patients' teeth will not occlude properly, and patients may sometimes present with symptoms of headaches, temporomandibular joint pain (the TMJ is the joint between the upper and lower jaw), and tooth pain. Crowded teeth that are in malocclusion are difficult to clean, and patients can suffer from an increased caries rate (cavities) and possibly gingivitis and periodontitis leading to lost bone and loose teeth.

The orthodontist analyzes each case by scrutinizing the shape of the head, jaws, and mouth. A number of diagnostic X-ray images are obtained, because by measuring certain landmarks visible on those images, it is possible to determine how much more the jaws are likely to grow. The timing of orthodontic treatment is patient specific, but in most cases it will begin during the late "mixed dentition" stage of tooth development, a time when most of the permanent teeth have erupted but some of the deciduous ("baby") teeth may still be present. Most children who undergo orthodontic treatment begin in the 10–12-year-old range.

Tooth movement is accomplished by applying a "moment" to a tooth. A moment is the product of force and distance. That moment is provided by the arch wire, which is fixed at one bracket, and connected to a slot at another bracket. The fact that the wire is bent, and has a tendency to straighten, is the force needed to define the moment. As a moment is exerted on a tooth, for example, to pull it toward the cheek, the periodontal membrane and jaw bone on the cheek side of the tooth are compressed, and the periodontal membrane and bone on the tongue side of the tooth are placed in tension. Bone, as we have already seen, is a tissue which responds to forces placed on it, and it will resorb where it is compressed, allowing the tooth to move in that direction (toward the cheek). At the same time, the space provided by the moving tooth is filled in with newly deposited bone. This dynamic process continues until the desired extent of movement has occurred. Combinations of wires, o-rings, and elastics may be used not only to move teeth but to rotate and straighten teeth.

Calculating the proper amount and direction of the force applied to a tooth is crucially important to the success of orthodontic treatment. If the force is high because rapid movement is wanted, it's likely that the patient will complain of pain. In a worst-case scenario, the roots of the teeth may begin to resorb (get smaller) due to excessive force. Too low a force and movement will take too long to reorient the teeth. The amount of force may be calculated knowing the modulus of elasticity of the wire, the wire dimensions, and the cross-sectional shape of the wire (square or round). Wires are made of cobalt–chromium, nickel–titanium, and titanium–molybdenum alloys. All have different moduli of elasticity, yield strengths, and frictional coefficients. This latter property is significant when the wire has to be able to slide freely through the slots on a bracket.

Children having orthodontic treatment are sometimes embarrassed by the appearance of wires and brackets on their teeth, and their shyness is revealed when they avoid smiling. Adults may also be reluctant to have co-workers know that they are undergoing orthodontic treatment. For these reasons, a variety of more esthetic approaches have been developed. Brackets may be made from ceramic materials that can be white, transparent, or an off-white color that seeks to match the color of the patient's teeth. Arch wires are typically silvery metallic in color, but metal wires that are coated with white epoxy are available, as are wires made from polymers or polymer composites. Also, if it is desired to completely hide the fact that orthodontic treatment is going on, a new system called "lingual orthodontics," or orthodontics done on the tongue side of the tooth, provides brackets and wires that are cemented and placed behind the teeth and, therefore, invisible to an observer. Still another option is offered by Invisalign™, which

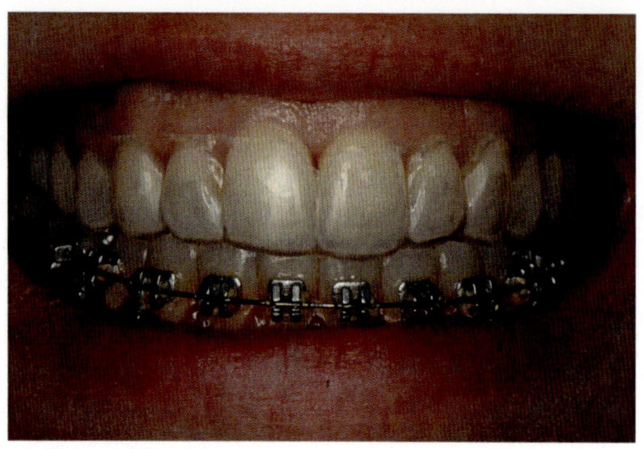

Fig. 13.30 Facial view of a patient showing traditional orthodontic brackets on the lower teeth and Invisalign™ "invisible braces" on the upper teeth. Image courtesy of Dr. Kenneth Boberick

uses a design similar to a tooth protector (called an "aligner") made from clear plastic that snaps over the teeth. New aligners must be made as teeth move and the treatment progresses. Because the "aligners" are removable, this system may be preferred by adults who will choose not to wear them in certain social situations. The orthodontist uses a computer program to design a series of "aligners" which when worn in proper sequence will provide the necessary force required to achieve the desired degree of movement in the proper amount of time. Figure 13.30 shows a patient with traditional orthodontic brackets bonded to the lower teeth and the Invisalign™ appliance worn on the upper teeth.

The best result with orthodontic treatment is obtained just at completion. After the brackets, wires, and other devices are removed, the teeth tend to start drifting back to their earlier positions. Almost everyone who has orthodontic treatment is asked to wear a retainer indefinitely to keep their teeth in their new positions. The retainer can be "permanent," in the form of a wire bonded to the lingual surfaces of the anterior teeth to keep them from moving, or it can be a removable appliance made either for the top or bottom arch. Teeth are held in correct position by a polymer acrylic material on the inside of the teeth and a wire on the outside of the teeth (Fig. 13.31).

13.8 Summary

While most people would not routinely describe a visit to the dentist as fun or enjoyable, recent advances in dental technology have reduced the incidence of dental decay through prevention, eliminated much of the discomfort, and produced new materials that allow the dentist to create beautiful highly esthetic long-lasting restorations which preserve natural tooth structure. Fluoride treatment of water has markedly reduced the rate of decay in children's teeth, and with attention to cleaning and flossing, there is no reason why teeth cannot last a long time. As patients age, however, the teeth may become quite brittle and fracture; treatment of the elderly dental patient is an evolving problem.

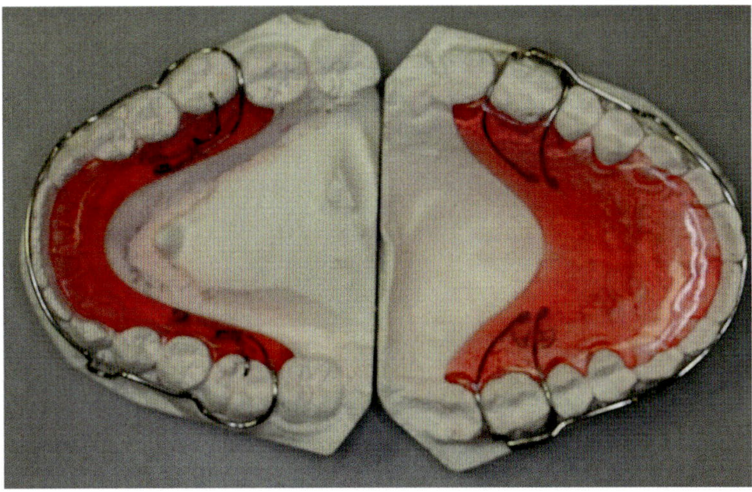

Fig. 13.31 Removable orthodontic retainers placed on a model of a patient's jaws. Image courtesy of Dr. Kenneth Boberick

13.9 Foundational Concepts

- The addition of fluoride compounds to the drinking water supply is an example of positive outcomes of public health policy. The fluoride combines with hydroxyapatite in the tooth to form a fluorapatite that resists tooth decay.
- A tooth consists of a hard outer coating of dental enamel containing 96 % hydroxyapatite. The enamel covers the dentin, a porous substance with less mineral, and the dental pulp lies deep within dentin. The pulp is a living tissue with nerves and a blood supply. The roots of the tooth are anchored in bone and covered with a thin layer of cementum. The structure of enamel consists of rods that lie perpendicular to the outer surface of the tooth, and differences in rod composition are exploited by acid etching the tooth to provide a mechanically retentive surface for sealants.
- Tooth decay usually begins in the pits and fissures of the chewing (occlusal) surfaces of teeth in the back of the mouth (posterior), so sealing these features with a liquid polymer reduces the chances for decay to begin.
- Oral bacteria colonize the surfaces of teeth and, if not periodically cleaned off, can lead to a disease of the gums that may eventually result in infection and loss of the tooth.
- Teeth that have some portions removed by decay or during a dental procedure may be restored with dental amalgam (an alloy consisting of silver, tin, copper, and mercury) or a dental composite (consisting of a polymer matrix with additions of micron-sized particles of glass or ceramics).
- Severely damaged teeth may require a crown to be fabricated and cemented over the remaining tooth structure. Crowns may be made from only metal, from metal-fused-to-porcelain, or from a ceramic.

- Missing teeth may be replaced with dental implants or with fixed or removable partial dentures.
- Orthodontic treatment seeks to align and organize the teeth so that the patient can chew properly and to enhance appearance. However, teeth tend to drift back to their original positions after therapy, and a retainer worn overnight is often needed to keep the teeth in place.

Acknowledgement Figures 13.4 and 13.16 reprinted from The Journal of Prosthetic Dentistry, volume 81, by A.M. Diaz-Arnold, M.A. Vargas, and D.R. Haselton: "Current Status of Luting Agents for Fixed Prosthodontics", pages 135–141, 1999, with permission from Elsevier.

References

1. Griffin, S., Jonkes, K., & Tomar, S. (2001). An economic evaluation of community water fluoridation. *Journal of Public Health Dentistry, 61*, 78–86.
2. Alvarez, L. (2011). Looking to save money, more places decide to stop fluoridating the water. *The New York Times*. New York.
3. Scheid, R., & Weiss, G. (2011). *Woelfel's dental anatomy*. Philadelphia: Lippincott Williams and Wilkins.
4. Kinane, D., & Bouchard, P. (2008). Periodontal disease and health: Consensus report of the sixth European workshop on periodontology. *Journal of Clinical Periodontology, 35*, 333–337.
5. Bharti, R., Wadhwani, K., Tikku, A. & Chandra, A. (2010). Dental amalgam: An update. *Conservative Dentistry, 13*, 204–208.
6. van Meerbeck, B., de Mumck, J., Yoshida, Y., Inoue, S., Vargas, M. & Vijay, P. (2003). Adhesion to enamel and dentin: Current status and future challenges. *Operative Dentistry, 28*, 215–235.
7. Strub, J., Rekow, E., & Siegbert, W. (2006). Computer-aided design and fabrication of dental restorations: Current systems and future possibilities. *Journal of the American Dental Association, 137*, 1289–1296.
8. Wostmann, B., DBuditz-Jorgensen, E., Jensen, N., Mushimoto E., Palmqvist, S. & Sofou, A. (2005). Indications for removable partial dentures: A literature review. *The International Journal of Prosthodontics, 18*, 139–145.
9. Porter, J., & von Frauenhofer, J. (2005). Success or failure of dental implants? A literature review with treatment considerations. *General Dentistry, 53*, 423–432.

Rehabilitation Technologies 14

"Rehabilitation is to be a Master Word in Medicine."

Dr. William Mayo

A walk around any shopping mall will provide encounters with folks who are actively using rehabilitation aids. Their needs may have arisen as the result of war injuries and amputations or hereditary conditions. However, a noticeable proportion of those in wheelchairs are diabetes patients, the obese, or those suffering from emphysema.

You may have noticed that the wheelchairs are quite sophisticated, and the patients can often operate the chair by themselves. Technology has entered into the mainstream of rehabilitation, and as long as the funding is available to pay for assistive devices, the medical device industry will continue to develop and market tools that enable the disabled to live more "normal" lives. In this chapter, we will learn about the stimulus for the growth of rehabilitation medicine (the American Disabilities Act), survey the types of devices currently available, and look into the future to catch a glimpse of the new devices in development.

14.1 Introduction

The human body is a complex machine capable of learning, adapting, healing itself, and performing many precise tasks. Most people can independently perform the basic functions of everyday life otherwise called "activities of daily living" (ADLs), such as walking, dressing, eating, seeing, hearing, and bathing. In addition, humans are expected to perform "instrumental activities of daily living" (IADLs) such as housework, learning, shopping, observances, sports, transportation, and using technology. If you think about it, all this requires remarkable coordination between the brain and various organs/tissues such as the liver (energy supply), muscles (motors),

G.R. Baran et al., *Healthcare and Biomedical Technology in the 21st Century: An Introduction for Non-Science Majors*, DOI 10.1007/978-1-4614-8541-4_14,

nerves, and tendons. Individuals who cannot perform some or all of these activities because of physical problems can be considered disabled.

Disability is a physical or mental condition that restricts a person from performing activities of daily living (ADLs), gainful occupation, or leisure activities. People become severely disabled for many reasons including genetic or birth defects, developmental factors, diseases, old age (e.g., senility, Alzheimer's disease), pain, accidents, violence, self-harm, or psychological/mental problems. In the past, attempts to restore lost physiologic function have not met much success. Current efforts or advancements in technologies aimed at restoring lost physiologic function can be primarily attributed to increased funding for research, mobility and daily function aids, laws protecting the disabled, advances in surgical techniques, and anesthesia and infection control. These stimuli, combined with advances in engineering and manufacturing sciences, have helped bring technologies to market that improve the lives of disabled individuals.

According to the 2010 US census data, there were approximately 56 million Americans who had some sort of serious disability (http://www.census.gov/people/disability/). The definition of disability varies among individuals, different government agencies, advocacy groups, or cultures and changes depending on medical advances. For example, the US government's Social Security Disability Insurance program narrowly defines disability as a condition that prevents an individual from engaging in any substantial gainful activity or employment for a certain duration. An example of an advocacy group's attitude which might conflict with the view of the general public is that many members of the deaf community believe that deafness should not be considered a disability [1]. In the USA, the American Disabilities Act (ADA, passed originally in 1990 and amended in 2008) promises civil rights protection to all Americans with disabilities and guarantees equal opportunity in public accommodation, communication, employment, and transportation. The ADA requires public entities such as schools, hospitals, stores, and mass transit to provide improved access such as wheelchair-accessible ramps or lifts, parking spaces for the handicapped, Braille signage, and installation of full-length bathroom mirrors. The opening statements of that act are shown in Table 14.1.

Currently, many disabilities cannot be cured by drugs, surgeries, or regenerative therapies. However, the quality of life of people with disabilities can be improved by employing a combination of biotechnologies that includes drugs, surgery, therapy, and various assistive or prosthetic technologies such as computers, wheelchairs, dentures, knee implants, magnifying glasses, robotic limbs, or hearing aids. The duration of therapy or treatment needed to restore lost function often depends upon the cause of disability, the extent of the disability, and the current state-of-the-art medical technology. This can be demonstrated by comparing the treatment required to restore missing function in cataract patients versus stroke patients. Until the last century, vision loss caused by cataracts doomed the patient to blindness until death. However, once the surgical procedure for removal of the diseased lens was developed, blindness caused by cataracts can be cured with a single and safe operation without the need for additional glasses or rehabilitation.

Table 14.1 Provisions of the American Disabilities Act

Findings	Purpose
Physical or mental disabilities in no way diminish a person's right to fully participate in all aspects of society, yet many people with physical or mental disabilities have been precluded from doing so because of discrimination; others who have a record of a disability or are regarded as having a disability also have been subjected to discrimination	To provide a clear and comprehensive national mandate for the elimination of discrimination against individuals with disabilities
Historically, society has tended to isolate and segregate individuals with disabilities, and, despite some improvements, such forms of discrimination against individuals with disabilities continue to be a serious and pervasive social problem	To provide clear, strong, consistent, enforceable standards addressing discrimination against individuals with disabilities
Discrimination against individuals with disabilities persists in such critical areas as employment, housing, public accommodations, education, transportation, communication, recreation, institutionalization, health services, voting, and access to public services	To ensure that the federal government plays a central role in enforcing the standards established in this chapter on behalf of individuals with disabilities
Unlike individuals who have experienced discrimination on the basis of race, color, sex, national origin, religion, or age, individuals who have experienced discrimination on the basis of disability have often had no legal recourse to redress such discrimination	To invoke the sweep of congressional authority, including the power to enforce the fourteenth amendment and to regulate commerce, in order to address the major areas of discrimination faced day to day by people with disabilities
Individuals with disabilities continually encounter various forms of discrimination, including outright intentional exclusion; the discriminatory effects of architectural, transportation, and communication barriers; overprotective rules and policies; failure to make modifications to existing facilities and practices; exclusionary qualification standards and criteria; segregation; and relegation to lesser services, programs, activities, benefits, jobs, or other opportunities	
Census data, national polls, and other studies have documented that people with disabilities, as a group, occupy an inferior status in our society and are severely disadvantaged socially, vocationally, economically, and educationally	
The nation's proper goals regarding individuals with disabilities are to assure equality of opportunity, full participation, independent living, and economic self-sufficiency for such individuals, and the continuing existence of unfair and unnecessary discrimination and prejudice denies people with disabilities the opportunity to compete on an equal basis and to pursue those opportunities for which our free society is justifiably famous and costs the USA billions of dollars in unnecessary expenses resulting from dependency and nonproductivity	

In contrast, a stroke (a disruption of blood supply to a portion of the brain) can cause permanent neurologic damage (e.g., paralysis, speech loss) and pain; in extreme cases, a stroke patient will need to relearn or regain skills related to activities of daily living such as walking and speaking. The loss of motor function in stroke patients often requires extensive rehabilitation by a multidisciplinary team of physicians, nurses, physical therapists, occupational therapists, speech therapists, psychologists, and social workers, and rehabilitation can take anywhere from months to years. This chapter will focus on technologies that help people with physical disabilities lead more normal lives.

14.2 History of Rehabilitation Medicine

Archeological finds have shown Egyptians using nonfunctional wooden prosthetic limbs or toes after amputation. There is also plenty of archeological evidence that shows ancient Romans, Egyptians, or Persians made and used artificial eye prostheses (also called ocular prostheses) for cosmetic reasons. Most eye prostheses were worn outside the eye socket and attached to a cloth or facial skin. Eye prostheses or glass eyes that could be worn inside the eye socket (which were of course very uncomfortable) were first manufactured by the Venetians during the sixteenth century (Fig. 14.1). Other simple assistive devices such as crutches or walking canes that improve balance and mobility have been used for centuries.

Wars and the resulting increase in disabled individuals have in general spurred interest in developing technologies that can replace lost limb function. The need for rehabilitation technologies increased dramatically during World Wars I and II. It should be noted that during those wars, the severely injured for the most part did not survive, and so the development of extensive rehabilitation technologies was not an urgent need. The situation has changed dramatically during the modern wars fought in Asia, Africa, and the Middle East; advances in body armor, combat medicine, and rapid evacuation protocols have meant that 90 % of the soldiers survived severe injuries that required sophisticated and lifelong rehabilitation. The twentieth and twenty-first centuries have also seen tremendous improvements in medical

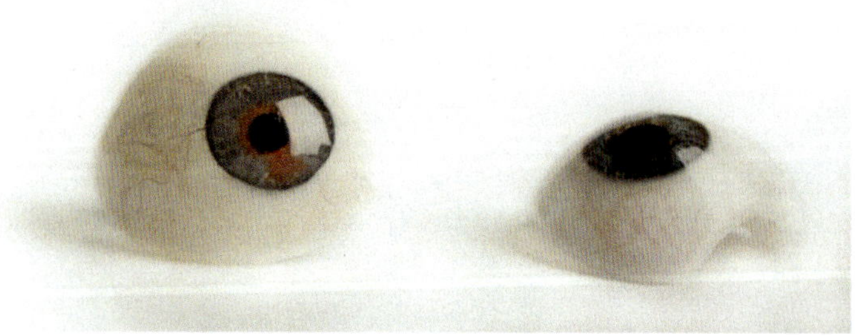

Fig. 14.1 Artificial eye prostheses made from glass or polymers

technologies to effectively treat deadly infections, diseases, or decrease child mortality. As a result, humans in general are living longer, even with various chronic disabilities, and to meet this demand, research and development of new and cost-effective technologies that can improve the quality of life of both civilians and military personnel has flourished.

14.3 Rehabilitating Musculoskeletal Disabilities

The musculoskeletal system consists of muscles, bones, tendons, ligaments, cartilage, and associated tissues that move the body and maintain its shape. The functioning of this system can be affected by many factors including trauma due to accidents or sporting activities, poor ergonomics, unexplained pain, and systemic diseases. Many times there are no definitive cures to treat musculoskeletal problems, and the course of treatment often prescribed is rehabilitation. In some cases a less serious musculoskeletal condition that is left untreated can lead to serious chronic disabilities later. For example, low-level back pain which affects more than 80 % of the adults in the USA can encourage them to follow a sedentary lifestyle, which in turn may lead to serious conditions such as heart disease or diabetes.

14.3.1 Musculoskeletal Pain

Pain is a complex physiologic process controlled by both the central (brain and spinal cord) and peripheral nervous (any nerve outside the brain and spinal cord) systems. A modern theory of pain, called the gate control theory, was developed by Ronald Melzack and Patrick Wall in the 1960s to explain how the sensation of pain is perceived by the brain. According to this theory, the perception of pain is a complex interplay between the central and peripheral nervous systems. For example, when someone injures his or her toe, the pain signals travel along the peripheral nervous system to the spinal cord and to the brain. However, before the pain signal from the toe reaches the brain, it encounters "nerve gates" in the spinal cord. For as yet unknown reasons, if the nerve gate is open, the individual will feel pain; if the nerve gate is closed, the pain signal will not reach the brain. External stimuli such as electrical current, heat, cold, or massage can override pain signals by causing the nerve gates in the spinal cord to close. Interestingly, opioids (e.g., morphine) or even distracting brain signals (e.g., reading a book, rhythmic breathing, listening to music) can block pain signals from passing through the nerve gates.

What do you think? Have you ever tried these "tricks" to distract yourself when you are in pain and did they work?

Pain can devastate a person's social and economic life. Individuals suffering from either acute or chronic musculoskeletal pain may experience impairment in mobility, activities of daily living, sleep, and depression; these patients account for

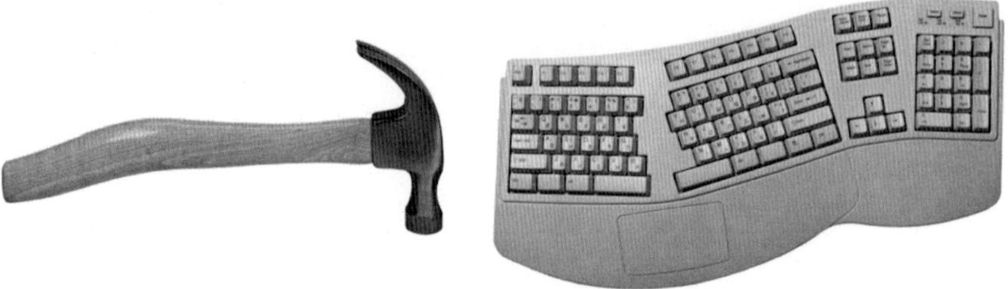

Fig. 14.2 Ergonomically designed hand tools and implements

25 % of doctor visits in the USA. The most common causes of musculoskeletal pain include arthritis, low back/neck vertebral disc herniation, muscle sprains/strains, tendonitis/bursitis, plantar fasciitis, carpal tunnel syndrome, fractures, tumor, sports injuries, and rotator cuff injuries. In the USA, a primary-care physician or physical therapist initially examines the patient suffering from pain. Note that in most states in the USA (not in Michigan, Indiana, and Oklahoma), patients can directly see a physical therapist without a physician's prescription, thanks to the "Direct Access" (DA) law. The argument that opponents of this measure made was that because therapists cannot order diagnostic tests, the proper therapy may not be identified.

When a patient presents with acute or chronic pain, the first step is to diagnose or find the cause. This can be done with general quality of life surveys, physical examinations, radiology (to rule out fractures), MRI (magnetic resonance imaging) to detect tumors or soft tissue injuries, EMG (electromyography) to detect neurologic issues, etc. Depending on the findings, the primary-care physician determines the next course of action, which may include a course of anti-inflammatory drugs or analgesics, orthoses, or sending the patient to a specialist (e.g., physical therapist, orthopedic surgeon). Acute pain with a well-known cause can often be alleviated by simple treatment options such as rest, removing the source of pain (e.g., using an ergonomic chair), or by using mild analgesics (e.g., over-the-counter pain medications such as aspirin, acetaminophen, ibuprofen, naproxen sodium), cold or heat compresses. Patients suffering from arthritis or other dexterity issues can also benefit from the use of assistive devices that may reduce pain during ADLs. Examples of such devices include larger-diameter pens or toothbrush handles, electric jar openers, raised toilet seats, and helpful devices for gripping/grabbing (Fig. 14.2).

If medication and therapy do not provide adequate relief, electrical stimulation techniques to alleviate neuromuscular pain symptoms that work on the principle of gate control theory may be the next step. In general, signals from large-diameter nerve fibers can inhibit or modulate signals from the smaller sensory nerve fibers which transmit pain impulses. Therefore, stimulation of the large fibers by external electrical pulses can override the small fibers' pain signals. Nonsurgical (e.g., transcutaneous electrical nerve simulators, Fig. 14.3) and surgically implanted electrode peripheral nerve stimulators may be used when pain cannot be controlled by standard therapies such as drugs (analgesics, anticonvulsants, muscle relaxants,

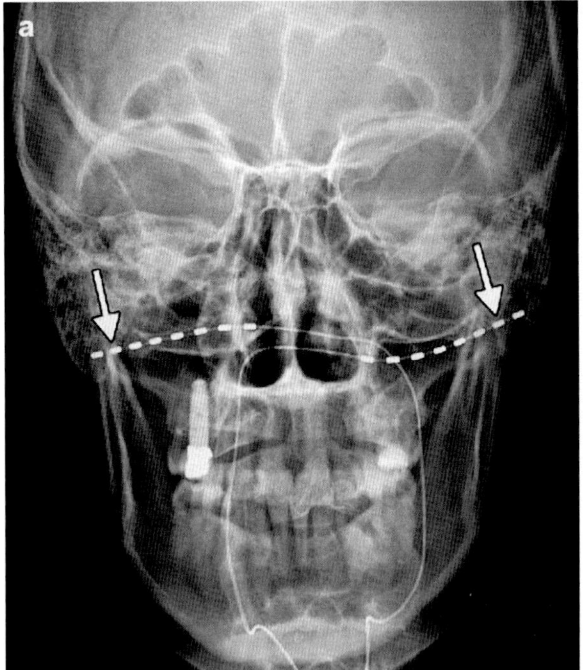

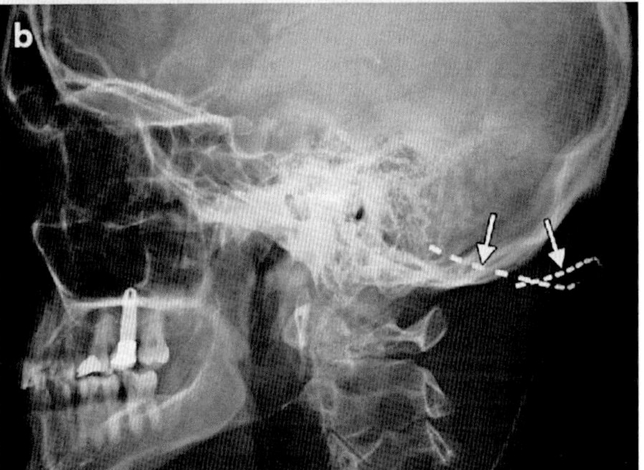

Fig. 14.3 Radiographs showing implanted electrodes for treatment of severe migraines. Copyright Springer Science+Business Media B.V.

antidepressants, topical anesthetics, and nerve blocks). It is interesting to note that the idea of using electricity to control pain was first thought of in the first century. A Roman physician named Scribonius Largus observed that gout pain can be relieved by coming in contact with a torpedo fish (an electricity-producing fish similar in appearance to an eel).

Sometimes, the source of pain is due to a serious condition such as a bone fracture, a tumor, degeneration of joint surfaces, soft tissue damage, or tissue tears (e.g., herniated intervertebral disc or meniscal tears in the knee joints). Many of these conditions may require treatment by surgical interventions or implants. Orthopedic surgeons and some neurosurgeons are trained to treat such musculoskeletal conditions. However, surgery is only the first step toward regaining full function. After surgery, the patient usually needs to undergo physical or occupational therapy to strengthen muscle function and to relearn how to perform the activities of daily living.

14.3.2 Physical Therapy and Orthoses

Physical therapy can help a wide range of individuals, ranging from those suffering from very low-level pain/disability to those suffering with severe disabilities. Physical therapists or physiotherapists utilize noninvasive tools to help patients regain strength, mobility, and fitness. Many specialize in areas such as pediatric care, geriatric (elderly care), cardiopulmonary rehabilitation, neurologic or stroke rehabilitation, or sports therapy. Physical therapy interventions can be classified as passive or active treatments. Passive treatments consist of electrical stimulation for pain, ice, massage (to release tension in the muscles), heat, myofascial techniques, ultrasound, and mobilization and manipulation. Active treatments include various types of exercises (e.g., strength training, aquatic therapy, orthotic training) and electrical stimulation for strength. Patients who undergo physical therapy may also need to see occupational therapists. These therapists can help the patients prevent further injuries at work/leisure and assist them with speaking, writing, and occupational skills.

Orthoses are medical devices (e.g., braces, wraps, ankle/foot orthotics, and insoles) used to support a weak or deformed body member (Fig. 14.4). A well-known example of an orthosis is a brace worn by children suffering scoliosis (abnormal curvature of the vertebral column) to prevent further worsening of spinal curvature. Orthoses can also be used to eliminate or restrict motion in an injured body part. For example, knee braces are worn to reduce pain caused by mild ligament sprains, strains, or other knee instabilities. Orthoses are different from splints

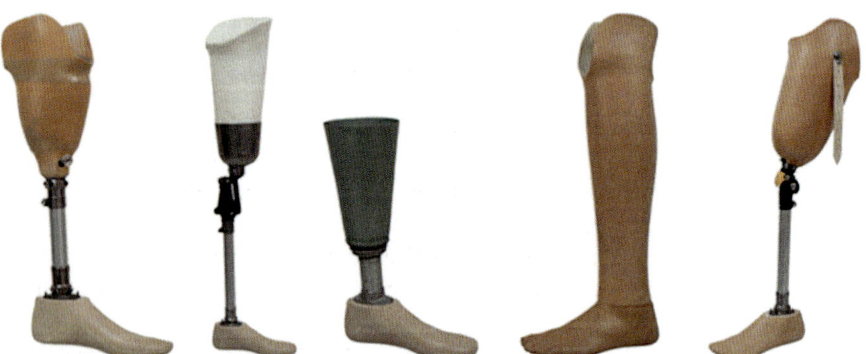

Fig. 14.4 Leg orthoses

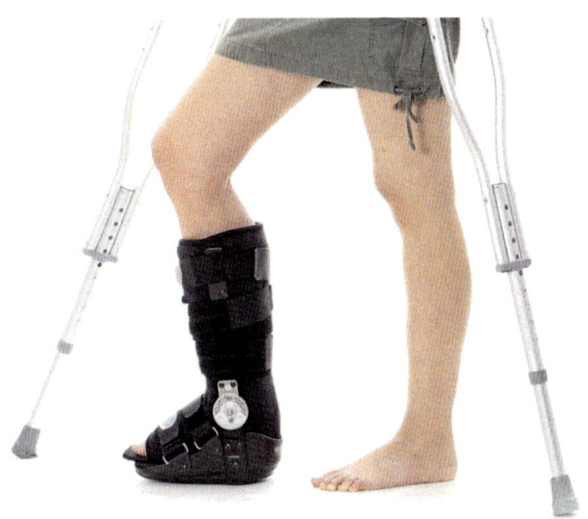

Fig. 14.5 An active lower-leg orthosis

(e.g., casts) which are used in the treatment of bone fractures or joint dislocations, and should not be confused with prostheses. Patients who have lost a limb partially or completely are sometimes fitted with artificial limbs known as prostheses.

Active or powered orthoses (Fig. 14.5) can help patients suffering from mobility challenges due to stroke, spinal cord injury, multiple sclerosis, weak quadriceps, or cerebral palsy to increase their ambulatory ability or stand and lead independent lives. In general, active orthoses include a power supply in the form of batteries, hydraulic/pneumatic actuators, direct current motors, sensors, and gait analysis software, all to provide extra power/energy to the wearer. Active orthoses called "exoskeletons" can also be worn by people with no disabilities (e.g., soldiers) to augment their walking or load-carrying abilities.

14.4 Amputation

Amputation is defined as the removal of a limb or limb portion from the body and has significantly deleterious impacts on the quality of life. After amputation, an individual may experience a threefold loss of function, sensation, and body image. The success of postoperative rehabilitation depends on the functional and psychological status of the patient. As of 2012, there are approximately two million people in the USA living with an amputated limb, mainly caused by diabetes, peripheral vascular disease, or war-related wounds.

Successful medical amputation is a relatively new phenomenon. The era of modern limb amputations began after the pioneering work by a renowned French military surgeon named Ambroise Pare in the 1500s. At least two major advancements in amputation surgery are credited to Pare: (1) use of a mild dressing instead of boiling oil and (2) ligature (blood vessel closure) for hemostasis (stopping the loss of blood) in amputations. Amputation techniques became more advanced after the discovery of anesthesia and infection-control techniques. In ancient times, amputations were rare, and many amputations were due to religious rituals, punishment, trauma, leprosy, or frostbite. Many of the injured preferred to die with their limbs intact for fear of living in the afterlife without limbs. The nonavailability of anesthesia, antibiotics, and techniques to stop bleeding required the amputation procedures to be rapid and complicated recovery and rehabilitation.

The upper and lower limbs (or extremities) are commonly referred to as the arms and the legs. In anatomical terms, the "arm" specifically refers to the segment between the shoulder and elbow, and the term "forearm" refers to the segment between the elbow and wrist. Both the upper and lower extremities are complex structures composed of bones, muscles, cartilage, tendons, ligaments, nerves, etc. For example, there are over 30 different muscles that are involved in the movement of the forearm, wrist, and fingers. The human hand consists of 27 different bones (e.g., ulna, radius, phalanges) and at least 18 joints. The upper and lower extremities are primarily organs of mobility. The lower extremities are specialized for two-legged locomotion (i.e., they enable us to walk or run). The arms and hands help us to reach, grasp, or manipulate objects. Both upper and lower limbs are essential for humans to perform normal daily activities and occupations.

Humans may lose limb function for a variety of reasons, including birth defects, pain, work-related injury, paralysis, or amputation. The loss of limb function can be both physically and emotionally devastating. The treatment or rehabilitation options depend on the severity of limb function loss. For example, an individual who is unable to move the arms may be suffering from arthritis or spinal cord impingement (back pain) and can be treated by drugs, surgery, or physical therapy. In contrast, the individual whose limb was amputated during an automobile accident or during warfare may need a prosthesis or mobility device and further rehabilitation [2].

Clinically, amputation is considered the last option when treatments such as limb salvage surgical procedures (done under anesthesia) or chemotherapy fail. The five common types of limb amputations are transtibial, transfemoral, transradial, transhumoral (or through the tibia, femur, radius, and humerus bones), and disarticulation (amputation through a joint). During amputation surgery planning, the orthopedic or vascular surgeon will try to save as much of the limb as clinically possible; toe amputation is better than a partial foot amputation, which in turn is preferred over a transtibial amputation. The need for a prosthesis and the type of prosthesis depends on the level of amputation and the patient. Usually, no prosthesis is needed after toe amputation.

14.4.1 Lower-Extremity Amputation

Patients who successfully recover after a lower-limb amputation often need a prosthesis for walking. In the Middle Ages, leg prostheses of wood and iron were made by armorers for knights, though they were too heavy to be of much use for walking. Modern amputations are painless in most cases, and the use of imaging tools allows the surgeon to determine the best level of amputation that will heal. Optimal healing occurs when the amputation is done near healthy tissue with a good blood supply.

Fig. 14.6 An exoskeletal leg prosthesis

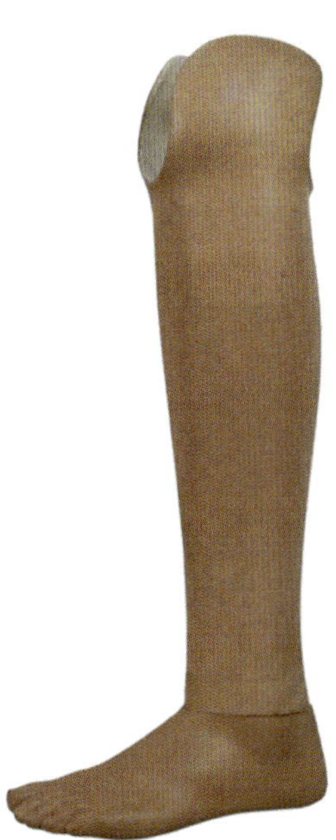

Advances in surgical techniques and post-amputation technologies such as wheelchairs also facilitate rehabilitation.

Wheelchairs are devices that provide wheeled mobility and seating support for patients with a walking disability, paralysis, or amputation. Even amputees who are fitted with prostheses are advised to have a wheelchair or other assistive devices such as canes, crutches, and walkers at hand. In many developing countries, a wheelchair is preferred over prosthetics because of lower cost and a lack of resources involved in prosthetic fitting. Wheelchairs can be either manually driven or powered by a battery and motor, with each type having its advantages and disadvantages. There are many manual wheelchair models/configurations: three wheelers, folding wheelchairs, hand-propelled tricycles, etc. Manual wheelchairs are simpler to operate and maintain and can be used by individuals with adequate upper-body strength. However, users can develop serious upper-body overload injuries, primarily in the shoulder and hand–wrist area. People without adequate upper-body strength can opt for an electric-powered wheelchair which contains batteries, motors, and control systems and is manufactured in different configurations (e.g., scooter, tilt, or reclining) to suit individual needs.

Leg prostheses are needed when a lower limb is lost. There are two types of designs: exoskeletal and endoskeletal. Exoskeletal prostheses (Fig. 14.6) have a hard outer plastic laminated shell or skin with a wood or urethane foam interior. The shell acts as the load-bearing component in this prosthesis. Lower-extremity exoskeletal prostheses generally have the following components: socket, knees, pylons, and feet. The socket is the portion of the prosthesis that fits around the residual limb and may be equipped with a liner for comfort. The knee components are used for transfemoral prostheses (above-the-knee amputations).

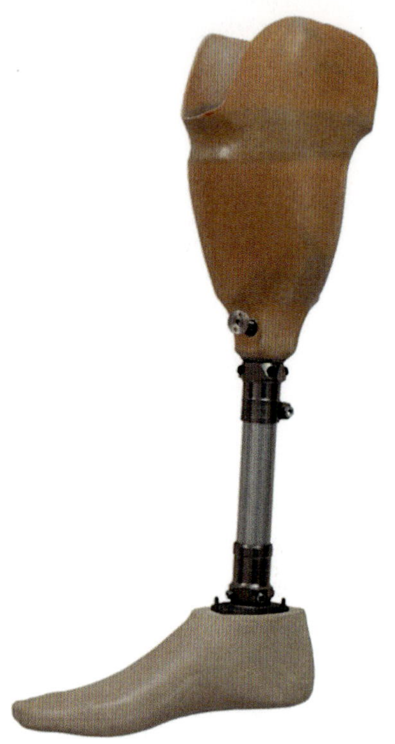

Fig. 14.7 An endoskeletal leg prosthesis

An endoskeletal prosthesis allows for sitting, standing, walking, or kneeling (Fig. 14.7). The knee component is made of stainless steel, titanium, or polymer composites and comes with different degrees of complexity (mechanical versus computerized). Pylons are the load-bearing unit in endoskeletal prostheses and transfer weight between the socket and the prosthetic foot.

There are probably hundreds of varieties of prosthetic feet available, and they are all designed to fit individual physiologic needs and to help amputees have as much of a normal gait as possible. Some prosthetic feet are designed specifically for athletes such as sprinters (Fig. 14.8). The J-shaped carbon composite prostheses are claimed to mimic the hind quarter of a cheetah and are used by many elite athletes, such as Oscar Pistorius. There is still a controversy about whether users of this J-shaped carbon composite prosthesis have an unfair advantage over athletes who compete in sports with natural legs [3].

After amputation, the patient undergoes several stages of rehabilitation to age the residual limb and prepare it for the prosthetic, which is fitted through a customized process often requiring the expertise of a skilled prosthetist and multiple visits to a clinic by the amputee. During this process, all the prosthetic components are brought into proper alignment to ensure comfortable locomotion. The fabrication of prosthetic devices is further complicated because of the prosthetic socket, the interface between the device and the residual limb; it is usually custom-made for each

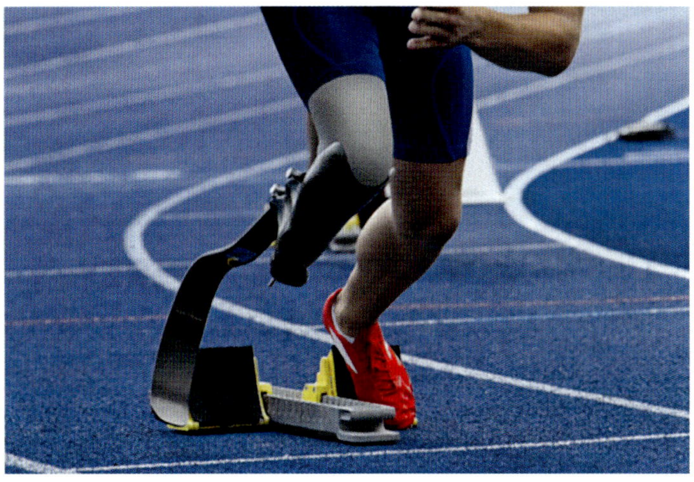

Fig. 14.8 A J-shaped prosthetic leg/foot used by athletes

individual, and poorly fitting sockets are a source of pain, discomfort, heat, skin chaffing, and ultimately a lower-quality of life.

Some leg prostheses incorporate artificial intelligence software that facilitates communication with various sensors, microprocessors, and sometimes even motors to supply assisted movement. These types of prostheses are commonly called "bionic" limbs (Fig. 14.9). The software is designed to analyze and provide real-time prosthetic movement adjustments for the user. This is based on feedback received from various sensors placed throughout the prosthesis and the residual limb and can sense body movement or electrical signals from the muscles (e.g., hamstrings) near the remaining limb. Bionic limbs are priced between tens of thousands to millions of dollars. Note that even though these prostheses are very advanced, the signals used to control the prosthesis are not optimal. Natural limb movement is a complex process controlled by various parts of the brain. Although researchers are working on the idea of controlling prosthesis by thought, currently the technology of the brain–machine interface is inadequate to permit building a prosthesis or orthosis that is directly controlled by the brain. That would require implantation of sensors (electrodes) directly in the brain which is currently not recommended outside of research environments.

To avoid problems related to socket fit, prostheses can be directly attached to the residual bone (into the intramedullary canal of a femur) of the amputated limb. This method is based on the principle of osseointegration. By directly attaching the prosthesis to the bone, a stable fit that avoids the problems related to socket-type prostheses is achieved. However, an osseointegrated prosthesis has its own set of problems; the implant system is ready to use only after two surgical sessions done 6 months apart. Other disadvantages include superficial infections at the implant–skin penetration area, pain during loading, mechanical complications, deep bone infections, risk of bone fractures, and implant loosening.

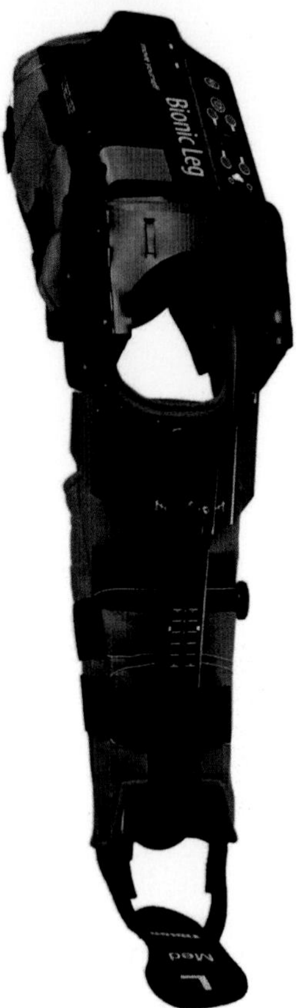

Fig. 14.9 Robotic leg orthosis. Tibion™ bionic leg orthosis and shoe insert with foot sensor. Creative Commons Attribution License Copyright by Nancy N. Byl, in: Mobility training using a bionic knee orthosis in patients in a post-stroke chronic state: a case series. Journal of Medical Case Reports July 2012, 6:216

14.4.2 Upper-Extremity Amputations

The incidence of major upper-extremity amputation is relatively low when compared to lower-extremity amputations. Almost 90 % of upper-extremity amputations occur due to trauma in the younger civilian population or soldiers. Many of these amputations occur at the thumb or finger level. The surgeon will first attempt to replant or revascularize (ensure that blood vessels are still functioning) the digit before considering amputation. Other reasons for upper limb amputation include burns (e.g., high-voltage electrical burns), infections, malignant tumors, birth defects, psychological conditions, or peripheral vascular disease. In the case of major upper-extremity amputation (e.g., transhumeral or wrist disarticulation), the patient undergoes pre- and post-amputation rehabilitation, including psychological support, pain management, occupational readjustment, and prosthesis fitting. There are many different types of prostheses available for upper-extremity amputees. They include:

Cosmetic: Some amputees may prefer prostheses that look and feel like natural hands to help them interact more easily in social settings. Prostheses made of PVC or silicon may be used for this purpose. These cosmetic prostheses, also called "cosmeses," are considered passive.

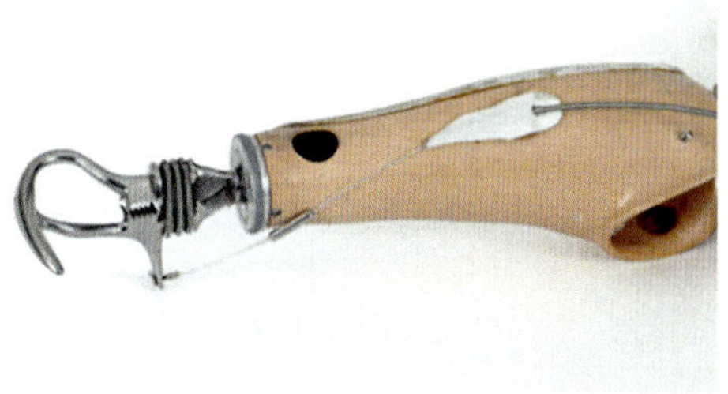

Fig. 14.10 An older version of a mechanical arm prosthesis showing cable control of one of the grasping hooks

Mechanical: Despite technological advances, most upper-extremity prostheses worn by amputees are controlled mechanically. These prostheses may be operated by "Bowden cables," which were first used in the bicycle and aircraft industry to control brakes or throttles. The amputee operates the Bowden cable(s) using gross muscle and shoulder movements to open/close a grabbing device (split hooklike) which simulates a thumb–finger pinch (Fig. 14.10). Large muscle movement and mental concentration is required to operate this device, potentially leading to muscle fatigue and loss of interest on the part of the patient. The advantages of this kind of prosthesis include simplicity of operation and easy maintenance.

Myoelectric prostheses: Externally powered prostheses may avoid the problems associated with mechanical control. They are equipped with an external battery that powers various motors, similar to the technology used to build hands in robots. Externally powered upper-extremity prosthesis can be controlled by physical switches, body movement, muscle activity signals, or signals directly from the brain. Currently, it is more practical to build prostheses that can be controlled by signals generated in the residual limb muscles (that's why this type of prosthesis is called a "myoelectric" prosthesis). When a muscle contracts, a small electrical signal in the range of a few to 30 mV is produced by the muscle cells. Electromyography (EMG), also referred to as myoelectric activity, is a technique of detecting, recording, and analyzing electrical signals produced during various muscle activities. In the case of a myoelectric prosthesis, these electrical signals are captured by multiple surface EMG sensors placed inside the prosthetic socket. While these prostheses use EMG measured on the skin surface, attempts have been made to surgically implant sensors directly into the residual muscles. The noisy EMG signals acquired from either surface or implantable sensors are then processed by an onboard computer and sent to different motors to produce a motion in a myoelectric hand, myoelectric elbow, or myoelectric hook ("Greifer") prosthesis. The major limitations to building a myoelectric prosthesis include size, weight (not more than 3 kg), tactile sensing, and battery life.

Hybrid prostheses: These prostheses contain both mechanical and electric control systems. An example of such a prosthesis is a body-powered locking elbow (mechanical) with a myoelectric wrist and hand.

Bionic arm prostheses: Systems in which hand and elbow function is directly controlled by the human brain are in the experimental stages of development (Fig. 14.11). Efforts are underway to lengthen human nerve cells so that they

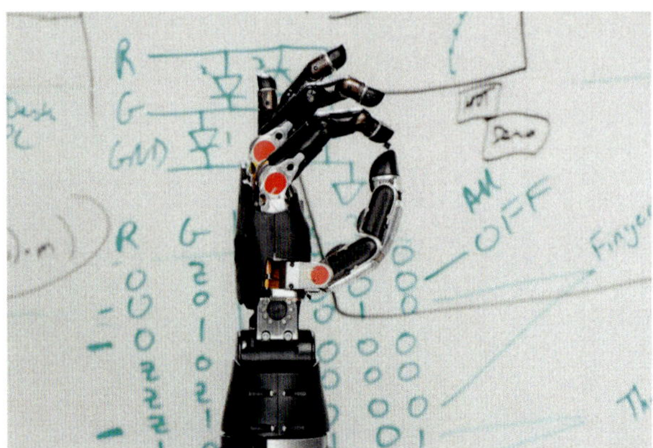

Fig. 14.11 Futuristic hand and arm prosthesis being developed with funding from DARPA (the Defense Advanced Research Projects Agency)

may more easily be connected to electronic circuitry and have proven successful in a laboratory setting [4].

Arm or hand transplantation: Even though there are many advances in artificial and robotic prostheses, some patients benefit from limb transplantation. During the past decade, surgeons have built on experience with kidneys, lungs, heart, and liver to perform face and limb transplantation. The scientific name for face and limb transplantation is "vascularized composite allotransplantation" (VCA). The required vascularized composite, face (not head) or limb, is usually harvested from a traumatic brain-dead donor. Recent recipients of VCA include individuals who lost their limbs through traumatic incidents such as roadside bombs, gun shots, or severe burns. As of 2012, less than 100 people have participated in vascularized composite allotransplantation (face or hands). Limb transplants are superior compared to any artificial prosthesis in terms of their ability to restore near-normal function. However, the surgical techniques are relatively new and challenges such as nerve regrowth and immune reaction remain.

14.5 Rehabilitating Hearing

Sound is a mechanical wave (also called a "material wave") that travels as tiny vibrations through gases, liquids, and solids. Humans can hear sound waves through a sophisticated organ called the ear. Human hearing begins in utero (in the womb). Human ears can normally process sound waves with frequencies between 20 and 20,000 Hz (audible frequency range), though the exact audible frequency range depends on individual factors such as age. The 2010 statistics compiled by the National Institute on Deafness and Other Communication Disorders (NIDCD) indicate that 36 million US adults suffer from some degree of hearing loss. Factors that cause hearing loss or deafness include heredity, infections, trauma, medications, aging, exposure to loud music, occupational exposure to loud noise (e.g., construction, firearms, airline ground maintenance), or earwax. Possible treatments for hearing loss include hearing aids, cochlear implants, special training, medication, and

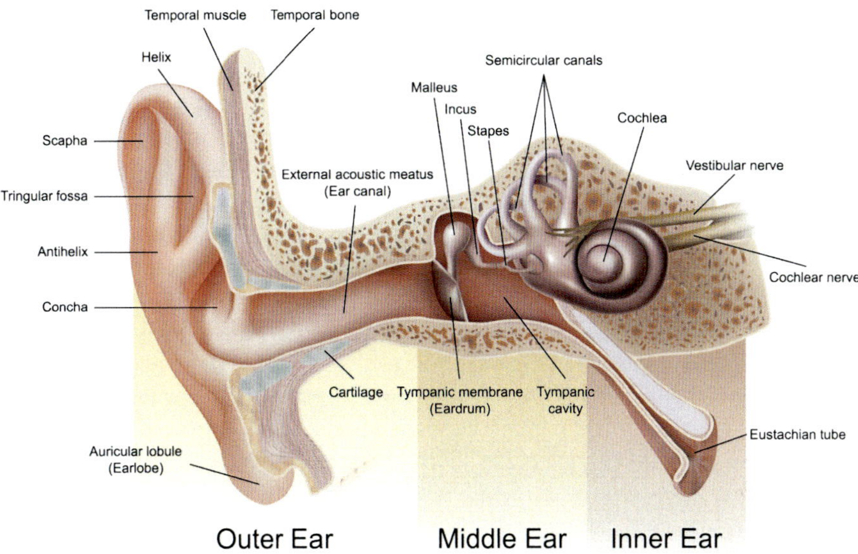

Fig. 14.12 Diagram of ear anatomy

surgery. Doctors who specialize in hearing loss treatments are called otolaryngologists or ENT (ear, nose, and throat) physicians.

The human ear is divided into three distinct sections: the outer, middle, and inner ear (Fig. 14.12).

The outer ear is composed of the pinna and the ear canal. Pinna, a cartilaginous tissue covered with skin, helps collect sound waves. The ear canal is lined with hair follicles and glands that produce a waxy substance called cerumen (commonly known as earwax). Earwax protects the skin of the ear canal against dust, irritants, or bacteria. The ear drum (tympanic membrane), a thin conical-shaped membrane, separates the ear canal from the middle ear. The middle ear is composed of three tiny bones, called the malleus, incus, and stapes (acting as "hammer," "anvil," and "stirrup," respectively). The inner ear is enclosed in dense bone and is composed of two specific parts: (1) the organ of hearing (the cochlea) and (2) the organ of balance (the vestibular labyrinth). The cochlea is a spiral-shaped fluid-filled tissue and contains specialized cells called the hair cells. The hair cells can transform fluid vibrations caused by the ear ossicles into electrical/nerve signals (there are a few thousand hair cells in each cochlea). These signals then travel via the auditory nerve to the brain, where the electrical signals are processed by the part of a brain called the auditory cortex. The vestibular system contributes to balance and sense of spatial orientation.

In summary, sound enters the external ear (pinna) and travels through the ear canal. The sound causes the eardrum and its tiny attached bones (ossicles) in the middle portion of the ear to vibrate. The vibrations then travel through the spiral-shaped cochlea and are converted by hair cells into electrical signals, which are processed by the auditory cortex located in the brain. It is also interesting to note that humans can hear through a secondary mechanism called bone conduction. The skull bone acts as a collector of sound waves (bypassing the middle and external ear) which are then processed via the cochlea and the auditory cortex. Hearing loss can occur when something goes wrong either in the outer, middle, or inner ear. Hearing loss can occur either in one ear or both ears. When left untreated, hearing loss can lead to many secondary problems, including isolation and loneliness.

In the outer or middle ear, infections, abnormal bone growths, benign or malignant tumors, earwax buildup, or ruptured eardrums (tympanic membrane perforation) can cause hearing loss. Infections are usually treated with antibiotics. Earwax can block the ear canal and prevent conduction of sound waves. Conductive hearing loss caused by earwax buildup can be restored with earwax removal. A ruptured eardrum (tympanic membrane perforation) can be caused by infections, loud blasts of noise, sudden changes in pressure, or trauma. Perforated ear drums that don't heal on their own are repaired using "myringoplasty" (the perforation is glued/filled using film paper or gelatin) or tympanoplasty (connective tissue grafting). Tumors are usually treated by surgical removal followed by radiation or chemotherapy.

Aging, heredity, and prolonged exposure to loud noise may cause wear and tear to the hairs or nerve cells in the cochlea. When these hairs or nerve cells are damaged or missing, electrical signals are not transmitted as efficiently, and hearing loss occurs. Damaged hair cells usually mean muffled higher pitched tones and difficulty picking out words against background noise. This type of hearing loss is known as "sensorineural" hearing loss and is permanent.

If hearing loss cannot be treated medically, the patient may need a hearing aid. Hearing aids have been used to improve hearing since the seventeenth century. Ear trumpets and cones were used as instruments to amplify sounds. The manufacture of modern electrical hearing aids began with the invention of the telephone. Early analog hearing aids used a carbon microphone and electric amplifier to increase the loudness of the incoming signal. Modern digital hearing aids use microcomputers to process incoming sound signals and adjust or eliminate any background noise. Patients can obtain a hearing aid from otolaryngologists, audiologists, and other hearing aid specialists after an audiology exam (or hearing test). Even though modern technology can miniaturize hearing aids, it should be kept in mind that elderly patients may have difficulty wearing extremely small hearing aids due to hand dexterity problems (or ergonomics).

14.5.1 Cochlear Implants

The notion that an electric current applied to the cochlea or to the auditory nerve might be perceived by the brain as sound is not new. It had its beginnings in the late eighteenth century, and Benjamin Franklin may have suggested the possibility 200

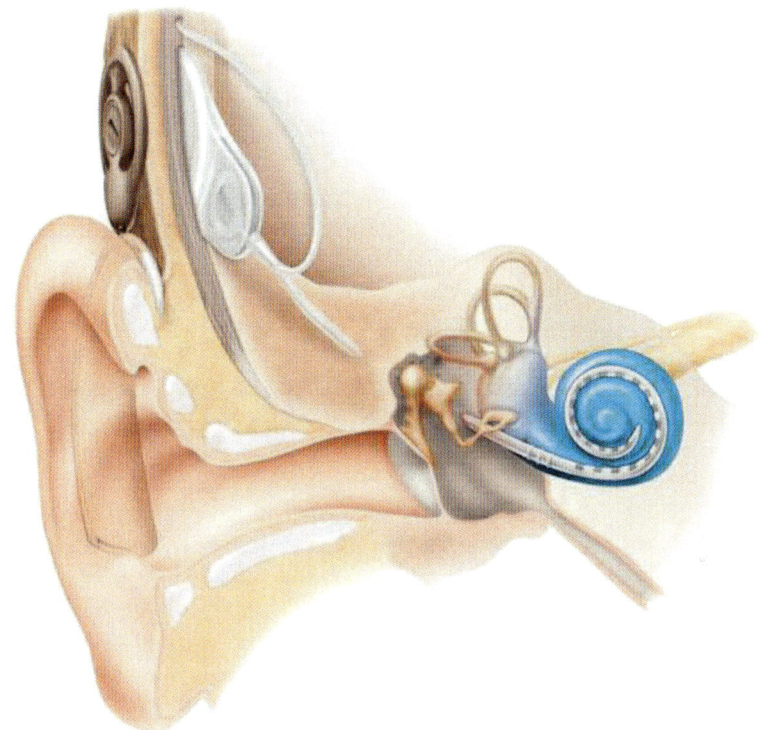

Fig. 14.13 A cochlear implant. Copyright by Springer-Verlag GmBH Berlin Heidelberg

years ago. Alessandro Volta, an Italian physicist who invented the "modern version" of a battery was the first to stimulate his own auditory system electrically. He connected a 50 V battery (direct current) to two metal rods and inserted them into his external ears—not something we advise the reader to emulate! He received the sensation of a boom within the head followed by a sound similar to that of the boiling of thick soup. Others tried different methods to use electric signals to aid hearing, but the idea did not become a clinical reality until the 1950s. In 1957, Djourno and Eyries in Paris implanted a rudimentary single channel electrode into the auditory nerves that were exposed during an operation. The patient was having surgery to eradicate a cholesteatoma (middle ear cyst) in his only hearing ear. By stimulating the electrode with an external current generator, they could produce a perception of sound that the patient likened to crickets chirping.

A cochlear implant (Fig. 14.13) is an electronic device that is inserted into the inner ear of a totally deaf person to introduce or restore the perception of sound [5]. The cochlear implant has been the result of research in many disciplines, including surgical anatomy, surgical pathology, biology, biophysics, neurophysiology, psychophysics, speech science, engineering, surgery, audiology, rehabilitation, and education. This implant is quite different from a simple hearing aid which merely amplifies sound.

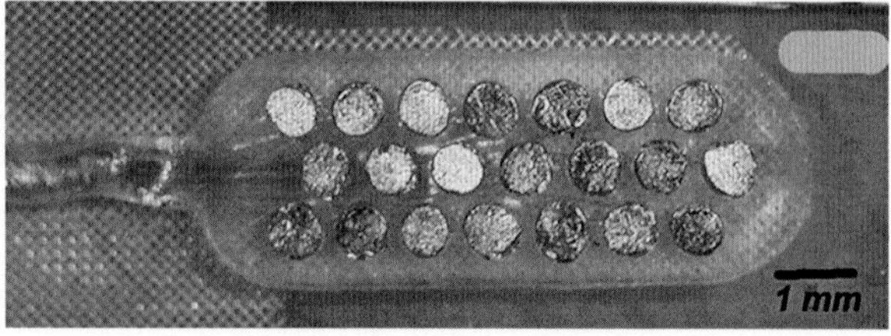

Fig. 14.14 The electrode component of an auditory brainstem implant. Copyright by Springer Science and Business Media LLC

The cochlear implant contains external and internal parts. The external detachable component comprises a microphone, a small battery-powered device for processing the signal, and an induction coil that transmits the refined signal through the skin to the implant. The external component gathers and processes sound using a microphone and a microprocessor. The internal component uses an electrode array implanted inside the cochlea that simulates the hair cells. The electrodes are usually made of gold, platinum, iridium, or their alloys. The electrical signals transmitted by the electrodes then continue normally to the brain through auditory nerves. These implants typically have between only 4 and 22 electrodes, less than 1 % of the number of hairs present in the cochlea. The implant surgery takes approximately 2 h and is done under general anesthesia. Hearing through a cochlear implant takes time to learn or relearn. Currently, cochlear implants are used by more than 200,000 patients worldwide. Patients who undergo cochlear implantation have a higher risk of developing meningitis (inflammation of the thin tissue that surrounds the brain and spinal cord, called the meninges) after surgery.

14.5.2 Auditory Brainstem Implant (ABI)

People with damaged or nonexistent auditory nerves due to disease (e.g., neurofibromatosis or von Recklinghausen's disease), trauma, or birth defects still cannot hear even if they have a fully functioning ear. These patients can benefit from auditory brainstem implants (ABI, Fig. 14.14). These devices can enable humans to hear without ears by bypassing the natural hearing process. Auditory brainstem implants process sound and send sound signals directly to the brain through penetrating electrodes placed in the brainstem. Similar to cochlear implants, the auditory brainstem implant contains an external receiver, processor, and implantable electrodes. A simple surgery is needed to implant the electrodes. Auditory brainstem implants placed on the surface of the cochlear nucleus are not as effective as cochlear implants because of tonotopic complexity (the locations in the brain where sounds of different frequency are processed are next to each other). A penetrating version implanted in the inferior colliculus (the midbrain nucleus of the auditory pathway) replicates sound better because it uses microelectrodes to more accurately deliver frequencies to appropriate nerves.

14.6 Rehabilitating Vision Loss

The human eye is a complex visual sense organ (Fig. 14.15). Different tissues in the eye work together in a way similar to a camera's functioning.

The cornea is a transparent tissue with a highly organized group of living cells and proteins and is responsible for gathering light into the eyes. The cornea contains no blood vessels, and the corneal cells are highly dependent on the tear film for nutrients and oxygen. The pupil, surrounded by the iris, is the round black circle in the eye that adjusts its diameter depending on the intensity of the surrounding light. The iris and pupil act like the aperture of a camera. The iris contains pigments that determine the eye color, an inherited trait. The light that is partly focused by the cornea passes through the pupil and is then further focused by the lens. The lens focuses the light onto a membranous tissue called the retina (situated in the very back of the eye). The retina acts like a camera film and contains specialized photoreceptor nerve cells (rods and cones) that convert light signals to electrical impulses and send them through the optic nerve to the brain where an image is constructed. The central area of the retina is called the macula. The macula is responsible for the most detailed central vision. As one can see (pun intended), the eye is a complex organ containing many components. Vision can be affected (e.g., refractive errors) or completely lost (e.g., blindness) when one of these components fails to function properly. According to World Health Organization statistics, worldwide there are 285 million people suffering from a visual impairment. The reason for failure could be genetic, a disease, infection, aging, occupation, or trauma. There are various

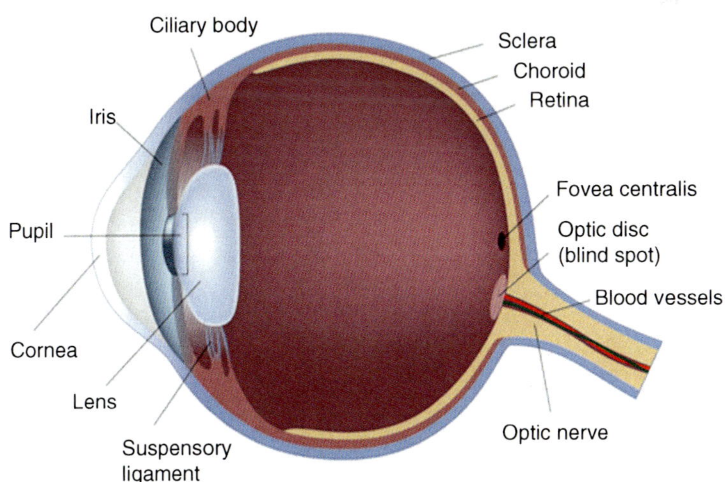

Fig. 14.15 Diagram of a human eye

technologies available to rehabilitate diverse degrees of vision loss. Eye doctors who can perform eye exams as well as surgeries are called ophthalmologists; optometrists test eye properties and prescribe corrective lenses.

Anophthalmia (the absence of one or both eyes) and microphthalmia (one or both eyes are abnormally small) are rare birth defects caused by genetic mutations, abnormal chromosomes, or environmental factors. This is different from another extreme birth defect called cyclopia where a child is born with one eye and other head and facial defects. Cyclopia children rarely survive after birth. Children with anophthalmia are fitted with an artificial eye. Even though the prosthetic eye does not restore vision, it is used for cosmetic purposes, to promote socket growth and avoid facial deformity.

14.6.1 Rehabilitating Refractive Errors

Every year millions of individuals around the world suffer from blurry vision or refractive errors. During childhood, the first sign of blurred vision is the inability to see small letters on the blackboard. This condition is caused by the eye's inability to focus light sharply on the retina. Contrary to popular belief, refractive errors are not usually caused by nutritional or vitamin deficiencies but typically occur for one of three reasons: (1) the corneal curvature is flatter or steeper than usual, (2) changes in the power of the lens, and (3) the overall length of the eyeball (distance from cornea to retina) is longer or shorter than normal. There are four common types of refractive errors sometimes called blurred vision: myopia (nearsightedness), hyperopia (farsightedness), presbyopia (difficulty focusing close up), and astigmatism (blurry and distorted images). An individual's refractive error is measured in diopters (the unit of measurement of the power of a lens) by a special instrument called a "phoropter." To measure refractive error, the individual is asked to read an eye chart placed at optical infinity (20 ft or 6 m for nearsightedness and 16 in or 40 cm for farsightedness) through different phoropter lenses. Individuals with farsightedness usually have difficulty reading books or words on computer screens. Individuals with shortsightedness usually have difficulty seeing distant objects. The most common method used by ophthalmologists or optometrists to correct refractive errors is to prescribe contact lens or glasses, which help refocus the light sharply on the retina. Individuals with extreme farsightedness may also need additional aids such as magnifying lenses or computers with zoom function software installed.

Many individuals do not like wearing contact lenses or glasses and may opt for surgical correction of vision errors. Refractive errors such as myopia (nearsightedness) can be treated by LASIK, or "laser-assisted in situ keratomileusis." This procedure was accidentally discovered in 1974 by a Russian scientist, Svyatoslav Fyodorov, who was asked to remove glass particles from the eye of a boy who had an accident and shattered his eyeglasses. During the surgery, Fyodorov made several incisions in the eye to remove the glass and after the cornea healed, discovered that the child no longer needed glasses! His nearsightedness had been cured.

The first paper describing the use of a laser to perform the specific type of eye surgery called radial keratotomy was published in 1985. In this procedure, incisions are made in the cornea in a radial or bicycle spokes-like pattern. The incisions allow the sides of the cornea to bulge out; the central portion of the cornea flattens, and the focal point of the eye changes. Prior to 1985, the surgery was performed using a diamond knife, but the laser was to eliminate the need for much of the cutting. The LASIK procedure, patented in 1989, uses a highly specialized laser, a cool ultraviolet light beam to "ablate" (remove) microscopic amounts of corneal tissue to reshape it. After local anesthesia, consisting of numbing eye drops and an intravenous drug to relax the patient, an ultrathin corneal flap is created on the eye's surface by a thin blade (microkeratome) or a laser (this option is taken in a procedure called "All-laser LASIK"). After laser energy is applied to reshape the cornea, the corneal flap is put back in place, to serve as a type of natural bandage. Normal corneas usually heal or regenerate within a matter of days.

The two types of lasers used in this surgery are the conventional LASIK and wavefront LASIK. The wavefront-guided process adds a measurement of subtle distortions or aberrations of the cornea beyond only those causing near- and farsightedness and astigmatism, though these additional distortions are responsible for no more than 10 % of the total refractive error in the eye. The wavefront-guided LASIK appears to yield slight superior results when compared with traditional LASIK.

What are the issues associated with this popular procedure? First, the FDA has approved it only for patients 18 years of age and older whose eye prescription has not changed for at least 1 year. There is no point to permanently changing the eye's focus point if the eye is still developing. The prospective patient should also not have any corneal abnormalities such as keratoconus, a condition where the cornea adopts a cone-like shape. The FDA and the American Academy of Ophthalmology have issued guidelines, which state that prospective patients should not be pregnant or breast-feeding; should not be taking the prescription drugs Accutane, Caradone, Imitrex, or oral prednisone; should not be nearsighted; and should be in good general health. Other contraindications for LASIK include blepharitis (an inflammation of the eyelids that causes crusting of the eyelashes), exceptionally large pupils, thin corneas (which do not leave much tissue for the LASIK procedure), and regular participation in contact sports that put the patient at risk of receiving shocks to the face and eyes. Also, LASIK unfortunately cannot correct vision for patients with presbyopia (a natural condition of aging eyes where near vision is compromised and normally resolved by wearing reading glasses) or help those with night driving problems. The latter are often another natural consequence of aging and may be improved by wearing glasses.

The most common risks include infection, scarring that will make it impossible to wear contact lenses, a decrease in contrast sensitivity, dry eyes (LASIK may worsen this symptom for patients already complaining of dry eyes), glare or haloes, and night driving problems.

Other laser-enhanced surgical procedures for the eyes include photorefractive keratectomy (PRK), which is similar to LASIK but intended for patients with a low to moderate degree of near- or farsightedness, or those with nearsightedness and astigmatism, but requires a longer healing time than LASIK. Laser epithelial keratomileusis (LASEK) is intended for patients with thin corneas. Vision may also be improved after implantation of synthetic lenses.

14.6.2 Blindness

According to World Health Organization statistics, worldwide there are 39 million people suffering from blindness. Blindness can result when any step of the optical pathway such as the retina, the optic nerve, visual cortex, or other cortical areas in the brain involved in the processing of vision sustains damage. The causes of blindness include cataracts, glaucoma, age-related macular degeneration, corneal opacity, diabetic retinopathy, childhood blindness, and retinitis pigmentosa (an inherited trait characterized by a damaged retina for which there is currently no cure). Currently, most cases of blindness caused by cataracts or corneal opacity can be treated.

Macular degeneration is a condition that affects more and more patients as they age, and the likelihood of developing this disease is related to the patient's genetic makeup. Treatment often involves injection of an anti-VEGF medication to prevent vascularization (blood vessel formation) in certain areas of the retina.

Corneal blindness can be treated by removing the damaged or diseased cornea and replacing it with a healthy cornea from a deceased donor. Almost anyone can be an eye donor after death. Eye donations actually refer to corneal donations, and a cornea from a deceased donor is usually transplanted within 7 days of donation.

The eye's natural crystalline lens is made primarily of water and protein and is normally clear. Cataract, painless clouding or opacification of the natural lens of the eye, is the most common cause of curable blindness in the world and generally comes on with age. Since a cataract affects the clarity of the lens, it prohibits the light from passing through the lens to the retina. The word cataract is derived from the Greek word meaning "white water falling." Around 300 BC, the ancient Hindus were the first to discover that within the eye there was a structure (the lens) and that if this structure became cloudy, sight would be lost. It is estimated that in the USA alone, there are over 24 million people suffering from cataracts. Throughout recorded history, various concoctions and eye drops were tried to cure cataracts but with little success. The only satisfactory treatment for cataracts available today is a surgery to remove the opaque lens and replace it with an artificial one. Other causes of cataract include injury, inflammation, diabetes, skin disease (atopic dermatitis), and occupational cataract (found among glassblowers, quarry workers, and steelworkers).

There are two types of surgical procedures to treat cataracts:

(1) Phacoemulsification utilizes a small incision on the side of the cornea to access the cataract with a tiny probe. Ultrasound energy is then used to break up the diseased lens for removal by suction. This is the most popular kind of cataract surgery.

(2) Extracapsular surgery requires a longer incision; the cloudy core is removed intact followed by removal of the remaining lens by suction.

The aphakic eye (eye without a lens) perceives a very blurred image of its surroundings. For clear vision, some sort of optical correction either internally or externally is

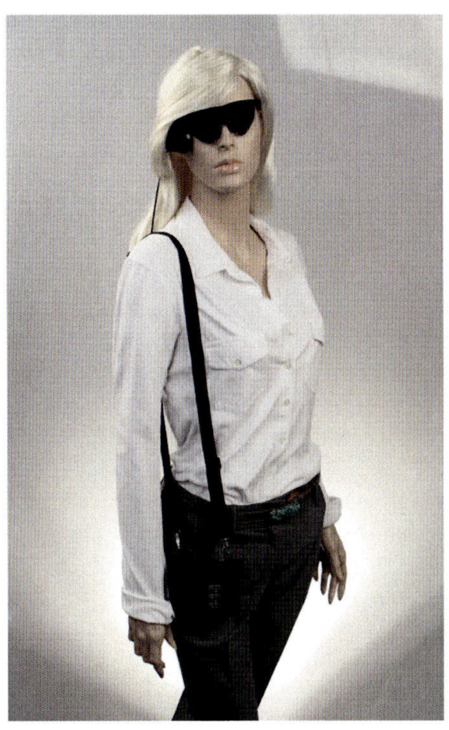

Fig. 14.16 The Argus II retinal prosthesis. Copyright © 2013 Second Sight Medical Products, Inc.

needed after the surgery. Until the advent of contact and intraocular lens implants, thick spectacles were the only means of achieving a finely focused image on the retina after a cataract surgery. An intraocular lens is a prosthetic device intended for replacing the natural lens of the eye. During the turn of the nineteenth century, an Italian surgeon tried to insert a glass lens after surgery, but due to its weight it immediately sank to the bottom of the eye. For another 150 years, surgeons tried different materials but without much success; everything they tried was toxic to the eye. During World War II, a British surgeon named Harold Ridley discovered that parts of Plexiglass™ from shattered aircraft canopies that penetrated into the eyes of pilots did not cause any harmful inflammation in their eyes. He used this discovery to create intraocular lenses made of poly(methyl methacrylate) or PMMA to fit inside an aphakic eye. Currently, many different models of hydrogel polymer intraocular lens implants are used to replace diseased lenses. The surgery normally takes less than an hour (diseased lens removal and intraocular lens implantation), and the patient needs no thick glasses for vision.

The retina is the rearmost part of the eye and contains specialized cells called photoreceptors. There are two types of photoreceptor cells: rods and cones. Rods are sensitive to low light levels, while cones are responsible for color vision and are much more concentrated in the central yellow spot known as the macula. Different models of retinal prostheses are being developed around the world [6]. Here, we will discuss a retinal prosthesis nicknamed "Argus II" (Second Sight Medical Products, Inc., Sylmar, CA; Fig. 14.16).

In February 2013, the US Food and Drug Administration (FDA) approved the first retinal implant for use in the USA as a humanitarian use device (HUD). According to the FDA, the HUD is a "medical device intended to benefit patients in the treatment or diagnosis of a disease or condition that affects or is manifested in fewer than 4,000 individuals in the United States per year." The Argus II consists of an external unit and an implantable unit. The external unit includes a miniature video camera, a wireless transmitter mounted on a pair of eyeglasses, and a video processing unit worn on the patient's belt. The scene captured by the camera is processed by the video unit and sent back to the wireless transmitter. The implantable unit consists of a wireless receiver (antenna) to receive the video signals and a 60-electrode array. The electrode array is mounted on top of the retinal membrane lining and emits small pulses of electricity which stimulate the retina's remaining photoreceptor cells. The remaining photoreceptor cells then transmit the digitized visual information along the optic nerve to the brain, creating the perception of patterns of light. After implantation surgery, a patient will undergo rehabilitation to learn how to interpret these visual light patterns. Argus II does not fully restore normal vision; however, it can improve a patient's ability to perceive images and movement. The cost of the Argus II has been quoted as approximately $150,000 excluding surgery and rehabilitation costs, but it will likely come down with time. It took 20 years of research and $200 million dollars of private and public funding to develop this device.

14.7 Speech Rehabilitation

Humans communicate with each other primarily by speaking and hearing. Every human being has a unique way of speaking by combining receptive or expressive language along with unique nonverbal cues, such as body language, facial expression, and gestures. The production of sounds or speech in humans is a complex process. Four different anatomic areas work together to produce speech or sound (Fig. 14.17). These include the oral cavity, nasal cavity, pharynx, and larynx (voice box). Three basic elements are necessary to produce speech: (1) a power source, (2) a sound source, and (3) a sound modifier. Air is the power source needed to produce a sound or speech. The respiratory system (e.g., lungs, rib cage, and diaphragm above the stomach) provides the air, which moves through the larynx (voice box) and trachea into the oral and nasal cavities. As the air travels through the trachea, the vocal cords in the larynx vibrate to produce sound. When the sound (voice) passes through the oral and nasal cavities, the tongue and lips move to modify the laryngeal sound to discernible speech. The voice and speech production process as well as timely nonverbal cues are coordinated by the brain.

Voice impairment can occur when the larynx in people with normal speaking skills sustains damage. The nerves controlling the larynx may be impaired because of an accident, a surgical procedure, a viral infection, or cancer. There are three major approaches used to restore voice after larynx damage or removal, including the use of an electrolarynx (a battery-powered vibrating equipment placed against the front of the neck while speaking), operative tracheoesophageal (TE) voice

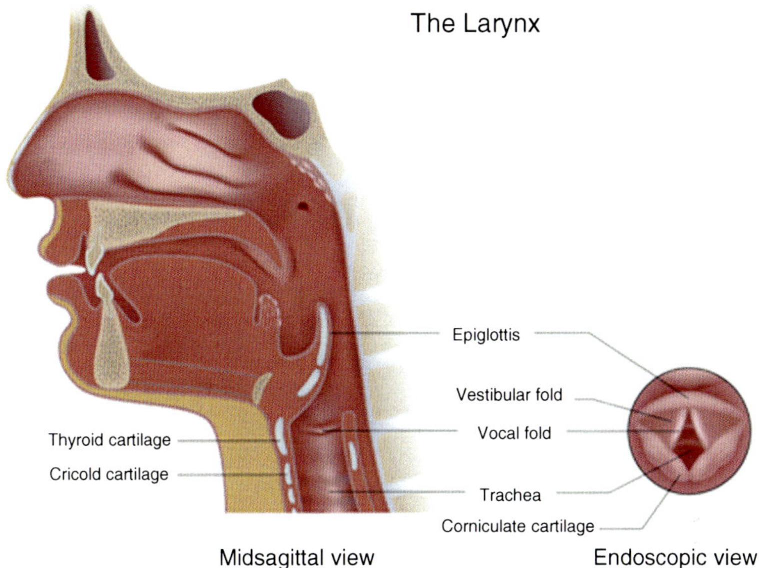

Fig. 14.17 Human voice production system

restoration (the patient covers an opening in the trachea with a finger, and a voice valve implanted in the airway permits some sounds to be made), and esophageal speech (speech produced through burping).

Aphasia is a medical term used to describe a loss of speech or language. The most common cause of speech loss in adults is damage of cerebral tissues responsible for speech and language. Brain damage can occur due to stroke (a common cause for speech loss), accidents, infections, and brain tumors. Speech language pathologists (SLPs) or speech therapists are trained to diagnose and help restore speech capabilities in these patients by employing strategies to improve cognitive skills, exercises for strengthening oral muscles, and teaching compensatory strategies.

14.8 Summary

Humans can become disabled in a single moment at any stage of life. The number of disabled individuals is greater now than at any other time in history, because more accident victims are surviving severe injuries (occupational and travel-related accidents, military-related trauma), because of poor health, and because of improvements in medical care. The financial and human costs of caring for the disabled are huge. Of course, humanity will be best served by taking proactive actions to prevent physical disability and to reduce the cost of medical care. These actions include educating the general public about preventive self-care (e.g., safety, exercise, avoiding obesity, smoking cessation programs); eliminating environmental causes of disability; upgrading occupational and travel safety; continued development of smart medical, engineering, and rehabilitation devices; and educating future rehabilitation service providers, physicians, engineers, or biomedical scientists. Even though we have come a long way in restoring lost function, more can be done to improve the quality of life of disabled individuals.

14.9 Foundation Concepts

- The American Disabilities Act passed in 1990 promises civil rights protection to all Americans with disabilities and guarantees equal opportunity in public accommodation, communication, employment, and transportation.
- Most disabilities cannot be cured by drugs, surgery, or tissue engineering methods. Relief is often provided by relying on other assistive technologies, including wheelchairs, crutches, orthoses, and prosthetic eyes and limbs. There is a growing incorporation of computer-aided or electronic controls into advanced limb prostheses such as bionic arms and legs, though the expense of these devices precludes their availability for all patients.
- Research is progressing to develop better ways to integrate arm and leg prostheses with the human body to allow more vigorous movement and to involve surviving elements of the nervous system to control prosthetic limb movement.
- Technological aids to improve hearing have continued to improve. Cochlear and auditory brainstem implants can now bring hearing to totally deaf patients, although it may be necessary to learn or relearn how to hear. Future improvements in implantable devices for the ear and eye will be made as scientists increase the number of connections to the central nervous system. This may be accomplished by decreasing electrode size and increasing electronic connection density.

References

1. Sparrow, R. (2005). Defending deaf culture: The case of cochlear implants. *Journal of Political Philosophy, 13*, 135–152.
2. Herr, H., Whitely, G., & Childress, D. (2003). Cyborg technology—biomimetic orthotic and prosthetic technology. In Y. Bar-Cohen & C. Breazeal (Eds.), *Biologically inspired intelligent robots*. International Society for Optical Engineering: Bellingham, WA.
3. Evelith, R. (July 24, 2012). Should Oscar Pistorius's prosthetic legs disqualify him from the Olympics? www.scientificamerican.com/article/cfm?id=scientists-debate-oscar-pistorius-prosthetic-legs-disqualify-him-olympics.
4. Cullen, D., & Smith, D. (2013). Bionic connections. *Scientific American, 308*, 52–57.
5. Moore, D., & Shannon, R. (2009). Beyond cochlear implants: Awakening the deafened brain. *Nature Neuroscience, 12*, 686–691.
6. Zrenner, E. (2002). Will retinal implants restore vision? *Science, 295*, 1022–1025.

Appendix A: A Proposal to the National Institutes of Health Under the Small Business Innovative Research Program

G.R. Baran et al., *Healthcare and Biomedical Technology in the 21st Century: An Introduction for Non-Science Majors*, DOI 10.1007/978-1-4614-8541-4,

OMB Number: 4040-0001
Expiration Date: 06/30/2011

APPLICATION FOR FEDERAL ASSISTANCE
SF 424 (R&R)

3. DATE RECEIVED BY STATE | **State Application Identifier**

1. * TYPE OF SUBMISSION
☐ Pre-application ☒ Application ☐ Changed/Corrected Application

4. a. Federal Identifier CA165492
b. Agency Routing Identifier

2. DATE SUBMITTED 08/22/2011
Applicant Identifier BC112599

5. APPLICANT INFORMATION
*** Organizational DUNS:** 057123100
* Legal Name: Cancer Therapeutics, LLC
Department: Division:
* Street1: 3711 Market Street
Street2: University City Science Center
* City: Philadelphia County / Parish:
* State: PA: Pennsylvania Province:
* Country: USA: UNITED STATES * ZIP / Postal Code: 191226027

Person to be contacted on matters involving this application
Prefix: * First Name: Eleanor Middle Name: M.
* Last Name: Brown Suffix:
* Phone Number: 215-205-5555 Fax Number: 215-205-5555
Email: ecicinsk@temple.edu

6. * EMPLOYER IDENTIFICATION *(EIN) or (TIN):* 231365982

7. * TYPE OF APPLICANT: R: Small Business
Other (Specify):
Small Business Organization Type ☒ Women Owned ☐ Socially and Economically Disadvantaged

8. * TYPE OF APPLICATION:
☒ New ☐ Resubmission
☐ Renewal ☐ Continuation ☐ Revision

If Revision, mark appropriate box(es).
☐ A. Increase Award ☐ B. Decrease Award ☐ C. Increase Duration ☐ D. Decrease Duration
☐ E. Other (specify):

* Is this application being submitted to other agencies? Yes ☐ No ☒ What other Agencies?

9. * NAME OF FEDERAL AGENCY: Dept. of the Army -- USAMRAA

10. CATALOG OF FEDERAL DOMESTIC ASSISTANCE NUMBER:
TITLE:

11. * DESCRIPTIVE TITLE OF APPLICANT'S PROJECT:
A novel targeting system for delivering chemotherapeutics to tumors

12. PROPOSED PROJECT:
* Start Date 01/01/2012 * Ending Date 01/31/2013

*** 13. CONGRESSIONAL DISTRICT OF APPLICANT**
PA-001

14. PROJECT DIRECTOR/PRINCIPAL INVESTIGATOR CONTACT INFORMATION
Prefix: Dr. * First Name: Mohammad Middle Name: L.
* Last Name: Kamali Suffix:
Position/Title: Chief Scientific Officer
* Organization Name: Cancer Therapeutics, LLC
Department: Division:
* Street1: 3711 Market Street
Street2: University City Science Center
* City: Philadelphia County / Parish:
* State: PA: Pennsylvania Province:
* Country: USA: UNITED STATES * ZIP / Postal Code: 19122
* Phone Number: 215-205-5555 Fax Number: 215-205-5555
* Email: mkamali@CTLLC.com

SF 424 (R&R) APPLICATION FOR FEDERAL ASSISTANCE — Page 2

15. ESTIMATED PROJECT FUNDING

a. Total Federal Funds Requested: 300,000.00
b. Total Non-Federal Funds: 0.00
c. Total Federal & Non-Federal Funds: 300,000.00
d. Estimated Program Income: 0.00

16. * IS APPLICATION SUBJECT TO REVIEW BY STATE EXECUTIVE ORDER 12372 PROCESS?

a. YES ☐ THIS PREAPPLICATION/APPLICATION WAS MADE AVAILABLE TO THE STATE EXECUTIVE ORDER 12372 PROCESS FOR REVIEW ON:
DATE:

b. NO ☐ PROGRAM IS NOT COVERED BY E.O. 12372; OR
☒ PROGRAM HAS NOT BEEN SELECTED BY STATE FOR REVIEW

17. By signing this application, I certify (1) to the statements contained in the list of certifications* and (2) that the statements herein are true, complete and accurate to the best of my knowledge. I also provide the required assurances * and agree to comply with any resulting terms if I accept an award. I am aware that any false, fictitious. or fraudulent statements or claims may subject me to criminal, civil, or administrative penalties. (U.S. Code, Title 18, Section 1001)

☒ *** I agree**

** The list of certifications and assurances, or an Internet site where you may obtain this list, is contained in the announcement or agency specific instructions.*

18. SFLLL or other Explanatory Documentation

Add Attachment | Delete Attachment | View Attachment

19. Authorized Representative

Prefix: Mr. * First Name: Robert Middle Name: W.
* Last Name: Walters Suffix:
* Position/Title: President
* Organization: Cancer Therapeutics, LLC
Department: Division:
* Street1: 3711 Market Street
Street2: University City Science Center
* City: Philadelphia County / Parish:
* State: PA: Pennsylvania Province:
* Country: USA: UNITED STATES * ZIP / Postal Code: 191226027
* Phone Number: 2152048691 Fax Number: 2152047486
* Email: rwalters@CTLLC.com

*** Signature of Authorized Representative**: Completed on submission to Grants.gov

*** Date Signed**: Completed on submission to Grants.gov

20. Pre-application

Add Attachment | Delete Attachment | View Attachment

OMB Number: 4040-0010
Expiration Date: 08/31/2011

Project/Performance Site Location(s)

Project/Performance Site Primary Location ☐ I am submitting an application as an individual, and not on behalf of a company, state, local or tribal government, academia, or other type of organization.

Organization Name: Cancer Therapeutics, LLC

DUNS Number: 0571231000000

* Street1: 3711 Market Street

Street2: University City Science Center

* City: Philadelphia County:

* State: PA: Pennsylvania

Province:

* Country: USA: UNITED STATES

* ZIP / Postal Code: 19122 * Project/ Performance Site Congressional District: PA-001

Project/Performance Site Location 1 ☐ I am submitting an application as an individual, and not on behalf of a company, state, local or tribal government, academia, or other type of organization.

Organization Name: Temple University

DUNS Number: 0571231920000

* Street1: 1947 N. 12th st.

Street2:

* City: Philadelphia County:

* State: PA: Pennsylvania

Province:

* Country: USA: UNITED STATES

* ZIP / Postal Code: 19122 * Project/ Performance Site Congressional District: PA-001

Additional Location(s) Add Attachment Delete Attachment View Attachment

Principal Investigator/Program Director (Last, first, middle): Kamali, Mohammad

424 R&R and PHS-398 Specific Table Of Contents

Principal Investigator/Program Director (Last, first, middle): Buerk, Donald

RESEARCH & RELATED Other Project Information

1. * Are Human Subjects Involved? ☐ Yes ☒ No

1.a If YES to Human Subjects

Is the Project Exempt from Federal regulations? ☐ Yes ☐ No

If yes, check appropriate exemption number. ☐ 1 ☐ 2 ☐ 3 ☐ 4 ☐ 5 ☐ 6

If no, is the IRB review Pending? ☐ Yes ☐ No

IRB Approval Date:

Human Subject Assurance Number:

2. * Are Vertebrate Animals Used? ☒ Yes ☐ No

2.a. If YES to Vertebrate Animals

Is the IACUC review Pending? ☒ Yes ☐ No

IACUC Approval Date:

Animal Welfare Assurance Number: none

3. * Is proprietary/privileged information included in the application? ☒ Yes ☐ No

4.a. * Does this project have an actual or potential impact on the environment? ☐ Yes ☒ No

4.b. If yes, please explain:

4.c. If this project has an actual or potential impact on the environment, has an exemption been authorized or an environmental assessment (EA) or environmental impact statement (EIS) been performed? ☐ Yes ☐ No

4.d. If yes, please explain:

5. * Is the research performance site designated, or eligible to be designated, as a historic place? ☐ Yes ☒ No

5.a. If yes, please explain:

6. * Does this project involve activities outside of the United States or partnerships with international collaborators? ☐ Yes ☒ No

6.a. If yes, identify countries:

6.b. Optional Explanation:

7. * Project Summary/Abstract 1234-MedVas Abstract.pdf | Add Attachment | Delete Attachment | View Attachment

8. * Project Narrative 1235-MedVas Summary Narrative.pdf | Add Attachment | Delete Attachment | View Attachment

9. Bibliography & References Cited 1236-Med Vas References_Rev1.pdf | Add Attachment | Delete Attachment | View Attachment

10. Facilities & Other Resources 1237-MedVas Facilities and Resources. | Add Attachment | Delete Attachment | View Attachment

11. Equipment | Add Attachment | Delete Attachment | View Attachment

12. Other Attachments Add Attachments | Delete Attachments | View Attachments ☐

ABSTRACT

The product that will be developed by Cancer Therapeutics, LLC is a drug targeting vehicle for cancer therapeutics used in combination with radiation therapy. The product uses a feature of ionizing radiation to match drug delivery selectivity with that of the radiation treatment. More than 50% of cancer patients receive radiation therapy, or chemotherapy, or a combination of both. While modern radiation therapy techniques are highly tunable to tumor locations, combination therapies are limited by the poor selectivity of most systemic chemotherapy strategies. We have recently patented a drug targeting system that selectively delivers chemotherapeutics to tumor endothelial cells using cell surface proteins that are upregulated by exposure to ionizing radiation. We have demonstrated that surface targets are significantly upregulated by exposure to radiation therapy, and that various molecules can be used to ensure that both core and peripheral cancer tissues are targeted. We have demonstrated that our system can be used to control tumor growth in a rodent model, and that multiple targeting ligands increase delivery efficiency. In this Phase 1 proposal, we intend to demonstrate proof-of-concept that a bifunctionalized format of our product can selectively deliver a vascular disrupting agent to endothelial cells, and more effectively and safely inhibit tumor growth in an animal model of disease.

NARRATIVE SUMMARY

This proposal will increase the effectiveness and safety of combined radiation and chemotherapies for cancer treatment. Current combined treatments are limited by the poor cancer-selectivity of drugs. The product being developed here will be the first drug delivery system that uses focused radiation to guide chemotherapeutic agents to cancer cells, while sparing normal tissues from side effects.

Appendix B: A Representative U.S. Patent

US005219899A

United States Patent [19]

Panster et al.

[11] **Patent Number: 5,219,899**

[45] **Date of Patent: Jun. 15, 1993**

[54] **PASTY DENTAL MATERIAL WHICH IS AN ORGANOPOLYSILANE FILLER COMBINED WITH A POLYMERIZABLE BONDING AGENT**

[75] Inventors: **Peter Panster**, Rodenbach; **Ralf Janda**, Bad Homburg; **Peter Kleinschmidt**, Hanau, all of Fed. Rep. of Germany

[73] Assignee: **Degussa Aktiengesellschaft**, Frankfurt am Main, Fed. Rep. of Germany

[21] Appl. No.: **963,045**

[22] Filed: **Oct. 19, 1992**

Related U.S. Application Data

[63] Continuation of Ser. No. 512,250, Apr. 20, 1990, abandoned.

[30] **Foreign Application Priority Data**

Apr. 22, 1989 [DE] Fed. Rep. of Germany 3913252

[51] **Int. Cl.**[5] **C08F 283/12**

[52] **U.S. Cl.** **523/118**; 523/115; 523/116; 523/117; 525/479

[58] **Field of Search** 525/479; 523/115, 116, 523/117, 118

[56] **References Cited**

U.S. PATENT DOCUMENTS

3,926,906	12/1975	Lee et al.	260/41
4,427,799	1/1984	Orlowski et al.	523/116
4,504,231	3/1985	Koblitz et al.	433/228
4,575,545	3/1986	Nakos et al.	526/242
4,690,986	9/1987	Sasaki et al.	525/479
4,717,599	1/1988	Merrill	525/479
4,728,709	3/1988	Klemarczyk et al.	528/15
4,826,893	5/1989	Yamazaki et al.	525/479
4,853,434	8/1989	Block	525/479
5,132,337	7/1992	Panster et al.	523/117

FOREIGN PATENT DOCUMENTS

0381961	8/1990	European Pat. Off. .
4002726	9/1990	Fed. Rep. of Germany .
2051842	1/1981	United Kingdom .

OTHER PUBLICATIONS

Chemical Abstract No. 53364 to Charles Mallon, vol. 100, 1984.

Primary Examiner—John C. Bleutge
Assistant Examiner—Margaret W. Glass
Attorney, Agent, or Firm—Beveridge, DeGrandi, Weilacher & Young

[57] **ABSTRACT**

A pasty dental material is disclosed which hardens to a high gloss polishable mass in the presence of an initiator. The mass is formed of a polymerizable bonding agent combined with an organosiloxane filler which contains units of the formula I

```
        |
        O
        |
   —O—Si—O—
        |
        O
        |
```

and which has been subjected to an after treatment which is a condensation in an autoclave for a period of time of 1 hour to 5 days at a temperature of 60° C. to 250° C. under a pressure which is the sum of the partial pressures at the given temperature.

12 Claims, No Drawings

G.R. Baran et al., *Healthcare and Biomedical Technology in the 21st Century: An Introduction for Non-Science Majors*, DOI 10.1007/978-1-4614-8541-4,

PASTY DENTAL MATERIAL WHICH IS AN ORGANOPOLYSILANE FILLER COMBINED WITH A POLYMERIZABLE BONDING AGENT

CONTINUING APPLICATION DATA

This application is a continuation of U.S. patent application Ser. No. 07/512,250, now abandoned, filed Apr. 20, 1990, which application is entirely incorporated herein by reference.

INTRODUCTION AND BACKGROUND

The present invention concerns a pasty dental material, which hardens to a high-gloss polishable mass in the presence of an initiator, formed of a polymerizable bonding agent and a finely divided filler as the essential components. The material contains as a bonding agent at least one polymerizable methacrylate and an optionally silanizable, new filler based on functional polysiloxanes. It may also contain initiators to trigger polymerization, other fillers, such as finely ground glass types, highly dispersed silicas or previously produced polymers, pigments and stabilizers. Other additives such as softeners or impact strength improvers may also be contained in the composition.

The term "dental material" as used herein means, for example, filling materials for carious defects or other dental defects in the mouth, inlays, crown and bridge materials, veneers, sealing and protective coatings, plastic adhesives to fix inlays or crowns and bridges, stump build-up materials, denture materials as well as masses for the production of artificial teeth.

Standard dental masses of the above mentioned type contain at least one monomeric ester of methacrylic acid, but in most cases a mixture of several of such esters. Suitable monofunctional esters of methacrylic acid are e.g. methylmethacrylate, ethylmethacrylate, isopropylmethacrylate, n-hexylmethacrylate and 2-hydroxyethylmethacrylate.

Recently, multi-functional esters of methacrylic acid with a higher molecular weight have also been used frequently, such as ethylene glycol dimethacrylate, butandiol-1,4-dimethacrylate, triethylene glycol dimethacrylate, dodecandiol-1,12-dimethacrylate, decandiol-1,10-dimethacrylate, 2,2-bis-[p(γ-methacryloxy-β-hydroxypropoxy)-phenyl]-propane, the diaduct of hydroxyethylmethacrylate and trimethylhexamethylene diisocyanate, the diaduct of hydroxyethylmethacrylate and isophoron diisocyanate, trimethylolpropanetrimethacrylate, pentaerythritetrimethacrylate, pentaerythritetetramethacrylate and 2,2-bis[p(β-hydroxy-ethoxy)-phenyl]-propanedimethacrylate (bis-GMA).

The materials for dental use may, depending on the application purpose, be hardened in different ways. Dental filling materials exist in the form of photo-hardening as well as self-hardening (autopolymerizing) masses. The photohardening masses contain photoinitiators such as benzoinalkylether, benzilmonoketals, acylphosphinoxide or aliphatic and aromatic 1, 2-diketocompounds such as e.g. camphorquinone as well as polymerization accelerators such as aliphatic or aromatic tertiary amines (e.g. N,N-dimethyl-p-toluidine triethanolamine) or organic phosphites and harden when irradiated with UV or visible light.

The self-hardening materials consist as a rule of a catalyst paste and a base paste of which each contains a component of a redox system and which polymerize when the two components are mixed. One component

of the redox system is in most cases a peroxide, such as e.g. dibenzoylperoxide, the other is in most cases a tertiary aromatic amine, such as e.g. N,N'-dimethyl-p-toluidine.

Other dental materials such as prosthesis plastics or plastic masses for the production of artificial teeth polymerize under heat application. The initiators in those cases are as a rule peroxides such as dibenzoylperoxide, dilaurylperoxide or bis(2,4-dichloro-benzoylperoxide).

Dental materials also contain as a rule pigments which—added in small amounts—act to match the color of the dental masses with the various shades of natural teeth. Suitable pigments are e.g. black iron oxide, red iron oxide, yellow iron oxide, brown iron oxide, cadmium yellow and orange, zinc oxide and titanium dioxide.

Dental materials further contain mostly organic or inorganic fillers in order to avoid a shrinking of the volume of the plastic mass during polymerization. Pure monomeric methylmethacrylate for instance shrinks during polymerization by about 20 vol %. By adding about 60 weight parts of solid methylmethacrylate-pearl polymer the shrinking may be reduced to about 5–6 vol % (see German Patent 24 03 211).

Other organic fillers are obtained by producing a polymer which consists essentially of esters of methacrylic acid and either is or is not cross-linked. This polymer optionally contains surface-treated fillers. If it has been produced as a polymer it may be added to the dental material in this form; if on the other hand it was produced by solventless polymerization in compact form it must be ground into a so-called splinter polymer before being added to the dental material.

Frequently used preformed polymers are in addition to the already mentioned filler-containing pearl and splinter polymers homopolymers of methyl methacrylate or, preferably non-cross-linked, copolymers of the methyl methacrylate with a low content of esters of the methacrylic acid or acrylic acid with 2 to 12 carbon atoms in the alcohol component, preferably in the form of a pearl polymer. Other suitable polymers are non-cross-linked products based on polyurethanes, polycarbonates, polyesters and polyethers.

Inorganic fillers are e.g. ground glasses or quartz with average particle sizes between 1 and 10 micrometers as well as highly dispersed silica with average particle sizes between 10 and 400 nm.

The glasses are preferably aluminumsilicate glasses which may be doped with barium, strontium or rare earths (see German Patent 24 58 380).

It should be noted in regard to the finely ground quartz or the finely ground glasses and the highly dispersed silica that the inorganic filler is as a rule silanized prior to the mixing with the monomers in order to achieve better bonding to the organic matrix. For this purpose the inorganic fillers are coated with silane coupling agents which in most cases have a polymerizable double bond for reaction with the monomeric esters of the methacrylic acid.

Suitable well known silane coupling agents for this purpose are e.g. vinyltrichlorosilane, tris-(2-methoxyethoxy)-vinylsilane, tris-(acetoxy)-vinylsilane and 3-methacryloyloxypropyltrimethoxysilane.

The initially mentioned, recently used monomers with higher molecular weight also result in a decrease of polymerization shrinkage. To these monomers the described inert inorganic finely ground glasses or organic fillers or mixtures thereof are added up to 85 wt %, which results in a further reduction of the shrinkage to ca. 1 vol %.

The inorganic fillers not only result in a decrease in polymerization shrinkage but in addition in a significant strengthening of the organic polymer structure.

This strengthening also shows itself in an improvement of mechanical characteristics and in an increase in wear resistance (R. Janda, Quintessenz 39, 1067, 1243, 1393; 1988). Good mechanical characteristics and high wear resistance are important requirements which must be fulfilled by a hard dental compound which is intended as a long-term replacement for lost hard natural dental substance.

But in addition to strengthening characteristics, the filling compounds also must fulfill other material parameters. An important parameter in this context is the polishability. High gloss polishability is of significant importance for filling materials and crown and bridge materials for at least two reasons:

- A high-gloss and completely homogenous surface must be required of the filling material for aesthetic reasons, so that the filling cannot be distinguished from the surrounding, absolutely smooth, natural tooth enamel. This high-gloss filling surface also must retain its characteristic for a long period.
- A highly smooth filling surface is also important so that plaque or discoloring media cannot attach themselves.

However, it has now been shown that the previously described finely ground quartz or glass fillers have good strengthening characteristics, but do not fulfill requirements in regard to their polishability. It has therefore been attempted to grind these fillers even finer in order to obtain more homogenous surfaces. However, physical grinding methods are limited, so that average grain sizes below 1 μm are hard to achieve.

When highly dispersed silica (average particle size 10 to 400 nm) was used as a filler in dental masses (German Patent 24 03 211) it was surprisingly shown that these fillers were able to achieve a significant improvement in polishability. Disadvantages of the highly dispersed silica result from its great thickening effect, so that today, as a rule, filling amounts above 52 wt % cannot be obtained, unless insufficient processing technology characteristics are tolerated.

The materials filled with highly dispersed silicic acid also showed clearly lower stabilities and hardness than those filled with quartz or finely ground glass.

SUMMARY OF THE INVENTION

It is an object of this invention to provide new photo-, heat- or self hardening dental materials containing a polymerizable organic bonding agent and a finely divided filler as essential ingredients, which on the one hand may be polished to high gloss and thus fulfill the aesthetic requirements of a dental material, but which on the other hand have better physical characteristics than the dental materials representing the present state of technology.

In attaining the above and other objects, one feature of the invention resides in new, pasty dental materials, which harden to a high-gloss polishable mass in the presence of an initiator, comprising a polymerizable bonding agent and a finely divided filler, which contains as a filler an organopolysiloxane which consists of units of the formula

$$\begin{array}{c} | \\ O \\ | \\ -O-Si-O- \\ | \\ O \\ | \end{array} \qquad (I)$$

and units of the formula

$$\begin{array}{c} R^1 \\ | \\ -O-Si-O- \\ | \\ O \\ | \end{array} \qquad (II)$$

wherein R^1 stands for a linear or optionally branched alkyl group with 1 to 6 carbon atoms bonded with an acrylate or methacrylate residue or for a single olefinic unsaturated, preferably end-positioned unsaturated linear, optionally branched hydrocarbon residue with 2 to 8 carbon atoms or for a cyclic, single olefinic unsaturated hydrocarbon residue with 5 to 8 carbon atoms or for a linear, optionally branched alkyl group with 1 to 8 carbon atoms, a cycloalkylene group with 5 to 8 carbon atoms, a phenyl group or an alkylaryl group and/or units of the formula

$$\begin{array}{c} R^1 \\ | \\ -O-Si-O- \\ | \\ R^2 \end{array} \qquad (III)$$

wherein R^2 represents a methyl, ethyl or phenyl group, and the free valences of the oxygen atoms bonded with the silicon atoms in the units (I), (II), (III) are as in the silica structures saturated by a silicon atom of a same or different unit whereby the ratio of silicon atoms of the units of Formula (I) to the sum of silicon atoms of units (II) and (III) is 3:1 to 100:1.

The units according to Formulas (I) to (III) may naturally be present in different forms in respect to each other, i.e. they may be present in the form of a statistical copolycondensate or in the form of a block-copolycondensate or in the form of a so-called mixed copolycondensate. According to the invention, the fillers of the new dental materials may in respect to the units according to Formulas (I) to (III) be present in any of the mentioned forms and their mixtures.

This means that in the case of a pure statistical copolycondensate which contains units of the Formula (I), (II), and/or (III) a pure statistical distribution of the components according to the molar ratios of the starting products is given.

In the case of a so-called block-copolycondensate, blocks of identical units according to Formula (I) and (II) and/or (III) form. Finally, a so-called mixed copolycondensate possesses structures of a statistical copolycondensate as well as of a block-copolycondensate.

The fillers according to the invention are used in the dental masses in an amount from 20 to 90 wt %, preferably 50 to 85 wt %. The unsaturated organic residue R^1 possibly also present at the units according to Formula (II) may in particular act to achieve a stronger bond between the polysiloxane filler and the polymer matrix which is later produced from the polymerizable organic bonding agent.

Organic residues R^1 in which a double bond is sterically readily accessible and in particular relatively easy to polymerize are therefore especially suitable. This applies in particular for the group

$$-(CH_2)_3-O-\overset{\overset{O}{\|}}{C}-\overset{\overset{CH_3}{|}}{C}=CH_2$$

since it is known that it is especially easy to polymerize and since the polymer matrix to which the filler is to be added is as a rule a methacrylate system, as well as for linear hydrocarbon residues with end-positioned double bond, such as e.g. the vinylbutenyl- or octenyl residue. However, cyclic hydrocarbon residues with polymerizable double bonds are also suitable. But in many cases R^1 may be one of the organic residues without double bonds also mentioned under Formula (II) in claim **1**.

DETAILED DESCRIPTION OF THE INVENTION

A particularly advantageous filler composition which is characterized by being readily obtainable and easily prepared especially by technical availability of the starting materials uses an organopolysiloxane as filler which consists only of the units of Formula (I) and the specific units of Formula (II)

$$-O-\underset{\underset{\underset{|}{O}}{|}}{\overset{\overset{|}{\overset{O}{|}}}{Si}}-(CH_2)_3-O-\overset{\overset{O}{\|}}{C}-\overset{\overset{CH_3}{|}}{C}=CH_2$$

whereby the molar ratio of the units of Formula (I) to the units of Formula (II) is 3:1 to 100:1. Such a filler is characterized by the fact that it principally no longer requires silanization before being added to the methacrylate matrix, i.e. it no longer requires treatment with a methacrylsilane, since these methacryl groups are already present in the filler in a homogeneously distributed form.

But this does not exclude that in individual cases, in view of a further water-repellant finishing with further strengthening of the bonding between the organopolysiloxane filler and organic polymer matrix, an additional silanization of the filler is performed.

During the realization of the invention it was surprisingly discovered that very good mechanical characteristics and polishability of the dental material may also be achieved if the organopolysiloxane filler used contains no unsaturated, but only saturated residues R^1.

This applies for fillers which contain units according to Formula (I), (II) and (III) as well as for fillers which contain only units according to Formula (I) and (II). Such organopolysiloxane fillers without functional double bonds should, prior to their addition to the organic polymer matrix, be treated with a suitable organosilane compound, preferably 3-methacryloyloxy propyltrimethoxy- or 3-methacryloyloxy propyltriethoxysilane.

This applies analogously also for a filler composition according to the invention which is advantageous for reasons of especially ready availability of the starting materials and in which the polysiloxane is made up of units of Formula (I) and the specific units of Formula (III)

$$-O-\underset{\underset{CH_3}{|}}{\overset{\overset{CH_3}{|}}{Si}}-O-$$

whereby the molar ratio of the units according to Formula (I) to the units of Formula (III) is 3:1 to 100:1.

The monomeric elements of the fillers according to the invention are principally known compounds, e.g. $Si(OC_2H_5)_4$ as monomeric element for a unit of Formula (I), a compound

$$(H_3CO)_3Si-(CH_2)_3-O-\overset{\overset{O}{\|}}{C}-\overset{\overset{CH_3}{|}}{C}=CH_2 \text{ or}$$

$$(H_3CO)_3Si-CH_2CH_2CH_3$$

as monomeric elements for units of Formula (II) and a compound $(H_3C)_2Si(OC_2H_5)_2$ as monomeric element for units of Formula (III).

The compositions of the dental filling materials that may be produced from them may be described e.g. by formulas for a particular polymer unit such as

$$40\ SiO_2.CH_2=\overset{\overset{CH_3}{|}}{C}-\underset{\underset{O}{\|}}{C}-O-(CH_2)_3SiO_{3/2}.(CH_3)_2SiO_{2/2}$$

$$10\ SiO_2.C_3H_7SiO_{3/2}.(H_5C_2)_2SiO_{2/2}$$

$$50\ SiO_2.(H_3C)_2SiO_{2/2} \text{ or}$$

$$30\ SiO_2.CH_2=\overset{\overset{CH_3}{|}}{C}-\underset{\underset{O}{\|}}{C}-O-(CH_2)_3SiO_{3/2}.$$

A typical acidic catalyst is e.g. hydrochloric acid or acetic acid, while amines are in addition to ammonia the typical basic catalysts.

In view of the physical characteristics the fillers of the composition according to the invention are particularly well suited for use in the dental materials according to the invention if they have a specific surface of about up to 200 m^2/g, preferably about up to 100 m^2/g, and a particle size from 0.01 μm to 100 μm, preferably 0.1 μm to 30 μm.

The fillers contained in the dental material according to the invention may be obtained according to various methods. One of these methods achieves this by dissolving an alkoxysilane of the general formula

$$Si(OR^3)_4 \qquad (IV)$$

whereby R^3 is a linear or branched alkyl group with 1 to 5 carbon atoms, and an alkoxysilane of the general formula

$$R^1-Si(OR^3)_3 \qquad (V)$$

in which R^1 has the same meaning as in Formula (II), and/or an alkoxysilane of the general formula

$$(R^2)_2Si(OR^3)_2 \qquad (VI)$$

in which R^2 has the same meaning as in Formula (III) in a mostly water-miscible solvent which, however, dissolves the silanes according to Formula (IV), (V) and (VI), and by adding to the solution while stirring an amount of water which is at least sufficient for the complete hydrolysis and condensation, then by precondensing the reaction mixture during continued stirring at a certain temperature ranging from room temperature to 200° C., by stirring the forming solid matter, optionally after addition of additional solvent or water, for 1 to 6 more hours at 60° C. to 200° C., at normal pressure or under a pressure which corresponds to the sum of partial pressures at the respective temperature, then post-treating the formed organopolysiloxane, optionally after a change of the medium and/or pH value, for another 4 hours to 5 days at 60° C. to 250° C. in the liquid phase, then separating according to standard methods from the liquid phase, optional washing, drying at room temperature up to 200° C., optionally in a controlled atmosphere or in vacuum, optional subsequent tempering for 1 to 100 hours at temperatures from 150° C. to 250° C. in a controlled atmosphere or in vacuum, optional grinding and/or classification, whereby the organopolysiloxane which has been separated from the liquid phase and optionally washed is prior to or after one of the phases of drying, tempering, grinding, classification treated in water, a water/alcohol mixture or in pure alcohol, in the presence of an acidic or basic catalyst, preferably in presence of ammonia, for a period of 1 hour to 5 days at temperatures from 60° C. to 250° C. under a pressure which corresponds to the sum of partial pressures at the respective temperature.

The advantageous application oriented technical characteristics of the new fillers are also based on the acidic or basic thermal treatment prior to or after the drying or in another of the optionally used treatment phases, since this results in particular in a strengthening of the polymer structure.

As a principle the corresponding halide or phenoxy compounds may be used in place of the alkoxy compounds as starting materials for the process. However, their use offers no advantages, but may e.g. in the case of chlorides result in problems because of the hydrochloric acid released during hydrolysis.

The hydrolysis of the monomers must be performed with an essentially water-miscible solvent which however dissolves the starting materials. Alcohols which correspond to the alkoxy groups at the monomeric starting materials are preferred.

Particularly suitable are methanol, ethanol, n- and isopropanol, n- and isobutanol and n-pentanol. Mixtures of such alcohols may also be used as solvents during the hydrolysis.

It is naturally also possible to use other polar solvents which are essentially water-miscible, but this is not very logical for reasons of process technology because of the solvent mixtures produced with the hydrolytically separated alcohol.

The hydrolysis is preferably performed with an excess of water above the stoichiometrically required amount. The amount of water required for hydrolysis depends on the hydrolysis speed of the respective monomer in such a manner that with an increasing amount of water the hydrolysis speeds up. However an upper limit may be given through segregation and forming of a two-phase system. As a rule hydrolysis is preferred in a homogenous solution.

Because of the mentioned aspects, in practice that maximum amount of water (in weight) is used as is used overall at silane monomers.

The polycondensation may be performed at different temperatures. Since the polycondensation is fastest at higher temperatures it is preferably performed at reflux temperature or slightly below. In principle the hydrolysis and polycondensation may still be performed at still higher temperature than reflux temperature, i.e. under pressure.

During polycondensation the reaction mixture may congeal into a solid mass. For this reason it is useful to add a corresponding amount of solvent or water for dilution.

As a rule, the solvent here will be the same as the one already used during hydrolysis of the silanes, i.e. preferably a lower alcohol with 1 to 5 carbon atoms.

As an alternative to the dilution with a solvent, it is naturally also possible to dilute with water. Whatever is used in the individual case depends on which physical characteristics are desired in the copolycondensate to be produced.

This may also be influenced by the duration and temperature of after-treatment in the liquid phase or in dry form. An after-reaction at higher temperature always results in a strengthening of the polymer structure and in an improvement of the mechanical properties.

The separation of the formed solid matter may be performed according to standard methods, such as filtration, decantation, centrifugation or distilling off of the liquid phase. The washing of the formed solid matter is preferably performed with the solvent used during the separation or with water.

The dried or tempered product may be ground in the usual devices and may be classified into various grain size fractions. Depending on the circumstances, one or the other of the finishing measures washing, drying, tempering, grinding and classification may be foregone, or they may be performed in a different sequence.

A classification may e.g. also be performed at the wet product which may have been optionally dried or tempered before.

The duration of the hydrolysis depends on the hydrolysis suitability of the starting materials and on the temperature. The hydrolysis temperature depends in particular on the alkoxy groups located at the silicon whereby the methoxy group hydrolyzes fastest and the process is slowed down with increasing chain length or increasing branching.

Hydrolysis and polycondensation may be accelerated by addition of organic or inorganic bases, e.g. ammonia or amines, or organic or inorganic acids, e.g. hydrochloric acid, or by the standard condensation catalysts, e.g. dibutyl tindiacetate.

In order to compensate for different hydrolysis and polycondensation characteristics of the monomeric components of a statistical copolycondensate, the monomeric components according to Formula (IV), (V) and/or (VI) may be precondensed according to one production version. For this purpose the monomeric components—with or without the use of a solvent dissolving the starting materials, preferably linear or branched alcohols with 1 to 5 carbon atoms corresponding to the alkoxy groups—are precondensed in the presence of an amount of water insufficient for complete hydrolysis, preferably 1 to 100 mol % of the amount required for it, for a period of 5 min to 5 days at room temperature to 200° C.

In order to promote this precondensation effect an acidic or basic condensation catalyst may be added to the process. Preferred catalysts are e.g. hydrochloric acid, acetic acid, ammonia, soda lye or caustic potash solution which are used in gas form or dissolved in water or in an organic solvent.

After the precondensation has been performed the complete hydrolysis and polycondensation, after optional addition of further water and optional addition of further solvent, is performed as described.

According to a different method so-called block copolycondensates are obtained in which blocks of identical units according to formula (I) and (II) and/or (III) have been formed. In this method the monomeric components according to Formula (IV), (V) and/or (VI), respectively independent from each other, are precondensed with or without the use of a solvent dissolving the starting materials, preferably a linear or branched alcohol with 1 to 5 carbon atoms corresponding to the alkoxy groups, in the presence of an amount of water insufficient for complete hydrolysis, preferably 1 to 100 mol % of the amount needed for this, for a period of 5 min to 5 days at room temperature to 200° C., the obtained condensates are combined and then, after optional addition of additional water and/or optional addition of additional solvent, the complete hydrolysis and polycondensation is performed as described.

Naturally, it is also possible to use one of the above mentioned condensation catalysts in the production version according to the invention.

According to another method so-called mixed copolycondensates are obtained in which a partial formation of blocks of identical units according to Formula (I) and (II) and/or (III) is present, but in which at least one monomeric component is always not precondensed and at least one monomeric component is precondensed.

This method is characterized by precondensing from the monomeric components according to Formula (IV), (V) and/or (VI) at least one monomer, but no more than 2 monomers, independent from each other, with or without use of a solvent dissolving the starting materials, preferably a linear or branched alcohol with 1 to 5 carbon atoms corresponding to the alkoxy groups, in the presence of an amount of water insufficient for complete hydrolysis, preferably in the presence of 1 to 100 mol % of the amount required for this, for a period from 5 min to 5 days at room temperature to 200° C., by combining the obtained precondensate or the obtained precondensates and at least one unprecondensed component with each other, and by then performing—after optional addition of additional water and/or optional addition of additional solvent—the complete hydrolysis and polycondensation as described.

The use of an acidic, basic and/or metal-containing condensation catalyst for precondensation is also feasible in this production version and the further treatment of the formed polycondensate takes place as in the other described production processes.

During the performance of the precondensation the amount of water used depends on the oligomerization degree to be obtained, i.e. which block size is to be attained. If more water and a longer precondensation time are used for precondensation this results naturally as a rule in larger units than if less water and a shorter reaction time are used. The duration of the precondensation depends, as already described above, in general naturally also on the hydrolysis readiness of the monomeric components and on the temperature.

The fillers for the new dental materials are characterized in particular by the quantitative hydrolysis and condensation yield and elementary analyses. In purely optical respects there is no difference between the copolycondensate obtained according to the various production processes. Depending on the treatment the fillers according to the invention have surfaces of about 0 to 200 m^2/g. The desired particle size diameters of 0.01 μm to 100 μm may be set without difficulty by using standard grinding techniques.

Another object of the invention is the use of the dental material for the production of dental fillings, inlays, dental sealants, coatings to protect tooth surfaces, crowns, veneers, bridges, dentures, artificial teeth, bonders for the attachment of inlays, crowns and bridges and for the building up of tooth stumps.

The invention is further explained by the following illustrative examples.

1. Preparation of Filling Materials to be Used in Accordance with the Invention

EXAMPLE 1

1,465.2 g (7.03 mol) $Si(OC_2H_5)_4$ and 34.8 g (0.234 mol) $(CH_3)_2Si(OC_2H_5)_2$ were dissolved in 750 ml ethanol. The solution was heated to reflux temperature and then 525 ml of 10% aqueous ammonia solution was added. It was first stirred for 30 min with reflux, then the formed solid matter was diluted with 750 ml of water. After another 2 hours of stirring the suspension was cooled with reflux to room temperature and the formed white solid matter was filtered off the liquid phase and washed with a total of 500 ml of water. 700 ml of 2% NH_3 solution were added to the solid matter and it was then transferred into an autoclave. After treatment of the autoclave content for 24 hours at 150° C. the solid matter was dried for 24 hours at 120° C. in the dryer in N_2 atmosphere and then ground for 24 hours in a ball mill.

The yield was 437.2 g (99.4% of theoretical yield) of a dental filling material, consisting of polymer units of the formula $(CH_3)_2SiO_{2/2}.30\ SiO_2$.

	Specific surface: 22 m^2/g		
Analyses:	% C	% H	% Si
Theory:	1.28	0.32	46.4
Actual:	1.12	0.40	45.6

EXAMPLE 2

1,456.5 g (6.99 mol) of $Si(OC_2H_5)_4$ and 43.5 (0.175 mol) of methacryloyloxy propyltrimethoxysilane were combined in 750 ml of ethanol. The solution was heated in a 6 l Woulff bottle (3 neck flask) with KPG agitator and reflux condenser to reflux temperature while stirring and 500 ml of 5% NH_3 solution was added to it at boiling point. After ca. 30 min of stirring with reflux the formed white solid matter was diluted with 750 ml of water. Stirring was continued for another 5 h with reflux; then the suspension was cooled to room temperature and the solid matter was filtered off from the liquid phase. 500 ml of 5% ammonia solution was added to the solid matter and it was then transferred to an autoclave.

After stirring the autoclave contents for 48 h at 130° C. the ammonia was washed off the solid matter and it was then dried for 24 h at 100° C. in N_2 atmosphere and then ground for 12 h in a ball mill. The yield was 450 g (99.6% of theoretical yield) of a dental filling material consisting of units of the formula

$$H_2C{=}C(CH_3){-}C({=}O){-}O{-}(CH_2)_3{-}SiO_{3/2}\cdot 40\ SiO_2$$

Specific surface: 23 m^2/g

Analyses:	% C	% H	% Si
Theory:	3.26	0.43	44.6
Actual:	3.12	0.34	44.0

EXAMPLE 3

1,431.8 g (6.87 mol) of $Si(OC_2H_5)_4$, 42.7 g (0.172 mol) of methacryloyloxy propyltrimethoxysilane and 25.5 g of $(CH_3)_2Si(OC_2H_5)_2$ were combined in 750 ml of methanol. The solution was heated to reflux temperature and then 400 ml of 5% ammonia solution were added to it. After following the procedures analogous to Example 2, 450 g (98.6% of theoretic yield) of a dental filling material consisting of units of the formula

$$CH_2{=}C(CH_3){-}C({=}O){-}O{-}(CH_2)_3{-}SiO_{3/2}\cdot(CH_3)_2SiO_{2/2}\cdot 40\ SiO_2$$

were obtained.

Specific surface: 32 m^2/g

Analyses:	% C	% H	% Si
Theory:	4.07	0.64	44.4
Actual:	3.82	0.59	43.4

EXAMPLE 4

722.9 g (3.47 mol) of $Si(OC_2H_5)_4$, 14.3 g (0.0867 mol) of $n{-}C_3H_7{-}Si(OCH_3)_3$ and 12.9 g (0.0867 mol) of $(CH_3)_2Si(OC_2H_5)_2$ were dissolved in 375 ml of ethanol. The solution was heated to reflux temperature and 200 ml of ln-HCl solution were added to it. After 1 h the solid matter formed and was diluted with 400 ml of methanol, and was then stirred for another 30 min with reflux. The solid matter was subsequently filtered off, 500 ml of 10% ammonia solution were added to it, and it was stirred for another 15 h in an autoclave at 150° C. After further processing according to Example 2 the yield was 220.0 g (98.6% of theoretic yield) of a dental filling material consisting of units of the formula

$$n{-}C_3H_7SiO_{3/2}\cdot(CH_3)_2SiO_{2/2}\cdot 40\ SiO_2$$

Specific surface: 56 m^2/g

Analyses:	% C	% H	% Si
Theory:	2.3	0.51	45.9
Actual:	2.1	0.40	44.8

EXAMPLE 5

727.8 g (3.49 mol) of $Si(OC_2H_5)_4$ and 22.2 g (0.1165 mol) of $CH_2{=}CH{-}Si(OC_2H_5)_3$ were combined with

each other. 3 ml of 0.1 n acetic acid solution was added to the mixture and it was stirred for 3 h at 80° C.

After this precondensation 400 ml of ethanol and 200 ml of water were added to the mixture and it continued to be stirred. After 2 h of reflux the solid matter formed and was filtered. After washing with a total of 1 liter of water it further processed analogous to Example 4. The yield was 216.0 g (98.5 % of theoretic yield) of a dental filling material consisting of units of the formula

$$CH_2{=}CH{-}SiO_{3/2}\cdot 30\ SiO_2$$

Specific surface: 22 m^2/g

Analyses:	% C	% H	% Si
Theory:	1.28	0.16	46.3
Actual:	1.17	0.20	45.8

EXAMPLE 6

To 727.8 g (3.49 mol) of $Si(OC_2H_5)_4$ 2 ml of 1% aqueous ammonia solution were added and it was stirred for 2 h at 100° C. At the same time 5 ml of ethanol and 0.5 ml of 2% aqueous ammonia solution were added to 19.0 g (0.07 mol) of $(C_6H_5)_2Si(OC_2H_5)_2$ and it was stirred for 10 h at 100 C. The two precondensates were then combined and 500 ml of ethanol as well as 150 ml of 2% aqueous NH3 solution were àdded, and it was stirred for an additional 3 h with reflux. The formed solid matter was filtered off and was after washing with 500 ml of ethanol further processed analogous to Example 4.

After a concluding 24 h tempering at 150° C. in N_2 atmosphere 220.0 g (98.1% of theoretical yield) of a dental filling material consisting of units of the formula

$$(C_6H_5)_2SiO_{2/2}\cdot 50\ SiO_2$$

were obtained.

Specific surface: 31 m^2/g

Analyses:	% C	% H	% Si
Theory:	4.50	0.31	44.7
Actual:	4.40	0.26	43.9

EXAMPLE 7

To 17.3 g (0.087 mol) of $(C_6H_5)Si(OCH_3)_3$ 0.2 ml of 2% methanolic NH_3 solution were added and it was first stirred for 5 h at 60° C. Then the precondensate was combined with 727.8 g (3.49 mol) of $Si(OC_2H_5)_4$. After further processing analogously to Example 7 216.3 g (98.2% of theoretic yield) of a dental filling material consisting of units of the formula

$$(C_6H_5)SiO_{3/2}\cdot 40\ SiO_2$$

were obtained

Specific surface: 48 m^2/g

Analyses:	% C	% H	% Si
Theory:	2.85	0.20	45.5
Actual:	2.95	0.31	45.8

II. Preparation of the Dental Materials According to the Invention

To produce the dental masses according to the invention the filling materials of Examples 1 to 5 were ground with a ball mill to an average grain size of between ca. 3 to 7 μm. The fillers were then according to standard procedures silanized with 3-methacryloyloxy propyl-trimethoxysilane.

The fillers were in amounts from ca. 70 to 73% (m/m) added to a monomer matrix as it is usually used for dental plastics. Then initiators were added and the masses were kneaded into homogeneous pastes.

A number of physical characteristics was determined with the help of hardened test bodies prepared from the various pastes and were compared to those of commercially available products and laboratory test products (Table 1).

Testing and Evaluation of Polishability

Test bodies with a diameter of 15 mm and a thickness of 3 mm were produced from all materials. The surfaces of all test bodies were first evenly sanded with fine sanding paper (600 grit). Then they were polished on a cotton cloth under water with superfine aluminum oxide (average particle size 0.04 μm).

The polishability was evaluated visually and graded with the help of a point scale ranging from 1 to 5 with 1=dull and 5=high gloss. Examples of dental masses according to the invention

1. Heat-Hardened Dental Masses According to the Invention.

The production of the test bodies of the heat-hardened dental masses according to the invention took place in such a way that the masses were pressed into the respective test body molds and were then hardened at 90° C. for 30 min in a water bath at 6 atmospheres above atmospheric pressure.

The following examples use these abbreviations:

Example 9 (numbers in weight parts):
73.0 filler according to Example 1
18.2 bis-GMA
8.5 TEDMA
0.3 dibenzoylperoxide
Example 10 (numbers in weight parts):
70.0 filler according to Example 2
20.3 bis-GMA
9.4 TEDMA
0.3 dibenzoylperoxide
Example 11 (numbers in weight parts):
70.0 filler according to Example 3
20.3 bis-GMA
9.4 TEDMA
0.3 dibenzoylperoxide
Example 12 (numbers in weight parts):
71.0 filler according to Example 4
19.6 bis-GMA
9.1 TEDMA
0.3 dibenzoylperoxide
Example 13 (numbers in weight parts):
73.0 filler according to Example 5

-continued

18.2 bis-GMA
8.5 TEDMA
0.3 dibenzoylperoxide

bis-GMA: 2,2-bis-[p-(methacryloyloxy-β-hydroxypropoxy)-phenyl]-propane
TEDMA: tirethyleneglycoldimethacrylate

2. Optically Hardening Dental Masses According to the Invention

The optically hardening dental mass according to the invention consists of a white paste which is hardened through irradiation with a dental halogen lamp (Translux, Kulzer Company). Irradiation time 100 sec.

Example 14 (Number in weight parts):
70.0 filler according to Example 2
19.0 bis-GMA
8.7 TEDMA
0.2 camphorquinone
0.1 N,N-dimethyl-p-toluidine

Commercially available products with which the dental masses according to the invention are compared in Table 1:

Conventional composites (Estilux, Kulzer Company):

The filler is a silanized lithium aluminum glass with an average grain size of ca. 4 μm. The filler content is ca. 75% (m/m). Hybrid composites (Degufill H, Degussa):

The filler is silanized barium aluminumsilicate glass with an average grain size of ca. 2 μm, which is however 100% finer than 5 μm, as well as silanized, highly dispersed SiO_2. The filling degree of glass is ca. 70% (m/m), that of highly dispersed SiO_2 ca. 11% (m/m). This results in a total inorganic filler content of ca. 8% (m/m).

Microfiller composites (Durafill, Kulzer & Co., GmbH):

The filler is silanized, highly dispersed SiO_2 with an average grain size between 0.01 to 0.04 μm. The filling degree is ca. 50% (m/m).

The hardening of all masses was performed with the Translux lamp (Kulzer Company) and an irradiation time of 40 sec. Heat-hardening laboratory test products=VP (Numbers in weight parts):

VP1:	17 bis-GMA
	7.7 TEDMA
	75 bariumaluminumsilicate glass, silanized (average grain size ca. 4 μm)
	0.3 dibenzoylperoxide
VP2:	35 bis-GMA
	14.7 TEDMA
	50 highly dispersed, SiO_2, silanized (average grain size 0.01–0.04 μm)
	0.3 dibenzoylperoxide

The hardening of these pastes took place analogously to the heat-hardening masses according to the invention.

TABLE 1

Characteristics of the Dental Masses According to the Invention in Comparison with Commercially Available Products and with Conventional and Microfilled Heat-Hardening Dental Masses

Beispiel[1]	9	10	11	12	13	14	Estilux	Durafill	Degufill H	VP1	VP2
Biegefestigkeit[2]	125	130	80	118	120	90	100	62	110	140	65

TABLE 1-continued

Beispiel[1]	9	10	11	12	13	14	Estilux	Durafill	Degufill H	VP1	VP2
	Characteristics of the Dental Masses According to the Invention in Comparison with Commercially Available Products and with Conventional and Microfilled Heat-Hardening Dental Masses										
$[N/mm^2]$ DIN 13											
Biegemodul[3] $[N/mm^2]$ DIN	8500	9000	10700	7500	8000	7600	9700	322	8000	11000	3900
Druckfestigkeit[4] $[N/mm^2]$	435	400	450	460	470	280	300	350	320	350	410
Vickers Harte[5] HV 5	1100	860	750	780	820	830	660	290	680	660	330
Polierbarkeit[6]	5	5	5	5	5	5	1	4	3	1	4

Key:
[1]example
[2]flectional strength
[3]flexion module
[4]pressure resistance
[5]pyramid hardness
[6]polishability

We claim:

1. A pasty dental material able to harden to a high-glass polishable mass in the presence of an initiator, comprising a polymerizable bonding agent which is a monofunctional or multifunctional ester of methacrylate acid or mixtures thereof, and a fine particle filler, wherein the filler is an organopolysiloxane which consists of units of formula I

$$\begin{array}{c} | \\ O \\ | \\ -O-Si-O- \\ | \\ O \\ | \end{array} \qquad (I)$$

in combination with at least one member selected from the group consisting of: units of formula II and units of formula III, wherein the units of the formula II are as follows:

$$\begin{array}{c} R^1 \\ | \\ -O-Si-O- \\ | \\ O \\ | \end{array} \qquad (II)$$

wherein R^1 stands for a linear or branched alkyl group with 1 to 6 carbon atoms bonded with an acrylate or methacrylate residue, or for a single olefinic unsaturated, linear, optionally branched hydrocarbon residue with 2 to 8 carbon atoms, or for a cyclic, single olefinic unsaturated hydrocarbon residue with 5 to 8 carbon atoms, or for a linear, optionally branched alkyl group with 1 to 8 carbon atoms, a cycloalkylene group with 5 to 8 carbon atoms, a phenyl group or an alkyaryl group,

and the units of the formula III are as follows:

$$\begin{array}{c} R^1 \\ | \\ -O-Si-O- \\ | \\ R^2 \end{array} \qquad (III)$$

wherein R^2 represents a methyl, ethyl or phenyl group, and

the free valences of the oxygen atoms bonded with the silicon atoms in the units of formulas (I), (II), (III) are as in polymeric silicic acid $SiO_{4/2}$ saturated by a silicon atom of a same or different unit whereby the ratio of silicon atoms of the units of Formula (I) to the sum of silicon atoms of units of formulas (II) and (III) is 3:1 to 100:1, said organopolysiloxane having been heated in water or in water—alcohol mixture or in pure alcohol, in the presence of an acidic or basic catalyst at a temperature of 60° C. to 250° C. for 1 hour to 5 days under a pressure which corresponds to the sum of partial pressures at the respective temperature.

2. The dental material according to claim 1, wherein the filler is present as a random copolycondensate, block-copolycondensate or as a mixture thereof.

3. The dental material according to claim 1 wherein R^1 stands for the group

$$-(CH_2)_3-O-\overset{\overset{\large O}{\|}}{C}-\overset{\overset{\large CH_3}{|}}{C}=CH_2-.$$

4. The dental material according to claim 1 wherein an organopolysiloxane is used as filler which consists of units of Formula (I) and units of Formula (II) with the formula

$$\begin{array}{c} | \\ O \\ | \\ -O-Si-(CH_2)_3-O-\overset{\overset{\large O}{\|}}{C}-\overset{\overset{\large CH_3}{|}}{C}=CH_2 \\ | \\ O \\ | \end{array}$$

whereby the molar ratio of the Formula (I) units to the Formula (II) units is 3:1 to 100:1.

5. The dental material according to claim 1 wherein an organopolysiloxane is used as filler which consists of Formula (I) units and Formula (III) units with the formula

$$\begin{array}{c} CH_3 \\ | \\ -O-Si-O- \\ | \\ CH_3 \end{array}$$

whereby the molar ratio of the Formula (I) units to the Formula (III) is 3:1 to 100:1.

6. The dental material according to claim 1 wherein the filler has a specific surface of up to 200 m^2/g, and a particle size of 0.01 μm to 100 μm.

7. The dental material according to claim 6 wherein the surface is up to 100 m^2/g.

8. The dental material according to claim 6 wherein the particle size is 0.1 μm to 30 μm.

9. The dental material according to claim 1 wherein the filler is in the form of a random copolycondensate prepared by a process comprising dissolving an alkoxysilane of the formula

$$Si(OR^3)_4 \quad (IV)$$

wherein R^3 is a linear or branched alkyl group with 1 to 5 carbon atoms, and an alkoxysilane of the formula

$$R^1{-}Si(OR^3)_3 \quad (V)$$

in which R^1 has the same meaning as in Formula (II), and/or an alkoxysilane of the formula

$$(R^2)_2Si(OR^3)_2 \quad (VI)$$

in a water-miscible solvent which, however, dissolves the silanes according to Formula (IV), (V) and (VI), and by adding to the solution while stirring an amount of water which is at least sufficient for the complete hydrolysis and condensation, then by precondensing the reaction mixture during continued stirring at a certain temperature ranging from room temperature to 200° C., by stirring the forming solid matter, optionally after addition of another solvent or water, for 1 to 6 more hours at 60° C. to 200° C., at normal pressure or under a pressure which corresponds to the sum of par-

tial pressures at the respective temperature, then post-treating the formed organopolysiloxane, optionally after a change of the medium and/or pH value, for another 1 hour to 5 days at 60° C. to 250° C. in the liquid phase, then separating according to standard methods from the liquid phase, optional washing, drying at room temperature up to 200° C., optionally in a controlled atmosphere or in vacuum, optional subsequent tempering for 1 to 100 hours at temperatures from 150° C. to 250° C. in a controlled atmosphere or in vacuum, optional grinding and/or classification, whereby the organopolysiloxane which has been separated from the liquid phase and optionally washed is prior to or after one of the phases of drying, tempering, grinding, classification treated in water, a water/alcohol mixture or in pure alcohol, in the presence of an acidic or basic catalyst, preferably in presence of ammonia, for a period of 1 hour to 5 days at temperatures from 60° C. to 250° C. under a pressure which corresponds to the sum of partial pressures at the respective temperature.

10. A method of using the dental material according to claim 1 comprising shaping the composition into a dental filling, inlay, veneer, seal, crown, bridge, denture or artificial tooth.

11. The method of using the dental material according to claim 1 as an adhesive comprising applying said material to an inlay, crown or bridge and adhering the inlay, crown or bridge to a structure underlying said inlay, crown or bridge.

12. The pasty dental material according to claim 1 wherein R^1 is a single olefinic end positioned unsaturated linear hydrocarbon residue of 2 to 8 carbon atoms.

* * * * *

Appendix C: An Informed Consent Form Used in a Human Clinical Trial

G.R. Baran et al., *Healthcare and Biomedical Technology in the 21st Century: An Introduction for Non-Science Majors*, DOI 10.1007/978-1-4614-8541-4,

Page 1 of 3

INFORMED CONSENT FORM

TITLE: Interactions between red blood cells and
Principal Investigator: Dr....
Date of preparation: February 13, 2004
Address: Department of Biomedical Engineering

1. INTRODUCTION:

   1) Statement. You are being offered participation in a research study.

   2) Purpose. If you consent to participate, blood, after collection from you, will be used in experiments that study the interactions between red blood cells and model drug carriers coated with antibodies against endothelial adhesion molecules. Blood contains three primary types of formed elements, the white cells, the platelets, and the red cells, which give its red color. Red blood cells may have an effect on adhesion of model drug carriers to irradiated endothelium. The adhesion of model drug carriers to irradiated endothelium may provide a new way to deliver chemotherapeutic drugs to tumors without damaging normal tissues.

   3) Number of subjects. 10 subjects per year will be enrolled into the research project at this institution. The estimated duration of this project is three years.

   4) Locations: Department of Biomedical Engineering

   5)Anticipated duration of subject participation. 10-20 minutes per subject for drawing blood.

2. PROCEDURES TO BE FOLLOWED:

A standard venipuncture technique, performed by a trained phlebotomist, will be used to collect the blood. No drugs will be administered as a part of the procedures. Blood will be collected no more than twice a week. Collections will take 10-20 ml of blood. The amount of blood drawn during any eight-week period will not exceed the amount drawn on healthy donors at the blood bank. Hematocrits will be monitored; donors with a significant reduction of hematocrit will be discontinued from participation. There are no additional or extra procedures will be performed on you because you are participating in a research study.

3. RISKS ASSOCIATED WITH PARTICIPATION

The risks of venipuncture include: commonly, the occurrence of discomfort and/or bruise at the site of puncture; infection and less commonly, the formation of a small blood clot or swelling of the vein and surrounding tissues, and bleeding from the puncture site.

4. BENEFITS ASSOCIATED WITH PARTICIPATION:

YOU WILL RECEIVE NO HEALTH RELATED BENEFIT FROM YOUR PARTICIPATION. The society may benefit from the new method to deliver drug carrier to tumors without damaging normal tissues.

Initials of Subject Acknowledging Reading This Page ___________________

TITLE: Interactions between red blood cells and …
Principal Investigator: Dr.…
Date of preparation: February 13, 2004

5. ALTERNATIVES TO PARTICIPATION:

You may decline to participate. If you decline to participate, you will not undergo the venipuncture.

6. CONFIDENTIALITY:

In this study subject-specific records will be maintained and the records will be identified by the names of subjects. Under federal privacy regulations, you have the right to determine who has access to your personal health information (called "protected health information" or PHI). PHI collected in this study may include your medical history, the results of physical exams, lab tests, x-ray exams, and other diagnostic and treatment procedures, as well as basic demographic information. By signing this consent form, you are authorizing the researchers at the University of … to have access to your PHI collected in this study. The Institutional Review Board (IRB) at the University of … Health Science Center may review your PHI as part of its responsibility to protect the rights and welfare of research subjects. Your PHI will not be used or disclosed to any other person or entity, except as required by law, or for authorized oversight of this research study by other regulatory agencies, or for other research for which the use and disclosure of your PHI has been approved by the IRB. Your PHI will be used only for the research purposes described in the Introduction of this consent form. Your PHI will be used until the study is completed.

You may cancel this authorization in writing at any time by contacting the principal investigator listed on the first page of the consent form. If you cancel the authorization, continued use of your PHI is permitted if it was obtained before the cancellation and its use is necessary in completing the research. However, PHI collected after your cancellation may not be used in the study. If you refuse to provide this authorization, you will not be able to participate in the research study. If you cancel the authorization, then you will be withdrawn from the study. Finally, the federal regulations allow you to obtain access to your PHI collected or used in this study.

7. COMPENSATION AND TREATMENT FOR INJURY:

I understand that I am not waiving any legal rights or releasing the hospital or its agents from liability and negligence. I understand that in the event of physical injury resulting from the research procedures, the University of … does not have funds budgeted for compensation either for lost wages or for medical treatment. Therefore, the University does not provide for treatment or reimbursements for such injuries. If any injury occurs, study sponsor will provide medical treatments and compensation.

8. QUESTIONS:

If you have any question about the research study, you can contact Dr. … at…. If there are any research-related injuries, you can contact Dr. … at … (24 hours). You may contact Dr. …, IRB Chairman at … if you have any questions about your rights as a participant in this study or your rights as a research subject.

Initials of Subject Acknowledging Reading This Page ____________________

Page 3 of 3
TITLE: Interactions between red blood cells and....
Principal Investigator: Dr. ...
Date of preparation: February 13, 2004

9. PAYMENT FOR PARTICIPATION:

   There is no payment for donors.

10. COSTS OF PARTICIPATION:

   There are no additional costs to you that may result from participation in the research.

11. PREMATURE TERMINATION:

   Under rare circumstances, your participation may be terminated by the investigator without regard to your consent.

12. VOLUNTARY PARTICIPATION:

   The participation is voluntary and the refusal to participate will involve no penalty or loss of benefits to which the subject is otherwise entitled. You may discontinue participation at any time without penalty or loss of benefits to which you are otherwise entitled. If you are a student or an employee of University of ... Health Science Center, your academic or employment standing will not be affected by choosing not to participant in the study.

13. CONSENT OF SUBJECT:

   I have read or have had read to me the description of the research study as outlined above. The investigator or his/her representative has explained the study to me and has answered all of questions I have at this time. I have been told of the potential risks, discomforts, side effects and adverse reactions as well as the possible benefits (if any) of the study.

   I freely volunteer to participant in the study. I understand that I do not have to take part in this study and that my refusal to participant will involve no penalty or loss of rights to which I am entitled. I further understand that I am free to later withdraw my consent and discontinue participant in this study at any time. I understand that refusing to participant or later withdrawing from the study will not adversely affect my subsequent medical care.

____________________________ ____________________
Signature of Research Subject or Legally Authorized Representative — Date

____________________________ ____________________
Signature of Person Conducting Consent Interview — Date

____________________________ ____________________
Signature of Witness — Date

____________________________ ____________________
Signature of Principal Investigator — Date

Index

G.R. Baran et al., *Healthcare and Biomedical Technology in the 21st Century: An Introduction for Non-Science Majors*, DOI 10.1007/978-1-4614-8541-4,

Printed by Publishers' Graphics LLC
ASO140902.19.35.3